# Science at the Bedside

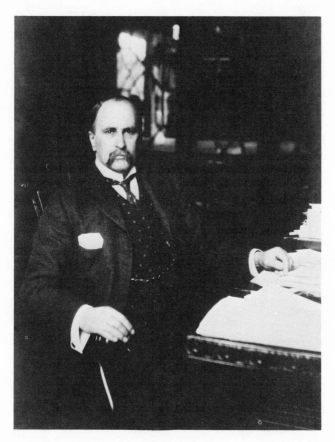

William Osler

# Science at the Bedside

## Clinical Research in American Medicine, 1905–1945

A. McGehee Harvey, M.D.

Distinguished Service Professor of Medicine
The Johns Hopkins University School of Medicine

The Johns Hopkins University Press
Baltimore and London

The Johns Hopkins University Press, Baltimore, Maryland 21218
The Johns Hopkins Press Ltd., London

Frontispiece: Photo, courtesy of Alan M. Chesney Archives,
Johns Hopkins Medical Institutions.

Library of Congress Cataloging in Publication Data

Harvey, Abner McGehee, 1911–
Science at the bedside.

Includes bibliographical references and indexes.
1. Medical research—United States—History—20th century.
2. Medicine, Clinical—Research—United States—History—20th century.
I. Title. [DNLM: 1. Academic medical centers—History—United States.
2. History of medicine, 20th century—United States.
3. Physicians—United States—Biography.
4. Research—History—United States.
WZ 70 AA1 H3s]
R854.U5H37      610'.72073      80-28786
ISBN 0-8018-2562-8

To wrest from nature the secrets which have perplexed philosophers in all ages, to track to their sources the causes of disease, to correlate the vast stores of knowledge, that they may be quickly available for the prevention and cure of disease—these are our ambitions. To carefully observe the phenomena of life in all its phases normal and perverted, to make perfect the most difficult of all the arts, the art of observation, to call to aid the science of experimentation, to cultivate the reasoning faculty, so as to be able to know the true from the false—these are our methods. To prevent disease, to relieve suffering and to heal the sick—this is our work.

WILLIAM OSLER

# Contents

꧁

**Part III**
**The Professionalization of Clinical Science: Full-time**
**Professorships      131**

**Part IV**
**The Pattern of Development in Selected**
**Medical Centers      189**

# Preface

❧

If the science of Medicine is not to be lowered to the rank of a mere mechanical profession, it must preoccupy itself with its history.

EMILE LITTRÉ, 1801–1881

In 1850 Thomas King Chambers began his Gulstonian Lectures as follows:

Mr. President,—The time spared by us from the active duty of applying our knowledge to the benefit of mankind cannot, I think, be better spent than by engaging our minds in a retrospect of the advances made in science by those whose mission it is to search out pure truth, and to whom pure truth is a final object to live for. To us, knowledge, how good and lovely soever it be for its own sake, must always be a by-end, a step merely towards the still better and lovelier goal of "good-will towards men."

Our object, then, in reviewing these researches, and in adding to them such observations as our own sphere of action supplies, should be to deduce from them rules of practice, to gather from the tree of knowledge fruit for the solace and refreshment of mankind.[1]

Both benefit and pleasure accrue to the student of medical history. Comparing the present state of our knowledge with that of the past can have a stimulating effect and produce a feeling of satisfaction in one's own scientific accomplishments. There are, of course, other rewards from the analysis of medicine from a historical viewpoint. One cannot fully appreciate the present state of medical knowledge unless one knows something of its genesis; one cannot effectively assess the future if one is ignorant of the past.

History is often presented as a straightforward chronological catalog of important events. The essential facts of history can be vitalized by dressing them up in the roles of the men and women concerned in their development. This applies especially to medical history even though progress in medicine is determined to a major degree by political, social, and economic influences. Even though a biographical approach to medical history can be overemphasized, each epoch in its evolution can be studied effectively by analyzing the important contributions to medical science and the institutions in which new men and women of stature have worked and new ideas of scientific value have been forged.

In the study presented in this volume the answers to a number of questions about the evolution of clinical science in the United States have been sought. Who were the clinical scientists and what were their aims and motives? What techniques (observational, instrumental and experimental) were available for their use? Where did they do their work and what facilities did they have at their disposal? How were these clinical scientists trained and selected? How were their results made available to other scientists and to the general body of physicians? How was their research supported? How did learned societies and other medical organizations influence the conduct and direction of clinical investigation?

The objective of this study is to document the history of clinical science in the United States and the emergence of the clinical scientists whose accomplishments were primarily responsible for the creation of the scientific basis of medical practice. In the period emphasized (1905 to 1945) medical research made possible the advances that permitted medicine to gain its present prestige. It was during this period that medical research became established in this country on a scale and of a quality that surpassed the accomplishments in the best European centers.

# Acknowledgments

I am deeply indebted to Jerome Bylebyl, Victor McKusick, and Owsei Temkin for reading various chapters and offering useful criticism.

I have received a great deal of help in constructing the chapters related to individual schools and institutions. Without this help, a reasonably complete and accurate account would not have been possible. I wish to thank the following colleagues for their help with various individual chapters: Edward C. Atwater, Gert Brieger, Charles C. Carpenter, William B. Castle, John E. Deitrick, Robert Ebert, Roberto Escamilla, Maxwell Finland, A. Stone Freedberg, Halsted R. Holman, Rudolph Kampmeier, Attallah Kappas, Gordon Meiklejohn, Raymond D. Pruitt, Paul Reznikoff, William D. Robinson, David Rytand, John de C-M Saunders, C. H. Smith, Wesley Spink, R. G. Sprague, Donald Tapley, Alvin Tarlov, George Thorn, Malcolm S. M. Watts, Francis Carter Wood, and Lawrence Young.

I wish to express my deep appreciation to Joseph T. Wearn, Isaac Starr, Cecil J. Watson, the late Tinsley R. Harrison, William B. Castle, and Nolan Kaltreider for providing special information about their research careers and clinical science at their respective schools.

The research involved in the preparation of this book was made possible by a grant from the Commonwealth Fund. Publication has been aided by a grant from the Burroughs-Wellcome Fund.

# Introduction

The last half of the nineteenth century may well be called the era of experimental medicine. Important events developed along three lines: one, the discovery of the functions of organs; two, the discovery of the causes of many infectious diseases; and three, the discovery of new methods of treatment. In one generation there was a complete realignment of the outlook on physiology, pathology, and practice, all of which came from a recognition that experiment is the very basis of science. It was at this developmental stage that clinically trained individuals began to apply the methods of the basic sciences to the study of human disease. As William Osler pointed out, the realization came that there must be clinicians who kept in close touch with physiology, pathology, and chemistry and who were prepared to transfer to the wards, through proper channels, the knowledge of the laboratory. He stated:

> The organized medical clinic is a clearing house for the scientific traders who are doing business in all parts of the body corporate, and the application of new facts to medicine must come through it, or through that small but happily increasing group of men who find time amid the daily cares of practice. . . . In every country there must be found strong men like Weir Mitchell, Mackenzie, Meltzer, and Herter, who find it possible to combine experimental work with practice, but we must recognize the pressing need of organization if internal medicine is to keep in close touch with the rapid advances of the sciences.[1]

## Definition of Medical Research

The question is often raised as to whether there is such a science as *medicine* or whether this is simply a name used in reference to a group of sciences, certain features of which are utilized to form the base for the practice of medicine. It was Richard Shryock's opinion that medicine "may indeed be given independent status as the branch of biology which deals with disease; that is, in terms of pathology (including etiology) and of clinical medicine (including surgery and therapy). Even this definition may be viewed as too broad in that it includes both the study of disease as such and the treatment thereof."[2] Within the scope of this definition medicine borrows whatever knowledge it may need from related sciences in the accomplishment of its important purpose—improving the quality of medical practice. Clinical investigation is principally concerned with the application of the methods of science to the study of disease in man.

As Shryock pointed out, the term *research* is relatively modern. It means a more or less systematic investigation of phenomena with the purpose of adding to the sum total of knowledge in a given field. In this respect it implies planning, so that isolated observations that are unplanned trial-and-error improvements in the art are not to be viewed, in the opinion of some observers, as research. On the other hand, one cannot limit research to experimental studies. Simple observation using quantitative procedures has increased the extent of our knowledge in the various sciences. It has been suggested that the term *research* be applied by definition only to those investigations that involve new relationships and require "the use of imagination or other mental processes beyond those called for in simple observations."[3] An excellent description of medical research was given by Theobald Smith:

> Research is fundamentally a state of mind involving continual reexamination of the doctrines and axioms upon which current thought and action are based. It is, therefore, critical of existing practices. Research is not necessarily confined to the laboratory although it is usually associated with an elaborate technique and complex instruments and apparatus which require a laboratory housing. This is controlled research which endeavors to pick out of the web of nature's activities some single strand and trace it toward its origin and its terminus and determine its relation to other strands. The older type of research involving observation and study of the entire fabric of disease largely with the help of the unaided senses, such as was the practice of doctors a century ago, has had its day, but backed by experience and a keen, observant mind it even now occasionally triumphs over the narrow, controlled research of the laboratory. It is the kind used by Darwin and other early biologists in establishing on a broad comparative basis the evolution of plant and animal life.[4]

As time has gone on, research has become more experimental and less observational. It was Osler who noted: "Man can do a great deal by observation and thinking, but with them alone he cannot unravel the mysteries of nature. Had it been possible the Greeks would have done it; and could Plato and Aristotle have grasped the value of experiment in the progress of human knowledge, the course of European history might have been different."[5]

Thomas H. Morgan described the role of experiment in research:

> Physics has progressed because, in the first place, she accepted the uniformity of nature; because, in the next place, she early discovered the value of exact experiments; because, in the third place, she concentrated

her attention on the regularities that underlie the complexities of phenomena as they appear to us; and lastly, and not the least significant, because she emphasized the importance of the experimental method of research. An ideal or crucial experiment is a study of an event controlled so as to give a definite and measurable answer to a question—an answer in terms of specific theoretical ideas, or better still an answer in terms of better understood relations.[6]

In the following discussions, the principal concern will be the acceptance in clinical departments of medicine of a responsibility to apply the methods of science to the study of disease in man, the emergence of the full-time clinical scientist, and the influence of his activities on medical education and medical practice. These developments can be fully understood only if activities in other fields of science that led up to their implementation are considered. Clinical research has had an important impact on medical education and basic research as well as on activities in other sciences. It has had a significant effect on the attitude of the general public to physicians and to medicine in general. Thus, the developments in clinical investigation cannot be understood unless they are considered in relation to the economic, social, and intellectual circumstances in which they developed, as well as in relation to other sciences, medical education, medical practice, and public health.[7] As clinical investigation has developed and the availability of research laboratories close to the patient area in the hospital has become a reality, the definition and scope of clinical research have broadened.

## The Process of Clinical Research

Research begins with formulating a problem. Next comes devising an experiment to answer some specific question to be asked of nature. Here the need for imagination, insight, and ingenuity as well as for clear and consecutive thought is obvious. This is followed by performance of the experiment, which entails a sequence of observation, recording, study, comparison, analysis, and reasoning; all similar to the procedures of the observational method. Clinical investigation demands, above all, the gift of observation. In clinical study the investigator must see what others have not seen or cannot see; sometimes what he himself never expected. He must be able to visualize the experiments with which nature has provided him in terms of the physiological and biochemical abnormalities produced by disease. This is often the starting point for the better understanding of the normal mechanisms of human function. Medical research directly upon man is different from other forms of biological research. Man is highest in the order of evolution and psychologically more complicated than other species. In addition, the investigator is a man and frequently a physician responsible for the welfare of his patient. In these important respects, the kinds of experiments possible are not only limited but also subject to errors due to misinterpretation on the part of the observer.

Osler was well aware of the limits to which justifiable experimentation in man could be carried. As he pointed out, the final test of every new procedure, medical or surgical, must be made on man, but never before it has been tried on animals. Although some looked upon animal experimentation as unlawful, Osler believed that progress was not possible without it. In Osler's view, absolute safety and full consent were the conditions that made human experimentation allowable. He thought that a physician had no right to use patients entrusted to his care for the purpose of experimentation unless direct benefit to the individual was likely to follow. Once this limit was transgressed, the sacred cord that binds physician and patient snapped instantly. Risk to the individual had to be taken with his consent and full knowledge of the circumstances; Osler could not honor too highly the bravery of such men as the soldiers who voluntarily submitted to the experiments, under the direction of Walter Reed and James Carroll, on yellow fever in Cuba.[8]

## The Social Setting for Research

In dealing with clinical investigation one must recognize its setting in society. The appreciation of medical research as a source of new knowledge, and of medicine as a means of applying it, depends upon sociological and cultural factors that are elusive to clear definition because they are so pervasive. Medical research as a deliberate, well-supported activity is relatively new. There is no reference to it in the Hippocratic oath, which means that for two thousand years physicians were not reminded that it was their duty to go beyond simply finding a remedy for a complaint. If they did go further, their actions (like many others that were eventually proved valuable) were unrequired and unrewarded.

The last hundred years have witnessed, as a result of overt research efforts, important new findings in relation to essentially every recognized disease. Medical research has left the medical profession itself somewhat behind and at times rather resentful. Medical research, then, is in its youth; attentive, adaptable. It suffers from no unalterable traditions although it may now be in the process of accumulating them.

It is evident that the attitude of universities toward research has changed within the last fifty years. In 1929, upon the twenty-fifth anniversary of the initiation of the Carnegie Institution of Washington, Edwin G. Conklin recorded a striking reminder of this:

> Many colleges and universities that are now important centers of research made little provision for it 25 years ago. They were glad to say that their professors were conducting original work since this was good advertising, but those professors in general conducted their studies in the tag ends of their time and largely at their own expense. Most of us remember how

professors used to talk about their research as "my own work," whereas teaching and administration was "the university's work." It is only within recent times that this has changed and universities in this country have come to recognize that research is as important a part of the work of a university as teaching and that both must go forward together in order that education and information may properly advance.[9]

As George Rosen pointed out, an essential task of historical investigation is to develop concepts and generalizations. Medicine is, as mentioned, but one aspect of the general civilization of the period; it exists within a matrix at once political, economic, social, and cultural. This concept applies to that special area of medicine, young in its life history, clinical investigation, and to the activities of the full-time clinical scientist. Rosen emphasized that the historical approach is necessarily characterized by two fundamental attributes, human and temporal, since history is ultimately concerned with the behavior of men in time. Sometimes change is characterized by cataclysmic violence, at other times it is so slow as to be hardly perceptible. Every sudden transition and transformation in history is rooted in the past out of which it comes. This is abundantly true in medicine, as we shall see in this presentation. The bacteriological discoveries of the 1880s represent one case in point. Within two decades, largely between 1877 and 1898, the microbial causes of numerous human and animal diseases were revealed for the first time. Until the 1880s, microbes had been shown to be the probable or certain etiologic agents in only a few diseases. A similar type of development can be documented in the history of nutrition—the development of the concept of deficiency diseases and the discovery of vitamins. A crucial stage in the historical process is that of relative quiescence, in which dynamic forces exist and yet may not be able to make themselves felt. This stage is the link between the preexplosive and the explosive phases of the process and has been designated by Rosen as the "critical level." This concept has many important implications, including the idea that before attainment of a critical level a variety of interacting elements and forces have been producing changes.[10]

This concept can be clearly seen in the emergence of clinical investigation and of the full-time clinical scientist. In this volume an attempt will be made to depict the formative period in the century before the development of clinical investigation—a development that appears to be America's most important contribution to modern-day medicine. Special attention will be paid to the critical stage beginning, in 1905, with the establishment of the first full-time research divisions in a clinical department.

# Part I

❦

# Setting the Stage for Clinical Science

# 1

# Formative Influences

The history of medicine and the medical sciences in the United States can be divided into four periods.[1] In the first of these, which extended from the mid-eighteenth century to about 1820, British influence prevailed; in the second period, which extended from 1820 to 1860, French medicine held sway; whereas in the third period, from 1860 to 1900, German influence was dominant. After this period American medicine emerged on an independent level, although many young men still went to Europe for experience. These various stages of dependence were not peculiar to American scientific culture, and parallel examples can be found in the experience of other colonial countries. Before 1820, the development of medical research in this country lagged behind the developments in medical practice. In early America one survived by taking care of immediate problems; thus, there was neither time nor social advantage to be gained by scientific research. Each period of development brought changing conditions in this country, and migration to the cities, together with the accumulation of wealth in a variety of hands, enabled Americans to bring about improvements in various cultural and scientific activities and ultimately to gain independence. As Shryock pointed out, the lack of research in this early period is to be attributed not only to the underdeveloped character of the country, but also to the lack of various conditions and facilities that were essential to medical studies. The valuable contributions made in taxonomy were stimulated by the novelty of the New World's flora and fauna. A similar stimulus might have acted in relation to medicine even before schools and hospitals were available, if the observers had found equally novel forms of illness there. This was not the case, however, and physicians did not embark on original studies until institutions such as those already in operation in Europe became functional in the United States.[2]

3

## The British and Scottish Influence

### Trained European Doctors

The first step in the movement of medical culture to America was the migration of European doctors here; the second was the training of American physicians in Europe. Having received their education in Leyden, Edinburgh, and London, some of these individuals returned with the aim of establishing schools of their own.[3] The more able ones appear to have studied at Edinburgh University and were more impressed by this school than by the London hospitals.

### The Edinburgh Influence

J. Gordon Wilson has sketched the influence of Edinburgh on American medicine in the eighteenth century.[4] He traced the evolution and development of the school in Edinburgh from the experiences of the Monros and others at Leyden in the early eighteenth century.

There were many Edinburgh graduates in America before 1765, when the first medical school was organized in Philadelphia. These physicians were located chiefly in Pennsylvania, Maryland, and the Carolinas. One of the most distinguished was Cadwallader Colden (1688–1776) who received his M.D. degree in Edinburgh in 1705. After immigrating to America, he practiced in Philadelphia from 1708 to 1715 and then settled in New York in 1718. His best known medical work was on diseases prevalent in New York, including various "anginas" and "eruptive fevers." Another Edinburgh graduate (M.D., 1765) who settled in New York was Samuel Bard (1742–1821), who became the first professor of the theory and practice of medicine in King's College in 1769.

Some of these Edinburgh graduates, although isolated in the colonies, kept in touch with their Scottish professors. Thus, one finds John Lining, a physician in Charlestown, South Carolina, writing, around 1750 to Robert Whytt, professor of the Institutes of Medicine, an account of the anthelmintic virtues of the Indian pink (which was introduced to the English by the Indians), and about how the drug may best be prepared.[5] In 1753 (before Benjamin Rush wrote his classic account) Lining wrote, at the request of Whytt, an account of the 1748 yellow fever epidemic at Charlestown, comparing it with other epidemics observed.

An excellent illustration of the continued intercourse between Edinburgh and American physicians is the following letter, dated December 10, 1779, addressed to Professor William Cullen by Mr. James Clephan, a student at Edinburgh in 1757:

> It is now 22 years since I had the happiness of listening to your instructions, yet they have made such an impression on my mind as to make me strenuously wish to have your opinion of the few practical observations

which I have had the opportunity of making on the diseases endemic in fleets, hospitals and prisons. I have not attempted to touch on theory, as I felt myself unequal to the task. But I have endeavored faithfully to observe disease as she presented herself and if you think these observations can be of any use to mankind I shall feel myself highly pleased in having contributed ever so little to clear the intricate path which leads to the temple of health, and amply rewarded by having your approbation. . . . Your most obedient servant, James Clephan.[6]

Thus, some of these Edinburgh graduates brought with them the spirit of investigation through careful clinical observation, even though the facilities with which to indulge in research were minimal.

By the middle of the eighteenth century, American students were going to Edinburgh in increasing numbers. William Shippen and William Morgan—the founders of the first American medical school, the Medical College of Philadelphia—received their training there.

Morgan's inaugural address[7] at the opening of this school is, of course, a medical classic. In it he outlined "a scheme for transplanting medical science into the seminary and for the improvement of every branch of the healing art. . . . I propose to confine myself in practice to those cases which belong most immediately to the office of a physician, that I may prescribe for and attend such cases to greater advantage. I shall therefore avoid, all I can, interfering in the proper business of surgery." Thus, Morgan was probably the first to encourage specialization in the practice of medicine in the United States. In the concluding paragraph of his famous address he said: "Next year I desire to attempt a course of lectures upon the Institutes or Theory of Medicine which will be illustrated with practical observations. Possibly in a few years, more persons duly qualified may offer to undertake full and complete courses of every branch of medicine; and a plan may be adopted conformable to that which has followed in the, so justly celebrated, school of physic at Edinburgh."

Shippen and Morgan were joined in 1768 and 1769, respectively, by Adam Kuhn and Benjamin Rush, both graduates of Edinburgh University. At the same time Thomas Bond gave bedside instruction in the Pennsylvania Hospital and the faculty was on its way to being formally organized.[8]

Other American medical schools were begun in connection with the arts colleges already established at Columbia (1768) and Harvard (1783). These early American schools, which incorporated such recent innovations in medical education as the teaching of chemistry, were, in some respects, superior to the English schools. These new American institutions were, however, the training ground of only a small percentage of practitioners; the majority continued, until after 1820, to be trained primarily by apprenticeship. Thus, the rank and file of the profession had no contact with such research interest as the meager formal education available at that time could provide. There was essentially no concern for research in these new schools. Some of the young professors, including Benjamin Rush, returned from Europe with enthusiasm for original work, as may be attested to by the experiments on the physiology of digestion that he and his students performed (see chapter 3). The professional conditions in existence at that time, however, were not conducive to clinical research.

Most of the collegiate institutions of that day had a theological background, and, although science acquired a more prominent place, the early professors of "natural philosophy" were so concerned with explaining the new scientific outlooks that few of them had the time for or the inclination toward original contributions. It was understandable that they failed to transmit any enthusiasm for research to the medical faculties with which they were associated. Following the example of the Church of England, Protestant denominations maintained a strong influence over American colleges, and, by 1800, their intellectual climate was perhaps less favorable to scientific work than it had been a generation earlier. Private practice received almost exclusive attention in the schools, as well as in the subsequent careers of the graduates.

In that early period the separation of the various diseases was not far advanced. The need then was for simple observation in an effort to lay this basic groundwork, for one obviously cannot effectively study diseases that have not been distinguished from each other. Pathologic anatomy, although recognized in America as early as 1766, was not a general activity, since there was a strong popular aversion to human dissection. Theoretical pathologic systems such as Rush's revived the ancient "tension" theory ascribing all illness to "excessive action" in the walls of blood vessels, with the result that every condition could be treated by bleeding and purging to relieve this tension. It was just such a simplistic viewpoint, or "sure cure," that the laity wanted. It was also what the busy practitioners desired. If one cause and one remedy were known, then further research was simply unnecessary.

## The Paris Period (1820–1860)

### Louis and the Development of Clinical Medicine in the United States[9]

On a rainy autumn day in October 1905, a small group of men were crowded into the doorkeeper's house of the Montparnasse Cemetery in Paris. After a while the shower stopped, and the group came out and gathered at the door of a mausoleum—that of the "Famille Louis," where lay the remains of the great French physician Pierre-Charles-Alexandre Louis (1787–1872). Osler placed a wreath at the base of the mausoleum and made the following remarks:

> While not sitting with Bichat and Laennec on the very highest seats of our professional Valhalla, Louis occupies a seat of honor . . . with his friends,

Andral and Chomel, and with Bretonneau and Corvisart, with Bright, Addison and Hodgkin, with Skoda and Schönlein—among the men who gave to the clinical medicine of the 19th century the proper methods of work. Louis had special claims to remembrance as the introducer of the "numerical method," by which he made his works on typhoid fever and on phthisis . . .

Returning from a prolonged residence in Russia, he took up work at the Charité as a voluntary assistant to Chomel, and for 7 years he noted with the greatest accuracy and detail the chief symptoms in certain diseases and then correlated these with the postmortem appearances. It was an original attempt to introduce mathematical accuracy into the study of disease. . . . He took no private practice and allowed nothing to interfere with his daily routine.

. . . through his students he may be said to have created the American school of clinical medicine. Between 1830 and 1850 a group of young men from America studied here and came under his influence in a very special manner. Earliest to arrive and chief among them in his affection, was James Jackson, Jr., son of Professor James Jackson of Harvard. . . . To give the names of Louis' American students is to mention the men who, in the third quarter of the 19th century, occupied the most prominent position in our ranks: from Boston, Oliver Wendell Holmes, Henry I. Bowditch, George C. Shattuck; John T. Metcalf, Alonzo Clark, and John A. Sweet of New York; W. W. Gerhard, Alfred Stillé, William Pepper, Sr., and Meredith Clymer of Philadelphia; from the southern states, Power of Baltimore and Cabell of Virginia . . .

It is not too much to say that it was the direct inspiration derived from him that laid the foundation of accurate clinical methods in the United States.[10]

Present-day scientific medicine has important roots in the work of the Paris Hospital School in the first half of the nineteenth century.[11] For approximately sixty years physicians and students from all over the world traveled to Paris to attend this revolutionary school where many famous clinicians were creating a new approach to clinical medicine. It was a medicine based on new techniques and concepts. It relied on physical examination by eye, hand, and ear; on the concept of a thorough history of the disease being studied; on the anatomical location of a lesion.

Probably no one went further along these lines than Louis, the "inventor" of the numerical method.[12] Louis, the great admirer of observation and the founder of the Societé d'Observation Médicale, became its great systematizer. Systematic clinical examinations and systematic autopsies were analyzed using the numerical technique. Louis was by no means the first Paris clinician to use statistics, but he was the first to make them the basis of medicine.

In order to understand Louis and his contributions, one must have a clear picture of Paris and its hospitals in this era, which has been referred to as that of "hospital medicine," as contrasted to the earlier period of "library medicine" or "bedside medicine" or the later period of "laboratory medicine." The hospital was a doctor's fortress. Although Marie-François-Xavier Bichat and Louis were never professors, their hospital positions enabled them to exert a tremendous influence on future generations. The French Revolution, which had set out to abolish hospitals, actually strengthened them and made them the core of medicine.

The main diseases treated in these hospitals, and consequently the main objects of scientific observation, were listed by the American observer F. C. Stewart: phthisis, pneumonia, typhoid fever, cancer, eruptive fevers (especially smallpox), puerperal peritonitis, and heart disease; in the old, apoplexy, cancer, and diseases of the urinary tract; in children, pneumonia, phthisis, and meningitis. There was also a surprising prevalence of malaria, rheumatism, lead poisoning, and syphilis.[13] The Paris student of that day who wanted to become a practitioner was trained on the wards. Simon Flexner designated the French type of medical education as the "clinical type," as opposed to the "university type" or the "proprietary type," and he defined the Paris faculty as composed of hospital staffs engaged in teaching.[14]

One of the early eclectics was Auguste-François Chomel, who received his training at the Charité and succeeded René-T.-H. Laennec in 1827 as professor of clinical medicine at that hospital.[15] He allowed Louis to collect thousands of case histories and autopsy records on his wards in the Charité. Louis did clinical research on Chomel's wards for seven years, thus becoming the "ancestor of the full-time clinical investigator." Louis's great book on phthisis appeared in 1825. It contained 184 pages on pathological anatomy, twice that number on symptoms, and one-third more on therapy. Qualitatively, he did not add many new facts to what Laennec and Gaspard-Laurent Bayle had found, and yet Louis's quantitative approach and his extraordinary, almost painful thoroughness gave his statements a finality and certainty never before attained.

James Jackson described the plan of study that Louis employed:

> First, then, he ascertained when the patient under his examination began to be diseased . . . he went back to the period when the patient enjoyed his usual health and he also endeavored to learn whether that usual health had been firm or in any respect infirm. He noted also the age, occupation, residence and manner of living of the patient. Likewise, any accidents which had occurred and which might have influenced the disease then affecting him. He ascertained also as much as possible the diseases which had occurred in the family of his patients. Secondly, he inquired into the present disease ascertaining not only what symptoms had marked its commencement but those which had been subsequently developed and the order of their occurrence and recording those which might not seem to be connected with the principal disease as well as those which were so connected. Also measuring the degree or violence of each symptom with as much accuracy as the case would admit. Thirdly, he noted the actual phenomena present at his examination, depending for this not only on the

statement of the patient, but on his own senses, his eyes, his ears, and his hands. Under this and the preceding head, he was not satisfied with noting the functions in which the patient complained of disorder, but examined carefully as to all the functions, recording their state as being healthy or otherwise and even noticing the absence of symptoms which might bear on the diagnosis. Thus, all secondary diseases and those which accidentally co-existed with the principal malady were brought under his view. Fourthly, he continued to watch his patient from day to day, carefully recording all the changes which occurred in him until his restoration to health or his decease. Fifthly, in the fatal cases he exercised the same scrupulous care in examining the dead as he had in regard to the living subject. Prepared by a minute acquaintance with anatomy and familiar with the changes wrought by disease, he looked not only at the parts where the principal disorder was manifested but at all the organs. His notes did not state opinions, but facts. He recorded in regard to each part which was not quite healthy in its appearance, the changes in color, consistency, firmness, thickness and so forth, not contenting himself with saying that a part was inflamed or was cancerous or with the use of any general but indefinite return.[16]

Thus, Louis's methods form the basis of the modern technique of information-gathering from the patient, which is used every day in the clinic. It was Osler's appreciation of Louis's techniques that led him to incorporate them into the design of the medical clinic at Johns Hopkins.[17]

Louis is best known for his introduction of statistics into the analysis of medical observations. Strong objections were raised against his "statistical approach," however, even by such a methodologically sophisticated scientist as Claude Bernard. What is more important about Louis is that he was probably the first full-time clinical investigator, even though his principal tools were observation and numerical analysis of the gathered facts.

## The American Pupils of Louis

As powerful as was the effect of Louis's writings on American medicine, it cannot compare with the influence he exerted through his pupils, who "made him their model." Louis attracted hard-working, capable men. As his obituary in *Lancet* (1872) stated: "Year by year fresh bands of students came to imbibe from his lips the instruction which their predecessors had abandoned with reluctance till his academic progeny knew no distinction of race or even color but coalesced into a noble band of enthusiasts in the cause of medicine, of science, and of humanity."[18] In this academic progeny Louis's American pupils take an unusual position. The group of young men who studied under Louis in Paris between 1830 and 1849 gave an important impetus to the study of medicine in the United States. These men had, of course, to make their contributions largely through their clinical work in the hospitals.

One of Louis's most impressive students from Boston was James

Jackson, Jr., the son of Dr. James Jackson of Harvard, who along with Jacob Bigelow was instrumental in bringing about more rational ideas on the treatment of disease. After taking his A.B. degree in 1828, the younger Jackson attended the medical lectures at Harvard and in the spring of 1831 went to Paris, where he remained until the summer of 1832.

Two letters written by Louis to Jackson's father give an advanced view of the benefits of postgraduate study and service, now embodied in residency and research fellowship training. "I pointed out to him [James Jackson, Jr.] the advantage it would be for science and for himself if he would devote several years exclusively to the observation of diseases. . . .

"I believe that he would be well pleased to follow for a certain period the vocation for which nature has fitted him, but he has stated to me that there are many difficulties which would prevent his devoting himself exclusively to observations for several years. But can these difficulties be unsurmountable?" And again, "Let us suppose that he should pass four more years without engaging in the practice of medicine. What a mass of positive knowledge will he have acquired. How many important results will he have been able to publish to the world during that period?" In another letter the following year, written just before young Jackson left for home, Louis refers again to this subject and urges the father to allow his son to devote himself exclusively to observation for several years in Boston:

> Think for a moment, sir, of the situation in which we physicians are placed. We have no legislative chambers to enact laws for us. We are our own law givers or rather we must discover the laws on which our profession rests. We must discover them and not invent them for the laws of nature are not to be invented and who is to discover these laws? Who should be a diligent observer of nature for this purpose if not the son of a physician who has himself experienced the difficulties of the observation of disease, who knows how few minds are fitted for it and how few have at once the talents and information requisite for the task. . . . All this is united in your son.[19]

Young Jackson was one of the founders in 1832 of the Society of Medical Observation, which consisted of the ablest students of Louis, Chomel, and Gabriel Andral. During his stay in Paris, Jackson made an important study of cholera, which was published in this country in 1832. It was most timely, as it gave the American profession a clear description of the disease, with which it was inexperienced. Jackson made noteworthy studies of emphysema and was the discoverer of the prolonged expiration of early pulmonary tuberculosis. Osler stated that he knew of no young man in the profession who had given promise of such exceptional eminence. Young Jackson died prematurely, and his influence in extending Louis's methods and views throughout New England was chiefly through his father, who, though approaching his sixties, became an ardent follower of Louis and the numerical method.

Henry I. Bowditch, son of the celebrated mathematician Nathanial Bowditch, received an M.D. degree from Harvard in 1832. After a residency at the Massachusetts General Hospital (MGH), he spent two years training under Andral, Chomel, and particularly Louis.[20] He was one of the earliest advocates of sanitary science and was a founding member of the Boston Society for Medical Observation, which was organized in 1846.[21] The second State Board of Health in the United States was created in Massachusetts in 1869, and he was its president for ten years. Bowditch's chief interest was diseases of the chest and he worked on an improved method of removing an effusion from the pleural cavity.[22]

Of all the pupils of Louis, there was none whose name became more of a household word than Oliver Wendell Holmes. Soon after reaching Paris in April 1833, Holmes wrote: "I am more and more attached to the study of my profession and more and more determined to do what I can to give to my country, one citizen among others who had profited somewhat by the advantages offered him in Europe. The whole walls of the school of medicine are covered with notes of lectures the greater part of them gratuitous, the dissecting rooms are open and the lessons are ringing aloud through all the great hospitals."[23]

Louis had, in Holmes's view, the power to attract young men and to instill in them an ardent ambition. Holmes returned to America with high ideals and a large amount of professional knowledge and independence of thought. In 1836 he received his M.D. degree at Harvard.

Holmes's most important contribution was made in 1843, when he read an essay on the contagiousness of puerperal fever before the Boston Society for Medical Improvement. This was long before the nature of contagion was understood and several years before the studies of Semmelweiss. Holmes's rules for the guidance of physicians in midwifery practice need little revision today:

One, a physician attending cases of midwifery should never take any active part in the postmortem examination of cases of puerperal fever. Two, if a physician is present at such autopsies, he should use thorough ablution, change every article of dress and allow 24 hours or more to elapse before tending to any case of midwifery. Three, similar precautions should be taken after the autopsy or surgical treatment of cases of erysipelas. Four, on the occurrence of a single case of puerperal fever in his practice, the physician is bound to consider the next female he attends in labor unless some weeks at least have elapsed as she is in danger of being infected by him and it is his duty to take every precaution to diminish her risk of disease and death. Five, if within a short period, two cases of puerperal fever happen close to each other in the practice of the same physician, the disease not existing or prevailing in the neighborhood, he would do wisely to relinquish his obstetrical practice for at least one month and endeavor to free himself by every available means from any noxious influence he may carry about with him. Six, the occurrence of three or more closely connected cases in the practice of one individual, no others existing in the neighborhood, and no other sufficient cause being alleged for the coincidence, is *prima facie* evidence that he is the vehicle of contagion. Seven, it is the duty of the physician to take every precaution that the disease should not be introduced by nurses or other assistants by making proper inquiries concerning them and giving timely warning of every suspected source of danger. Eight, whatever indulgence may be granted to those who have heretofore been the ignorant causes of so much misery, the time has come when the existence of a private pestilence in the sphere of a single physician should be looked upon not as a misfortune but a crime and in the knowledge of such occurrences duties of the practitioner and his profession should give way to his paramount obligations to society."[24]

In 1847 Holmes was elected professor of anatomy and physiology at Harvard Medical School; he held this position continuously for thirty-five years, although the chair of physiology was separated in 1871. As a lecturer in anatomy he became immediately popular. Holmes emphasized two things that Louis had stressed: one, always make sure that you form a distinct and clear idea of the matter you are considering; two, always avoid vague approximations when exact estimates are possible.

Another Boston student of Louis was George Cheyne Shattuck,[25] who received his M.D. degree from Harvard in 1835. He and Alfred Stillé, of Philadelphia, read a paper before the Paris Society for Medical Observation in 1838, which was a landmark in pointing out the distinction between typhus and typhoid fevers. In 1849, he succeeded Holmes as visiting physician to the MGH and served in this capacity for thirty-six years.

Other Boston pupils of Louis were John Dicks Fischer[26] and Jonathan Mason Warren.[27] Fischer was the first to introduce formal education of the blind into this country. He conceived the plan of, and was connected with, the Perkins Institution for the Blind in South Boston, which was founded with state aid in 1829. He was a physician of the MGH, was present at the first administration of ether at that hospital, and was one of the first to use ether in childbirth.

Jonathan Mason Warren was the son of John Collins Warren and the grandson of Dr. John Warren. He arrived in Paris in the fall of 1832 and studied surgery under Guillaume Dupuytren, Jacques Lisfranc, and Philibert-Joseph Roux, and medicine under Louis. On October 16, 1846, he assisted his father in the operation that was the first public demonstration of surgical anesthesia. A few weeks later he substituted for Morton's apparatus the cone-shaped sponge, which was used to administer ether at the hospital for twenty years.

Perhaps the most distinguished of the Philadelphia pupils of Louis was William Wood Gerhardt.[28] In 1831 Gerhardt went to Paris and studied under François-J.-V. Broussais, Chomel, and Louis. In 1832, with Caspar Wistar Pennock, his lifelong associate, who was also a pupil of Louis, he published his observations on cholera. After returning to Philadelphia in 1834 he studied several hundred cases of typhus and typhoid fever, concluding that they were separate entities. While Shattuck of Boston, Robert Perry of Glasgow, and Lombard of Geneva simultaneously reached the same conclusions as Gerhardt, Osler assigned the credit for this discovery to Gerhardt, by virtue of his complete work and his publication in the *American Journal of the Medical Sciences*.[29] His *Diagnosis, Pathology and Treatment of Diseases of the Chest* (1842) was the first systematic treatise on chest diseases written by an American.

Alfred Stillé was house physician at the Blockley under Gerhardt in 1835. After his tutelage under Gerhardt and Pennock, he also studied under Louis. Stillé played a part in the differentiation of typhus and typhoid fever. He recalled this effort:

> The year 1836 is memorable for an epidemic of typhus which prevailed in the district of the city which is the usual seat of epidemic caused or aggravated by crowding, viz., south of Spruce and between 4th and 10th Street. A great many of the poor creatures living in that overcrowded region who were attacked with typhus were brought to the Philadelphia Hospital where I had charge of one of the wards assigned to them. . . . Every step of my study of typhus in the wards and postmortem revealed new contrasts between the two diseases so that I felt surprised that the British physicians should have continued to confound them.[30]

In 1854 Stillé was elected to the chair of medical practice in the Pennsylvania Medical College. In 1864 he succeeded Dr. William Pepper (primus) in the chair of medicine at the University of Pennsylvania. He was the first secretary of the American Medical Association and its president in 1867. He wrote an important monograph on cerebrospinal meningitis and another on cholera.

Caspar Wistar Pennock[31] received his M.D. degree from Pennsylvania Medical College in 1828, presenting his thesis, "Experimental Researches on the Efficacy and Modus Operandi of Cupping Glasses in Poisoned Wounds." In the spring of 1830 he went to Europe to study medicine, giving particular attention to the investigation of diseases of the heart. He attended the teaching sessions of Louis. Stillé recalled his training with Pennock: "Meanwhile I studied physical exploration and diagnosis with Dr. Pennock who . . . devoted himself especially to diseases of the heart. I had assisted him in some of the experiments on sheep which he performed to demonstrate the mechanism of the heart's action and at the hospital I was instructed by him in the clinical diagnosis of heart disease by physical methods."[32] Pennock's chief contribution to medical literature was an edition of James Hope's *Treatise on the Heart*, to which he added valuable information, including descriptions of the experiments he performed.

## The Period of German Influence

Early in the nineteenth century there was recognition in Germany of the new scientific trends progressing in France. German physicians became more aware of the contrast between the work of the French clinicians and physiologists and the "armchair theorizing" in their own land. They were particularly impressed with the systematic character of the hospital studies of Louis. Meanwhile, the school of "hospital medicine" in France was finding a competitor in the "laboratory school," which was advanced by the work of François Magendie (1783–1855) and then of Claude Bernard (1813–78), among others.[33] They added an experimental approach to the problems of medical science, believing that a causative analysis of both normal and abnormal physiologic processes would contribute more to the advance of curative medicine than mere careful clinical observation and correlation with pathological findings. Unfortunately, Magendie and Bernard could not establish a strong institutional base for experimental medicine in France. Although the French showed a great understanding of the value of and need for scientific research, they failed to expand the facilities for research and to recognize new fields for exploration.

France was, however, the pioneering country in the establishment of modern scientific facilities. The Polytechnique, organized in 1794, was the model academic institution in the natural sciences. Among its resources were the first academic research laboratories in chemistry, and, as pointed out, modern experimental physiology began with the work of Magendie in the physiological laboratory at the Collège de France.

Until 1830, the level of medical research in Germany was inferior to that in France. The network of German universities at that time retarded, rather than enhanced, the development of research. The biological sciences were under the domination of *Naturphilosophie,* which gave birth to much imaginative writing but little research.

Three conditions have been cited to explain the scientific superiority of Germany in the latter half of the nineteenth century: first, the relative excellence of laboratory and hospital facilities for research and the prompt recognition of new fields; second, the recognition of the university as the seat of original research and the development of organizational devices to foster it; and third, the existence of a network of academic institutions that made possible the mobility of teachers and students, leading to a substrate of scientific competition that did not exist elsewhere.[34] This decentralization of the German academic system stemmed from the political dismemberment of Germany that took place at that time. There were twenty independent universities in Germany proper, fostered by the princes of the numerous small states that comprised Germany in the eighteenth and nineteenth centuries, as well as German language universities in Switzerland (Zürich, Bern, and Basel), Austria (Vienna, Prague, Graz, and Innsbruck), and Dorpat, in the Baltic Sea Provinces of Russia. This decentralization led to academic competition, which forced universities to make decisions, which would not have been made otherwise. No single institution in Germany was able to lay down standards for such a system of decentralized institutions, in which scientists and students were relatively free to move from one place to another. Improvements in facilities for research and training and the opening of new fields of research had to be made by each university in order to attract the best scientists or to keep them. Decentralization also forced the institutions to correct mistakes and to do away with traditions that retarded scientific development.[35] As we shall see, Americans who studied in Germany were quick to recognize these conditions, and it was such competition within a decentralized system that played an important role in the rapid development of American clinical research in the first quarter of the twentieth century.

## The Establishment of Basic Science Laboratories

As mentioned, an important factor aiding the German effort was a university system that provided an effective framework for the organization and direction of systematic research. The eighteenth century had witnessed an increase in both the number and the activity of German universities and the dawn of the university as a teaching-research center. Young men with fresh scientific viewpoints gradually filled the chairs vacated by older men with philosophical tendencies.

The rapid development of the biological sciences in the latter half of the nineteenth century in Germany was to have a profound effect on clinical science. The laboratories that had the greatest effect on the development of university teaching and research were the investigator-student organizations that had their origins in the first half of the nineteenth century. Such laboratories were an outgrowth and expansion of the private laboratory. Private laboratories flourished in France at the beginning of the nineteenth century, and there was also a famous one in Stockholm presided over by Johann Jacob Berzelius. It was to these centers that ambitious young men from other countries, including Germany, went for their instruction. German science, its medical science particularly, was under the influence of the *Naturphilosophie* as expounded by Lorenz Oken and Friedrich von Schelling, and, while chemistry was affected to a lesser degree than medicine, the instruction was for the most part authoritarian even in that subject. There was a total lack of opportunity and no appreciation for experiment, the life blood of chemistry as well as the other fundamental sciences. The chemical approach to modern experimental physiology was initiated by Justus von Liebig (1803–73) and Friedrich Wohler (1800–1882) in Germany and by Antoine-Laureut Lavoisier (1745–94), Michel-Eugène Chevreul (1787–1889), and Jean-Baptiste Dumas (1800–1884) in France. Liebig was fortunate enough to have studied in Paris, where there were, in the 1820s, a few laboratories in which professor and assistant worked side-by-side. These very inadequate laboratories were labelled by Claude Bernard, who himself worked in a damp cellar, "the tombs of scientific investigators." Liebig was admitted to Gaultier de Claubry's private laboratory, where he completed a paper on explosives, which he presented before the Academy of Sciences. By chance, Alexander von Humboldt was present in the audience; he was impressed by the young chemist and arranged a meeting for him with Louis-Joseph Gay-Lussac, who gave him an opportunity to work in his laboratory. Von Humbolt was later instrumental in Liebig's appointment as professor in the small university of Giessen.

Liebig is credited with establishing one of the first teaching laboratories of modern times in Giessen in 1825. It was in this primitive laboratory, which consisted of one room in a deserted barracks, that the leading teachers of chemistry for all of Germany and for other countries as well were trained. Liebig was one of the principal founders of physiological chemistry and the chemistry of carbon compounds. He discovered hippuric acid, chloral, and chloroform, and his studies of uric acid compounds, as well as his mode of estimating urea, were important. Friedrich Wohler was associated with Liebig in his investigations of uric acid and in other work. In 1828 Wohler succeeded in effecting an artificial synthesis of urea. This was the first time that an organic substance had ever been built up artificially without any intervention of vital processes, and it soon became clear that there was no essential difference between the structural chemistry of life and that of inanimate nature. In 1842, Wohler confirmed a discovery that became the starting point of the modern chemistry of metabolism—the fact that benzoic acid taken orally appears as hippuric acid in the urine. Thus, these two workers were inaugurators of what Carl von Noorden called the qualitative period of metabolism research.

Liebig's laboratory had been anticipated by one year (1824) by the physiologist Johannes-Evangelista Purkinje (1787–1869), who outfitted a room in his own house in Breslau in which to instruct students. It was Johann Wolfgang von Goethe's influence that led to Purkinje's appointment in 1823 as a professor of physiology at Breslau, where he remained for twenty-seven years, exerting an influence on the development of physiology in Germany almost as great as that of Carl Ludwig a half century later. Purkinje was not provided with a university laboratory until 1842, but the one that he established at home became a wedge by means of which experimental science was extended in Germany and in other countries. Purkinje was the first to study the vertigo and rolling of the eyes produced by rotating the erect body in a vertical axis (1820–25). Although he did not connect the phenomenon with the semicircular canals, his description was the starting point of modern work on vestibular function. Rudolf Buchheim (1820–79), the pharmacologist and the teacher of Oswald Schmiedeberg, opened a laboratory in his own home in Dorpat in 1849.

Thus, the German medical scientists, first influenced by foreign training, benefited by organizing their private and university laboratories as research centers. The new approach, which the Germans acquired from the French, was particularly applied to subjects of human concern. Accompanying their scientific efforts was a tendency toward philosophical speculation. The concept of evolution elaborated by Herder, von Goethe, Shelling, and Hegel around the turn of the century favored embryological and hence microscopic studies. An example is found in the beliefs about the etiology of infections. Disease had sometimes been viewed by the philosophers of nature as a sort of living parasitic entity inseparably associated with man. This idea proved to lead somewhere when subjected to real investigation. The transition from theory to fact was first accomplished by Johann Lucas Schönlein, who showed the element of truth it contained when he demonstrated in 1839 that a human skin disease (favus) was caused by a living parasite. A year later, Jacob Henle presented his studies on miasma and contagion, in which he anticipated the germ theory of disease.

## The Influence of Johannes Müller

The transition from speculative philosophy to science is best illustrated in the career of Johannes Müller (1801–58). Beginning as a student of *Naturphilosophie*, he was primarily responsible for introducing the modern scientific spirit into Germany. He believed that the function of physiology was to study living phenomena as a whole. Müller credits Karl Rudolphi with demonstrating to him the importance of the experimental method.

In the 1820s, Müller employed both physical and chemical procedures in the investigation of human physiology. He was the first to demonstrate that each sense organ is related to its own peculiar sensation and to no other. The discovery of this law of "specific nerve energies" illustrated his ability to generalize. Müller's *Handbook of Human Physiology* (1834–40) was a landmark in the turning away from natural philosophy toward observation and experiment. He was one of the first to recognize the importance of using the new achromatic microscope, and he gave impetus to those histological studies that were so important a feature of German medicine. The histologists Theodore Schwann, Jacob Henle, and Rudolf Virchow were all trained under Müller, as were the physiologists Emil DuBois-Reymond, Hermann von Helmholtz, and Ernst Brücke.[36]

Shortly after the achromatic microscope became available in 1831, Robert Brown, an Englishman, discovered the plant cell nucleus. Its importance was emphasized by Schleiden of Hamburg; Schwann, Müller's prosector at Berlin, discovered nucleated cells in animal tissues. Following these discoveries there was, during the thirties and forties, an intensive study of cell structure that led to the conclusion that the cell was both the structural and physiological unit of all living organisms. This was Schwann's theory of 1839. Outstanding was the work of Jacob Henle (1809–85), who followed in Marie-Françirs Xavier Bichat's footsteps in investigating tissue structure. These discoveries were applied to pathology with a complete revolution in that science by Rudolf Virchow (1812–1902), who succeeded Müller as the dominating figure in German medicine. Virchow undertook studies in pathological physiology as a basis for improving therapeutics. He was the first to demonstrate the nature of leukemia. He also showed that all cell growth originated in preceding cells and thus threw light on the nature of tumors of all types. In 1856 he became the director of the first independent pathological institute.

Research in physiology received an important step forward in 1847, when Brücke, Ludwig, Helmholtz, and DuBois-Reymond came together in Berlin and set out to constitute physiology on a chemical-physical foundation. Helmholtz represented the complete scientist in that he persistently experimented, constantly sought improved instruments and techniques, and always attempted to measure his findings. He was one of the discoverers of the law of conservation of energy. After completing his work on nerve function with measurements of the velocity of nervous conduction and of reflex action he turned to the sense organs. In 1851 he invented the ophthalmoscope and a year later the ophthalmometer. These two instruments made possible for the first time observations of the interior of a living organ. The modern science of ophthalmology was born, as well as a motivation to search for other instruments with a similar purpose.

## German "Physiological Medicine"

Johannes Müller accepted Broussais's concepts of physiological pathology, and his disciples carried on these ideas with vigor. Müller's influence extended beyond physiology, and he demanded exactness and conciseness in pathology as well. As indicated, his importance for medical science in Germany is best exemplified by the men he trained.

Within a short period three periodicals were organized as outlets for the new endeavors in German medical science. In 1842, Carl Reinhold August Wünderlich and Wilhelm Roser started the *Archiv für Physiologische Heilkunde* at Wurzburg, and Henle established the *Zeitschrift für Rationelle Medizin* at Zurich in 1847. At Berlin, Ludwig Traube in 1846 began the publication of his *Beiträge zür Experimentellen Pathologie und Physiologie,* which in its early issues contained his own investigations on the results of cutting the vagus nerves and the pathogenesis of the resulting pneumonia, as well as Virchow's famous work on embolism and thrombosis. After one year the *Beiträge* was succeeded by the *Archiv für Pathologische Anatomie und Pathologische Physiologie und für Klinische Medizin,* which was founded by Virchow and Benno Reinhardt. All of these journals emphasized the scientific treatment of the problems in medicine, based on experience and experiment. The description of phenomena was no longer sufficient; instead, an attempt was made to understand their interrelations and their origin and development. The principle, enunciated by Magendie, that pathology is the physiology of the diseased individual was constantly emphasized.

The title that Carl Reinhold August Wünderlich (1815–77) had given to his *Archiv* led to the term *physiological medicine*,[37] which was soon accepted as the name of this new school of medical science. There was an intention to replace anatomical research with physiological investigation, to pass from the purely descriptive to a consideration of the relations existing between various morbid phenomena, and to establish a pathological physiology as had been suggested by John Hunter, Dupuytren, and Magendie. Although this was a great advance from the previous period in German medicine, there still prevailed rather narrow and limited views concerning clinical medicine. There was, in the beginning, resistance to any effort to establish definite clinical syndromes or to describe individual diseases.

Virchow's views of clinical research were expressed in the *Prospectus* contained in the first volume of his *Archiv* (1847): "The ideal we shall strive to realize ... is that practical medicine shall become applied theoretical medicine, and theoretical medicine shall become pathological physiology. Pathological anatomy and clinical medicine ... are essential to us as sources of new questions, the answering of which will fall to pathological physiology."

In a following article, he continued: "Pathological physiology takes its questions from pathological anatomy, partly from practical medicine; it creates its answers partly from observations at the bedside, and thus it is a part of clinical medicine, and partly from experiments on animals. The experiment is the ultimate and highest resort in pathological physiology."[38]

Experimental physiology received an enormous boost, and one physiological institute after another was organized. Under Virchow, pathological anatomy became a powerful and independent science. These great branches of science, physiology and pathological anatomy, now became emancipated from clinical medicine.

## The Development of Clinical Science in Germany

The result of these developments was the establishment of the clinical laboratory; not only for diagnosis, but also for the teaching of students and the conduct of research. Simon Flexner pointed out that the germ of this idea may be traced back to such men as John Hughes Bennett and Lionel Smith Beale in Great Britain and to Friedrich Theodor von Frerichs (1819–85) and Ludwig Traube (1818–76) in Germany, who applied microscopic, chemical, and experimental methods to the investigation of clinical problems.[39] The first cooperative investigation of a disease was, however, undertaken by Bright at Guy's Hospital in 1842. A complete clinical unit with consulting room and laboratory was provided.

It was natural that laboratories for the fundamental sciences should be developed before those for the clinic were established. Sixty years elapsed between Liebig and Purkinje's beginnings and the opening of the investigator-student laboratory in Hugo von Ziemssen's clinic in Munich in 1884.

Johann Lucas Schönlein (1783–1864) was trained under the influence of the prevailing natural philosophy, but at Würzburg in 1813 he found exceptional opportunities for medical study. In 1824 he established a clinic, in which auscultation and percussion were practiced, microscopic and chemical examinations of the blood and urine were carried out, and the diagnosis was checked at autopsy. The strength of the German school of medicine under Müller and Schönlein lay in the recognition of the natural sciences as the foundation of medicine. Nowhere else at that time, except in Germany, did the methods of physics, chemistry, physiology, and pathology penetrate the clinic. Experimental pathology came to life in the clinics, especially in those devoted to internal medicine.

Schönlein was succeeded by the brilliant Frerichs, and, later, Ludwig Traube also was given a clinic in Berlin. Traube's foundations were laid in physiology, whereas Frerichs's were laid in chemistry and pathology. Both of these men were experimentalists, using the laboratory to investigate clinical problems and bringing the knowledge that the laboratory and experiment had yielded into their clinical teaching.

Traube was taught by Purkinje, Müller, Skoda, Rokitansky, and Schönlein. He was a master clinical physiologist, investigating the pulmonary disorders occasioned by the section of the vagus nerve, the pathology of fevers, the effects of digitalis and other drugs, the relation of cardiac and renal disorders. He introduced the thermometer in his clinic as early as 1850. Frerichs is known for his discovery of leucine and tyrosine in the urine of patients with acute yellow atrophy of the liver, his pathological studies of cirrhosis of the liver, and his books on Bright's disease, diseases of the liver, and diabetes. He was the teacher of Paul Ehrlich, Bernard Naunyn, Ernst von Leyden, and Joseph von Mering, all of whom were important contributors to the development of modern medicine.[40]

Bernard Naunyn (1839–1925), who was Frerichs's assistant for nine years, discussed Frerichs's attitude toward his assistants:

> He accepted each one from the very first day as a man who unquestionably could and would do everything the position required of him. So confident was he, unfortunately, of this, that he never gave us any instructions as to how we should do anything; indeed, he scarcely said what he wanted done, and he actually managed to have everything done to his satisfaction without any such explanations. . . . It was just as much a matter of course that we should make scientific investigations and produce able pieces of work, as that we should perform our clinical duties to his satisfaction.[41]

Naunyn eventually became professor of medicine in Strasbourg in 1888. He developed his interest in the metabolic diseases from Frerichs, and his studies of liver function, icterus (jaundice), and diabetes occupied him throughout his career. His pupil Stadelman investigated the relation of beta-hydroxybutyric acid to diabetic coma, and Naunyn himself coined the term *acidosis* to describe the pathological condition present. Reflecting on conditions in the 1860s, Naunyn wrote: "Already a few German clinicians began to equip themselves with laboratories in which problems of clinical medicine were investigated experimentally according to those methods [i.e., of chemistry, physics, physiology, pathological and microscopic anatomy]. It was at that time that experimental pathology in the German clinics came to life, and it was this that foreigners came to learn from us."[42] Naunyn in turn had as his pupil Oscar Minkowski, whose work on the pancreas and diabetes was one of the preconditions for the discovery of insulin.

The laboratory that came to stand nearest to the clinic was the pathological, the first independent one being Rudolf Virchow's at the Charité in Berlin in 1856. It contained facilities for work in pathological anatomy, experimental pathology, and physiological and pathological chemistry; it was the model for pathological laboratories all over the world. It not only attracted pathologists from other countries, but also played a remarkable role in the training of biochemists. Willy Kühne was a chemical assistant of Virchow's, and Hoppe-Seyler was another assistant there before becoming professor of chemistry at Tübingen and professor of biochemistry at Strasbourg. A special feature of Virchow's laboratory was the study of disease structure as well as disordered function, and the employment of the methods of experiment as well as those of observation. Thus, it was in reality a laboratory of experimental medicine.

In 1873 Osler recorded his impressions of Virchow, Frerichs, and Traube. He returned for a second visit in 1884, at which time he wrote of the laboratories of Frerichs, Leyden, and Carl F. O. Westphal that "the wards are clinical laboratories utilized for the scientific study and treatment of disease, and the assistants, under the direction of the professor, carry on investigations and aid in the instruction. The advanced position of German medicine and the reputation of the schools as teaching centers are largely fruits of this system."[43] Flexner pointed out that such observations had led Osler to state that his "second ambition" was "to build a great clinic on Teutonic lines here in America... Lines ... which have placed the scientific medicine of Germany in the forefront of the world."[44]

It was against this background that the investigator-student laboratory in the clinic arose. Hugo von Ziemssen (1829–1902) was a pupil of Virchow's. Not himself a laboratory worker, his professional distinction was in the field of literature and the history of medicine. His encyclopedic knowledge was perhaps the best preparation for the innovation he was to introduce into the clinic. The investigator-student laboratory in Germany was not designed for the teaching of all medical students. It was not an elementary laboratory of instruction in methods of diagnosis, but rather a place in which advanced students and assistants primarily studied problems of human disease, but it did not exclude the study of more fundamental scientific subjects. Whereas the new university hospital in Munich was built in 1878, von Ziemssen had already provided a modern laboratory for the assistants at Erlangen in 1873. His later laboratory in Munich, which was more comprehensive, included three divisions (chemical, physical [physiological], and bacteriological), a library, and examination rooms. Such a laboratory was opposed on the grounds that it was a duplication of existing laboratories, it was uneconomical, and the students would be made too scientific. Despite these objections, the idea took root. A similar laboratory was introduced by Curschmann in his Leipzig clinic in 1892, and others soon appeared throughout Germany.

The strength of the new German medicine was its close association with physiology and the new pathological anatomy. Before the English and the French, the Germans knew how to turn to account the immense advances that were being made in anatomy and histology, in physiology and physiological chemistry. From the German laboratories came a series of valuable investigations, whose themes were chemical and pathological-anatomical and embraced experimental pathology.

From 1840 to 1870, however, during the early period of so-called "physiological medicine," clinical observations fared badly. In the concepts of tuberculosis and other diseases such as varicella and variola, confusing errors were made, principally through a failure to comprehend and respect the clinical, nosographical method. The attitude that characterized Virchow was that the function of clinical medicine was to raise questions; that of pathological physiology to answer them. During this period, pathological anatomy, physiology, and experimental pathology had an equal share in discouraging clinical medicine, which lost its standing in terms of its own problems and became, in large measure, reduced to a kind of accessory science subordinate to pathology and physiology. This loss in standing can be illustrated by the judgment pronounced on clinical medicine by Naunyn in a retrospective survey written in 1908: "Not until recently did German internal medicine take a share in the development of nosography, semiology and diagnostics, and that this occurred so late was due to the physiological school."[45] After the work of Müller, clinical medicine flattered itself with the name *physiological;* but the enthusiastic advocates of the new movement, in their zeal, sought to find in physiology not only the direction of their activities but also the decisive word in pathological and especially in clinical questions. The clinical "pictures" were only "recognized" insofar as they reflected physiological laws; the attempt was to interpret the separate symptoms in the light of these frequently very distorted physiological images. Often they were simply constructed instead of found by critical and impartial observation. Traube also made clinical medicine the servant of physiology, losing himself in petty details and subtleties in symptomatology in order to preserve the most intimate connection possible with physiology. Other clinicians did the same. The fault lay in an overwhelming pride in speculation and laboratory wisdom, as contrasted with an interest in living nature.

The next generation of German clinicians had a deep interest in clinical nosographical problems. Ernst von Leyden (1832–1910), who had replaced Ludwig Traube (1818–76), together with the aging Frerichs and a number of other prominent clinicians throughout Germany, inaugurated a new and more clinical era in medicine. On this subject Naunyn wrote:

> Not until after 1870 did we come into the full enjoyment of building up our complexes of symptoms, our clinical pictures empirically. The more earnestly we became absorbed in our cases the more did our interest in causistry increase, and now our training in the methods used in anatomy, physiology and chemistry made good. The demand for a thorough examination of the cases gained more and more ground as the condition for "a serviceable case." These endeavors soon bore ample fruit; in neurology, abdominal diseases, diseases of the blood, but above all and most brilliantly in the pathology of metabolism. In the works on metabolism in fever and diabetes German clinical medicine early asserted its superiority. We owe this to our physiological school, the Pettenkofer-Voit School at Munich. It was a very long time before the value of such investigations began to dawn on the mind of the French.[46]

Thus, we see how German "physiological medicine" was an important preparatory step to the new era of clinical science. It contributed to clinical medicine chiefly through the stimulus given to the introduction of new methods of investigation—graphic, microscopic, and chemical. Although these methods were developed chiefly by the physiologists and chemists, the clinicians also adopted them. One may mention, for example, the introduction in 1852 of methods for counting the hemocytes by the physiologist Karl Vierordt, and his use in 1855 of the sphygmograph for investigating the pulse; the measurement of the color of the blood by the anatomist Herman Welcher; and the invention of methods for the examination of the urine by the physiological chemists C. Trommer and Johann Florian Heller. Such discoveries opened the way for the application of the methods of science to the study of disease in man and to the birth of the modern-day clinical scientist.

Interest in clinical science was also awakening in France, where Gabriel Andral (1797–1876), one of the older members of the Paris School, advocated clinical thermometry in 1841 and began to determine the content of fibrin and corpuscles in the blood, and of albumin in serum by weight, which he introduced as a clinical method. The Paris physiologist Étienne-Jules Marey (1830–1904) greatly advanced clinical medicine by the development of various graphic methods. Not until this had been done could serviceable sphygmographs, cardiographs, and so forth be constructed. In Armand Trousseau (1801–67), France had a clinical observer of the first rank. His description of diphtheria in its various forms and stages is well known. He advocated the introduction of tracheostomy and thoracocentesis, and his studies on typhoid fever, scarlatina, and many other diseases were of great value. He repeatedly emphasized the importance of observations at the bedside. "To know the natural course of the disease is more than one half of medicine." It was in Germany, however, that momentum was greatest by 1870, and it was in this direction that prospective American scientists and physicians turned.

## German Training Centers of Particular Importance to American Medicine

The social setting in the United States at the end of the Civil War provided no incentive for research. Anyone who withdrew from his medical practice to do research would lose his position on the ladder leading to the key teaching positions and practice opportunities. Advancement came only with the decease of one's predecessor and not from any research contribution. There were no clinical research laboratories, no training in the research methods of the basic sciences, and no career opportunities for the clinician who might develop an interest in research. As migration to the cities increased, however, industry prospered, and money became available for philanthropic purposes. As soon as a few men realized the practical value of the new developments taking place in medical science in Germany, and as soon as they realized how deficient medical education and medical science were in the United States, an awakening took place, and a determined group of medical statesmen set out to change the situation.

America's slowness to create a cultural climate in which scientific medicine could flourish was one of the important factors leading to the great medical migration to study in Germany. This continued as long as America lacked laboratories and instructors for teaching modern medicine and the ways of research. The number of American physicians studying in Germany decreased in the 1850s, swelled in the 1870s and 1880s, and remained strong in the 1890s. It was, however, definitely on the decline in the decade and a half before World War I. This pattern was related closely to the conditions at home. In the beginning there was an awareness of the German achievements in medicine; then a concern to establish facilities and an intellectual climate here that would be conducive to real scientific work; finally, such rewarding developments as the establishment of the first research laboratories in America and the ultimate achievement by Americans of a reputation in scientific medicine. With the successes of the first postgraduate training opportunities in medicine and medical research, it soon became respectable to stay at home for advanced training.

Americans interested in ophthalmology were the first to migrate in large numbers to German universities. This migration stemmed from the important work of Helmholtz and Albrecht von Graefe, which focused the interest of the medical world on this specialty in the 1850s. Elkanah Williams of Cincinnati brought the ophthalmoscope to America in 1855 and around 1871 described a case of the Marfan syndrome. By the 1870s ophthalmology had become the first well-established medical specialty in the United States.

Leipzig exerted the strongest attraction on the graduate physicians whose interest was in one of the basic sciences, particularly physiology. Heidelberg, too, had its quota of famous names in the 1880s and 1890s, including Kühne, Wilhelm Erb, and Vierordt. Kühne conducted a well-attended course in practical physiology, which was popular with Americans, in which he demonstrated various tests and the use of instruments.

Many of those who went to Germany intending to do clinical studies, such as John J. Abel and Franklin Paine Mall, soon discovered the exciting world of original scientific work. Mall told William Henry Welch, for example, that it was his contact with Wilhelm His, and especially with Ludwig, that opened his eyes to the sciences of anatomy and physiology. In comparison with the thousands who went to Vienna or Berlin for special studies, those Americans who worked in the laboratories of the smaller universities were few in number, yet their influence on the course of American medicine and clinical research, as evidenced by such men as Welch, Mall, Graham Lusk, and Russell H. Chittenden, was immeasurable. As A. Magnus-Levy wrote:

> Between 1873 and 1890 one place outshone all the others because of the high standard of its faculty, the University of Strasbourg. When this university was established in 1871, the outstanding professors in their respective fields were recruited from the whole German Empire. The watchword of the time was "Science without prejudice and without preconception." Side by side with this belief was the idea of "academic freedom" and unrestricted liberty of movement from one university to another, which proved to be of great value both to professors and students. The majority of the scientists changed the place of their activity several times in their career and even full professors seldom remained permanently in the chairs to which they were first called. The ambition for a better and wider sphere of activity kept their passion for work alive; a new call compelled them to face new tasks, to adapt themselves to a new environment and inspired them in many ways through contact with new colleagues in their own field and in related departments.[47]

As already stated, the success of German medical science resulted from the competition among universities for the best scientists, the creation of new faculty positions, new training opportunities, new research facilities, and the development of new specialty fields of medical science. These factors, which made a great impression on men like Henry P. Bowditch, Welch, Abel, and Mall, influenced the creation of full-time posts in the preclinical departments in American medical schools and were a major basis for the drive to establish full-time clinical chairs. In the United States, the inability to choose men for clinical professorships from outside the local faculty was a restraining factor on motivation to clinical research in the midst of limited opportunity. One could not change location if it was necessary to rebuild a clinical practice. The Rockefeller Institute for Medical Research might well have been at Columbia University if the custom of appointing local men to clinical chairs had not been so firmly rooted at the latter institution.[48]

### Ludwig and His American Pupils

Carl Ludwig (1816–95) was one of the outstanding physiologists of the nineteenth century, the greatest teacher of this science, and the one most influential in stimulating the application of scientific methods to clinical research.[49]

Ludwig picked up the torch from Johannes Müller and began to explain vital processes in terms of physics and chemistry as early as 1842, when he offered his dissertation at Marburg on a physical theory of renal secretion. Ludwig supported his conclusions by physicochemical experiments, and his researches were the foundation of knowledge on diffusion through membranes. Robert Wilhelm Bunsen, who taught chemistry and physics at Marburg, had a great influence on him. Ludwig's ingenuity, resourcefulness, and knowledge of the physical sciences formed the basis for his work, which completely restructured the methodology of physiology.

Two major contributions of Ludwig's while at Marburg were his experiments on renal function and his invention of the kymograph in 1846.[50] In 1847, Ludwig visited Berlin and met DuBois-Reymond, Helmholtz, and Brücke. These four young scientists, who were to shape the future of physiological thought for decades to come, were known as "The 1847 Group." Because of their individual and combined efforts, German physiology entered a remarkable period of scientific discovery dominated by the physicochemical approach.[51]

When the new chair of physiology was inaugurated at Leipzig in 1865, Ludwig created a model physiological institute there. Lombard stated that, in a building which had the form of a capital E, "the main portion was arranged and equipped for the study of physiological processes from the physical side. One wing was devoted to histological work, the other to physiological chemistry. Ludwig divided the work on the basis of his ability to judge the capabilities of the students. He found something for each worker to do and he himself cooperated in the experimentation and in the publication of the results."[52]

Ludwig's importance as a teacher equalled his achievement in research. Osler, in a visit to Ludwig's laboratory in 1884, recorded his impressions:

> Probably the most notable figure in medical Leipzig is Professor Ludwig, Director of the Physiological Institute and the nestor of German physiologists. Indeed, he has a higher claim than this, for when the history of experimental physiology is written his name will stand preeminent with those of Magendie and Claude Bernard. . . . He has the honor of having trained a larger number of physiologists than any other living teacher; his pupils are scattered the world over, and there is scarcely a worker of note in Europe—bar France—who has not spent some time in his laboratory.[53]

Thus, Ludwig created a modern physiological laboratory and made an extraordinary contribution in terms of the pupils who worked in it. This can be clearly illustrated by Ludwig's remarks to Mall when the latter thanked him for the stimulating influence he received during his period in Ludwig's laboratory. Ludwig simply replied: "Pass it on."[54] Through the group Ludwig trained, including Henry P. Bowditch, Charles S. Minot, William Henry Welch, Franklin Paine Mall, John J. Abel, Frederic S. Lee, and Warren P. Lombard, he had a significant influence on the evolution of clinical science and the emergence of the clinical investigator in America.[55]

### Carl Voit and the Development of Medical Science in the United States

Carl (von) Voit[56] established a school of physiology in Germany,[57] and, through the men he trained, he had a significant influence on clinical investigation in the United States. Voit had studied under a number of notable German professors, including Albert von Kolliker and Virchow, but most importantly Liebig. After this he joined the laboratory of Max von Pettenkofer. In 1863 Voit accepted the chair of physiology at the University of Munich, where he aimed at a better understanding of the metabolic processes through the use of preciser techniques of analysis. He developed reliable methods of investigation for measuring intake and output of human subjects. He discovered that the total nitrogen in food could be recovered in the urine and stool. In collaboration with Pettenkofer, he constructed the famous open-circuit metabolic apparatus for the analysis of gas-exchange in man, together with a calorimeter to measure heat loss. These instruments enabled them to explore the metabolic turnover in the organism and trace the pathways of individual substances. Voit's distinguished students included Max Rubner and three Americans—Graham Lusk, Wilbur O. Atwater, and Francis G. Benedict.

Lusk also studied under Ludwig, from whom he learned the "physical side" of physiology, but Voit made the greatest impression upon young Lusk, who received his Ph.D. degree from Munich in 1891. Lusk became the American apostle of the Voit-Rubner doctrines of nutrition. No other American who studied in Germany subjected himself more thoroughly to the influence of German science than did Lusk, who returned home with the highest academic ideals and a crusading spirit. Along with John S. Billings, David Linn Edsall, Mall, Welch, Flexner, Lewellys Franklin Barker, Rufus I. Cole, and others, Lusk helped to promote the development of effective investigative work in clinical departments.

Max Rubner (1854–1932),[58] whose name is closely connected with the development of the quantitative calorimetric method and the energy aspect of metabolism, studied medicine in von Ziemssen's clinic before coming to Voit's laboratory. His discoveries included the law of isodynamics, as well as proof that energy principles could be applied to metabolism through the use of combined direct and indirect calorimetry and metabolic balances. Lusk's work was intimately tied up with questions similar to those that Rubner worked on.

Otto Frank was Carl Voit's successor as professor in Munich. Frank pioneered in the exact mathematical and physical analysis of the circulation. In 1891, Frank worked in Ludwig's laboratory. This shows the interdigitation of the schools of physiology in Europe, which were to have such an important influence on clinical science in America. In 1894, Frank became Voit's assistant; he established the foundations for an exact calculation of cardiac work and the precise criteria for the construction of manometers. Finally, he enunciated a method for the determination of cardiac stroke volume in man and animals on the basis of the wave and air chamber theories. One of his important pupils was Carl J. Wiggers. Later, Wiggers and John R. Murlin were associates in Lusk's laboratory in New York. Thus, Lusk's influence was spread to other areas when Murlin went to the University of Rochester and Wiggers became professor of physiology at Western Reserve.

### Friedrich von Müller: Clinician–Investigator

At Munich the great clinical teacher was Friedrich von Müller, a pupil of Voit's. Beginning in 1902 he influenced many outstanding Americans, including E. Cowles Andrus, Lewellys Franklin Barker, Eugene F. DuBois, William S. McCann, Basil McLean, Ralph Major, George Canby Robinson, Warren Sisson, Cecil J. Watson, and others. Of von Müller, Robinson said in 1909 that few medical teachers in America even aimed at his high ideals, which Robinson identified as the establishment, through rigorous study and preparation, of clinical medicine as a science; the devotion of more attention to pathology and the basic sciences; and the dedication of one's life to clinical teaching and research.[59] Barker spoke for all of von Müller's students when he said: "In von Müller I found a great clinical teacher—one of the best Germany has ever produced. He exerted a profound influence upon me. An accurate diagnostician and a reliable therapist, he recognized the importance of clinical laboratories in which physical, chemical, and biological methods could be applied to the study of the patients in his wards."[60]

This statement was made during a visit to von Müller's clinic in the late fall of 1903, almost two years before Barker was to set up similar research laboratories in the department of medicine at Johns Hopkins. In commenting later, Barker spoke as follows:

> But through my experience in Friedrich von Müller's clinic in Munich I had learned that the work of a clinical laboratory could be advantageously extended by securing investigators trained in the so-called pure sciences of physics, chemistry, and biology who would devote themselves to the special application of the methods and principles of those sciences to the solution of the special problems of diagnosis and therapy. Von Ziemssen had recognized this need and clinical research laboratories had been established in the hospital at Munich. Later von Müller also regarded these as essential for the work of a university medical clinic.[61]

Such experiences of Americans abroad created great dissatisfaction with the conditions at home. "Where in America," demanded Lusk, "is there to be found a Müller, a Noorden, Minkowski, Krehl, Kraus, His, Levy, or Mortiz? When I have spoken with distinguished and powerful clinicians about imitating the German methods, I have always been told that that kind of thing was impossible here."[62] One explanation of America's backwardness in clinical science came in the same year from Samuel James Meltzer of the Rockefeller Institute. America's "lack of progress," he said in a speech to the newly created Association for the Advancement of Clinical Research, was due to the fact that at that time teaching was "mostly still in the hands of men who received their medical training nearly exclusively in this country."[63]

As we shall see, virtually all of the men associated with the move to establish scientific medicine in America had been trained abroad. Lusk's ideal model for the organization of a medical clinic was Friedrich von Müller's clinic. In his article entitled "The Reorganization of Departments of Clinical Medicine," Lusk quoted Müller's description of his own clinic's activities as follows:

> At half past eight I go to my institute, at ten to the wards. My clinic (at 9 A.M.) is in the theatre . . . I show the patients . . . examine and explain them. This takes an hour, and then I go with a part of my students . . . to the wards and instruct them personally. This takes another hour. Then I go around the wards with my assistants and it is one or half past one when I have finished. . . . I go to my institute in the afternoon and give a general lecture . . . upon the diseases of the brain, . . . the respiratory system and so on. . . . I have one assistant in biological chemistry, another in physiology, one working on nervous diseases, one doing bacteriological work and making a vast number of tests, Wasserman tests and so on. . . . Research work I do . . . in connection with my assistants. . . . I have my own laboratories. . . . Would it not be possible to conduct the school for the common practitioner in the old established manner? No. The general

practitioner has always . . . to deal with the highest good, with the health of his fellow creatures and . . . he must be an educated man. . . . He must have some ideal which elevates him above the daily . . . disappointments of life and he will find his refuge in his science. Only a good scientific education will enable him to follow the progress of medicine with critical understanding. Without a good scientific training he would sink into the mere routine.[64]

Thus von Müller and, following his example, Lusk, saw that the development of clinical science in departments of medicine, where the practitioners of the future were taught, was the most effective way to build a scientific base for medicine and so improve the practice of medicine.

As will be described later, the scientific accomplishments of Lusk and his research associate at Bellevue Hospital and Cornell, DuBois, were a vital force in the advancement of clinical science.

# 2

cy/ゆ

# Programs for Training Premedical Students
in the Basic Sciences

Before any of the new approaches to medical science that were so successful in Germany could be effectively transferred to the United States, an army of physicians trained in the research methods of the basic sciences had to be developed. In the 1860s, there were no requirements for knowledge in the basic sciences for admission to medical schools, and there were no laboratory facilities for teaching the techniques of the basic sciences to premedical or medical students. The part-time instructors in physiology and chemistry did no research and therefore could not stimulate the students in this area.

## Studies Preparatory to Medicine

One of the events that played a significant role in changing this situation took place at Yale University in 1869, when the Sheffield Scientific School initiated a course entitled "Studies Preparatory to Medical Sciences." At a meeting of the governing board, held on October 21, 1868, the following action was taken: "Voted, that a course of study preparatory to medical studies be arranged and announced and that Messrs. Johnson, Eaton, Verrill and the secretary of the school [Daniel Coit Gilman] be a committee to adjust the same."[1] Thus was started a course in biology preparatory to medicine, probably the first in the United States. It gave recognition to the principle, not then generally understood, that the study of medicine should rest upon a knowledge of the sciences, particularly those now designated as biological. Perhaps equally important was the training such a course of study offered in the scientific method for men who aimed to be proficient in both the science and the art of medicine.

31

For the freshman and sophomore years this course was composed of a judicious admixture of mathematics, physics, chemistry, and botany, followed in the junior year by qualitative and quantitative analysis, organic chemistry (with some reference to its physiological and medical bearings), botany, and zoology, as well as history, English, modern languages, and other subjects. In the senior year, the work was more specialized, embracing special topics in botany, zoology, and comparative anatomy—particularly embryology, the laws of hereditary descent, physiological botany, and medicinal plants. The first graduates (1872) of the new course were T. Mitchell Prudden[2] and Thomas Hubbard Russell. The former eventually became a distinguished professor of pathology at the College of Physicians and Surgeons of Columbia University and later a director of the Rockefeller Institute for Medical Research; the latter, a professor of materia medica and therapeutics at Yale Medical School. After 1874 the course was reorganized and its scope broadened; it attracted an increasing number of students, whose conspicuous success in their medical studies emphasized the value of the training.

Who were the members of the committee that designed this far-reaching venture at Yale? Daniel C. Eaton and Addison E. Verrill received their appointments in the department of philosophy and the arts at Yale on July 26, 1864; Eaton as professor of botany, Verrill as professor of zoology. Easton was a graduate of Yale whose interest in botany led him to Harvard University, where he studied under Asa Gray. Verrill became preeminent as an investigator in invertebrate zoology. Trained at the Lawrence Scientific School of Harvard, he worked as Louis Agassiz's assistant from 1859 to 1864.

Samuel W. Johnson was elected professor of analytical chemistry in 1856. In 1852 Johnson studied chemistry at Leipzig and the following year with Liebig at Munich. In 1856 Johnson was appointed chemist to the Agricultural Society of the State, and his first report concerned the various ways in which chemistry could be of service to farmers. After the Civil War, Johnson became chemist to the State Board of Agriculture. He fostered interest in the establishment of experimental stations. In 1875 the Connecticut legislature appropriated money for experiments in agriculture under the direction of Professor Wilbur O. Atwater of Wesleyan University, who had studied chemistry under Johnson in 1869. (Atwater was a product of the Voit school in Germany; see p. 27.)

On July 28, 1863, the Yale corporation appointed Daniel Coit Gilman as a professor of physical and political geography. Gilman graduated from Yale College in 1852 and, after study at Berlin, became assistant librarian at Yale in 1856. In that year he wrote an important article entitled "Scientific Schools in Europe." After 1865 he gave all his energies to the work of the Sheffield Scientific School. Gilman voiced many ideas vigorously held by the colleagues on the governing board, relative to the character of the curriculum of a technical or scientific school. In

"Our National Schools of Science," an article published in the *North American Review* in October 1867, he pointed out that such schools were in a formative state, that no one could foretell exactly what they would become, but that "they were a very significant indication of the spirit of the age, a manifestation of the desire for an advanced education on some other basis than the literature of Greece and Rome." Gilman was a major force in the creation of sound ideas regarding the nature and position of a true scientific school in the educational scheme.

## Physiological Chemistry

In 1882, a new professorship was established at the Sheffield Scientific School, announcement of which was made in the annual statement of the governing board for 1882–83:

> The school has been fortunate during the past year in adding to the corps of its permanent officers Russell H. Chittenden as occupant of the newly founded chair of physiological chemistry. Mr. Chittenden was a graduate of the Institution in the class of 1875. After graduation he remained, pursuing a course of special study in physiological chemistry; and on account of the proficiency he displayed in this particular subject, was almost immediately made instructor in it and had the main charge of the laboratory of physiological chemistry until 1878. He then went to Germany and studied chemistry and physiology in the University of Heidelberg. On his return, he resumed charge of the physiological laboratory, and in 1880 received from Yale College the degree of doctor of philosophy. In the summer of 1882 he went to Germany to carry on an investigation in physiological chemistry with Professor Kühne of Heidelberg.[3]

Thus, Chittenden became the director of the first laboratory of physiological chemistry in this country, as well as the first candidate to receive the degree of doctor of philosophy in physiological chemistry.

It was undoubtedly the vision of Professors Johnson, Brewer, and Brush that led to the establishment of the laboratory of physiological chemistry in 1874. The laboratory consisted of a small room on the second floor of Sheffield Hall. A year or two later an additional room was renovated to meet the needs of the department, an expansion that continued gradually until, in 1886, a large part of the entire second floor of Sheffield Hall was occupied by the laboratory. Soon there were two groups of students pursuing physiological chemistry side by side: regular undergraduates of the biological course and graduate students doing advanced degree work.

The success of the Scientific School students entering on the study of medicine became so clearly recognized that students in the college who were expecting to study medicine began to clamor for admission to some of the course offerings. The governing board agreed to furnish an optional course of instruction in the biological sciences to the junior and senior classes of the academic department and to provide and equip suitable laboratories for such instruction. The courses offered to the academic students were physiology, with demonstrations and illustrative experiments, by Chittenden, one hour a week through the year; elementary biology, covering the rudiments of biology and the elements of the morphology of animal tissues, by S. I. Smith, eight hours a week in the laboratory for one-half year; physiological chemistry, by Chittenden, eight hours a week in the laboratory for one-half year; a short course of lectures by Smith on embryology; and a somewhat longer course by Chittenden on experimental toxicology. The number of academic students desiring to take these courses quickly exceeded the number (twenty) allowed by the agreement.

Even the members of the governing board were surprised at the results that followed the establishment of the biological course. They had, of course, realized that the prospective medical student needed a better preparatory training, but they had not expected such a dramatic response to their efforts, a response that showed itself not only in the increasing number of students who applied for admission, but also in the quality of the applicants.

The board expressed its opinion regarding the educational value of a chemical-biological training for prospective medical students:

> In one sense any course of study inasmuch as it is disciplinary is a preparation for medical as well as for other studies, but no argument is needed to show that purely mental training, which may be the best preparation for theological or legal studies, for instance, is a very imperfect preparation for the study of medicine. As a rule, the student while at the medical school has very little time or opportunity for the training of the senses and the acquisition of the power of accurate observation which are so evidently requisite in the practice of medicine or surgery.... The study of the methods of modern scientific investigation and their practical application in the laboratory, unquestionably furnish the best and readiest means for this kind of training. A still more apparent advantage of this class of study is that they may readily be made to furnish the best groundwork for the special medical education. As an illustration, a thorough acquaintance with the elements of physics and chemistry is essential for the understanding of the first principles of physiology, and yet neither physics nor chemistry has properly any place in the curriculum of the medical school, and cannot well be taught the student already grappling with subjects presupposing a knowledge of them. The elements of these important studies should be mastered before the medical school is entered, and when studied practically in the laboratory as only they can properly be studied, they also give training in scientific method and manipulation, which is so essential both to the student and practitioner of medicine.[4]

In 1869 this course of study was generally looked upon as an unnecessary luxury for the prospective medical student. Within a few years, however, as graduates of the school made outstanding records at medical school, a decided change of attitude became apparent. These students not only had an increased knowledge in chemistry and biology, which made them superior medical students, but had also sharpened their mental skills by cultivating habits of observation, by learning to draw logical deductions from observed facts, and by training in the methods of scientific investigation.

The number of Scientific School undergraduates pursuing the biological course up to 1892 was usually about thirty-five to forty juniors and seniors each year, with twenty to twenty-five Yale College seniors taking the courses in comparative anatomy and physiological chemistry and twenty to forty college juniors taking the course in physiology. Some years later the course in physiology was attended by as many as two hundred college students.

Of even greater significance was the number of graduates and other advanced students taking graduate work in physiological chemistry and doing research in this subject. For years physiology had been confined largely to the study of physical functions, while the chemical functions were more or less neglected. The best minds in medicine and in physiology were beginning to realize that in the study of function the chemical aspects could not be ignored. This was particularly true of certain branches of physiology, notably nutrition and the processes of digestion, secretion, and excretion. Facts were being brought to light that made it clear that important new knowledge in medicine and physiology was destined to come through physiological chemistry. Among the Yale graduates who took these courses were many who made outstanding contributions to American medicine, including Joseph A. Blake, Lewis Atterbury Conner, Harvey Williams Cushing, John Staige Davis, John A. Hartwell, John F. Howland, Theodore Caldwell Janeway, Elliott Proctor Joslin, Alexander Lambert, Samuel Waldron Lambert, Bertin Lee, A. N. Richards, Richard Pearson Strong, Howard C. Taylor, W. Gilman Thompson, and H. Gideon Wells.

The reorganization of Yale University on a departmental basis in 1919, followed by the construction of the Sterling Hall of Medicine—in which, in 1923, the corporation installed the administrative offices of the school of medicine and the departments of anatomy, physiology, physiological chemistry, and pharmacology—resulted automatically in the abolition of the Sheffield Laboratory of Physiological Chemistry, after a period of nearly fifty years of valuable contributions.[5]

## Preparation for Medical Research

### Daniel Coit Gilman

A vital step in the development of clinical science in America was the appointment of Daniel Coit Gilman[6] as president of the Johns Hopkins University in 1875. Gilman's great contribution to the advancement of learning, the development of the first true university graduate school in this country, is well known. His interest in medical education and his efforts to raise it to the same high academic level are not so generally recognized. It was this aspect of his beliefs which was, however, responsible for further training in the basic medical sciences.

Gilman's ideas had a warm reception during his short period as president of the University of California,[7] and by the time of his arrival in Baltimore his ideas were well crystallized. In his inaugural address at Johns Hopkins University on February 22, 1876,[8] he sharply criticized the educational standards of the existing medical schools and then said:

> We need not fear that the day is distant . . . which will see endowments for medical science as munificent as those now provided for any branch of learning, in schools as good as those now provided in any other land. . . . It will doubtless be long, after the opening of the university, before the opening of the hospital; and this interval may be spent in forming plans for the Department of Medicine. But in the meantime we have an excellent opportunity to provide instruction antecedent to the professional study of medicine.

He then discussed a course of undergraduate study that would "train the eye, the hand and the brain for the later study of medicine." In 1878, he presented a report prescribing a premedical course that included the study of chemistry, biology, and physics, modern and ancient languages, and other subjects leading to a Bachelor of Arts degree and that was far in advance of the admission requirements of existing medical schools.

## The Chemical-Biological Course and Research Training in the Department of Biology at Johns Hopkins

Johns Hopkins decreed in his will that the university and hospital should cooperate in the promotion of medical science. Consequently, Gilman and the original faculty gave much thought to medical education, and a thorough foundation for the medical course was provided by instruction in physics, chemistry, and biology. Prominence was given to biology because of its fundamental relation to medicine. Henry Newell Martin, the professor of biology, was familiar with the methods employed in the best physiological laboratories in England and on the continent. An associate professor was responsible for morphology and comparative anatomy, leaving Martin free to teach and do research in physiology in accordance with his own personal training. Three of the university fellowships (there were twelve available) were allotted to students of biology. Thus the stage was set to attract young men who were interested in obtaining a suitable foundation for the subsequent study of medicine.

In University Circular #9 (1881)[9] a description of the graduate instruction and opportunity for research was given. A few key areas of biology and physiology were selected to begin with, and the very best facilities possible were provided for their study. The choice was deter-

mined by two considerations: first, the founder of the university especially desired cooperation with the Johns Hopkins Hospital in advancing
medical science; and second, the general policy of the university. According to that policy, with which, when a choice was possible between
two subjects in which to afford special facilities for advanced study and
research, the one selected was that in which such facilities were less
commonly provided elsewhere in the United States. In this way an attempt was made to complement, rather than to rival, the work of other
institutions of higher learning.

The university allowed the student to select his plan of study from one
of several schedules described in the university catalog. Among the subjects that could be taken up after studying physics and chemistry was
biology, and this study was recommended to those preparing themselves
for the study of medicine.

Physiology was thought to be a subject having special claims on Johns
Hopkins:

> Notwithstanding a small number of brilliant physiological discoveries
> made in the United States, and the fact that several distinguished
> physiological investigators are found here, it can hardly be said that
> America has taken her fair part in contributing to the modern advance of
> physiology. The costliness and variety of accurate instruments required for
> modern physiological research almost preclude any but a well endowed
> institution from obtaining them: hence the majority of medical students,
> even had they time, have not the opportunity of acquiring that practical
> knowledge of the methods of physiological inquiry which is so valuable an
> auxilliary in those therapeutical and pathological researches, which, con-
> ducted on the modern experimental method, have added so much in late
> years to the list of remedial agents at the disposal of practicing physi-
> cians. . . .
>
> For the reasons briefly stated, animal physiology has formed one of the
> subjects for special advanced study selected by the Johns Hopkins Univer-
> sity; and of its subdivisions, more attention is given to what is commonly
> known as experimental than to chemical physiology, the latter being al-
> ready fairly well provided for in several colleges. The chief endeavor has
> been to provide special facilities in the so-called experimental physiology
> and the instruments brought together for advanced study and research in
> that branch of knowledge are believed to be more numerous and to cover a
> wider ground than those to be found elsewhere in this country. . . .
>
> Students who follow this course will acquire a knowledge of the method
> of using all the chief instruments employed in physiological research and
> so it is hoped will be qualified to carry out afterwards scientific investiga-
> tions on the physiological action of drugs in experimental pathology.[10]

As J. G. Adami stated in 1901, what Henry Newell Martin did in Baltimore was of basic importance in laying the foundation for medical science in America.[11]

# 3

❦

# The Importance of the Basic Sciences in the Training of Clinical Scientists in the United States

Before there were facilities in clinical departments for research, both students and faculty did their investigative studies in anatomy, physiology, chemistry, and pathology laboratories. Here many who later became outstanding clinical scientists received their early training and, most important, their stimulus to a research career. In the next chapters the role played by these basic science departments in the evolution of clinical science will be described.

## The Origins of Physiological Research in America

Physiology was the first of the experimental medical sciences. In the United States two laboratories of physiology were developed in the 1870s, the first in Boston and the second in Baltimore. The history of American physiology may conveniently be divided into the pre- and post-laboratory periods.[1]

John Richardson Young's thesis at the University of Pennsylvania in 1803 was entitled "An Experimental Inquiry into the Principles of Nutrition and the Digestive Processes." He introduced a small frog into a large frog's stomach, pulling the former out with a string when he wished to examine it. He found that digestion was the formation of a true solution without the appearance of putrefaction. Young tested the gastric juice chemically and concluded that the acid present was phosphoric. Thus, he narrowly missed the discovery of hydrochloric acid, which was made by Prout in 1824.[2]

Other physiological work in the same field was done at the University of Pennsylvania. In 1803 Oliver H. Spencer presented his study, "Experiments and Observations on Digestion," reaching conclusions similar to those of Young. In 1805 Thomas Ewell submitted his thesis entitled "Notes on the Stomach and Secretion." In a dog he had isolated, with ligatures, some two feet of the ileum and into this had injected some well-boiled meat saturated with a pig's gastric juices. The intestine was returned to the abdomen, and in three hours the animal was killed. The autopsy showed that one-third of the material had been absorbed and that the lymphatics contained chyle. This was probably the first vivisection experiment made in America.

Little other physiological research appeared until Beaumont's work almost three decades later. Beaumont, who carried out 238 experiments on a patient, Alexis St. Martin, published the results in 1833 in a volume entitled *Experiments and Observations on the Gastric Juice and the Physiology of Digestion.* He described many important observations, including the length of time it takes various foods to digest in the stomach; that animal foods are digested more easily than vegetable; that oily substances retard digestion and delay the passage of foodstuffs from the stomach; the first accurate description of gastric juice; and that mental disturbances have a profound influence on the secretion of gastric juice and on digestion. Beaumont's work gave physiologists a method of studying gastric phenomena in animals. His studies were the inspiration of the "miniature stomach" method of Rudolf P. H. Heidenhain and Ivan Petrovich Pavlov. However meaningful Beaumont's work seems now, its immediate influence on the development of physiology and medicine in the United States was negligible. No university offered him a professorship, no medical school invited him to lecture. The American medical world was clearly not ready at that time for science.

There were others who made important contributions to physiology in the prelaboratory period, including Robley Dunglison, Charles-Edouard Brown-Séquard, H. F. Campbell, Austin Flint, Jr., William Hammond, S. C. E. Issacs, and S. Weir Mitchell. Among these, Mitchell probably provided the strongest impetus toward the development of the experimental physiological laboratory. He often turned to the laboratory for the solution of his clinical problems, as illustrated by his researches on the venom of poisonous serpents, on the knee jerk and its reinforcement, and on the function of the cerebellum.[3]

John Call Dalton, who was the first American to devote his time exclusively to physiology, took his M.D. degree at Harvard in 1847 and learned to experiment under the guidance of Claude Bernard. Dalton must be given the credit for establishing, at the College of Physicians and Surgeons in New York, the first permanent physiological laboratory in America. It was, however, essentially a private laboratory; it was not for students and did not attract a body of workers or produce a series of investigations, such as characterized the laboratories organized later at Harvard and Johns Hopkins. It was not until 1887 that Dalton's old laboratory was expanded and organized in the modern sense. John G.

Curtis, who succeeded Dalton, expanded the activities in the laboratory and Samuel James Meltzer did his physiological experiments there before he joined the Rockefeller Institute for Medical Research (see chapter 6).

## The Laboratory of Physiology at Harvard

The first university facility for experimental physiology in America was developed in Boston in 1871,[4] with Ludwig's pupil Henry Pickering Bowditch (1840–1911) as its director. Bowditch entered Harvard College in 1857 and four years later matriculated at the Lawrence Scientific School in Cambridge to study chemistry. In 1868 he received his M.D. degree from Harvard. No one played a greater role in the development of basic science in this country than did Henry P. Bowditch. From his simple beginning at the Harvard Medical School there evolved, "facilitated by numerous other individuals, institutions and circumstances," a new medical educator—the biomedical scientist who devoted his career to teaching and research and refrained from the private practice of medicine.

A number of changes took place in the faculty of the Harvard Medical School in the 1860s. From the viewpoint of experimental science, none was more important than the 1864 appointment of Brown-Séquard to the newly created chair of physiology and pathology of the nervous system. Unfortunately, Brown-Séquard remained for only a short period, giving a sporadic series of lectures from 1865 to 1867. In his brief stay he did, however, stimulate faculty interest in experimental physiology. His major contribution was to synthesize the experimental physiology of Magendie and Bernard and the pathological studies and clinical correlations pioneered by Louis. Perhaps his greatest accomplishment at Harvard was his influence on Henry P. Bowditch, who attended his lectures. Henry P. Bowditch, the nephew of Henry I. Bowditch, was particularly influenced by two of his other teachers—Oliver Wendell Holmes and Jeffries Wyman, both of whom devoted their careers to the scientific side of medicine. Bruce Fye's studies indicate that without these influential friends and his uncle's prominent stature at Harvard, young Henry Bowditch would have pursued a traditional medical career rather then devoting himself to physiology.[5]

In 1868 Henry P. Bowditch journeyed to France to study with Brown-Séquard, who, having only recently returned to Paris, could not accommodate him as a graduate student. Brown-Séquard suggested that Bowditch enroll in the courses of Claude Bernard and his student Louis-Antoine Ranvier. Bowditch was able to do experimental work with Ranvier and acquired enthusiasm for experimental physiology. He found, however, that the facilities for research in Paris were poor. Willy Kühne, who was in Paris during 1869, advised Bowditch to work first with Max Schultze and then to enter Ludwig's physiological institute for his intensive training.

In contrast to Bernard's laboratory, Ludwig's institute seemed to Bowditch to be both stimulating and well-equipped. Bowditch's first work on the innervation of the heart, which appeared in 1871, marked him as a productive experimental physiologist. More important was Bowditch's appreciation of the value of the German scientific approach to medical research and education.

In 1870, Bowditch was nominated to the Harvard corporation as assistant professor of physiology. He decided to remain in Ludwig's laboratory for an additional year, however, so that he would be qualified to incorporate research with his other responsibilities.

When Bowditch received another offer from President Charles W. Eliot in 1871, he accepted on the condition that physiology would be a separate department, and that he have a voice in the affairs of the school. His conditions were agreed to, and Bowditch then turned to the acquisition of the necessary apparatus for his new department. He received a financial commitment from his father for the purchase of the necessary laboratory equipment. He also acquired specialized European literature devoted to experimental medicine as the foundation for his library. An expenditure of $7,000 was made to remodel two rooms in the attic of the medical school as laboratories, which assured Bowditch of at least a modest facility for his research, where students could also participate in experimental physiology. Thus, Bowditch returned to the faculty at Harvard prepared to introduce the German concept of the basic medical scientist to America. Unlike his predecessors, who had divided their time between clinical and laboratory pursuits, Bowditch was to devote his entire time to physiology. He would not have to rely upon income from the practice of medicine to support his research activities. The position of Bowditch at Harvard was a small beginning, but it represented the initial stage of university support of the full-time basic medical scientist, whose recognized role was to combine teaching and research in his specialized area. It also represented the professionalization of physiology in the United States.

It would be five years later, with the opening of the Johns Hopkins University in 1876, before the first deep institutional commitment to original research by the preclinical faculty would become a reality. This was not the case at Harvard when Bowditch returned from Europe. Although President Eliot made some attempt to facilitate the research efforts of his faculty, he made it clear that their primary responsibility was to teach. There was no suggestion that Bowditch should consider himself as having a responsibility to organize a program for the replication of his own career training in terms of the development of future physiologists.

On November 19, 1871, Bowditch initiated a series of experiments concerning the rate of transmission of the nerve impulse and soon returned to the study of ciliary motion, which had interested him earlier. With no assistants, no graduate students, no mechanic to help arrange and maintain the experimental apparatus, and no one to deliver lectures to medical students but himself, he soon appreciated the advantages for scientific work that had been available to him in Germany. He began a campaign to make the medical community of America aware of the fruits of the German research effort. Beginning in 1873, and for the next decade, he published a periodic "Report in Physiology" in the *Boston Medical and Surgical Journal*.

The circumstances surrounding a career in medical science in this country when Bowditch returned in 1871 are depicted in a letter written by William Henry Welch to his sister in 1878: "I was often asked in Germany how it is that no scientific work in medicine is done in this country, how it is that many good men who do well in Germany and show evident talent here are never heard of and never do any good work when they come back here. The answer is that there is no opportunity for, no appreciation of, no demand for that kind of work here."[6]

Thus, at that time, any student who elected to train under Bowditch for a career in experimental physiology would find no positions available for him. Although Bowditch did not emphasize training advanced workers in physiology during his early years at Harvard, he did offer medical students firsthand experience in experimental physiology. In the Harvard University catalog of 1872–73 it was noted for the first time that "to third class students opportunities are given for original investigations in the laboratory," and it was announced that a "course of study for graduates" had been introduced.[7] The new approach at Harvard led to more laboratory instruction, a practice that soon extended to other schools. This was an important step, because students received instruction in the techniques of science, which they could later apply in their clinical research. Joseph W. Warren published a detailed description of the physiological laboratory and enumerated its apparatus in 1884.[8] Productive work was soon the hallmark of this new "institute," but equally important was the attraction to it of interested young men seeking training. Work was done in essentially every phase of experimental medicine, including physiology, general biology, pharmacology, experimental pathology, psychology, and experimental surgery. Among Bowditch's disciples were Walter B. Cannon, G. Stanley Hall, William James, Warren P. Lombard, Charles S. Minot, and William T. Porter.

During Bowditch's early tenure, reform of medical education at Harvard Medical School progressed steadily. The course in physiology consisted of an excellent combination of lectures and demonstrations. In 1883 he became dean of the medical faculty, and, during his ten years in that position, the four-year course of study was instituted and bacteriology was recognized as a required medical subject.[9]

An excellent example of the influence that this laboratory had on clinical investigation is illustrated by the following story of Cannon, who became Bowditch's successor in 1905, and his fellow student Albert Moser. They asked Bowditch to assign a research problem to them. Bowditch suggested that they use the newly discovered x-ray and an opaque contrast medium to test Kronecker and Meltzer's theory of the nature of swallowing. The method of study, although primitive—and, unknown to them, dangerous—was available and adequate. The problem, which rapidly enlarged to encompass all the mechanical factors of digestion, was ripe for study and, as the flood of definitive results showed, well within their powers. Horace Davenport pointed out that this is a classic example of the right suggestion to the right students at the right time.[10]

On December 9, 1896, Cannon and Moser began the work that was to lead to "the application of roentgen rays to the study of the mechanical factors of digestion in man." In the first experiments, the animal was held in front of the x-ray tube; in later experiments, the tube was beneath a tabletop, on which the animal and the screen were placed. Cannon crouched over the tube, receiving the x-ray burns from which he was to suffer for the rest of his life. Cannon and Moser first fluoroscoped a dog lengthwise while the dog swallowed a pearl button. The movement was described as "irregular," which meant that the button was not squirted down the esophagus, as Kronecker and Meltzer[11] had said liquids were. Realizing that they needed a better contrast medium, they used bismuth subnitrate, which became the contrast medium of roentgenologists for the next fifteen years. On December 29, Cannon and Moser gave, before the ninth annual meeting of the American Physiological Society, the first demonstration of gastrointestinal fluoroscopy.[12]

Reviewing a list of staff members, research fellows, and graduate students in the department of physiology at Harvard from 1871 to 1971,[13] one becomes aware of the enormous contribution that this department made to clinical science. The list includes such distinguished clinical investigators as Henry K. Beecher, Douglas D. Bond, William B. Castle, Stanley Cobb, Arthur R. Colwell, E. C. Curnen, Vincent P. Dole, Jacob Fine, Reginald Fitz, Sheppard I. Franz, William J. German, Carl Gottschalk, Alfred Kranes, Eugene M. Landis, Harold D. Levine, R. L. Levy, Robert R. Linton, Champ Lyons, Rustin McIntosh, Monroe McIver, Jonathan C. Meakins, Hugh Montgomery, Gordon S. Meyers, Louis H. Newburgh, Joseph H. Pratt, Oscar Ratnoff, Paul Reznikoff, J. F. Ross, Richard S. Ross, Stanley J. Sarnoff, E. B. Schoenbach, Arnold N. Seligman, L. Hollingsworth Smith, Eugene A. Stead, Joseph T. Wearn, and J. E. Wood III.

## The British Influence on American Physiology

We have seen how young Americans went to Germany for training in physiology and chemistry; how the schools of Ludwig and Voit were major contributors to the evolution of medical science in America; and how Bowditch established the first laboratory of physiology in the United States. Great Britain also contributed significantly to the development of physiology in the United States, but in a different way.

In the middle of the nineteenth century, certain British anatomists and clinicians dealt with physiology as a sideline, and there were no useful laboratories in existence. Beginning in 1836, William Sharpey (1802–80), of the University College in London, became a major force in improving physiologic teaching and research in Great Britain. In 1866, Sharpey made the astute decision to bring Michael Foster, then only thirty years of age, to teach physiology at University College. Foster, who had great organizational talents, was a superb teacher and was intimately acquainted with physiology in Germany. He created the first physiological laboratory in the British Isles[14] and was instrumental, with Sharpey and Sir John Burdon-Sanderson among others, in founding the Physiological Society of Great Britain in 1876.

When Foster left London for Cambridge in 1870, Burdon-Sanderson became his successor. Four years later, he succeeded Sharpey as Jodrell Professor of Physiology and finished his career as Regius Professor of Medicine at Oxford. As a young man, Osler had studied in Burdon-Sanderson's laboratory, making his observations on blood platelets there.

It was, however, Foster who had the greatest influence on physiology in America, in the form of his student Henry Newell Martin.[15] Martin was only twenty-eight years old when he took up his duties in 1876 as a professor of biology at the Johns Hopkins University. In addition to his work with Foster, he had also had contacts with Thomas Henry Huxley. A unique course of laboratory work, designed to give a broad view of living forms and functions, had been introduced by Huxley in 1873. Martin helped to import the course to Cambridge and, under Huxley's direction, prepared the famous textbook on practical biology that was published in 1876. Martin was the first to take the degree of Doctor of Science in physiology while at the same time qualifying in medicine in London. In 1874, the call to America came.

Like Bowditch, and, indeed, in cooperation with him, Martin was actively interested in stimulating research among those interested in physiology. Martin's outstanding students included William T. Councilman, George Sternberg, Henry Sewall, William Henry Howell, John J. Abel, W. T. Sedgwick, T. H. Morgan, Ross G. Harrison, Frederic S. Lee, and Walter Reed. Seven of the original twenty-four members of the American Physiological Society had been students of Martin's.[16] Sewall, one of Martin's most promising students, was recruited by the University of Michigan, where, in 1887, he offered an optional laboratory course in physiology, the first of its kind ever given in an American medical school.

Martin was an active investigator. His method of perfusion for the isolated mammalian heart ranks among the greatest contributions ever made in an American physiological laboratory. Sewall tells of the morning, in 1880, when Martin arrived at the laboratory remarking: "I could not sleep last night and the thought came to me that the problem of isolating the mammalian heart might be solved by getting a return circulation through the coronary vessel."[17] By the close of the day he had made the experiment successfully. Excellent papers on the influence of variations in temperature and pressure on heart rate and on the effect of drugs on the isolated mammalian heart followed.

### William Henry Howell

William Henry Howell became the first professor of physiology in the Johns Hopkins University School of Medicine. Howell enrolled in the "Chemical-Biological" course at Johns Hopkins in 1879. Upon graduation he was awarded a scholarship, which enabled him to continue his training. Howell later remarked: "In this way my original intention to become a practitioner of medicine was diverted and I entered upon the career of a teacher and investigator." Physiology was the keystone of Martin's department of biology and it was in that environment that Howell, at twenty-four years of age, began his career as a teacher. During this period his interest in the coagulation of the blood developed.

Howell accepted the chair of physiology at the University of Michigan in 1889, when Henry Sewall left for Colorado. In 1891 the laboratory course in physiology at Michigan became a requirement for all medical students; it was the first such course to be required in any medical school in the country.

In 1892 Howell accepted an appointment as associate professor of physiology under Henry P. Bowditch at Harvard. His stay there was short also, as, in 1893, Gilman offered him the professorship in Baltimore. Howell was the only one of the four full-time heads of the preclinical departments at Johns Hopkins who had not had experience in foreign laboratories.[18]

During his Ann Arbor–Harvard period, Howell published a description of particles in red corpuscles that take nuclear stains, known as Howell-Jolly bodies. While at Johns Hopkins, Howell was the first investigator to suggest that the two lobes of the pituitary gland are functionally different, and he described experiments showing that the circulatory effects of extracts of the pituitary gland are the result of substances derived entirely from the posterior lobe. Howell's interest in salt action suggested to him the possibility that cardiac slowing resulting from vagal stimulation might be caused by release of potassium. Guided by this hypothesis, he demonstrated the liberation of potassium during vagus stimulation, in amounts sufficient to stop the heart.[19] Howell was, therefore, among the first to suggest the chemical nature of the neural influences affecting heart rate. After 1909, Howell's interest was devoted almost exclusively to the study of blood coagulation. It was a student collaborator, Jay McLean, who discovered heparin. During his career Howell had many students who made significant contributions to clinical science or became clinical scientists, including E. Cowles Andrus, W. W. Duke, Joseph Erlanger, Arthur D. Hirschfelder, L. Emmett Holt, Reid Hunt, George Minot, and Arnold Rich, among others.

Thus, there were two great schools of physiology that helped establish the foundations of clinical science in the United States: one begun by Bowditch in Boston, which was inherited by Walter B. Cannon; and the other, with its British heritage, begun by Martin in Baltimore and continued with distinction by Howell. Many important clinical investigators had their training either in these laboratories or in those headed by students trained by Philip Bard, Henry P. Bowditch, Walter B. Cannon, William H. Howell, Eugene Landis, and Henry Newell Martin.

## Physiological Chemistry as a Background for Clinical Investigation

In his Harvey Lecture of 1908,[20] Otto Folin pointed out that clinicians in hospitals had in their possession valuable material for biochemical investigations. None of them were, however, trained at that time either to do or to direct such chemical work: "Without adequate provision for the thorough sifting and critical investigation of the observations of the clinicians, most of their impressions must remain hopeless mixtures of the correct, the probable and the impossible."

Folin stated that biological chemistry was a recognized independent branch of experimental science. It was preeminently a field of research for which a large body of men should be specifically trained, yet it was still one into which most of the workers had drifted by chance after their student years were over. He pointed out that universities were still turning out doctors of philosophy in chemistry who also knew physics and geology, but few who were familiar with any branch of biology; and that the medical schools were still graduating only physicians. The schools doubtless believed, he said, in the importance of the medical sciences, but they were "just beginning to understand that the development of those sciences demands suitably trained specialists; specialists who cannot grow up in sufficient numbers on the basis of personal initiative alone." As an indication of the infancy of that specialized scientific field, he pointed out that the first physiological chemist, Chittenden, was still in his early fifties.

It was useless to dream that chemical problems would be solved in hospitals unless the hospitals had trained men, suitable equipment, and an effective demand for such research. Folin believed that the most direct and important aim of biochemical investigation had to be the advancement of the ability to differentiate between the physiological and the pathological, which could be done only when the investigator was as alert for new points or false teachings in the domain of the physiological as in that of the pathological. Folin recommended, to achieve maximum service for the advancement of biological chemistry, providing a well-equipped hospital laboratory, even if necessarily a small one, some current literature, and one or two assistants; then giving the worker freedom, which he should have earned in order to get the position.

### The Development of Physiological Chemistry in the United States

In 1870 physiological chemistry in America had not achieved a significant place for itself. There was as yet no appreciation of the important role chemistry might play in the expanding field of medical science, and, as a result, so-called "physiological chemistry" was hardly more than a name. Even as late as 1900 there was no agreement as to whether physiological chemistry should be under the jurisdiction of the department of chemistry or of physiology. In these early years "medical chemistry" was largely confined to the determination of the composition of animal and vegetable tissues and fluids, together with some testing for abnormal or pathological constituents. The experimental method was limited to the "physical" aspects of physiology, as exemplified by the interest in nerve-muscle physiology. The potential of "chemical physiology" was either unrecognized or ignored as being of little practical importance.

In the 1870s any American student wanting to make progress in physiological chemistry went to Germany for the knowledge and experience he needed. Otherwise, he might be well-trained in chemistry according to the standards of that date, but he would be lacking in the knowledge of research methods and in the proper ways of approach to the study of physiological problems. Early developments of importance came at Yale when, in the 1870s, the Sheffield Scientific School began to function actively.[21] In 1874 Chittenden, an eighteen-year-old Yale undergraduate, was chosen to be director of a laboratory of physiological chemistry, and in 1880 he received the first Ph.D. degree to be awarded in that subject in America (see chapter 2).

There was not a special instructor in physiological chemistry at Harvard until 1898, when Franz Pfaff served in the double capacity of instructor in pharmacology and physiological chemistry. In 1904 Carl L. Alsberg became an assistant in physiological chemistry, and in 1905 he and Lawrence J. Henderson were appointed instructors in biological chemistry.

In the last decade of the nineteenth century, physiological chemistry gained recognition both as an educational tool and as a basic contributor to the knowledge of science and medicine. At that early date, however, anyone who ventured to prophesy that the most important advances in the scientific medicine of the next generation would come from the use of chemical methods of research would have found few adherents.

Professor Chittenden's laboratory was the intellectual birthplace of two others of the first group of great experimental biological scientists to teach at Yale, Professors Lafayette B. Mendel and Yandall Henderson.[22] These men were soon joined by Ross Granville Harrison, from Johns Hopkins, as professor of biology.[23] It was Harrison who first devised (in 1907) the method of tissue culture for animal cells that has been so essential in medical research.

With Chittenden, Mendel became one of the founders of the science of nutrition. Chittenden had done basic work on enzymes in digestion, and perhaps his greatest achievement was the establishment of the protein requirements of man. In collaboration with Thomas Burr Osborne, of the Connecticut Agricultural Experiment Station, Mendel made the fundamental discovery that some proteins were nutritionally inadequate since they lacked amino acids that could be synthesized by the body. These he christened "essential amino acids." As early as 1910 he found an important growth factor in milk residue, which contained a water soluble substance later known as vitamin B. Three years later he discovered that a serious eye disease, xerophthalmia, developed in rats lacking the fat-soluble vitamin A.

Mendel was the most influential of all of Chittenden's pupils. He studied also with Heidenhain at Breslau and with Eugen Baumann at Freiburg in 1895 and 1896. When he returned, he became closely associated with Chittenden, and, after Chittenden became director of the Sheffield Scientific School, Mendel was in charge of the graduate program.

One of Mendel's outstanding pupils was Stanley R. Benedict who had an important influence on the relationship of chemistry to medical research.[24] Benedict received his Ph.D. degree under Mendel in 1908. The great teacher Mendel was then at his height, and no other physiological chemist had so great an impact upon the medical profession until Folin and Benedict reached their prime.

The rapid development of physiological chemistry in America after 1890 was, to some extent, due to the growth of interest in the scientific method. The conviction that students could acquire firsthand knowledge of scientific principles only by personal experience in the laboratory was bringing about radical changes in the educational system of the country.

It is important to trace the early period of this expansion in experimental work and to discuss the laboratories in which the work was done. At this stage, there were no research laboratories in clinical departments; many of the workers who contributed to the development of clinical investigation had their early research training in physiological chemistry departments and did their work there.

### Studies of Nutrition

In the evolution of physiological chemistry in America studies in nutrition stand out. One of the pioneers was Wilbur O. Atwater, who took his doctorate at the Sheffield Scientific School at Yale in 1869 under Professor Samuel W. Johnson. He then studied under Voit at Leipzig; he became professor of chemistry at Wesleyan University in 1873.[25] Atwater studied dietary habits and between 1894 and 1897 worked out the "Atwater Standard Diet" for a man of 70 kilograms doing light work: 100 grams of protein per day, with fats and carbohydrates sufficient to make a total of 2,700 calories. Atwater's ambition was to learn more about the metabolic processes of the body under different physiological conditions; to emulate Rubner's work with the respiration-calorimeter; to determine the heat value of different foodstuffs; to measure heat production in man; and to confirm the general laws of metabolism in the human organism. Between 1892 and 1897 a calorimeter was built at Wesleyan University, largely through the skill of E. B. Rosa, the professor of physics.

Francis G. Benedict, professor of chemistry at Wesleyan, worked with Atwater in these studies. A graduate of Harvard (1893) and a student of chemistry at Heidelberg in 1895, Benedict became, in 1907, the director of the newly established Nutrition Laboratory of the Carnegie Institution, which was located in Boston (see chapter 12).

### Otto Folin and Stanley R. Benedict

When the University of Chicago opened in the autumn of 1892, Otto Folin was one of the Minnesota graduates of that year accepted for advanced study.[26] He chose chemistry as his major. His teachers included J. U. Nef, then professor of chemistry; Jacques Loeb, professor of physiology; and Julius Steiglitz, a young member of Nef's staff who was Folin's faculty adviser. In August 1896, Folin went to Europe to study with Olof Hammarsten at Uppsala, Ernst Salkowski at Berlin, and Albrecht Kossel at Marburg. While in Marburg, Folin learned of the technique of colorimetry (used in the brewing industry), which led to his first colorimetric method, that for the determination of creatinine. After receiving his Ph.D. degree from Chicago in 1898, he was eager to begin an academic career in physiological chemistry, but he could find no opening except as a chemist in a commercial laboratory. In 1899 he was offered an assistant professorship of chemistry at West Virginia University. There he discovered one of his most distinguished students, Phillip A. Shaffer, who later became professor of biochemistry at Washington University.

In the spring of 1900, Folin was offered a newly created position when Edward Cowles, medical superintendent of McLean Hospital for the Insane at Waverly, Massachusetts, decided to establish a research laboratory for physiological chemistry. Cowles hoped that studies using that approach might in time contribute to the better understanding of mental diseases. Folin was invited to plan, equip, and conduct that laboratory and to formulate his own program. He accepted promptly, realizing that it provided an opportunity to carry out the kind of studies that he was eager to embark upon.

While at McLean Hospital, Folin studied the protein metabolism of normal versus mentally disturbed individuals, by measuring all of the known nitrogenous and other products excreted in the urine. He hoped thereby to learn the normal range of variation in the partition of the total nitrogen and then to consider possible variations. First he had to devise better quantitative methods.

In 1905 Otto Folin published three papers that attracted wide attention.[27] These described a new system for the analysis of urine for urea, ammonia, creatine, creatinine, and uric acid. His new procedures were regarded as so great a step forward that Harvard University created a professorship of biochemistry for him, providing research laboratories in the newly completed medical school buildings. In laboratories in the United States and abroad, Folin's new techniques were quickly applied to the study of various human disorders and of pathological states produced in animals. Folin directed his attention to refining and improving these analytical methods for the constituents of urine and also modified them for use with small samples of blood. He appears to have been the first to realize the importance of knowing which products of metabolic activity the kidneys fail to excrete, as well as how much of these products clear the kidneys.[28]

The extent of protein digestion in the alimentary tract, the nature of the products absorbed, and the manner in which they are disposed of after absorption were important unresolved issues. Folin secured data on the concentration of urea and ammonia in deproteinated samples of blood taken simultaneously from branches of the mesenteric veins, the portal vein, the liver, systemic blood and muscle, and organ extracts. The nonprotein, nonurea, nonammonia nitrogen was correctly judged to consist largely of amino acids. These data afforded an explanation of the course of events in protein digestion and the distribution of amino acids to the tissues during and after the absorption period.

This was the state of the art when Stanley R. Benedict entered research in physiological chemistry.[29] He worked at Syracuse University for one year, and then joined Cornell's division of clinical pathology. Two years later (1912) he became head of the newly organized department of physiological chemistry at Cornell—an appointment for which Graham Lusk was responsible.

Benedict soon found, on critical study, that a number of Folin's methods could be improved upon, including those for uric acid, creatine, creatinine, total sulfur, and sugar. It was inevitable that the regular appearance of such critical studies should irritate Folin (although the two men always remained on good terms). Yet Benedict's contributions to analytical chemistry did not detract from the great eminence accorded to Folin by chemists, physiologists, and clinicians.

Especially important were Benedict's studies on methods for the determination of glucose in blood and urine. Other reducing substances exist in blood and urine, so that the older methods for sugar estimation gave results that were too high. Benedict's untiring efforts brought improvements that had great significance in the study of normal and abnormal carbohydrate metabolism.

It had been known for years that the uric acid metabolism in dogs was different than in man; in the latter, allantoin was excreted as the end product in the urine. Benedict observed that certain dogs did excrete uric acid. He soon discovered that this unusual pattern of purine metabolism was only present in the Dalmatian coach dog. This breed lacks the enzyme that converts uric acid to allantoin. Benedict was one of the earliest investigators to disturb the metabolic processes of tumors in an attempt to cause regression. Among his collaborators was John R. Murlin, who later became a professor at the University of Rochester, where he was the first to describe glucagon.

Thus, Folin and Benedict did much to lay the foundations for the development of clinical science. Henry A. Christian said of Folin:

> I speak with the authority of one who daily in my care of patients now for many years has utilized the methods that Dr. Folin perfected both for a better understanding of what ails sick humanity and as a guide to their therapeutic management. You, my younger colleagues and students, cannot envision medicine without the methods of blood analysis perfected by Folin and his pupils and those inspired by Folin's own accomplishments, so completely have these micromethods of quantitative analysis become a factor integrated into the web and woof of the fabric of clinical, medical and surgical work.[30]

Folin encouraged an interest in biochemical research among medical students, graduates, and physicians. Three of his students became Nobel laureates. Walter R. Bloor, one of his first graduate students, wrote as follows: "Folin was much interested in the medical students' laboratory and spent the whole time there when the class was in session. He did not circulate a lot but took one student or a group and worked intensively with them, doing a piece of research with the exercise they were working on."[31] There were some distinguished students in those first groups: George R. Minot, W. W. Palmer, Francis R. Rackemann, Elliott Proctor Joslin, and many others.

### *Lawrence J. Henderson*

It was Lawrence J. Henderson who established our knowledge of the acid-base equilibrium of the blood and who served as a mentor for many distinguished clinical investigators.[32] After receiving his M.D. degree from Harvard in 1902, Henderson went to Franz Hofmeister's laboratory in Strasbourg. When he returned to the United States he became a lecturer in biological chemistry at Harvard, where he remained throughout his career, serving as a professor of biological chemistry from 1919 until 1934 and as Abbott and James Lawrence Professor of Chemistry from 1934 until 1942.

During Henderson's long professional career his research developed in fairly distinct stages. The first was devoted to the application of physical chemistry to explain the maintenance of neutrality in body fluids, especially in the blood.[33] Out of this interest there evolved thoughtful consideration of the relations of organisms to their surroundings, which led to the publication of two volumes: *The Fitness of the Environment* (1913) and *The Order of Nature* (1917). As a result of his exhaustive examination of the blood as a complex multifunctional system, he published a treatise, *Blood, a Study in General Physiology*, in 1928. In a second stage he was concerned with the more complex social relationships of human beings. His book *Pareto's General Sociology; A Physiologist's Interpretation* shows the breadth of his intellectual interest. Many of the men who were influenced by him, including Dickinson W. Richards, W. W. Palmer, Louis H. Newburgh, James L. Gamble, Arlie Bock, and J. H. Talbott, later became notable contributors to clinical science. Other collaborators were A. Forbes, Henry L. Field, Jr., E. F. Adolph, W. O. Fenn, L. M. Hurxthal, E. B. Dill, and John S. Lawrence.

### Other Major Contributors

When the Johns Hopkins University School of Medicine opened in 1893, physiological chemistry was a part of pharmacology, and John J. Abel immediately advocated an independent chair.[34] This was established in 1908 under Walter Jones, who is famous for his work in nucleic acid chemistry. Jones stimulated many young men in research, including Charles R. Austrian, Milton C. Winternitz (later dean at Yale), and George Whipple.[35]

Although working almost a generation later than Abel, Edward C. Kendall performed hormone research that had valuable consequences in the field of clinical investigation. Kendall received his Ph.D. degree in chemistry from Columbia in 1910. He then accepted a position as research chemist for a large company and was asked to isolate the essential hormone of the thyroid gland. He soon found that close contact with clinical investigation was necessary for the success of his work, and, through the efforts of Nellis Barnes Foster, Kendall became head of the biochemical laboratory of St. Luke's Hospital in New York. In short order, he developed a new method for the determination of iodine, later hydrolyzed the thyroid proteins, and prepared a fraction with the then phenomenal concentration of 33 percent iodine. The conditions for work were less than ideal in New York, so he wrote to Louis B. Wilson at the Mayo Clinic, asking whether the clinic would be interested in a chemist who wanted to study the thyroid gland. Kendall went to Rochester in February 1914. On December 5, 1914, he isolated the crystalline thyroid hormone.[36] (For further reference to Kendall's contributions, see chapter 21).

Phoebus A. Levene immigrated to the United States in 1891, after receiving an M.D. degree at St. Petersburg.[37] After working for several years at Columbia's College of Physicians and Surgeons, he joined the staff of the newly formed Rockefeller Institute. He was the first to determine the formula of nucleic acid. He also worked on the chemistry of the mucoproteins and was the first to find the chemical formula for chondroitin sulfuric acid.

Of Levene's many well-known pupils, the one who was to contribute most to the development of physiological chemistry in relation to clinical medicine was Donald D. Van Slyke.[38] When, in 1910, Van Slyke began to study amino acids, Levene realized that Van Slyke had found a field of his own and left him free to explore it. In the pursuit of this research, Van Slyke showed a particular talent for devising ingenious laboratory procedures, by first developing a method for the quantitative determination of amino acids. Rufus I. Cole, director of the Hospital of the Rockefeller Institute (HRI), who spent a year in Levene's laboratory while the hospital was being built, recognized Van Slyke's unusual talents. In 1914, Van Slyke and his associate Glenn Cullen moved from their corner in Levene's laboratory to new and larger facilities in the hospital.[39]

A. Baird Hastings, a pioneer in clinical biochemistry, provided training in his laboratory for numerous young physicians who later pursued careers in clinical research.[40] Hastings received his Ph.D. degree under Professor Frederic S. Lee (a former student of Henry Newell Martin) at Columbia. Here he began his scientific studies in physiology and biochemistry and developed an interest in clinical investigation. With Harry Murray, a house physician, he studied problems relating to pH, chloride, and $CO_2$ content of the blood in parathyroid disease and in gastric tetany. While working for his doctorate, he was also doing experiments for the U.S. government on the physiology of fatigue. These experiments involved studies of acid-base balance in fatigue, which paralleled those in diabetes that Cullen and Van Slyke were carrying out at the HRI. After Hastings graduated from Columbia, he joined forces with Van Slyke. Van Slyke described the stimulating experience of working with Hastings: "Now that he had only one job, sixteen hour's work a day seemed to Hastings a simple life."[41] It was during these years and, according to Van Slyke, largely due to Hastings's drive and inspiration, that the laboratory conducted its work on the gas and electrolyte equilibria of the blood, which established hemoglobin as one of the main anions of the blood and revealed the quantitative role of Donnan's equilibrium in the distribution of chloride and bicarbonate ions between blood cells and plasma.

In 1926 Hastings was made professor of physiological chemistry at the University of Chicago. In 1928 he changed titles and laboratories and became professor of biochemistry. He was the first director of the Lasker Foundation and moved his laboratories to the department of medicine. There he developed a close relationship with the members of the departments of medicine and surgery, whose clinical services had opened in 1927. Many students from other schools flocked to his laboratories in the summertime, and his first two students, Richard Capps and Henry Harkins, later became professors of medicine and surgery, respectively. In 1930 Hastings became a visiting professor of biochemistry at Peking Union Medical College in China and later served as head of the department of biochemistry at Harvard. He was a great emissary for biochemistry and particularly for its application to clinical science. Whether the activity was research, teaching, or practice, he stimulated his assistants and students to independent research, epitomizing in his teaching the best existing thought, but always suggesting the unsolved problems for the future. Just before reaching retirement age at Harvard, Hastings became director of the division of biochemistry of the Scripps Clinic and Research Foundation in La Jolla, California, and later head of the laboratory for metabolic research there.

## The Influence of Experimental Pathology: William Henry Welch

Another great American medical statesman who trained under Ludwig was William Henry Welch (1850–1934). After entering the College of Physicians and Surgeons in New York, Welch realized that he needed further scientific training and returned to Yale. Here he came under the spell of two gifted chemists, Oscar H. Allen and George Frederick Barker.

In 1872 Welch reentered the College of Physicians and Surgeons. Its status in Welch's student days serves to highlight the enormous changes that Welch later stimulated in pathology and in medical education. The major part of the three-year program consisted of didactic lectures. The practical work was restricted to anatomy, medical chemistry, and a primitive course in clinical instruction. Emphasis was on producing practitioners, and the preceptorial system was utilized. From the preceptor, the student obtained his practical training by accompanying him on rounds and assisting in his office. There was no required course in pathology, although Francis A. Delafield provided a voluntary course with demonstrations. There was no opportunity for the student to study histology or to use a microscope. Welch became a prosector to the professor of anatomy and also devoted special time to autopsy work, which allowed him to acquire some technical skill.[42]

In 1876, after a year's internship, Welch went to Strasbourg to study histology under Wilhelm Waldeyer.[43] He spent part of his time in Felix

Hoppe-Seyler's physiological chemistry laboratory. He then went to Leipzig to study with Heubner, since Welch considered neurology as a possible field of practice. Heubner had shifted his interest to pediatrics; therefore Welch attended Wagner's course in pathological anatomy. Welch then decided to study physiology and was accepted in Ludwig's laboratory. Welch's work in Leipzig was ostensibly to prepare him to study under Virchow. Ludwig convinced him, however, that he should work instead with Julius Cohnheim (1839–84) in Breslau. This advice was critical in Welch's development, since Cohnheim's approach was functional rather than morphological. Among the group in Cohnheim's laboratory were Paul Ehrlich and Carl Weigert, who were beginning to use aniline dyes to stain microscopic sections. Cohnheim had a high opinion of Welch and later recommended him for the professorship of pathology at the Johns Hopkins University.[44]

While with Cohnheim, Welch investigated the pathogenesis of acute pulmonary edema. He concluded that its cause was primarily mechanical and that edema developed because of a disproportion in the work of the right and left ventricles. While at Breslau, Welch witnessed Koch's demonstration of his studies on anthrax to Cohnheim and Ferdinand Cohn.

On his return to New York in the spring of 1878, Welch received two offers to teach pathology. Delafield, at the College of Physicians and Surgeons, suggested that he give a series of lectures on pathological anatomy. Welch declined because there was no opportunity for laboratory work. The second offer, from Bellevue Medical College, included the use of a laboratory converted from small rooms. Welch worked intensively there for six years and established the foundation for the teaching of pathology in the United States. This was probably the first laboratory of experimental medicine in the United States—a small but very significant beginning.

In 1884 Welch accepted the professorship of pathology at the new Johns Hopkins University. Since the pathological laboratory was under construction, he set out for another year of European study. The new science of bacteriology was evolving at a rapid pace, and Welch recognized its significance. With Frobenius in Munich he learned the techniques of bacteriology, and he also worked with Max von Pettenkofer, who stimulated his interest in public health and hygiene. Acting on Robert Koch's advice, Welch then went to Goettingen to work with Flügge (1847–1923), who contributed greatly to Welch's bacteriologic background. This was followed by several weeks working under Koch himself.

In September 1885, Welch returned to Baltimore to begin work in a temporary laboratory on the top floor of the biology building. Soon he occupied the building on the hospital lot that had originally been intended as a "deadhouse," but was converted, according to his specifications, to house a laboratory of experimental medicine as well.

Welch's laboratory was a beehive of activity and had a tremendous influence on the progress of medical research in the United States. Many important investigators were trained in this laboratory, including William T. Councilman, William Stewart Halsted, Franklin Paine Mall, A. C. Abbott, Walter Reed, Simon Flexner, Lewellys Franklin Barker, George Nuttall, and James Carrol.

Welch's subsequent career, of course, had much to do with the development of clinical science in the United States. He founded the *Journal of Experimental Medicine* and was chairman of the Board of Scientific Advisors for the Rockefeller Institute and its research hospital. To a large degree, he was the implementor of the full-time system in clinical departments.

# Summary

During the period of British influence on American medicine, which prevailed from the mid-eighteenth century to about 1820, medical research in the United States lagged behind medical practice. In early America, survival meant taking care of immediate problems at hand, so that there was little time for other activities and no social advantage to be gained by medical research. The country was still underdeveloped, and the conditions and facilities for such research were virtually nonexistent. The situation might have been different if observers had found novel forms of illness in the United States, but this was not the case. In this early period, the separation of various diseases was not far advanced, and theoretical pathological systems, such as the ancient "tension" theory expounded by Benjamin Rush, ascribed all illness to "excessive action" in the walls of blood vessels, with the result that every condition could be treated by bleeding and purging to relieve the tension. If one cause and one remedy were known, then further research was unnecessary.

The Paris period (1820–1860) had an influence through the many Americans who studied in Paris under Louis. In the city's hospitals there emerged strong clinical traditions, and the leaders tended to have little interest in laboratory concepts and techniques. The methods that Louis developed in his study of various diseases were those that formed the basis of the modern techniques of clinical information-gathering that we use every day in the practice of medicine. Louis was probably the first full-time clinical investigator, even though his principal tools were observation and numerical analysis of the data. Two of the outstanding contributions of his American students were the essay of Oliver Wendell Holmes on the contagiousness of puerperal fever, which was published several years before the studies of Semmelweiss; and the contributions of Stillé, Shattuck, and particularly Gerhardt in clearly separating typhus fever and typhoid fever as distinct diseases. There were still no clinical research facilities in the United States, nor did any of the clinicians have the basic training that would equip them for work in experimental medicine.

Although France was the pioneering country in the establishment of modern scientific facilities, the importance of the innovative efforts in that country was quickly recognized in Germany, and the university system there proved an effective framework for the organization and direction of systematic research. Physiology as a science and the concept of experimental medicine both received more sympathy in Germany than in France. The man who did most for the introduction of physiology to Germany, Johannes Müller, was a generalist. Pressure for the separation of the disciplines by the younger generation of scientists was soon evident, however, and, when Carl Ludwig was offered a professorship in 1849 at Zürich, he accepted only on the condition that a separate teacher be appointed for anatomy. From then on the recognition of the new discipline proceeded rapidly, leading to a complete transformation of the scientific career in Germany. Science became a specialized and regularized occupation. Once a new and fruitful field was pointed out in one university, strong pressures led other universities to follow suit, thereby creating more opportunities for those desiring to work in the new field. Thus it became possible to concentrate after graduation on one well-defined and promising field of research, with a definite aim of a scientific career.

This mechanism was also responsible for the development of facilities for research and the introduction of new scientific methods. By the  1860s even clinical chairs were given almost exclusively to people with attainment in research rather than to outstanding practitioners, and from the middle of the century even public hospitals were increasingly staffed by doctors both interested in and trained in research. Thus, medicine became an applied science in Germany much earlier than it did elsewhere. What came to be known as *physiological medicine* developed rapidly and was an important preparatory step to the new era of clinical science. It contributed to clinical medicine chiefly through the stimulus given to the introduction of new methods of investigation. These methods were developed primarily by the physiologists and chemists, but the clinicians also adopted them, and soon every clinic had its laboratory, in which the methods of the basic sciences were being used to study the manifestations of disease in man.

At the end of the Civil War, there were no clinical research laboratories in the United States, no training in the research methods of the basic sciences was given either in premedical courses or in medical school, and no career opportunities existed for the clinician who might develop an interest in research. As the migration to the cities occurred and industry prospered, money became available for philanthropic purposes, and the situation changed. As soon as a few men realized the practical usefulness of the new developments taking place in Germany and as soon as it was realized how deficient medical education and medical science were in the United States, an awakening occurred, and a determined group of medical statesmen set out to change the situation.

The first need was for physicians who had some knowledge of the basic sciences. Steps were taken to create such a cadry of individuals with some ability and training for clinical investigation by the introduction at Yale of studies preparatory for medicine, in which students were trained in physics, chemistry, and biology. A similar step was subsequently taken at Johns Hopkins. In 1871 the first full-time professor of physiology in the United States was appointed at Harvard, and, five years later, a physiologically trained Englishman was made a professor of biology, at Johns Hopkins, setting the stage for the introduction into medical school of adequate courses in the basic sciences. Such courses provided, among their other accomplishments, opportunity for medical students and graduates to engage in laboratory research as a background for later participation in clinical science. A third laboratory for this purpose was organized in New York by William Henry Welch and moved in 1866 to Baltimore, where Welch was to become the first professor of pathology in the new medical school at Johns Hopkins. During the latter quarter of the nineteenth century, both physiology and biochemistry developed rapidly in the United States, and better opportunities became available for research and research training in these areas. Clinicians desiring training and the opportunity to do research worked in these laboratories since there were no facilities available for investigation in most clinical departments.

Shortly after the middle of the nineteenth century, therefore, American educator-scientists and administrators displayed increasing interest in the organization of medical science in Germany. Scientists and intellectuals who visited that country returned home enthusiastic about German academic life, and soon German university training became a standard preparation for scientific careers. The Land Grant Act, passed in 1862, and other circumstances brought about a large increase in the number of American colleges and universities between the sixties and eighties. The most important events were the rise of graduate schools in the seventies and, in the following decade, the establishment of the Johns Hopkins University School of Medicine, which was directly influenced by the German example.

Carl Ludwig, the Leipzig physiologist, had a major influence on the men who trained under him, including William Henry Welch, Franklin Paine Mall, Henry P. Bowditch, and John J. Abel. Ludwig had picked up the torch from Johannes Müller, and he instilled his American pupil Mall with the idea that medicine could not advance until the knowledge and methods of the basic sciences were applied to the study of human disease. Another major German scientist who established an important school of physiology was Carl Voit. Through the men he trained, notably Graham Lusk, he had an important influence on the development of clinical investigation in the United States.

As one looks at the subsequent developments, it is clear that the United States provided a milieu similar to Germany's, where competition within a decentralized system encouraged the establishment of specialized research roles and facilities. The usefulness and the necessity of such roles and facilities in the clinical field was not generally recognized at the beginning of the twentieth century, and, in the United States, such roles and facilities were strongly resisted. At that time, like medical scientists in general, clinicians were still thought of primarily as practitioners, and only secondarily as scientists. The problem of transforming the practitioner-amateur role into a scientific career in the clinical fields was to prove similar to the earlier problem of creation of scientific roles and the professionalization of the basic sciences.

Thus, the rapid rise in America's accomplishments in medical research starting from the 1880s can be attributed to the extent to which the possibilities inherent in the rapid developments in science were exploited through enterprise and organizational measures, in the recognition of new disciplines, in the creation of specialized scientific jobs and facilities for research, and in the introduction of large-scale systematic training for research. Competition determined many of the crucial decisions concerning all of these developments. Successful scientists were rewarded with university chairs and facilities. Their success encouraged others to take up science and incidentally transformed the pursuit of science into a regular professional career, first in the basic sciences and later, as we shall see, in the clinical area. This created pressure for further expansion of facilities and training and exposed the inadequacies of current institutions. The continuous growth that was set in motion created a situation in which research became a regularly established career. During the early period, after professionalization of the basic sciences, clinicians had to utilize the facilities developed there for what investigative work they did. In the next section we shall see how facilities and institutional arrangements for clinical science were developed.

# Part II

❧

## Creating the Facilities and Institutional Arrangements for the Development of Clinical Science

# 4

# Important Innovations at the Johns Hopkins University School of Medicine and Hospital

The reforms in medical education in America in the last quarter of the nineteenth century were highlighted by the strengthening of the basic sciences. A major change took place at Johns Hopkins, where, in 1893, the professorships of anatomy, physiology, pharmacology, and pathology were placed on a full-time basis. With the resulting improvement in both teaching and research productivity in the basic sciences, students preparing for a career in clinical medicine learned more of the research methods in the sciences basic to medicine. Undergraduate and graduate students began to take advantage of these new opportunities for research in Bowditch's laboratory of physiology in Boston, in Henry Newell Martin's laboratory of biology, and in Welch's laboratory of experimental medicine in Baltimore. Clinical medicine was, however, still founded on the study of pathology and not on physiology and chemistry. Among the role models for young men training for the medical profession were William Osler (1849–1919) and Austin Flint, Jr. (1812–86). Both had phenomenal powers of observation; both enlarged their clinical acumen by studying diseases at the autopsy table. Osler, of course, had training in physiology with Burdon-Sanderson in England, but concentrated on microscopy, since he had no talent for physiological research. He made several significant innovations, however, in his organization of the medical clinic at Johns Hopkins, that had a bearing on the development of clinical investigation.

## Osler's Medical Clinic at Johns Hopkins

Perhaps Osler's[1] most important innovation was the creation of an upper resident staff whose tenure of office often lasted several years, and who devoted all their time to the clinic.[2] He also introduced the

British system of clinical clerks and established facilities, as an integral part of the clinic, where students were taught laboratory methods of diagnosis—the examination of excreta and secretions, study of the blood, and performance of specific immunological tests. These changes had a profound influence on every medical clinic in the country in the ensuing years.[3]

## Another Important Contributor to the Development of Clinical Science: Franklin Paine Mall

One of the first to emphasize the need to put clinical departments on a university basis was Franklin Paine Mall (see chapter 7). Mall knew that medicine must change, that disease was the price of ignorance. He knew that medicine had to apply all that science could give to the development of greater skill in diagnosis and toward the discovery of specific rather than symptomatic treatments in disease. He was fully aware that the better-prepared student in the basic sciences, where the fruits of research were becoming evident, would find a disappointing difference when he reached the clinic, and that such well-trained students would not long accept an attitude toward disease that would seem static.[4] This situation is documented in James H. Means's recollections of his student days at Harvard.[5]

George E. Vincent, who later became head of the Rockefeller Foundation, recalled at the University of Chicago (1892–93), discussions led by Mall and Jacques Loeb on the application of scientific methods to the study of disease in man. In 1893 Mall accepted the professorship of anatomy at Johns Hopkins and, in Baltimore, continued to advocate full-time positions in the clinical departments. Osler placed major emphasis, on the other hand, on teaching students the techniques and skills necessary for observing and interpreting the manifestations of disease in patients; less on investigation of the underlying disease processes. His belief that pathology was the basic science of clinical medicine reflected the teachings and precepts of Pierre Louis's school, which Osler held in high esteem. In part, Osler's attitude may be attributed to the lack of adequate facilities for such study; but he, together with most of his contemporaries in America, did not fully comprehend how rapidly physiology and chemistry were progressing or the potential they had to form the base for important advances in clinical medicine. His introduction of laboratory methods at the bedside was for diagnostic purposes rather than to develop new knowledge.[6]

Assisting Mall in the course in neuroanatomy at Johns Hopkins was Lewellys Franklin Barker,[7] who was to assume the post of professor of medicine when Osler left Baltimore, in 1905, to become Regius Professor of Medicine at Oxford. After spending a year in Osler's clinic, Barker became a fellow in pathology under Welch. He then joined Mall in the anatomy department, where he rose to the position of associate professor, and in 1899 he was appointed associate professor of pathology as well. Thus, for eight years he worked in close association with Osler, Mall, and Welch. In 1895 he spent six months in Leipzig working under Max von Frey, making a detailed study of the localization of the sensory points in the skin of the arm.[8] He accepted the position of professor of anatomy at the University of Chicago in 1899, and, in 1903, he was given a leave of absence to work in Munich with Friedrich von Müller and in the chemistry laboratory of Emil Fischer. He had thus seen the vigorous pursuit of research both in the clinic and in the laboratory, a joint endeavor characteristic of German medicine.

Barker articulated Mall's ideas about the application of science to clinical medicine in an address, delivered on February 28, 1902, entitled "Medicine and the Universities,"[9] in which he proposed that clinical departments should rank with the basic science departments of the university and should emphasize research in the problems of human disease. In this address, Barker described vividly the transition in which the subjects of the first two years were taught by professors who gave their whole time to teaching and investigation. As a result of this change, students had obtained a thorough scientific training in those branches fundamental to clinical work. Now, he continued, students accustomed to the well-regulated work of the basic science courses complained, on entering the clinical years, of a lack of system in the teaching, of unsuitable arrangements of studies, of imperfect departmental relations, and of insufficient attention to sequence of subjects. In some institutions, students found that clinical professors often were not aware of the modern work in anatomy, physiology, physiological chemistry, and pathology.

Barker pointed out that "a modern university must be a center of original research, as well as a place of instruction . . . made up of scholars who are not only familiar with the results of previous investigations, but who, skilled in the methodology of their respective sciences, invade new territories, searching diligently for new facts."

In this forceful address Barker advanced his ideas of the necessary framework to promote clinical science. An exchange of letters between Mall, Flexner, Welch, and Barker provides documentation of these important events.[10]

## Barker as Professor of Medicine at Johns Hopkins

Barker succeeded Osler at Johns Hopkins in 1905. There were no funds to implement the full-time plan that he had outlined in his famous talk; however, Barker promptly made a significant move in the direction of putting the medical department on a university basis by organizing research divisions headed by full-time scientists in order to provide opportunities for clinical investigation.[11] Barker knew firsthand that von

Ziemssen in Germany had recognized the need for application of the fundamental sciences to the solution of the special problems of diagnosis and therapy and had founded clinical research laboratories first in Erlangen and then in Munich.

Barker was the first to organize full-time research divisions in a clinical department in the United States. There were three such divisions; the biological laboratory, under the direction of Rufus I. Cole; the physiological laboratory, under the direction of Arthur D. Hirschfelder; and the chemical laboratory, under Carl Voegtlin. There was also a general clinical laboratory for instruction and general research, under the direction of Thomas R. Boggs.[12] A psychopathological laboratory was projected, but no funds were available.

The following paragraph appeared in the annual report for 1907 of Henry Hurd, the director of the Johns Hopkins Hospital:

### Clinical Laboratory

During the past year the clinical laboratories in the Surgical Building have been thoroughly reorganized, and the work which is now being done there is of the highest order. A portion of these laboratories is devoted to special chemico-physiological problems under the direction of Dr. C. Voegtlin, an expert chemist; with him is associated Dr. J. H. King; the other rooms are given over to the study of new problems in the chemistry and bacteriology of the blood, under the direction of Dr. Rufus I. Cole, graduate of the Johns Hopkins Medical School, and ex-resident of the Hospital. As assistants he has had Drs. C. Deutcher, J. C. Meakins, R. Cecil, H. Klein, W. L. Moss, F. F. Russell and W. Gibson.

There is no doubt of the value of the work being pursued in these laboratories, and that it is as good work as is done in similar institutions in Europe.[13]

The difference between the British-type clinical teacher, represented by Osler, and the new era of young men interested in clinical investigation, represented by Barker, was succinctly stated by Cole, who served as resident physician under both professors:

Under Osler the opportunities for careful observation were never better and the importance of careful study of the more superficial aspects of disease never more insisted upon. But there existed in the clinic no great incentive to learn more about the fundamental nature of disease and facilities for making the necessary investigations were lacking. The belief was general that medicine was basically different from biology or chemistry or anatomy and could only be studied by different methods. From time to time doubts about this point of view were expressed but chiefly by workers in the underlying sciences and they usually held the opinion that the real investigations must be carried out by workers in their laboratories since clinicians neither had the necessary time nor did they have the adequate training for these more complicated researches ... Dr. Barker on the other hand felt that a primary function of the university department of medicine should be the encouragement of research and accordingly that the professor of medicine should be free from the burdens of a private practice and allowed to devote his time to his own investigations and those of his staff.[14]

## Cushing's Laboratory for Experimental Surgery and Medicine

Yet another important research facility was in the process of development at Johns Hopkins at just this time—the Hunterian Laboratory for Experimental Surgery and Medicine.[15] The erection of this laboratory resulted from the need for space for teaching third-year students. In a letter to Dr. William Henry Welch, the dean, William Stewart Halsted, the professor of surgery, wrote: "I should be sorry to have it forgotten that I initiated the operative course on animals. Courses in experimental surgery were given to the first class in their third year (1895). One of the inducements offered to Cushing to return to us was the transference of these courses to him."[16]

The building was completed in the summer of 1905.[17] Half of the space was allocated to the department of pathology and the other half to that of surgery, but clinical scientists in the new divisions organized by Barker had access to these laboratories. In them, a variety of problems, both basic and practical, were studied. Hirschfelder conducted experimental studies of cardiac lesions produced in dogs, and Voegtlin, with William G. MacCallum, carried out his important experiments on the relationship of calcium to the parathyroid gland.[18] Observations of natural diseases of dogs led to some interesting experimental studies. For example, valvular lesions due to endocarditis were found in dogs. Efforts were then made to reproduce these diseases in normal animals, as illustrated by the opening sentence in a paper by Harvey Williams Cushing and his colleague J. R. B. Branch: "We wish to mention briefly some attempts which have been made in the Hunterian Laboratory to reproduce chronic valvular lesions; to record certain cases of spontaneous valvular disease in the dog which have come under our observation; and finally to comment on the possibilities of future surgical measures in man directed toward the alleviation particularly of the lesion characterizing mitral stenosis."[19] Little did Cushing foresee, in December 1907, the ultimate attainment of this goal some forty years later.

## Barker's Clinical Research Divisions

### The Physiological Laboratory

In October 1905, the physiological laboratory, organized by Barker, began to study diseases from the standpoint of disturbance in function. The facilities consisted of a laboratory, in the new surgical building of the hospital, for the clinical study of patients. The special methods in use in physiological laboratories—particularly the graphic methods—were also used in this clinical study. A second laboratory, where diseases seen in the medical wards could be reproduced in animals and studied by physiological methods, was available. It was the aim in this laboratory "to bring the studies upon the patient as closely as possible into relation with the findings upon animals and mechanical models and to turn these results to practical use."

In 1907 the *Bulletin of the Johns Hopkins Hospital*[20] published a series of papers that emanated from the research laboratories organized by Barker. Three of these papers came from the physiological division and were presented by its director, Arthur D. Hirschfelder. A 1903 graduate of the Johns Hopkins University School of Medicine, Hirschfelder had studied abroad at the Pasteur Institute in Paris and at the University of Heidelberg. He served as resident house officer in Baltimore for a year and then returned to his home in San Francisco, where his father was a member of the faculty of the Cooper Medical College. After one year there, he came back to Johns Hopkins as a voluntary assistant in medicine and was soon placed in charge of the new research laboratory.

Barker outlined, in a paper before the Alabama State Medical Association in 1909,[21] the work of Augustus Waller and William Einthoven in developing the electrocardiograph, pointing out that Edelmann in Germany had developed and manufactured a complete instrument for the recording of the electrocardiogram in man. Barker ordered one of these instruments for the Johns Hopkins Hospital and designated George G. Bond to put the Edelmann "heart station" into operation when it arrived in October 1909. Walter Belknap James, who had studied physiology under Henry Newell Martin in Baltimore, and Horatio B. Williams at the Presbyterian Hospital in New York, had one of these instruments, as did Alfred E. Cohn at Mount Sinai Hospital in the same city. According to Bond's information, these two instruments did not become operative until several months after the one at Johns Hopkins did. In addition to taking electrocardiograms, Bond and Hirschfelder also devised a method of recording heart sounds and were able to obtain good tracings. After serving on the staff of the Johns Hopkins University for six years, Bond became assistant professor of medicine in the University of Indiana School of Medicine. In 1936 he was made professor of cardiology at Indiana.[22]

## The Chemical Laboratory

The chemical laboratory was under the direction of Carl Voegtlin, a native of Switzerland, who obtained his Ph.D. degree in chemistry from the University of Freiburg in 1903, studied in England, and then immigrated to the United States to take a position at the University of Wisconsin. Voegtlin did not have a technician or a secretary and washed his own glassware. The laboratory, which was located in a large room on the second floor of the surgical building, was modeled after the one in the First Chemical Institute in Berlin.

Voegtlin, in collaboration with MacCallum, discovered the role that the parathyroid gland plays in the control of calcium in the animal body.[23] After two years in the chemical laboratory, Voegtlin transferred to the department of pharmacology, in order to fill the post vacated by Arthur Loevenhart. J. M. Johnson, who had just obtained his Ph.D. degree in chemistry from the Johns Hopkins University in June 1908, was appointed to take his place.

## The Biological Laboratory

The biological division occupied three small rooms in the southeast corner of the second floor of the surgical building. The equipment included a small centrifuge and a larger one, which revolved 25 cc. tubes at a speed of 3,000 revolutions per minute, a speed necessary in precipitating bacteria from suspension. Sterilizers and all the apparatus necessary for routine bacteriological and biological investigation were at hand, and there was space for a limited number of small animals.

Rufus I. Cole, the director, was the first to employ blood cultures in Baltimore (1902).[24] Cole's pioneer studies of typhoid bacilli in the blood stream constituted one of the first systematic clinical laboratory studies done at the Johns Hopkins Hospital. At that time there was interest in the "opsonic" theory as an explanation of the ability of the body to recover from the invasion of disease-producing microorganisms. Among other areas of study was the treatment of infection by the use of specific vaccines. Frederick F. Russell, who was then an officer in the Medical Corps of the United States Army and who later introduced the practice of vaccination against typhoid fever in the army, began his work with typhoid vaccine in Cole's laboratory. Russell also studied opsonins and treated cases of osteomyelitis with autogenous vaccines, but without remarkable results.

A series of papers published in the *Bulletin of the Johns Hopkins Hospital,* respresenting work conducted in these clinical research laboratories, clearly indicates that the concept of training young men not only clinically, but also in the application of the methods of science to the study of human disease, was getting underway. It was in this setting that Cole realized the importance of this approach, which he implemented so successfully when he became the director of the HRI. Of the men appointed as directors of these research laboratories, only Cole fit the pattern in which clinical research was to be done by physicians who had sound clinical training, as well as experience in the techniques of basic research; he was the only one who had sufficient clinical expertise to gain the full respect of the hospital's part-time practicing physicians. Hirschfelder had had only a year as a resident house officer, whereas Voegtlin did not have an M.D. degree.

The importance of the in-depth clinical training that Cole had, in contrast to Hirschfelder and Voegtlin, may be seen by reviewing the further careers of the latter two men. Hirschfelder became professor of pharmacology at the University of Minnesota. In 1908 Voegtlin became an associate of John J. Abel in the department of pharmacology at Johns Hopkins. In 1913 he became chief of the division of pharmacology at the U.S. Hygienic Laboratory and, in 1937, was appointed director of cancer research in the Public Health Service. In January 1938, Voegtlin became the first chief of the National Cancer Institute.

After the departure of Cole in 1908, Paul W. Clough and then Arthur L. Bloomfield, who was later professor of medicine at Leland Stanford University School of Medicine, were active in Barker's bacteriological laboratory. After the departure of Voegtlin and Johnson, Andrew Watson Sellards was made temporary director of the chemical laboratory. Following his graduation from Johns Hopkins in 1909, Sellards went to the Philippines, where he became interested in Asiatic cholera and in amebic dysentery. He recognized that dehydration and acidosis were factors of great clinical importance in all of the dysenteries. On his return. Sellards studied the acid-base balance of the blood and did some of the first studies on acidosis in human diseases. In 1913 Walker and Sellards produced amebic dysentery in four human volunteers, by feeding them material derived from the stools of carriers.[25] Sellards became a member of the tropical medicine department at Harvard in 1914.

## Barker's Resignation

Barker resigned as chairman at Johns Hopkins in 1913, when full-time clinical professorships were established. He entered private practice in association with several younger men, who would do the primary gathering of the facts about the patients. It was Barker's great talent to take all of the information gathered by his associates and synthesize it in an effective way. Thus, he organized what might be called a "group practice."

There is controversy regarding Barker's achievements as professor of medicine at Johns Hopkins. Of interest is the impression of Barker expressed by a Johns Hopkins medical student, Dana Atchley, who later emerged as a good clinical scientist:

> Hopkins had appointed Lewellys Barker who had never been a practitioner of medicine. He held the M.D. degree but he taught neuroanatomy at the University of Chicago. He was considered a very promising man. He had written books on the subject and carried on extensive investigations; so Hopkins had appointed him to a professorship in medicine hoping that he would continue his research. They had made a

mistake. When he arrived they found that he knew no medicine and never had known any medicine. He built up a huge practice, got some bright young assistants who did all the diagnostic work and would merely come in and lay on his hands. He had a charming personality. He soon had earnings in the six figure bracket which was a great deal in those days. Barker encouraged no real scientific work for he didn't know anything about science. He organized a clique that took a vested interest attitude toward the professorship. They believed that the professor should be an active practitioner and they began to feel themselves being crowded out by somebody who knew something.[26]

(The last statement refers to the arrival of Theodore Caldwell Janeway, the first full-time professor of medicine, a subject that will be discussed later. Atchley's appraisal is probably biased, because it was given after the bitter experience that he—as well as Palmer and others—had at Johns Hopkins.)

In another evaluation of Barker, Charles R. Austrian wrote as follows:

His clinics at the bedside or in amphitheatre were models presented with a completeness, clarity and ease of expression seldom rivaled. He practiced and taught industry, system, honesty in work, brevity and unity in presentation. He made at least three real contributions to medicine in this country—first, he established here, as had von Müller and von Ziemssen in Germany, special research laboratories as integral parts of the medical clinics; second, he recognized and treated the individual as a unit—a psychobiological unit; and third, he emphasized the importance of group diagnosis.[27]

The importance of the establishment of research divisions by Barker cannot be underestimated. As pointed out by Cole, scientific investigation in departments of internal medicine did not begin with the opening of these research divisions, but the institution of laboratories for this specific purpose started a movement that was to influence greatly the character of university clinics.[28]

## Clinical Investigation in Surgery: Halsted's Innovative Ventures in General Surgery and in the Surgical Specialties

William Stewart Halsted was a pioneer in the founding of modern surgery in the United States and a potent stimulus to scientific investigation.[29] While studying medicine at the College of Physicians and Surgeons in New York City, he became interested in anatomy, and, after graduation in 1877, he spent two years in Europe attending courses in anatomy, as well as visiting the clinics of Theodor Billroth, Johann von Mikulicz, Ernst von Bergmann, Karl Thiersch, and Richard von Volkmann. In Germany he observed the implementation of Lister's antiseptic surgery.

On his return to New York in 1880, he worked with Welch in pathology at Bellevue, and, at Roosevelt Hospital, he inaugurated the first surgical outpatient department in New York. He became interested in Koller's discovery that the cornea could be anesthetized with cocaine. He experimented on himself and found that, by injecting this drug into a sensory nerve, he could render the whole area supplied by its branches insensitive to pain. Thus, he observed for the first time that nerve block could be utilized to obtain anesthesia for surgical purposes, a discovery promptly utilized in dental practice. He also demonstrated the blocking of the spinal cord with anesthetic drugs.

When Halsted was making these experiments on himself in 1885, it was not known that cocaine was a habit-forming drug. He sought hospital treatment for his addiction and came to lead a more thoughtful and leisurely existence, with time for reflection and the study of surgical problems; a life far more fruitful for medical science than if he had continued his strenuous pace in surgical practice. As he resumed his life in New York, however, he continued to have difficulty with his addiction.

Welch invited Halsted to Baltimore to live with him and to work in his laboratory, and Halsted spent the next three years, from 1886 to 1889, immersed in experimental work. Most importantly, he collaborated with Franklin Paine Mall and they become close friends. William T. Councilman, Welch's principal assistant at the time, noted:

> The entry of Mall into the laboratory marked a period of brilliant activity. Mall's first work here was on the structure of the intestinal canal, and in the course of this he demonstrated the peculiar character of the submucosa. The two men [Halsted and Mall] were very congenial and they worked together in the large south room of the laboratory, each receiving from and giving to the other. Halsted made full use of the work of Mall in the development of his method of intestinal suture . . . Halsted, of course, was already an ardent experimentalist and he had this drive reinforced by association with Mall.[30]

Florence Sabin spoke of their friendship in her biography of Mall: "The companionship of these two men was very close and only after Mall's death did I realize how closely they had followed each other's work; for then Halsted used to come over to the anatomical department and talk to me about his research just as he said he had always done with Mall."[31]

Councilman further commented:

> It is difficult to think of surgery more carefully conducted than was this experimental surgery by Halsted. The dog was treated as a human patient. There was the same care in anesthesia, the same technique in operation and in the closure of the wounds. These meticulous studies of Halsted's led him to realize the importance of careful handling of tissues, the necessity of controlling bleeding with a minimum of crushing of tissues with forceps, and the value of transfixing vessels and ligating them with the finest silk.[32]

Insight can be gained into Halsted's ability as a surgical technician by reading his paper, illustrated by Max Broedel, in the *Journal of the American Medical Association* in 1913.[33] Halsted contributed many important technical improvements and approached this work as true clinical investigation by attempting to understand the physiological basis involved. For example, in the autumn of 1887, at the suggestion of Welch, Halsted began experiments on extirpation and transplantation of the thyroid in dogs. The experiments resulted in the discovery, among other things, of the striking histological changes that signify hyperplasia and hyperactivity of this gland and that are similar to those found in Graves's disease.[34]

Halsted had an unusual approach to the development of the department of surgery. At an early stage he suggested to his fourth resident surgeon, Joseph C. Bloodgood, that he should undertake, in a more systematic manner than had hitherto been done, the study of all tumors and other tissues removed in surgery. Thus, surgical pathology was the first subspecialty established in Halsted's department. Later, in his apparently casual way, Halsted steered F. H. Baetjer into roentgenology; Harvey Williams Cushing and then Walter E. Dandy into neurosurgery; Hugh H. Young into urology; William S. Baer into orthopedics; and Samuel T. Crowe into otolaryngology. There is evidence to suggest that Halsted's apparent casualness was actually a well-designed plan for the development of clinical investigation in surgery. It seems reasonable to asssume that Mall and Halsted must have talked frequently about the development of the department of surgery and for the need to identify promising young surgeons who had the curiosity and originality to apply the methods of science to the study of the problems of surgery.[35] Halsted's innovative ideas may well have been to a large degree inspired by Mall, just as Mall had inspired Barker to begin full-time research divisions in the department of medicine.

## Harvey Williams Cushing
## and the Development of Neurosurgery

Harvey Williams Cushing matriculated at Yale College in 1887. While there, he decided on a career in medicine, primarily because of a course in physiological chemistry taught by Russell H. Chittenden. An early  clue to Cushing's innovative talent was the development, with Amory Codman, a fellow student at the Harvard Medical School, of the procedure of "continuous recording," which enabled both the anesthetist and the surgeon to tell at a glance a patient's condition during an operation by his pulse and respiration.[36]

During his period as house pupil at the MGH, Cushing, again in collaboration with Codman, helped to inaugurate the clinical use of x-rays. Wilhelm Konrad Roentgen's discovery of a new kind of ray had been announced in Germany on December 28, 1895. When Cushing became assistant resident in surgery under Halsted in 1896, he began taking x-rays. He has given his own account of this experience:

> No x-ray photos had been taken at the Johns Hopkins Hospital when I came down in the fall of 1896. Codman and I had been fooling with some exposures at the MGH using an old static machine and he continued for about ten years more until they had obviously affected his physical condition. We had, of course, no idea of burns or ductless gland disturbances and so forth. There was a large static machine in Ward C in Baltimore at the time and I got a 4″ tube and began making exposures, spending many an hour in a temporary dark room off the old amphitheatre with Rodinal as a developer. . . . I did all the x-ray work until I became resident succeeding Bloodgood.[37]

Cushing, soon an ardent disciple of Halsted's, spoke of him as follows:

> A man of unique personality, shy, something of a recluse, fastidious in his taste and in his friendships, an aristocrat in his breeding, scholarly in his habits, the victim of many years of indifferent health, he nevertheless was one of the few American surgeons who may be considered to have established a school of surgery comparable, in a sense, to the school of Billroth in Vienna. He had few of the qualities supposed to accompany what the world regards as a successful surgeon . . . when health permitted, working in clinic and laboratory at the solution of a succession of problems which aroused his interest. He had that rare form of imagination which seized upon problems and the technical ability combined with persistence that enabled him to attack them with the promise of a successful issue. Many of his contributions, not only to his craft but to the science of medicine in general, were fundamental in character and of enduring importance.[38]

Cushing displayed his own creative talents by research contributions that were important to medicine as well as to general surgery. These include: first, the introduction of the sphygmomanometer into clinical use in this country; second, the application to surgical care of the studies of Sidney Ringer on "physiological" saline;[39] and third, the establishment of the Hunterian Laboratory for Experimental Surgery and Medicine.

The investigations in the Hunterian Laboratory had several distinctive features. First, the same excellence of performance demanded by Halsted in the operating room was required of the workers in the laboratory. Every detail of his meticulous surgical technique was applied to the operations on animals. Second, the majority of the problems studied were basic in nature. Third, a spirit of thoughtful inquiry and creative scholarship pervaded the laboratory. Their experience here deeply affected students, fellows, and visitors from the United States and abroad during this critical period in the evolution of clinical science.

In this laboratory, Cushing began his studies (1908–12) of the normal functions and clinical disorders of the pituitary gland and the surgical treatment of its tumors. This work led to important milestones in endocrinology. In 1909 he introduced the terms hypopituitarism and hyperpituitarism. In a paper presented before the American Medical Association in June of that year he concluded:

> Two conditions: one due to a pathologically increased activity of the pars anterior of the hypophysis (hyperpituitarism), the other to a diminished activity of the same epithelial structure (hypopituitarism), seem capable of clinical differentiation. . . .
>
> Experimental observations show not only that the anterior lobe of the hypophysis is a structure of such importance that a condition of apituitarism is incompatible with the long maintenance of life, but also that its partial removal leads to symptoms comparable to those which we regard as characteristic of lessened secretion (hypopituitarism) in man. A tumor of the gland itself, or one arising in its neighbor, and implicating the gland by pressure, is naturally the lesion to which one or the other of these conditions has heretofore been attributed, though it is probable that oversecretion from simple hypertrophy, or undersecretion from atrophy, will be found to occur irrespective of tumor growth when examination of the pituitary body becomes a routine measure in the postmortem examination of all cases in which the condition suggests one or the other of the symptom-complexes described. . . . When the anterior lobe of the pituitary exhibits increased activity and enlargement in adults, the bones of the extremities become heavy, as do the viscera, since after adolescence the long bones cannot increase in length, the growing points at the ends of the bones have become fixed and incapable of further growth (acromegaly). If, however, cells in the anterior pituitary become excessively active before the long bones have stopped growing then they become longer and longer and a human giant may be the result. Gigantism then is a condition akin to acromegaly, but the onset occurs earlier in life.[40]

He later described the polyglandular syndrome resulting from excessive activity of the basophil cells in the presence of a basophilic adenoma of the hypophysis.[41] It is remarkable that Cushing, from clinical observations alone, was able to deduce a whole new concept in endocrinology, that is, that of a master gland, the pituitary, which influenced the level of function of other endocrine glands such as the thyroid, the gonads, and the adrenals.

Cushing was the pioneer neurosurgeon in this country, and, in November 1904, he gave his first report on the special field of neurological surgery in an address before the Academy of Medicine at Cleveland.[42] He described the physiological work of Sir Charles Sherrington on the motor area and stated that reports of removal of such tumors in the motor area were becoming more frequent. In a footnote, Cushing added prophetically: "It is not impossible that a diseased pituitary body may someday be successfully attacked."

Cushing's chief contributions during his first six years of work in this field were mainly technical. In addition to the use of blood pressure recordings during operations, he had developed a number of ingenious ways of diminishing hemorrhage, including a special cranial tourniquet. He improved the burrs and saws for opening the skull and devised electrodes for applying stimuli to the exposed surface of the brain. He laid the groundwork for gaining information on the natural history of brain tumors. His success was undoubtedly due to the fine basic training in general surgery that he received from Halsted.

## Walter E. Dandy

Walter E. Dandy, who began his training under Cushing, was one of the most imaginative clinical investigators in the history of neurosurgery. At the age of twenty-seven, Dandy, in association with Kenneth Blackfan, published the first of a series of ten classic papers on hydrocephalus and the circulation of the cerebrospinal fluid.[43] Prior to that time no satisfactory explanation of either existed.

Louis Pasteur made the oft-quoted statement: "In the field of observation chance favors the prepared mind." An excellent example is Dandy's discovery of ventriculography, in which accident played a considerable part.[44] On January 3, 1917, a patient whose abdomen was about to be explored for intestinal perforation was sent for a chest x-ray on the way to the operating room.[45] F. H. Baetjer, the hospital radiologist, recognized the presence of free air under the diaphragm. Dandy, then surgical resident, operated on the patient and confirmed the presence of intraperitoneal air, as well as the perforated typhoid ulcer through which it had escaped. This case probably crystallized for him what had been turning over in his mind as a result of the frequent comments by Halsted on the remarkable power of intestinal gases "to perforate bone," and his attention was finally drawn to its practical possibilities in the brain. From these and other clinical and pathological demonstrations of radiographic properties of air, as well as his earlier laboratory studies on hydrocephalus, it was but a small step for this genius to conceive of injecting air into ventricles, thus revolutionizing neurosurgery.

## Samuel J. Crowe and Otolaryngology

Pasteur once stated that, had he been steeped in the traditions and discipline of classical medicine, he would have had little chance to develop his original ideas. Perhaps the same can be said of the third of Halsted's innovators, Samuel J. Crowe.[46] Crowe entered otolaryngology superbly trained to observe, to experiment, and to utilize the physiological, pathological, and surgical approaches then being developed, yet he was untrammeled by the rigid blinds that had gradually been drawn in otolaryngology at that time. Crowe was intern, assistant resident, and research student for five years under Halsted. He came to investigation via surgery, where his mentor was the dynamic perfectionist Cushing. Crowe had planned a career in brain surgery with Cushing at Harvard when, "out of the blue," he was invited by Halsted to assume the directorship of a newly planned division of otolaryngology, a subject about which he knew nothing. He began this independent career at the age of twenty-nine. Among his farflung accomplishments were:

the creation of the first great clinic of otolaryngology in this country; conceived in the grand perspective of general surgery, pervaded by the spirit and example of its head, an oasis in a desert of medical practice; the first penetration into the terra incognita of deafness in the human being coincident with the founding of the Otological Research Laboratory which was accomplished through painstaking correlations between specific defects in hearing and the corresponding anatomical defects in the organ of Corti of the inner ear; the first to recognize as a major cause of deafness in children—lymphoid ingrowths about the Eustachian tubes—and the development by him of a method for prevention and treatment through radium implants. His attack on the problems of deafness was one of the most innovative and productive areas of research developed in any surgical specialty.[47]

5

# The Development of the Rockefeller Institute for Medical Research and Its Hospital

## The Rockefeller Institute for Medical Research

In 1901 there were, in France, Germany, England, Russia, and Japan, well-equipped and endowed institutions for research in medical science. In America, the laboratories that existed were mainly for the instruction of students and had only primitive equipment. A pioneering step in the correction of this situation was the establishment of the Rockefeller Institute for Medical Research.

On June 14, 1901, this institute was formally incorporated.[1] At the first meeting a pledge of $200,000 was made to the Board of Scientific Directors. During the ten-year period of preliminary work, this money was to be drawn upon at their discretion. The board decided not to centralize work in a single place, but to create fellowships to be distributed in existing laboratories throughout the country. The purpose was multifold: first, to enlist the cooperation of investigators in different places; second, to aid some promising lines of research that, for lack of funds, could not be continued; and third, to discover who and where the persons were who desired to undertake research work and what their qualifications were. Twenty-three grants were made to eighteen different laboratories in the United States, and three men were sent abroad—two to Ehrlich's laboratory in Frankfurt and one to Koch's Institute in Berlin. There were talented men and women in America eager to devote themselves to medical research, but few possessed the breadth of education, combined with the technical requisites, necessary for independent work. The directors were, therefore, unanimous in their feeling that, although many important investigations might be fostered by continuing the plan of grants, real progress would not be possible without centralizing the most important lines of work in a permanent, well-equipped place, under a competent head or series of heads. Their conclusions were placed before John D. Rockefeller, who, at the second meeting in June 1902, made another and larger gift to the institute, enabling the board of directors to erect a laboratory building in which to begin work along these broader lines. It was decided that the institute should be located in New York City. There was consultation with Columbia University, but, because the heads of the departments there were selected from local individuals, it was decided that the institute should be established as an independent organization.

Theobald Smith was the first choice as director, but he took himself out of the competition. After looking over the entire field in America and Europe, the directors selected Simon Flexner, who resigned his position as professor of pathology at the University of Pennsylvania in order to accept the post.[2] Flexner began his work July 1, 1903, and spent the following year in Europe, studying various institutions for research. Final plans for the new institute were adopted on June 13, 1904, and, on December 3 of the same year, the cornerstone was laid.

In order to assemble the nucleus of a laboratory staff, a building at the corner of Lexington Avenue and Fiftieth Street was fitted for temporary use. Work began in October 1904, and continued until the completion of the new building eighteen months later.[3] Each year's experience reinforced the conviction that the institute should train its own staff, selecting promising young applicants, from the United States and abroad, for careers in medical research. A number of resident scholarships and fellowships were therefore created.

In order to have a vehicle for publishing its studies, the institute, in February 1905, took over the *Journal of Experimental Medicine*, which had been started at the Johns Hopkins University, under the editorship of Welch.

## The Hospital of the Rockefeller Institute

A key individual in the development of the Rockefeller Institute and, subsequently, its hospital, was Christian Archibald Herter.[4] Herter received his M.D. degree from the College of Physicians and Surgeons in 1885. Thereafter, he worked for a year with Welch in Baltimore and with August Forel in Switzerland. Herter's interest soon turned to the relation of the laboratory sciences to medicine. He established his own laboratory, where chemistry, bacteriology, pathology,[5] and pharmacology were brought together by a few men whose combined skills embraced all of these fields. Over the last seventeen years of his life, Herter produced, in collaboration with his colleagues, some five books and seventy papers.

According to R. M. Hawthorne, Jr.,[6] Herter recognized two dominant approaches to medical research. The first was that of "men who look at the problems of medical science largely from the standpoint of structure and arrangement . . . they represent anatomy, embryology, pathological anatomy and histology." The second approach was that of "men whose interest lies in the study of function, rather than structure, and whose minds, far from being dismayed by the speculative aspects of their studies, invite such speculation so long as it is severely controlled by frequent appeals to facts won by experiment. . . . They are essentially experimentalists . . . Claude Bernard, Helmholtz, Pasteur and Ehrlich are the unexcelled prototypes of investigators of life-phenomena in medicine." Herter clearly belonged to the second group, because he recognized the need for research in physiological chemistry early in his career.[7] He was among America's pioneer investigators, who in only a decade or two built the science of biochemistry from virtually nothing to one of great importance to clinical science.

Herter's own work included researches concerning uric acid, autointoxication, the toxic properties of indol, uremic intoxications, acidosis, adrenalin glycosuria, bacterial infections of the digestive tract, intestinal infantilism, and a variety of other subjects. His most intriguing discovery was on the effect of toxins produced by the bacteria that inhabit the digestive tract. Normal intestinal flora are, of course, necessary for digestion, but abnormal and foreign bacteria can produce toxins that have the most profound effects on the body. One of these presumed effects was a variety of physical infantilism in children up to ten years of age, observed by Herter and the celebrated pediatrician L. Emmett Holt, and described by Herter in his book *On Infantilism from Chronic Intestinal Infection.* This condition, then known as "Herter's infantilism," would probably correspond to today's designation of celiac disease. Herter founded, with John Jacob Abel of Johns Hopkins, the *Journal of Biological Chemistry,* and the well-known Herter Lectures were endowed in his name.

When the temporary laboratories of the institute were in operation, Herter turned his attention to an associated hospital. Such a hospital was planned from the beginning, but it was Herter, with his special conviction that medical research should always be associated with patients, who pushed the plan to completion. It was originally intended that Herter should direct the hospital, but by 1908, when it was finally under construction, myasthenia gravis had so weakened him that this was no longer possible.

## Rufus I. Cole—The First Director

The establishment of the HRI represented an expansion of the original program, to include the study of disease in patients.[8] The members of the hospital staff, like those working in the laboratories, were to devote their full time to the institute, conducting research and operating the hospital. There was at that time no other hospital in the world devoted entirely to medical research, and the connection of such a hospital with laboratories for the study of the medical sciences was also unique.

As indicated earlier, the founders of the Rockefeller Institute for Medical Research had in mind from the beginning that the institute would be associated with a hospital of its own. Herter implied as much to Welch in a letter on May 15, 1901, in which he broke the news of Rockefeller's intention to found the institute. In January 1902, Flexner, not yet appointed head of the laboratories, wrote to Herter as follows: "We shall be closely watched by other hospitals in this country as well as by the general profession at home and abroad. Everything will lead to bring the institute and hospital into prominence; their close association; the large and growing endowments; the ideals for which they stand, and the good beginning made by the Institute. I think that we can start well. We shall be without traditional hindrance and shall have the world's experience, gathered at first hand, as a heritage."[9]

Herter and Flexner continued to exchange ideas about the hospital during the spring of 1902. When Flexner drafted his plan for the organization of the institute he suggested the type of hospital needed and emphasized that the institute should never lose sight of the immediate problems of human disease. "In order that these problems be not neglected," he wrote, "there should be attached to the Institute a hospital for the study of special groups of cases of disease. This hospital should be modern and fully equipped, but it need not be large. It should attempt to provide only for selected cases of disease." When the board of directors submitted to Rockefeller their plan for the institute, Flexner's statement on the hospital was included. No immediate action followed, since it was Rockefeller's policy to see one phase of an enterprise well underway before starting another, and, until 1907, the directors were busy with the organization of the laboratories. During this period, however, Herter continued to urge upon his fellow directors the importance of the hospital. His intense desire to be the director was evident in December 1902, when he wrote to Flexner that he still hoped "to try the experiment of looking after the hospital if the Board feels it to be a desirable thing for the Institute."[10]

In the "Estimate for the Endowment of the Rockefeller Institute" that the board of directors presented to Rockefeller early in 1907, they repeated their plea for a hospital:

> At the present time the conditions prevailing in the hospitals where large numbers of patients must be cared for, are such that adequate individual study of patients is impossible. The hospitals are of necessity places where traditional methods are applied rather than where new methods are originated. In a hospital affiliated with the Rockefeller Institute patients could be studied with an unprecedented degree of thoroughness. . . . Treatment, instead of being largely experimental, would gradually become a matter of certainty. The principles of treatment thus established by the thorough

study of a few patients would become applicable to the many.... At the present time there probably exists nowhere in the world a most advantageous affiliation of laboratories and hospitals such as is proposed.[11]

Then, in February 1907, Rockefeller authorized the preparation of plans. By June 1907, the outlines of a fifty-bed hospital, equipped with laboratories independent of those already existing in the institute, were presented.

When it was found that Herter could not undertake the directorship, two individuals of conspicuous ability, Theodore Caldwell Janeway of New York and Rufus I. Cole of Baltimore, were considered by the board. Welch certainly believed that Cole best represented the new era of the laboratory study of disease. Herter and the other directors concurred, and Cole was offered the position. On October 10, 1908, he was elected a member of the Rockefeller Institute, in charge of scientific and medical conduct of the hospital and, on November 28, was named director of the HRI.[12]

The responsibilities of the directorship, as offered to Cole, indicated a concept different from that which the board had envisioned earlier. Herter had proposed that attending physicians, representing the best medical talent of the city, should direct the care of patients, but should not be full-time members of the institute, although expected to give it priority over their private practice; and that a resident staff of young physicians perform the routine ward work and live in the hospital.[13] Presumably the scientific study of disease, for which the hospital was created, would be led by Herter himself and the staff of the existing laboratories, of whom at least two—Meltzer and Alexis Carrel—looked forward to testing and applying their ideas clinically. This scheme made research and patient care separate functions exercised by different sets of physicians.

Cole visualized, in the activities of the HRI, an opportunity to develop a program of intensive medical investigation in an environment pervaded by the research spirit, free from the ordinary routines of practice and of the teaching of medical students. Here he could train young men and women who would later carry the new methods and the new scientific approach to clinical medicine to other medical schools and hospitals. In retrospect, it seems an important quirk of fate that Cole, rather than Herter, was to have the opportunity to plan the program in the new hospital.[14]

Thus, the plan that Cole presented to the board of directors concerning the organization of the hospital staff called for a resident staff of young physicians capable of doing independent research, rather than being simply assistants to the physician-in-chief and his senior associates. Each would have full control of a group of patients suffering with a disease in which he was particularly interested. Each resident would be provided with enough assistants to leave him time for research, and adequate facilities for laboratory tests and animal experimentation would be at his disposal. The new hospital would be an independent department in which Cole and his staff would be an organized group comparable to the existing departments of the institute.[15]

The directors voted unanimously, in January 1909, to approve Cole's plan,[16] and, one month later, John D. Rockefeller, Jr., announced that his father would provide for the proposed salaried hospital staff in the general endowment of the new hospital.

The HRI was officially opened on October 17, 1910. Cole took a monumental step in advancing the concept that the diagnosis and treatment of disease should go hand in hand with their study in the laboratory—the ultimate basis for the principle of full-time academic medicine in clinical departments. In Cole's words:

> As soon as the work was underway, I realized that owing to conditions then existing in medical teaching, the hospital should have at least one other function besides the investigation of disease. The idea of so-called university departments of medicine was in the air and it was evident that this idea would soon reach concrete expression in a number of places. The new hospital appeared to be the logical place in which leaders of this new movement could be trained, be given opportunities to work and be fired with the spirit of investigation which could thus be disseminated throughout the projected clinics. It seemed that the hospital should not adopt a policy of splendid isolation but should play its part in the reorganization of medical teaching in this country.[17]

Under Cole's direction, the HRI became a potent force in setting an example and providing training for research on diseases in patients—that is, clinical investigation. His activities in developing this new concept constitute his outstanding contribution to American medicine.

Cole urged that the hospital be developed as a true research laboratory, with the closest possible connection between it and the institute laboratories.

## The Organization of the Hospital

The director of the hospital served as physician-in-chief, being responsible for the medical service. The hospital staff consisted of the physician-in-chief, several part-time specialists, including surgeons and a radiologist, and a limited number of nonresident physicians with proven research ability. Among them was to be a well-trained chemist who would make some of the more complicated examinations, oversee the work of the physicians who might not have special training in chemistry, and assist in directing the younger men in the chemical aspects of their investigations. The physician-in-chief was to have full charge of the admission and care of patients, as well as general supervision of the research work. He was also to have sufficient time for independent research, so that his efforts might serve as an example and stimulus to those associated with him.

Cole placed a special emphasis on the resident physicians, because he thought their contribution would be most important in determining the hospital's contribution to medical knowledge. In view of their responsibility for the immediate care and treatment of patients, it was necessary for all members of the resident staff to have excellent clinical experience.

The diseases for study were to be more or less regulated by the special interests of the residents. The resident staff was to be headed by a senior resident physician, qualified to supervise all of the patients. He was to retain his position as long as he desired and as long as he continued to be productive in research. Cole anticipated that most senior residents would embark on careers in academic medicine.

Cole, demonstrating an unusual ability in the selection of staff members for the hospital, found excellent clinical investigators. The first resident physician was George Canby Robinson, whose appointment began on September 1, 1910.[18] Robinson attended the Johns Hopkins University School of Medicine from 1899 to 1903. After two years in pathology at Pennsylvania Hospital, he became a resident physician there for a similar period. He then spent a year in Friedrich von Müller's clinic. When he returned, he practiced briefly in Philadelphia before assuming the residency at the HRI in 1910. George H. Draper began his duties that year as the first assistant resident physician to be appointed to the staff.[19] Within a few weeks, Homer Fordyce Swift and Henry Marks arrived from Europe, and Alphonse Raymond Dochez moved to the hospital from the institute laboratories, to complete the roster of the initial resident staff. Francis McCrudden[20] took over the direction of the chemical laboratories; Arthur W. M. Ellis from England and Francis W. Peabody from Boston joined the resident staff a short time later. Another early member of the staff was Florentin Medigreceanu,[21] who worked in the chemical laboratories.

The hospital, overlooking the East River, had eleven floors, three of which were below the ground level. In addition to the usual hospital facilities and living quarters for staff and nurses, there were four floors (with 60 beds) for patients in the main building. The two upper floors housed the laboratories and an operating room. Adjoining the main hospital was a small building that had nine rooms, separated by glass partitions, for patients with communicable diseases, and an autopsy room, with facilities for pathological work. The arrangement of beds was such that small groups of patients with the same disease could be housed together. The laboratories for chemical, bacteriological, and physiological research were extensive in relation to the bed capacity of the hospital.

Robinson's first task was the organization of the medical service, which included designing the clinical record forms, temperature charts, and admission slips, and handling all of the other details necessary to ready the hospital for its official opening. In order to facilitate the admission of patients and to secure the types of patients necessary for the planned research, a statement was published by the Rockefeller Institute, explaining that the hospital planned to study disease as it actually appears in human beings, under conditions equally favorable to treatment and to scientific observation. A common motive actuates the Institute as a whole. Namely, that of advancing knowledge and of securing more perfect means of preventing and healing disease. Thus the work of the laboratories and hospital is unified. Their common aim . . . admits of the same problems being studied both in their biological and pathological and in their clinical aspects. . . . The principle has been recognized that the ultimate purposes of medical research and discovery may be greatly served by the study of biological and chemical problems. . . . Special work in chemistry, pathology, bacteriology and physiology reinforce the clinical staff in the investigations carried on in the hospital. . . .

The subjects chosen for research in the first year are lobar pneumonia, acute anterior poliomyelitis, syphilis, and certain types of cardiac disease. Patients are admitted only by the resident physician to whom cases are referred by physicians or hospitals, or by direct application.[22]

Excellent cooperation was given by physicians attached to some of the leading hospitals. Many of them were interested in clinical research, but were without facilities to pursue it.

The early days at the HRI were recalled by Robinson in a letter written in 1928:

Life in the hospital was full of joy. A few patients in whom we had special and intensive interest; laboratories such as none of us had ever before seen in any clinics; varied interests both within and without the realm of medicine; the East River with its great span of light at night, and its laughing waters; a blazing hearth about which we gathered after dinner—all these things gave a setting in which friendship deepened and true sympathy thrived.[23]

## The Staff and Its Research[24]

### *Pneumonia*

Cole chose the study of acute lobar pneumonia as his special problem. The goal of the research was to discover a means of reducing the existing mortality rate of 25 percent. Dochez and Marks worked with Cole. Dochez graduated from the Johns Hopkins University School of Medicine in 1907 and soon joined the staff of the Rockefeller Institute in pathology and bacteriology, where he spent three years before transferring to the hospital staff.[25] The work in pneumonia was greatly enhanced by the addition of Oswald T. Avery to the staff in 1913.[26] Dochez worked closely with Avery until 1919, when he resigned to become an assistant professor of medicine at Johns Hopkins, where he began his classic studies of scarlet fever.[27] Dochez was called, in 1921, to Columbia University's College of Physicians and Surgeons, where he had a brilliant career as a professor of medicine and, for a time, as head of the department of bacteriology.

Henry Marks worked as Cole's direct assistant on the pneumonia service. He was a Harvard graduate who, after an internship at the MGH, spent two years abroad studying pathology. After one year with Cole he worked for a year in the institute laboratory.[28]

In January 1911, Francis W. Peabody joined the resident staff and began his studies of the chemical effects of pneumonia on the blood.[29] Peabody was a Harvard graduate who had interned at the MGH. He spent two years on the resident staff in medicine and pathology at the Johns Hopkins Hospital, followed by six months in Germany, working with Emil Fischer and Georg Fresenius. In 1913 he became the first resident physician of the newly built Peter Bent Brigham Hospital, where he worked closely with Henry A. Christian to establish it as an important research hospital of the Harvard Medical School. Peabody later became a professor of medicine at Harvard and the first director of the Thorndike Memorial Laboratory of the Boston City Hospital.

Cole's aim was to produce an immune serum against the pneumococcus by inoculating horses with gradually increasing quantities of pneumococci. Cole, Dochez, and Marks ran into an unexpected problem. As others had already discovered, the pneumococci isolated from patients by the Rockefeller group represented several strains, which differed in virulence. These strains differed sufficiently in their chemical nature to elicit different antibodies in the host's blood, therefore necessitating a different serum against each of the four identified types. By the end of 1912 Cole and Dochez had developed a serum for use against Type I.

To ascertain the type present in a given case of pneumonia, the patient's sputum was injected into the peritoneal cavity of a mouse, where the pneumococci multiplied and caused an inflammation that filled the cavity with fluid. When the fluid, laden with pneumococci, was placed in a vessel that contained immune serum of the type corresponding to the patient's pneumococcus, it showed a telltale clumping of the bacteria. Selective treatment based upon this "typing" lowered the mortality rate.[30]

Cole placed the chemical investigation of the pneumococcus in the skilled hands of Avery, who came from the Hoagland Laboratory in Brooklyn, where he spent seven years in a variety of investigations.[31] Avery and his associates soon located the specific immunity-inducing substances in the capsule, composed of polysaacharides, that surrounds the bacterium. They aimed their main attack at the unique capsule of the bacterium.[32] Avery's first step, taken with Dochez, was to show that the germ-free blood serum and urine of pneumonia patients contained a substance having the same specific immune reactions as those produced by the intact bacilli. This substance could also be recovered from the capsular material of cultures of virulent pneumococci. To follow up on this exciting lead, an experienced chemist was needed, and, in 1922, Michael Heidelberger,[33] who had participated in the institute work on

Tryparsamide was transferred to the hospital staff in order to begin the new work. Two years later W. F. Goebel joined the group.

By extracting the chemical ingredients of the capsule and testing them separately for their immunological reactions, Avery and his colleagues found that the differences in virulence and in immune reactions characteristic of the four known types of pneumococci depended upon the presence of specific substances in the capsule. Up to this time it had generally been assumed that proteins alone determined immunological specificity. When Avery, Heidelberger, and Goebel identified the specific substances of the pneumococcus capsule, however, to their surprise they found them to be carbohydrates.

Though this totally unexpected finding was at first greeted by wide skepticism, strong support came from Karl Landsteiner.[34] The active carbohydrates of the pneumococci closely fitted the description of Landsteiner's haptens. Although incapable themselves of stimulating the formation of antibodies when injected into animals, the haptens reacted specifically with the immune serum produced by injecting an animal with the whole organism. In short, the specificity of the antigens of the pneumococcus was that of the polysaccharides in the capsule.

Goebel and Avery succeeded in building up compounds of proteins and simple sugars that possessed antigenic properties similar to those of the more complex natural protein-polysaccharide compounds. They were finally able to produce an artificial antigen by combining a common protein with a specific pneumococcus polysaccharide. Their work provided an explanation of virulence and immunity in terms of chemical components of the invading organism. These contributions of Avery and his group stand, side by side with Landsteiner's discoveries, as foundations of the modern science of immunochemistry. They demonstrate how clinical investigation may lead to important basic scientific discoveries.

The attack on lobar pneumonia, begun by Cole and carried on by Avery and others, was one of the most elegant performances, from the standpoint of both theory and technique, in the history of medical science. As far as the cure of the patient is concerned, much of this work was made obsolete by the sulfonamide drugs and the antibiotics, both of which fortunately attack all strains of pneumococci with equal vigor.

*Work on Pneumonia and World War I*   The study of lobar pneumonia, led by Cole, had reached a stage of direct use to the nation by the onset of World War I. There was reason to believe that pneumonia would be a major cause of death in army camps. Cole and his team—Dochez, a resident physician, 1914–15; Henry T. Chickering, a resident physician, 1915–17; and Avery—prepared a monograph setting forth all they had discovered from practical experience about the existence of several types of pneumococci.[35]

Cole headed, with William G. MacCallum, a professor of pathology at

Johns Hopkins, a commission for the study of pneumonia (1918). Of the eight other members, two (Avery and Dochez) were from the HRI; Francis G. Blake had worked there, and Thomas M. Rivers, then at Johns Hopkins, later began a long career at the institute.

In July and August 1918, Eugene L. Opie, a former member of the institute, with Blake and Rivers, studied epidemics in several army camps.[36] Blake participated in experiments in which Opie's group produced lobar pneumonia in monkeys for the first time, by injection of pneumococci into the trachea. Later, working at the Army Medical School in Washington, D.C., with Russell L. Cecil, who was to become a professor of medicine at Cornell University Medical College, Blake continued his study of experimental pneumonia in monkeys, which helped to prove that the pneumococcus is the specific cause of lobar pneumonia.

After the war, Cole's pneumonia workers continued their efforts to produce effective curative sera against types of pneumococcus other than Type I. From 1924 until 1930, Louis A. Julianelle classified another organism often associated with pneumonia, Friedlander's bacillus, according to immunological types.[37] Julianelle later became chief of a division of the New York City Public Health Research Institute. Ernest G. Stillman, who joined the hospital staff in 1915, studied experimental pneumococcus infections in mice and rabbits.[38]

*Other Work on Pneumonia*    While the laboratory studies went on, patients with pneumonia presented problems that the hospital was well equipped to explore. Alfred E. Cohn and R. A. Jamieson studied the best ways of using digitalis to combat heart strain resulting from impaired blood flow through the congested lungs. John Staige Davis, Jr., a resident, studied the use of morphine in pneumonia. Alan M. Chesney, an assistant resident physician (1913–17), investigated treatment of the disease with ethylhydrocuprein (Optochin). Chesney later became dean of the Johns Hopkins University School of Medicine. Robert L. Levy, a resident physician (1919–20), made a study of the dilatation of the heart in lobar pneumonia.[39]

William C. Stadie identified the functional cause of the cyanosis that characterized grave cases of bronchopneumonia in the historic influenza epidemic of 1918,[40] and he developed the principles of controlled oxygen therapy that have since become a basic part of medical practice.[41] Van Slyke described this work as follows:

> The 1918 epidemic was characterized by large numbers of cases of bronchopneumonia with a high mortality. Cyanosis was a common sign. To find whether the cyanosis was due to deficient pulmonary oxygenation or to peripheral stasis it was necessary to determine the degree to which the arterial blood was oxygenated. Analysis of arterial blood as a diagnostic procedure had never been practiced. It was feared that puncture of an artery would lead to hemorrhage. However, Stadie . . . found one publica-

tion in which a German physician, Hurter, described arterial puncture on patients and outlined the technique. Stadie tried it on animals, then on himself and some of his colleagues, and finally applied it to patients. In the cyanotic patient the arterial blood was incompletely oxygenated showing that the cause of the cyanosis lay in the lungs. In normal arterial blood the hemoglobin is 95% or more saturated by oxygen. . . . In some of Stadie's more severely cyanotic patients the saturation was as low as 60%.

Being an engineer before he became a physician Stadie was able to design a chamber in which oxygen content, temperature, and humidity could be controlled and in which the patient could live as long as might be necessary.[42]

Stadie succeeded in restoring the oxygen saturation to 90 percent or above, by having the patient breathe air with 50 to 60 percent oxygen saturation.

In discussing his work at the Rockefeller Institute, Stadie said:

He [Rufus Cole] helped me get a grant of $2,000 for the construction of an oxygen chamber. I was unable to buy a Beckman spectrophotometer . . . I used a Dubosque colorimeter and my eye. I was even forced to dispense with the services of a consulting statistician. The grant, however, enabled me to indulge my besetting weakness for gadgetry. I devised a machine which every 15 minutes removed a sample of air from the chamber, analyzed it for oxygen, recorded the answer on a revolving roll of paper and if the oxygen had fallen down below a given value opened up the valve to admit fresh gas. Thanks to this Goldbergian device, my sleep was uninterrupted by analytical demands.[43]

Some years later Carl A. L. Binger refined this technique with the study of a much larger series of cases.[44]

By 1930 Avery and R. J. Dubos were making a promising attack on Type III pneumonia, against which Cole's group had not been able to make a potent serum. Dubos grew a harmless soil bacillus in the presence of the polysaccharide from Type III pneumococcus capsules. The soil bacillus, adapting itself to this compound, produced a specific enzyme that could digest it, and, this enzyme, in turn, had a remarkable protective effect against living Type III pneumococci in mice, rabbits, and monkeys.

With Glenn Cullen, Avery studied the enzymes of the pneumococcus. With Theodor Thjötta and Hugh J. Morgan, he investigated the nutrition of various bacteria and their need for accessory growth substances. With J. M. Neill, he looked into the oxidation-reduction powers of pneumococci. William S. Tillett and Thomas Francis, Jr., were active in the study of the carbohydrates. Almost all of those men who worked with Avery went on to professorships of bacteriology or medicine, or to full memberships in the Rockefeller Institute. Avery ascribed the success of his laboratory to the fact that "Cole picked these men and all I had to do was to pick their brains."[45]

## Syphilis

Homer Fordyce Swift initiated a study of syphilis and its treatment by "Salvarsan," Paul Ehrlich's remarkable new discovery known as "606."[46] Swift and Arthur W. M. Ellis, while resident physicians, applied the drug directly at the site of disease through the spinal canal. Known as the Swift-Ellis method, it was used for many years in the treatment of neurosyphilis.[47]

Swift,[48] a graduate of the New York University and Bellevue Hospital Medical College (1906), interned at the Presbyterian Hospital in New York (1906–8). He spent two years teaching pathology and dermatology (1908–10) and had a short period of study abroad before joining the resident staff of the HRI (assistant resident physician, 1910–12; resident physician, 1912–14). In 1914 he became an associate professor of medicine at Columbia University. After World War I he returned to the HRI and devoted his life to the study of rheumatic fever, with emphasis on the relation of streptococci to the disease.

Ellis[49] became a professor of medicine in the London Hospital School of Medicine, heading its new clinical research unit. Later he became Regius Professor of Medicine at Oxford. Ellis wrote in 1943, soon after his Oxford appointment:

> I can never be sufficiently grateful for the luck which brought me to the Rockefeller and to the companionship and friendship of the group that Robinson and Rufus Cole had collected. They were good days in every way and the . . . subsequent record suggests that we did not waste our time. I have often thought what a remarkable act of faith it was that we should all have been there consciously attempting to fit ourselves for full-time posts in medicine when no such jobs existed anywhere.[50]

## Biochemist to the Hospital

Flexner and Cole saw clearly that internal medicine was moving rapidly ahead along chemical lines. They sought an experienced chemist to conduct research of his own while acting as advisor to the staff on chemical problems. America had few biochemists qualified to fill such a role, and, in 1913, Flexner offered the position to Franz Knoop, an internationally known German biochemist. When Knoop declined the invitation, it dawned upon the director that the right man was already at hand.

Donald D. Van Slyke had come to the institute in 1907, from the University of Michigan, to work on proteins and their components, at first as an assistant to Levene.[51] (See chapter 2.) Van Slyke soon showed his special talent for devising ingenious laboratory procedures by developing a method for the quantitative determination of amino acids. Cole, who spent a year in Levene's laboratory while the hospital was being built, was well acquainted with the young biochemist and, like Levene, recognized his promise.

In 1914 Van Slyke and his associate Glenn Cullen moved to the hospital. Neither had any conception of clinical problems. Their new comrades, however, took them into their closely knit group, eagerly sharing problems. They joined Edgar Stillman, an assistant resident physician working on diabetes with Frederick M. Allen, in an investigation of the pathophysiology of acidosis. These three were aided, from 1915 to 1917, by Reginald Fitz (later professor of medicine at Boston University), W. W. Palmer (later professor of medicine at Columbia University's College of Physicians and Surgeons) and Franklin C. McLean (later professor of medicine at Chicago).[52]

Van Slyke then went on to apply the concepts of physical chemistry to similar phenomena in other fields of internal medicine. He entered upon a lifetime study of the acid-base reactions of the blood, the respiratory gas exchange, the transport of oxygen and carbon dioxide in the blood stream, the distribution of these gases and of electrolytes in the tissues, and the physical chemistry of kidney secretion. The results have affected the thought of every physiologically minded physician.

Van Slyke and Cullen began by defining acidosis in chemical terms, so that this condition could be evaluated in a given patient by direct measurement of carbon dioxide and bicarbonate in samples of his blood. For that purpose, Van Slyke devised an apparatus for the exact measurement of oxygen and carbon dioxide in solution in blood and other fluids. This apparatus took a place at once in the equipment of clinical scientists all over the world.

In 1920 Lawrence J. Henderson of Harvard, in collaboration with McLean and H. A. Murray, began a study of the changes in the distribution of electrolytes between blood plasma and cells, resulting from changes in oxygen or carbon dioxide tension. Their investigations overlapped those of the HRI, and, in 1921, Henderson, McLean, and Van Slyke agreed to transfer the problem to the latter's laboratory. McLean moved to the HRI, joining a team that included Cullen, A. Baird Hastings, James Harold Austin, and John P. Peters, for the work required a number of investigators working at the same time on different portions of the same blood sample. Each man·executed one specific analytical procedure. One by-product of these investigations was the further development of the Van Slyke method of blood-gas analysis, which lent itself to the measurement not only of the two major blood gases for which it was originally intended, but of many other substances in the body fluids, including carbon monoxide, total and nonprotein nitrogen, amino nitrogen, calcium, and sugar. A second by-product was the development of a theoretical general equation expressing the relation of the concentrations of hydrogen ions (pH) and potassium ions (pK) of buffer solutions to their effects.[53]

McLean, who was on leave from Peking Union Medical College, returned in 1921 to his professorship of medicine there. Van Slyke joined him, in 1922, as a visiting professor, continuing the work on blood chemistry with the collaboration of the Peking chemist Hsien Wu. Their results showed that the distribution of electrolytes between red cells and plasma conformed to the Donnan equilibrium, and that the effects of oxygen and carbon dioxide on this distribution could be explained and predicted by physicochemical laws.

Christen Lundsgaard (later a distinguished professor in Copenhagen) joined Van Slyke, in 1917–18, to study lung volume in normal persons and in patients with tuberculosis and pneumonia; the two conducted an authoritative study of factors producing faulty oxygenation of the blood, as evidenced by cyanosis in various diseases.[54]

In about 1923 Van Slyke took up the investigation of nephritis in its various forms, systematically evaluating all the alterations of metabolism, blood chemistry, and urinary excretion that could be chemically measured. The hospital physicians who participated in this study between 1923 and 1935 were A. S. Alving, W. E. Ehrich, R. R. Hannon, G. C. Linder, Christen Lundsgaard, J. F. McIntosh, E. Möller, Irvine H. Page, H. A. Salvesen, and Edgar Stillman. From Van Slyke's laboratory, the workers included A. Baird Hastings, J. A. Hawkins, Alma E. Hiller, and J. Sendroy.[55]

Van Slyke and his colleagues examined the alterations of protein, fat, and carbohydrate metabolism in nephritis; they continued the study of the equilibria of the gases and salts (electrolytes) in the blood, and their modifications in acidosis, a frequent concomitant to renal disease; and they improved laboratory procedures for measuring nitrogenous substances in blood and urine.

In 1930, with nine of his colleagues, Van Slyke published a monograph on the clinical course of different types of Bright's disease and the corresponding changes in the kidneys, based on findings in sixty-seven cases studied in this comprehensive way.[56] From the time Van Slyke began this program until he retired in 1948, he and his group studied about six hundred patients, three hundred of whom were under observation long enough to yield valuable information.

One of the important contributions of this work was the urea clearance test, a method of estimating the performance of the kidneys, introduced by Austin, Stillman, and Van Slyke.[57] Failure to excrete urea in sufficient amounts is the most characteristic physiological result of renal insufficiency. Van Slyke's previous studies had equipped him to measure urea in blood and urine; earlier, he and Cullen had worked intensively with urease, a ferment or enzyme that breaks down urea into ammonium carbonate. By a simple chemical procedure, the carbonate could be made to yield carbon dioxide gas; thus, Van Slyke could use his gas-analysis apparatus for determining the amount of urea in a sample of blood or urine.[58]

To the leader of this work—the biochemist without medical training, who in 1914 was not sure he could be useful to medical science as chemist to the HRI—the Association of American Physicians in 1942 awarded its prized Kober Medal for his contributions to clinical medicine.[59]

## Cardiovascular Research

George Draper and George Canby Robinson began research on the heart and circulation, focusing their attention on electrocardiography.[60] The instrument in the HRI was put in operation on March 5, 1911.

Alfred E. Cohn joined the staff soon after the hospital was opened. He was a Columbia graduate who had his clinical training in the Mount Sinai Hospital in New York and then spent several years studying pathology and clinical medicine in Germany and London. When Robinson ended his service as chief resident, in July 1912, Cohn was put in charge of research on diseases of the heart. Robinson continued on the staff, however, as an associate in the physiological division (with John Auer). In 1913 Robinson became an associate professor of medicine at Washington University in St. Louis, where he played an important role in the reorganization of the medical department and of the school.[61] As a result, he was asked to reorganize the Vanderbilt University School of Medicine (see chapter 15).

## Diabetes Mellitus

In 1914 Cole recruited Frederick M. Allen,[62] who was then engaged in diabetes research at Harvard Medical School. Allen's first goal was to produce experimental diabetes in order to better understand the human disease. It was known that dogs could be made diabetic by total removal of the pancreas, but the diabetes thus induced led to death so rapidly that it did not closely resemble the chronic human disease. Allen found that, by leaving just enough of the pancreas to support minimum utilization of sugar, he could produce diabetes that progressed slowly enough to permit long-term studies.

Allen concluded that not only the metabolism of carbohydrates is disturbed, but also the utilization of fats and proteins. He reasoned that the diabetic patient must be placed on what he called the "fasting or undernutrition treatment," calculated to provide only the minimum amount of carbohydrates to keep him alive, and a low total calorie intake.[63]

## Poliomyelitis

A thorough clinical description of the disease in its initial stages, in order to make early diagnosis possible, was an important goal of the hospital's program for poliomyelitis. An opportunity for such study presented itself when an epidemic of the disease broke out in New York City in the summer of 1911. Poliomyelitis was being studied in the institute laboratories by Simon Flexner and Paul F. Clark, with special reference to its mode of transmission. In order to correlate the clinical studies of poliomyelitis with the laboratory studies, the isolation building was opened and, during the summer, was filled with children suffering from this disease, most of whom had severe paralysis. Peabody, Dochez, and Draper gave their full time that summer to the study of poliomyelitis.

During this investigation, a conflict in philosophy between Flexner and Cole came to the fore. A belief in the desirability of separate and distinct spheres of activity for clinicians versus laboratory medical scientists colored Flexner's thinking and his decisions in the early years of his directorship of the institute. The integration of these two functions was proceeding rapidly, right at his very doorstep, under the able direction of Cole, but Flexner held out for his own point of view.

An immediate result of Flexner's attitude was the limitation imposed on the team of investigators who undertook clinical studies during the epidemic of 1911. The result of these studies was a substantial monograph, based on the investigation of almost two hundred cases, published in 1912 by Peabody, Draper and Dochez.[64] The bulk of the monograph was detailed description of thirty-four patients. The report added new clinical data, but there were no attempts to elucidate the clinical virology of the disease, such as characterized the work in Sweden during an epidemic in the same year. John R. Paul believed that the reason for this lay in Flexner's rigid separation of the character of the work to be carried out in the HRI, as opposed to his own research laboratory in the institute.[65] Flexner supported clinicians to the limit of his own beliefs, but he clung to the idea that physicians were supposed to practice their craft at the bedside—not in the experimental laboratory. The hospital team was not allowed access to monkeys, which would have enabled them to perform clinical virological tests. Dochez tried in vain to persuade Flexner that, by 1912, a proper clinical investigative study called for attempts to isolate the virus from patients. Denial of this request was understandable, considering Flexner's insistence that his own special department in the institute would take care of the experimental aspects of polio virus work.

Nowhere is the case for the laboratory aspect of clinical investigation more succinctly expressed than in the correspondence that Flexner and Cole carried on in 1911. Corner described Cole's position:[66]

When in 1911 Cole's attitude was questioned in the Board of Scientific Directors he gave Flexner a forthright statement of his position. "Men who were studying disease clinically," he wrote, "had the right to go as deeply into its fundamental nature as their training allowed, and in the Rockefeller Institute Hospital every man who was caring for patients should also be engaged in more fundamental study." It had required some energy and effort, he continued, to get the men to adopt this view, but they were all now convinced of its soundness and he hoped that some of them, at least, might share in the revolution, or evolution, of clinical medicine that was bound to come. "Of course," wrote Cole, "collaborative studies by the hospital and institute laboratories might be extremely valuable but unless the hospital first accomplished something independently, the other laboratory would never respect its work. Cooperation must develop spontaneously."

Flexner got the best of the argument in relation to this particular project.

The HRI study of poliomyelitis started a new trend in clinical investigation. Peabody and his coworkers pointed the way to a style of teamwork in which a group of clinical investigators worked enthusiastically for a common cause in the academic atmosphere of a well-equipped and well-run institution. It was a kind of investigation peculiarly appropriate to the new organization of house staff physicians then being introduced into the best of American teaching hospitals. In this case, the objective was to examine the acute febrile and subacute stages of poliomyelitis in a more meticulous manner than had ever been done before. To accomplish this, the investigators organized their interns and residents for around-the-clock clinical observations and for the performance of simple laboratory tests. Since crucial events frequently happen with surprising rapidity in the severely ill, paralyzed patient, this exacting standard of observation was set by Cole's team; thus, an important tradition in clinical investigation was established.[67]

The young men of the hospital staff well knew that Cole had established their right to a place in the ranks of investigative science. When they went away to help build other centers of research and teaching, they took with them the inspiration his stand had given them. Thus, the HRI, probably more than any other institution, advanced that evolution of medical science in America that Cole first prophesied and then fostered.

### Further Research by the Hospital Staff

*Cardiovascular Studies*   In 1911 Alfred E. Cohn joined the hospital staff, bringing with him experience acquired abroad and in New York City in the use of the electrocardiograph.[68] Cohn was an explorer and recorder of phenomena, rather than a discoverer of principles. He belonged to that school of medical biological observers to whom quantitative observation tends to be an end as much as a means. He mapped the size of the heart with x-rays; studied the action of important cardiac drugs; wrote on the structure of the normal and aging heart muscle; classified heart diseases and compiled statistics of the various types. His interest in the effects of aging on the heart led him into a long experimental study of the changes with age in certain physiological characteristics. This investigation began with chick embryos; in its later stages the hearts of dogs were also studied.[69]

Alfred E. Mirsky, Cohn's associate, came to the Rockefeller Institute in 1927. Mortimer L. Anson came at the same time to join John H. Northrop's laboratory of general physiology.

Mirsky assisted in Cohn's study of aging by measuring the pH of the blood of embryo chicks at successive stages of development. For this work, Mirsky and Anson needed a highly sensitive pH meter; they took the newly introduced glass electrode and adapted it for the purpose. Only a short while later, Duncan MacInnes and Malcolm Dole, at the Princeton laboratory of the institute, also began to improve the glass electrode. In 1929 the two groups published their definitive papers only a month apart. Neither was aware of the other's pioneering work on a technique that came into worldwide use.[70]

Many physicians who were associated with Cohn made their mark in clinical cardiology and other branches of medicine. Among these are Robert L. Levy, J. M. Steele, Jr.,[71] and Harold J. Stewart[72] of New York; Sir Francis Fraser of London; R. A. Jamieson of Toronto; and Fritz Lange of Munich. After two years at the HRI, Fraser[73] accepted an appointment at Columbia under Warfield Theobald Longcope. Subsequently he returned to London to become the first full-time professor of medicine in the medical school of St. Bartholomew's Hospital. He was appointed by the University of London to organize and direct postgraduate medical education in London, an accomplishment for which he was knighted.

*Streptococci and Rheumatic Fever*   Beginning in 1914, Homer Fordyce Swift[74] and Ralph A. Kinsella (later a professor of medicine at St. Louis University) attempted to classify the various streptococci by comparing their cultural characteristics with their immunological properties.[75] Like previous investigators, Swift was unable to recover consistently any one specific organism from patients with rheumatic fever or to reproduce the disease in animals with various organisms isolated from patients with the disease; but he patiently studied individuals for months, recording all of the clinical manifestations and the various laboratory tests in serial fashion.

Cohn and Swift found evidence of more serious disturbance in cardiac function than had generally been recognized.[76] After the acute symptoms had abated, electrocardiograms showed abnormalities for months. Cohn and Swift found that 90 percent of heart disease in young persons resulted from the endocarditis associated with rheumatic fever. Their emphasis alerted physicians to continue treatment much longer than had been customary, in order to avoid recrudescence of the endocarditis.[77]

In the laboratory, Swift and his associates continued the earlier work on streptococci. They found that the antigens of streptococci were not polysaccharides, like those found by Avery in pneumococci, but proteins.[78]

From 1928 to 1933, Rebecca C. Lancefield, of Swift's group, produced a classification of hemolytic streptococci into several groups, only one of which (group A) was pathogenic for man.[79] A close association was found between rheumatic fever, which could generally be traced to an antecedent infection of the tonsils, and Lancefield's group A hemolytic streptococci. Swift believed (1925) that the damage to the joints and lining of the heart in rheumatic fever resulted not from direct injury of tissues by the organisms, but from some sort of allergy-like hypersensitivity of the tissues to the streptococci. Christopher Andrewes, C. L. Derick, and Swift, following the clues of others on allergic reactions in tuberculosis, produced in rabbits a state of hyperallergy, as Swift called it, by sensitizing them with streptococci.[80] Between 1928 and 1932, Charles H. Hitchcock and Currier McEwen, of the hospital staff, worked actively with Swift in studies of the immunological relations of streptococci bearing upon the allergic theory of rheumatic fever. Although the precise nature of the disease process remained imperfectly known, the studies of Swift, Cohn, Lancefield, and their associates helped to define the preceding infection, the pathological process, the course of the disease, and the best methods of treatment available at the time.

Many of those who trained under Swift later made important contributions to clinical science and medical education. Andrewes was a member of the British team that isolated the influenza virus by transmitting the human disease to ferrets; C. P. Miller, Jr., did distinguished research in the infectious diseases and became a professor of medicine at the University of Chicago; Ralph H. Boots organized the Faulkner Clinic for the study of arthritis at Columbia, one of the first such clinics in the United States; and Derick returned to Peter Bent Brigham Hospital, where he was associated with Henry A. Christian throughout his career.

*The Virus of Rubeola*    In 1919 the virus of rubeola had not yet been cultivated, and there was great uncertainty whether the disease could be transmitted to animals. Francis G. Blake, who joined the hospital staff as an associate in 1919, and James D. Trask, a recent Cornell Medical College graduate who was an assistant resident physician of the hospital, reopened the question by trying a different method of infecting monkeys.[81] When they placed material from the nose and throat of a measles patient into the trachea of a monkey, the animal developed the disease. By passing the infectious nasopharyngeal drippings through a bacteria-retaining filter, they ruled out the possibility that one or another of the bacteria in the throat was causing the disease.

Later, they infected monkeys and showed that monkeys that had recovered from experimentally induced measles were immune to reinoculation. Blake and Trask, though not the first to show that the disease is caused by a filterable virus, were the first to provide a solid background upon which further research could proceed.

Blake was called, in 1921, to the chair of internal medicine at Yale. In 1924 the institute appointed him a member of the Board of Scientific

Directors, a post he retained until 1935. Trask accompanied Blake to Yale, as an instructor in medicine, and later became an associate professor of pediatrics.[82]


## The Hospital's Meaning to Clinical Science

Summarizing the hospital's work until the year 1930, Cole pointed out that such an institution contributes to the advance of medical science in two ways.[83] It may actually increase knowledge of disease, and it may, by example, influence medical thought and practice. He found it difficult to estimate the value of scientific contributions by the HRI. The new knowledge could be enumerated item by item, he said, but the sum total of reported work would omit what might well be the most valuable result—the use of the findings as starting points for new investigations and new generalizations. Cole thought that the HRI was especially likely to stimulate other medical investigators and to suggest new ideas to them, because it provided for thorough study of disease in the individual patient and in selected groups, at the bedside and in the laboratory, to an extent theretofore unknown.

Cole found it even more difficult to evaluate the influence of the HRI on medical practice. Obviously, there had been great advances in the previous two decades. When the hospital was founded, laboratory facilities in American medical clinics were almost nonexistent. By 1930 at least eight medical clinics had well-equipped research laboratories, and several of these had interchanged staff members with the institute. About thirty men formerly on the clinical staff of the institute were already occupying professorial chairs of medicine in the United States, England, Ireland, Denmark, and China.

The hospital was also influencing the American medical profession through staff members who went into private practice, giving to many communities medical care of the highest quality, as exemplified by the work of such men as Robert L. Levy, Henry T. Chickering, and Theodore J. Abernethy. To enumerate the many others would be misleading, because a sharp line cannot be drawn between medical scientists and private practitioners, many of whom also taught in medical schools and did research. As of 1953, about fifty men had gone from the hospital into private practice.

Cole felt that the leaven of science was already working in the American medical profession. There was a perceptible difference in the attitude of physicians; the best practitioners, not content with being skilled diagnosticians, were trying, more than in the past, to understand the diseases from which their patients suffered and to treat them by rational measures. Cole did not presume, of course, to distinguish between the influence of the Rockefeller Institute and that of the better medical schools in the creation of sounder medical practice in America; but, in retrospect, it is now clear that the institute's hospital, led by Cole, was in the forefront of this movement.[84]

## The Second Director of the Hospital of the Rockefeller Institute: Thomas M. Rivers

One of the most important appointments made by Cole was that of Thomas M. Rivers[85] (1922). Rivers had some research experience as a medical student at Johns Hopkins, and, during his internship in medicine there, he was involved in some of the early work on blood transfusion. After his internship, Rivers became a resident in pediatrics, where he had contact with John F. Howland, James L. Gamble, Kenneth Blackfan, and others active in clinical investigation.

In January 1918, Rivers entered the army. While Rivers was awaiting orders, Howland, on a visit to the surgeon-general's office in Washington, D.C., met Cole. Cole told Howland about the commission that the army had formed to investigate pneumonia following measles and mentioned that it did not include a single man who would know a case of measles if he saw it. This led to pediatrician Rivers being appointed a member of this commission. Rivers later joined the pneumonia board at Fort Riley in Oklahoma. In 1918 this board examined the occurrence of pneumonia, which proved to be postinfluenzal. As a result of their work, Opie, Blake, Small, and Rivers published a volume, in 1922, called *Epidemic Respiratory Diseases,* which described the pandemic of influenza.

Rivers's experience in the army turned his career goals from pediatrics to research, and, when he returned to Johns Hopkins after the war, he received a fellowship with MacCallum in pathology. It was during this period that he discovered the two types of influenza bacillus. He also met Charles E. Simon[86] and was imparted with Simon's enthusiasm for the study of filterable viruses. When Rivers joined the Rockefeller staff, Cole asked him to set up a laboratory in which to study viral diseases. Rivers chose to work on varicella—the object being to develop a vaccine for prevention of the disease.

His first discovery illustrates the importance of serendipity in medicine. Working with William S. Tillett,[87] Rivers wrote two papers on the probable isolation of the virus of chickenpox from rabbits.[88] Later, when they attempted to protect rabbits against the virus they had isolated, there was no protection. When they found that the serum from a patient who had recovered from chickenpox would neutralize the chickenpox virus, they were certain that they had not transmitted chickenpox. Their next step was to try infecting rabbits by inoculating the virus into their testes. After four or five passages, the rabbits developed signs of infection; however, they were not propagating the virus of chickenpox. At about this time Miller, Andrewes, and Swift, attempting to transmit rheumatic fever in the same way, encountered an active viral agent that Rivers recognized as identical to his. In short, both of these groups had isolated a hitherto unknown virus that occurs in apparently healthy rabbits. Rivers and Louise Pearce found that the new virus ("Virus III") had spontaneously infected the Brown-Pearce tumor, being carried along in the tumor cells as they were inoculated into fresh animals. This was an important discovery, because it made clear that one had to worry about natural viruses in experimental animals being used to isolate viral agents from man, and it gave the first hint that there were such things as "latent viruses."[89]

Between 1927 and 1933, Rivers gained experience with methods for producing smallpox vaccine by growing the vaccinia (cowpox) virus on a relatively large scale, using cultures of chick tissue to provide the living cells needed by the virus. The use of tissue cultures as hosts for the propagation of viruses had begun in Carrel's laboratory, the first thus cultivated having been the Rous sarcoma virus. The Rockefeller Institute's workers were, however, not the first to use the method for the cultivation of cowpox virus. As early as 1913, Edna Steinhardt, C. Israeli, and R. A. Lambert of Columbia University kept the virus alive for several weeks, probably without multiplication, in tissue cultures of the hanging-drop variety. In 1925 Frederick Parker, Jr., and Robert N. Nye of Boston grew vaccinia in similar cultures. Rivers and his associates grew vaccinia virus in flasks of culture fluid containing fragments of living tissue in sufficient amounts to justify their use of the word "fabrication" in the title of an article, published in French, describing their method. Subsequently, Rivers and C. P. Li reduced this method to its simplest form by the use of tissue fragments suspended in flasks of Tyrode's solution, a physiological solution containing only the necessary salts and a buffer substance to keep the proper balance of alkalinity. This method has since been extensively used for the cultivation of a variety of viruses and of organisms of the Rickettsia group.

The vaccinia virus cultivated by Rivers and his associates was successfully used for the vaccination of children, although it eventually became too attenuated to afford complete protection against smallpox. The work is historically important because it involved the first cultivation of a virus in tissue culture for use in human beings.

But the years Rivers spent working on vaccinia virus had more than this practical result. He was answering a major biological question: Could viruses grow in culture media containing no living cells? The whole theory of the nature of viruses hung upon this question. Even at the institute, it had been thought that viruses may not necessarily be dependent for their existence upon association with living cells of higher organisms. Flexner and Hideyo Noguchi had, for example, described the cultivation of "globoid bodies," thought to be living particles of poliomyelitis virus, in bacteriological media of the ordinary sort, free from living cells. Rivers failed, however, to confirm the experiments of workers who thought they were succeeding with cell-free culture media. In December 1926, he was ready to declare that the filterable viruses were obligatory parasites upon living cells. Realizing that he was about to contradict the previous work of the director and of a prominent member of his own institution, he took the manuscript to Noguchi, who made no comment upon it, and then to Flexner. After the director had read it, he returned the draft to Rivers, remarking, "this is a free country, Rivers; you must publish what you think is right."

The adage that chance favors the prepared mind was exemplified in 1935, when two cases of a previously unknown human virus disease occurred in the immediate environs of the Rockefeller Institute. For several weeks, two patients underwent illnesses resembling severe influenza, with symptoms indicating meningitis. Rivers and Thomas McNair Scott, of the hospital resident staff, obtained an infectious agent from the spinal fluid of both patients, with which they transmitted the disease to mice, proving the infection to be due to a virus. In a prolonged investigation that was a model of logic and precision, Rivers and Scott tested their virus against every procurable virus known to have similar characteristics. It differed from all except one, reported the previous year by Charles Armstrong and R. D. Lillie, from mice suffering with a disease called lymphocytic choriomeningitis. Consequently, Rivers and Scott were the first to recognize the existence of lymphocytic choriomeningitis as a human disease.

By the 1940s the Rockefeller Institute had become a world-renowned center of virological research. Its investigators dominated the field, and many virologists who were trained at the institute went to other institutions, where they made fundamental contributions to this science. Rivers, who assumed directorship of the hospital in 1937, was the key figure in this development. Among the clinicians who received their training in virology under him were Thomas McNair Scott, Francis Schwentker,[90] Joseph Smadel,[91] Charles Hoagland,[92] and Thomas Francis, Jr.[93] It was Francis who first isolated a human influenza virus that was totally unrelated immunologically to the earlier type A viruses. Francis designated this virus as type B, and he soon proved that it too was capable of causing widespread outbreaks of influenza in man. This work was a key factor in the consideration of any immunization program to control epidemic influenza, because it made investigators aware of the presence of two immunologically unrelated types of human influenza virus.[94]

In 1926 Rivers organized a symposium on viruses for the Society of American Bacteriologists and presented a paper in which he clearly distinguished viruses from bacteria. This paper was influential in establishing virology as a separate discipline. Two years later, he published a classic paper entitled "Some General Aspects of Pathological Conditions Caused by Filterable Viruses" and, in the same year, his book *Filterable Viruses* appeared. Prior to that time, the literature of virology was scattered through bacteriological publications or summarized in brief chapters in textbooks of bacteriology and preventive medicine. Rivers's book was unique in at least two respects: first, it was a cooperative venture; the participants included such pioneer investigators as Harold L. Amoss, Peter Olitsky, Ernest Goodpasture, Rudolph Glaser, Lewis Kunkel, and Jacques Bronfenbrenner; and second, it included information not only about animal viruses, but also about plant, insect, and bacterial viruses. Rivers clearly differentiated, for the second time, viruses from bacteria, stating that viruses, unlike bacteria, are obligate parasites that can live and multiply only in the presence of a living susceptible cell.

Rivers's textbook was dedicated to Charles E. Simon. Beginning in 1922, at Johns Hopkins, Simon conducted the first organized course for teaching the then known information about filterable viruses. He had three postdoctoral students, who were awarded a doctorate of science in filterable viruses. In 1927 he was made a professor of filterable viruses in the School of Hygiene and Public Health at Johns Hopkins. His department was the only one ever designated as a department of filterable viruses in this country. In 1927, at the time of his premature death, Simon was preparing his lectures as a textbook of filterable viruses (which would have preceded that of Rivers).[95]

Thus, Rivers had taken his place among the country's leaders in the virus field. He had trained several younger physicians for important places in bacteriology, internal medicine, and pediatrics: George P. Berry, at Rochester, New York, and later at Harvard Medical School as dean; Schwentker, at Johns Hopkins; Scott, at Pennsylvania; and, in later years, W. Paul Havens, at Jefferson Medical College; Smadel, at the National Institutes of Health; and Lewis Thomas,[96] at the Sloan-Kettering Institute.

## Diseases of the Blood-Forming Organs

In 1933 the hospital created a special service for the study of diseases of the blood-forming organs. Its director was Cornelius P. Rhoads, who had been at the institute since 1928, first in Flexner's laboratory, where he worked intensively on the virus of poliomyelitis, and later as pathologist to the hospital.[97] In 1931 he devised a method for explantation of the kidney in experimental animals, to make the renal vein accessible to procuring blood for chemical analysis. This was used effectively in Van Slyke's laboratory and elsewhere.

Rhoads was a member of a Rockefeller Foundation Commission, which made valuable contributions to the knowledge of two tropical diseases in which anemia is a characteristic feature. In Puerto Rico in 1931, the commission, led by William B. Castle of Harvard University, discovered that, in hookworm disease, the administration of iron cures the anemia whether or not the worms are removed. This finding had a great impact in the practical treatment of the disease. The commission's intensive study of tropical sprue reinforced the view that sprue is a deficiency disease, and it confirmed the curative value of feeding liver or a liver extract, which was first demonstrated by A. L. Bloomfield and H. A. Wyckoff of Leland Stanford University School of Medicine in San Francisco.[98]

When Rhoads took charge of the hematology service, he and a young assistant resident physician, David K. Miller, turned their attention to pernicious anemia, hoping to produce it in animals. They put several lots of pigs on Goldberger's black tongue diet. As the stomach lining deteriorated, the pigs developed a disease strongly resembling pernicious anemia, and also tropical sprue, in humans. At the time of death, their stomachs and livers contained no antianemia factor. Thus, the pig yielded information about the nature of human pernicious anemia that had not been obtained by previous experimenters using dogs.

Miller, Rhoads's associate in all this work, went to the University of Buffalo in 1937 and became professor of internal medicine there. Rhoads, with various assistants from the HRI staff, continued to study the anemias until 1940. He was then called to head the newly created and endowed Sloan-Kettering Institute, adjunct of Memorial Hospital, for the experimental study of cancer and kindred diseases.

# 6

❦

# Medical Societies and Progress in Clinical Science

The medical organizations of the western world have their roots in the guilds that dominated the economic life of the medieval towns and cities. In thirteenth-century Venice, for example, there already existed a guild of medical practitioners, and, by the fourteenth century, the guild had split into two groups; namely, a College of Physicians and a College of Surgeons. Comparable developments in the English-speaking world were, however, slower in coming. By the fourteenth century, the barber-surgeons and surgeons of London had been organized into separate guilds and they were amalgamated in 1540. It was not until 1518 that the physicians were incorporated, under the leadership of Thomas Linacre, as the Royal College of Physicians of London. Similarly, a joint guild of barbers and surgeons was founded at Edinburgh in 1505, but the surgeons succeeded in preventing the physicians from being chartered as a Royal College until 1681. The seventeenth century saw the emergence of new kinds of organizations to encourage the development of scientific (including medical) knowledge, of which the most important was the Royal Society of London, founded in 1662. The Society for the Improvement of Medical Knowledge was founded at Edinburgh in 1731, but this group soon expanded its interests beyond medicine to become, in turn, the Philosophical Society (1739) and the Royal Society of Edinburgh (1783). In 1737, however, a group of medical students organized the Medical Society of Edinburgh, for the specific purpose of furthering their medical knowledge.[1]

After the middle of the eighteenth century, a sprinkling of men from the United States went abroad to study medicine, chiefly in London and Edinburgh. They were instrumental in starting medical societies in this country. John Morgan organized the Philadelphia Medical Society in 1765. After three years, it merged with the Society for Promoting Useful Knowledge, which had been organized by Benjamin Franklin in 1743, to form the American Philosophical Society. Although doctors were active in the Philosophical Society, Philadelphia remained without a meaningful medical society until 1787, when the College of Physicians was organized. The college, whose real parent was the Edinburgh Medical Society, was dedicated to the exchange and publication of scientific reports. A number of lectureships were endowed, and a fine library was created. This society was representative of similar ones formed in other cities. Many of these "academies," as they were often called, also developed libraries. For example, the Academy of Medicine in New York, founded in 1847, has a large library, perhaps exceeded in size only by the National Library of Medicine.

## The Association of American Physicians

In the last quarter of the nineteenth century, medical science in Germany was the source of many advances in scientific medicine, which led to great improvements in the United States, such as the professionalization of the basic sciences. There was an increasing number of clinical teachers who saw the need for a forum in which the improvement of medical education and medical practice could be discussed without the distractions resulting from consideration of economic, social, and political questions. This need led to the formation of new societies, including the American Surgical Association in 1880, whose first president was the leading American surgeon Samuel D. Gross, and the American Climatological Association, founded in 1884.

For clinical science, the most important of these societies was the Association of American Physicians, founded in 1885, which was similar in size, structure, and organization to the American Surgical Association, after which it may have been modeled.

The spirit and ideals of this new association were well stated in the first presidential address, given by Francis A. Delafield:

> We all of us know why we are assembled here today. It is because we want an Association in which there will be no medical politics and no medical ethics; an Association in which no one will care who are the officers and who are not; in which we will not ask from what part of the country a man comes, but whether he has done good work and will do more; whether he has something to say worth hearing and can say it. We want an Association composed of members, each of whom is able to contribute something real to the common stock of knowledge, and where he who reads such a contribution feels sure of a discriminating audience.[2]

The initial steps in the formation of the Association of American Physicians took place on October 10, 1885, at an organizational meeting attended by Delafield, William H. Draper, and George L. Peabody of New York; Robert T. Edes of Boston; and William Pepper, William Osler, and James Tyson of Philadelphia.[3]

Francis A. Delafield, aged forty-four, had studied pathology in Germany. In 1876 he became an adjunct professor of pathology and the practice of medicine and, in 1882, a full professor at Columbia University's College of Physicians and Surgeons.

William H. Draper, at age fifty-five, was the first professor of dermatology at Columbia and one of the founders of the American Dermatological Association.

George L. Peabody was only aged thirty-five in 1885. After postgraduate study in Europe, he returned, in 1878, to become pathologist to the New York Hospital. From 1884 to 1887 he was a lecturer on medicine at Columbia; he later became a professor of materia medica and therapeutics.

Robert T. Edes, aged forty-seven, was Jackson Professor of Clinical Medicine at Harvard.

William Pepper, aged forty-two, had just succeeded Stillé in the senior chair of medicine at the University of Pennsylvania. From 1881 to 1894 he was provost of the University of Pennsylvania.

William Osler, a professor of medicine at Pennsylvania, was aged thirty-six.

James Tyson, aged forty-four, was secretary at the organizational and at the first annual meeting. He was an active participant in the medical department at Pennsylvania, becoming a professor of medicine in 1889.

Thus, the average age of these founders was forty-three years. All were experienced clinicians and had a strong foundation in pathology. All were in private practice, but also held academic positions on a part-time basis. Obviously, none could be classified as clinical investigators.

At the organizational meeting, a list of seventy-seven prospective members was prepared. Eighteen cities in the United States and Canada were represented. At a second organizational meeting, several men from the list of eligibles attended. These included Alfred L. Loomis, then aged fifty-four. Among the positions that Loomis held were those of professor of pathology and the practice of medicine at the University of the City of New York; physician to Bellevue Hospital; and lecturer on physical diagnosis at Columbia.

Francis Minot, aged sixty-four, was the oldest of the group of thirteen founding members. He was a visiting physician to the MGH and Hersey Professor of the Theory and Practice of Physic at Harvard.

George B. Shattuck, who studied in Paris and Vienna, was a visiting physician at the Boston City Hospital and, for many years, editor of the *Boston Medical and Surgical Journal.*

Frederick C. Shattuck, the thirty-eight-year-old younger brother of George B. Shattuck, graduated in medicine in 1883 and worked in London, Paris, and Vienna for three years. He was Jackson Professor of Medicine.

Reginald Heber Fitz was aged forty-two. After graduation from Harvard in 1868, he spent two years abroad with Rokitansky and Skoda in

Vienna and with Victor Cornil in Paris. He introduced cellular pathology into the United States. In his later years, he was a visiting physician at the MGH and Hersey Professor of the Theory and Practice of Physic at Harvard. In 1878 he became a professor of pathological anatomy at Harvard.

The last of the group was R. Palmer Howard, one of Osler's teachers. At age sixty-two, he was dean and professor of the theory and practice of medicine at McGill University.[4]

## The Initial Meeting

The first annual meeting was held in Washington, D.C., on June 17 and 18, 1886. About two-thirds of the original members came from four cities—New York, Philadelphia, Boston, and Baltimore. One of the important decisions made was to include not only distinguished medical men for membership, but also those in other clinical specialties, as well as outstanding basic scientists. At that time, pathology was the strongest basic science, but there were few full-time pathologists and almost none who encompassed the new cellular pathology of Virchow. "Experimental medicine" was represented, among the original members, by Welch. The specialties included were pediatrics, dermatology, neurology, and psychiatry.

The first scientific program of the association was an enormous success. A debate was held on the subject: Does the present state of knowledge justify a clinical and pathological correlation of rheumatism, gout, diabetes, and chronic Bright's disease? After papers were presented by Tyson and Draper, comments were given by Theodore Caldwell Janeway, Frederick C. Shattuck, Alfred L. Loomis, Horatio C. Wood, William Pepper, and Abraham Jacobi. The discussion reads like an early review of the "connective tissue" diseases.

A lively interchange took place around William T. Councilman's paper entitled "Certain Elements Found in the Blood in Cases of Malarial Fever."[5] Osler described the "ameboid" bodies, but he was still not certain whether they were areas of hyaline transformation or definite organisms. George Sternberg, then surgeon-general of the U.S. Army, believed that the bodies were malarial parasites, stating that the differentiation by staining excluded vacuoles.

The most important paper was that by Reginald Heber Fitz, entitled "Perforating Inflammation of the Vermiform Appendix."[6] He described the syndrome fully and made a vigorous plea for early diagnosis and prompt operation as the best treatment.

Experimental work was also presented, the most popular paper being that by Welch on experimental glomerulonephritis.[7] The first truly clinical investigation to be presented was a report by S. Weir Mitchell, on the tendon-jerk and muscle-jerk in disease.[8]

Some thirty years later, Osler called this meeting "the coming of age party of clinical medicine." Before this, clinical medicine in America had been "in bondage to tutors and governors—English, French and German. The fullness of time has brought the privilege of an heir—independence and a rich heritage."[9]

One who contributed greatly to the early success of the association was Herter. In 1900 Herter gave a paper on hyperoxaluria, one of the "inborn errors of metabolism" recognized some eight years later by Archibald E. Garrod.[10] Herter also discussed the pathology of acid intoxication,[11] which was an experimental biochemical investigation of acid-base balance; his study was a forerunner of the work of later investigators including Lawrence J. Henderson, W. W. Palmer, Andrew Watson Sellards, and James L. Gamble. A. N. Richards commented that, more than anyone else, Herter led the association on the pathway toward scientific medicine.

Welch's presidential address of 1901 was a keynote for what was to come in the twentieth century.[12] He pointed to the great progress made in establishing excellent laboratories for the experimental sciences and in placing these sciences on a full-time university basis. He then emphasized that no such facilities existed in clinical medicine and surgery. This was an early plea for more full-time career opportunities for those interested in clinical science (see chapter 7).

Members of the association soon recognized the wisdom of having basic scientists, as well as clinicians, as members. This was evidenced by Francis B. Kinnicutt's presidential address of 1907:

> The successive meetings of the Association have proved the wisdom and hopes of its founders. . . . Embracing as it does, in its membership, the pure scientist in medicine and the clinician in every field of its practice, this body has been an admirable example of the science and art of medicine walking hand in hand. . . . The one or the other leading for the moment, but always with the willingness and desire to have its steps corrected if perchance straying from the path of truth. . . . By such a union alone is secure progress in medicine attainable.[13]

The membership of the association has been composed, for the most part, of teachers of medicine. In the beginning, this teaching was done by the great practitioners of the day, who taught in terms of bedside medicine, which they based almost entirely on a foundation of morbid anatomy. They were the leaders of medicine before the era of modern scientific medicine began. Their academic status was gained by their success in practice. The membership was increasingly seeded with the newly developing medical scientists, whose approach was based on physiology and biochemistry. This process had much to do with shaping the character of the association and its continuing dedication to the development of new knowledge as the road to improvement in medical practice. The basic science members, always only a handful, have exerted an influence in terms of propagating research interest out of proportion to their numbers. The interdependence of the basic sciences and the clinical disciplines of medicine is clearly shown in the life history of the Association of American Physicians. The association is a prime example of the intellectual enrichment and growth that results from this type of scientific interaction.

The evolution of the association illustrates the three main eras in the development of medical education and research. The era of the great clinicians, the advent of university or full-time medicine, and the explosion in clinical science that began in the mid-1930s with the sulfonamides, grew rapidly during the war years, then at a logarithmic rate with the appearance of the National Institutes of Health and massive federal support for medical research.

## The Interurban Clinical Club and Its First Meeting[14]

Late one August afternoon in 1900, three distinguished American surgeons—Alton J. Ochsner, William J. Mayo, and Harvey Williams Cushing—were sitting on a bridge overlooking the river Seine. Paris was filled with physicians and surgeons attending the thirteenth International Medical Congress. All three men were completely bored with listening to the many papers presented at the congress, most of which were in languages they could ill understand. What had proved to be the chief attraction during that week was not a part of the congress. It was, instead, an operative clinic given each morning in the private hospital of an ambidextrous genius and showman, Eugène Doyen. Though these distinguished surgeons shuddered at his complete disregard for hemostasis and his emphasis on speed (for example, a mammary resection for cancer was performed in seven minutes), they visited his operating room every day. However they might disapprove of his surgical techniques, it seemed preferable to the boredom of the congress. Cushing suggested that opportunities of this sort were important, if only to see other surgeons display their true colors. His friends replied that this was exactly what they had been doing for a number of years—paying visits to other clinics in order to see the nature and quality of work there. The idea was put forth that it would be possible to observe more in a shorter time if a small group made such visits together and if the host clinic prepared a specific program for them.

Some eighteen months later, Cushing presented to George Crile the idea of organizing a small travel club of clinical surgeons who had an interest in "physiological pathology," as the recent work in laboratory investigation was called. At that time, plans for an experimental laboratory of medicine and surgery were underway in Baltimore, and, in Cleveland, an endowment had been secured for a laboratory of experimental medicine. Similar facilities were under consideration in other cities, so it appeared to be an ideal time for interested surgeons to join together and periodically pay visits to each other's home institution. A meeting was held in New York, on July 11, 1903, and George E. Brewer, George Crile, John Cummings Munro, Charles Harrison Fraser, and James G. Munford drew up a tentative list of charter members, nominated themselves to office, and designated Baltimore as the place of the first meeting.

It was a distinguished group that met in the House Officers' Assembly Room in the Johns Hopkins Hospital, on November 13, 1903, to conduct the first meeting of the American Society for Clinical Surgery. The program began with attendance at William Stewart Halsted's customary Friday morning exercise for third-year students. The members then moved to Howard Kelly's operating room, where J.M.T. Finney gave a demonstration of his newly devised pyloroplasty for ulcer. A demonstration of the teaching of operative surgery on animals to third-year students, which Cushing had organized, was held in his Hunterian Laboratory for Experimental Surgery and Medicine. Joseph C. Bloodgood explained his course in surgical pathology, and, at the end of the day, there was a demonstration of Hugh H. Young's new operation—perineal prostatectomy. All of the members felt they had started something that had the air of outstanding success. Osler obviously sniffed this air of enthusiasm and, by the ruse of asking the assembled surgeons to dine with him, got himself invited to the first dinner of the American Society of Clinical Surgery. The idea of such an interurban group was already in Osler's mind, but the surgical group was an inspiration for further progress.

With his knowledge of what the younger American clinicians were doing, Osler understood that such a club, organized for internists, would be a way to advance medicine in America in a unique way. On April 28, 1905, he called together a group of men, six from each of the four large cities of the east—Boston, New York, Philadelphia, and Baltimore—to form an interurban club patterned after the surgical club. Everyone invited received the following note:

> It is proposed to start among a few of the younger men in the eastern cities an interurban club on lines similar to the Society of Clinical Surgery. The number of members will be limited. The objects of the club will be: 1) to stimulate the study of internal medicine; 2) by mutual intercourse and discussion to improve our methods of work and teaching; 3) to promote the scientific investigation of disease; 4) to increase our knowledge of the methods of work in other clinics than our own. It is proposed to meet twice a year to have demonstrations and discussions. The program of each meeting is to be supplied by the men in the city in which the meeting is being held. It is proposed to hold the first meeting at the Johns Hopkins Hospital on April 28 and 29. The rules to govern the club will then be discussed and adopted. You are invited to become a member and to be present on that date.[15]

On the evening of April 28, the assembled group met for dinner and, with Osler as temporary chairman, officially organized the Interurban

Clinical Club, electing Richard Clarke Cabot as president and Thomas McCrae as secretary. Osler was elected the first honorary member. The charter members of the club, all but one (Barker) of whom were present at this inaugural meeting, were: Richard Clarke Cabot, Elliott Proctor Joslin, Edwin Allen Locke, Frederick Taylor Lord, Joseph Hersey Pratt, and Wilder Tileston of Boston; Charles N. B. Camac, Lewis Atterbury Conner, Walter Belknap James, Theodore Caldwell Janeway, Samuel Waldron Lambert, and Frank Sherman Meara of New York; David Linn Edsall, Aloysius Oliver Joseph Kelly, Warfield Theobald Longcope, David Riesman, Joseph Sailer, and Alfred Stengel of Philadelphia; Lewellys Franklin Barker, Rufus I. Cole, Charles Phillips Emerson, Thomas B. Futcher, Thomas McCrae, and William Sydney Thayer of Baltimore.

As one looks back over the past seventy-five years, the organization of the Interurban Clinical Club has perhaps had a more continuing influence than any other contribution that Osler made. Most of Osler's contributions were not truly original, whether one considers his clinical descriptions of disease, his relatively minor contributions in the laboratory, the origin of the basic concepts behind his "innovative" approaches to education, or the implementation of effective mechanisms for the exchange of ideas about education, research, and practice. But he often astutely picked up the ideas of others and was responsible for making them work. He had an intuitive sense of what was important, as well as the personality and character to promote successfully those ideas that appeared to him worthwhile. His ability to see a need clearly and to provide an impetus is well illustrated by the founding of the Interurban Clinical Club.

There can be no doubt of Osler's sound appraisal of the young men active in internal medicine in 1905, when one considers the careers of those he chose as charter members of the club. All proved to be outstanding physicians, and many made fundamental contributions to the creation of medicine's scientific base and to the application of scientific developments to medical practice in this country.

The program of the first meeting was dominated by Osler. Pratt recalled vividly Joseph Erlanger's presentation of his work on experimental heart block in the dog. All of those in attendance leaned forward in the little amphitheatre, trying to see the bundle of His encompassed by the special clamp that he had devised. The scene reminded Pratt of Rembrandt's group of surgeons at Dr. Tulp's anatomy lesson. Following this demonstration, Osler presented a patient with heart block. It was characteristic of Osler to bring together the laboratory and clinical aspects of a medical problem. The diagnosis of heart block was made on clinical grounds and confirmed by tracing the cardiac apex beat with the Marey cardiograph tracing and another of the venous pulsations with an air-filled tambour. The first electrocardiograms were not taken in this country until 1909.

The Interurban Clinical Club flourished and served an important role during the developmental period of the "new medicine." Osler's appreciation of its demands led to a chain of events that provided a helpful forum for teachers and investigators in the field of internal medicine during its logarithmic phase of growth. Other intercity organizations soon followed.

The Cosmopolitan Club was founded in 1911, at a time when the specialty of internal medicine was rapidly growing. Just as the limited size of the Association of American Physicians was to give rise to the impetus, in the first decade of the twentieth century, to the founding of the American Society of Clinical Investigation by a group of young internists, all of whom were members of the Interurban Clinical Club, so the limited size of the successful Interurban Clinical Club led a group of younger internists to establish a similar organization.

The Peripatetic Club grew out of discussions at a meeting of the Cosmopolitan Club. It was organized during the meetings of the Association of American Physicians in Washington, D.C., in May 1933; the first meeting took place on November 3 and 4, 1933, in New York City. This organization was successful due to the intense interest in it of Fuller Albright, who served as its secretary for many years.

The second interurban club was the Central Interurban Clinical Club, whose organizational meeting, under the leadership of Frank Billings and James B. Herrick, was held in Chicago on December 20, 1919.

Almost simultaneously with the beginning of the Central Interurban Clinical Club, internists from the cities in the lower Great Lakes region founded a similar organization. It was conceived by John R. Williams during a visit with Joslin in Boston in 1919, when the original Interurban Club was meeting in that city.

The Pacific Interurban Clinical Club was organized on June 29, 1923, during a meeting of the American Medical Association in San Francisco, by a small group of internists, including George Dock, Frank Pottinger, Nelson Janney, Albion W. Hewlett, Walter C. Alvarez, Eugene Kilgore, William Kerr, and Hans Lisser.

A similar club developed in the south, with members in New Orleans; Atlanta and Augusta, Georgia; Birmingham, Montgomery, and Fairfield, Alabama; Asheville, North Carolina; and Nashville and Memphis, Tennessee.

Thus, Osler's action stimulated a chain reaction. Details concerning the Interurban Clinical Club, including the programs of its meetings over the last three quarters of a century, and biographical sketches of its members, are available in the history of the club, published in 1978.[16]

## Societies for Experimental Studies

During the closing years of the nineteenth century, the study of disease by experimental methods was increasing rapidly; but it was done, for the most part, by those who were professionally trained in one of the basic medical sciences (e.g., physiology, pharmacology, pathology, biochemistry). A few physicians working in the university clinics and hospitals, and a small handful of men working independently, were also involved. One of those working independently was Samuel James Meltzer of New York.[17] Meltzer was unique in his emphasis on the value of societies for stimulating research. With a few of his contemporaries, in 1903, he organized the Society of Experimental Biology and Medicine, which quickly became known as the "Meltzer Verein." More importantly, Meltzer was the inspiration for the founding of the American Society for Clinical Investigation.

## Samuel James Meltzer

Samuel James Meltzer combined successfully the life of the practitioner and the experimental physiologist.[18] Born in northwestern Russia in 1851, he and his family moved, in 1876, to Berlin, where he studied medicine under Dubois-Reymond, Virchow, Helmholtz, and Friedlander. The one who exercised the greatest influence on his career, however, was the physiologist Hugo Kronecker (a student of Ludwig's).

Meltzer immigrated to New York City in 1883, where he found opportunities for his investigative work in the laboratory of Welch at Bellevue and in Curtis's and Prudden's laboratories at the College of Physicians and Surgeons. For a number of years he carried on his practice and investigations simultaneously. The majority of practicing physicians criticized the laboratory methods that were coming into use. Meltzer was, however, entirely in sympathy with the development of scientific medicine and was, at all times, the vigorous defender of experimental methods in medicine.

In the early years of Meltzer's work in New York, the leading physicians were Jacobi, Clark, the elder Flint, Delafield, and Edward G. Janeway, the scientific basis of whose training was mainly pathological anatomy. Later it was recognized that the study of function was essential to the making of a good physician, and Meltzer typified this idea when scarcely anyone else in the country did so. He held a unique position as an active member of important medical societies, both clinical and scientific, and as an able practitioner and a successful laboratory worker. He was thus able to stimulate younger men to undertake experimental work and to impress older men with the value and necessity of such work.

When he was asked, in 1904, to take charge of a department of experimental physiology and pharmacology at the newly established Rockefeller Institute, Meltzer did not hesitate in making his decision. He was the ideal man for the job—a genuine physiologist recognized by his peers, but whose interests were largely concerned with problems relating to practical medicine. Meltzer's major research contributions can be divided into three areas: first, the action of adrenalin upon the blood vessels and the pupillary muscle; second, the inhibitory action of magnesium sulfate and the antagonistic effects of the calcium salts; and third, the development of his method of artificial respiration by pharyngeal and intratracheal insufflation.[19] Another practical contribution was made in 1910, after Auer and Lewis, working in Meltzer's laboratory, had demonstrated for the first time that when anaphylactic shock is produced in guinea pigs by injecting them with a substance to which they are highly sensitive, death results, from intense constriction of the bronchi.[20] Viewing this observation in the light of his clinical experience, Meltzer proposed that bronchial asthma was a phenomenon related to anaphylaxis and was caused by exposure to a substance to which the individual was sensitive.

## Meltzer and the American Society for Clinical Investigation[21]

Although the date of the first annual meeting was May 10, 1909, the formation of this society was first suggested by Meltzer in June 1907, during a meeting of the American Medical Association at Atlantic City, New Jersey. While walking on the boardwalk with Longcope, Edsall, Tileston, and Pratt, Meltzer advanced the idea that the younger men interested in research who were not yet members of the Association of American Physicians should have the opportunity of meeting together to discuss their research. The same evening Meltzer invited this group, along with Christian and Cole, to his hotel room for further discussion of the idea. The outcome was the formation of a committee, consisting of Christian, Edsall, Pratt, and Tileston, which met in Boston on June 17, 1907. Before the next meeting, the committee was enlarged by the addition of Cole, Longcope, and Meltzer. Later Joseph A. Capps and Hewlett were added. These men, with the exception of Hewlett, met again in November 1907 and compiled a list of twenty-two men to invite to an organizational meeting.[22] The original title selected for the society was the American Society for the Advancement of Clinical Investigation. The word *investigation* was used instead of *research,* because there was another society composed of homeopaths known as the Society for Clinical Research.

Longcope recalled the meeting of November 7, 1907, at the Manhattan Hotel in New York City: "I remember . . . that we discussed at considerable length a list of names from which the membership of this new society should be recruited. As I recall the discussion, these men were selected because it was thought they would be interested in the new endeavor and were sympathetic with the idea of forming a society whose main object was to discuss the problems in clinical investigation in which each and every one was engaged."[23]

The society was formally organized, on May 11, 1908, at a meeting held in Washington, D.C. A constitution was adopted, and, since that time, the Society has held one meeting annually.[24] The first officers were

Meltzer, president; Edsall,[25] vice-president; Christian, secretary; Howland, treasurer; and Joseph L. Miller, Theodore Caldwell Janeway, and Hewlett, councillors. Letters of invitation were sent to thrity-four men, including the nine committee members. When the replies were in, thirty-two physicians indicated their desire to participate in the new society: B. K. Ashford, E. R. Baldwin, W. J. Calvert, J. A. Capps, H. A. Christian, R. Cole, D. M. Cowie, D. L. Edsall, C. P. Emerson, H. Emerson, M. Fischer, N. B. Foster, A. W. Hewlett, J. Howland, J. R. Hunt, T. C. Janeway, E. Libman, E. A. Locke, W. T. Longcope, E. J. McCarthy, S. J. Meltzer, J. L. Miller, W. E. Musgrave, J. H. Pratt, M. Richardson, E. C. Rosenow, J. Sailer, C. E. Simon, J. D. Steele, R. P. Strong, W. Tileston, and G. B. Wallace.

## The "Young Turks"[26] and the Emergence of Clinical Science

All the young men involved in the society were engaged in "clinical investigation," but in some instances, it was primitive in type, involving little more than the reporting of interesting cases. The concept of clinical science was a radical one at the turn of the century. When he arrived in the United States, Meltzer must have found the scientific atmosphere stifling. During that period, research received no adequate support from either government or commercial sources and very little from private subsidy. After Johns Hopkins set up his university, however, the principle of private subsidy began to gain favor. The founding of the Rockefeller Institute was a milestone. In 1901 the Board of Scientific Advisors received $20,000, to be distributed as grants for medical research. This concept of providing funds to assist individuals during the course of investigation was an innovation in striking contrast to the usual practice of rewarding researchers, if at all, at the termination of their work. By using private wealth to stimulate the initiation of scientific studies, the Rockefeller grants set a precedent for other philanthropists, the American Medical Association, private research foundations and, ultimately, the federal government. The opportunity was being created for qualified young men to enter research without the impediments that Meltzer had encountered. This involved not only the successful application of the techniques of science to the study of human disease, but also the conversion of the medical profession to the view that the mysteries of human illness needed to be explored and could best be solved by the use of scientific techniques. Mobilization of the needed investigators required in turn a drastic upgrading of the standards and methods of medical research as well as the opportunities for research training. These "Young Turks," who founded the American Society for the Advancement of Clinical Investigation, formed a corps dedicated to these tasks.

The formation of this society did not constitute an insurrection. Relations between the "Young Turks" and the Association of American

Physicians were entirely good natured. The new society was not formed in protest against the old, but in response to the needs of a younger generation that was already beginning to use methods in their studies unfamiliar to their elders.[27] In George Canby Robinson's words: "The idea of the Society was to bring together the men in the various clinics which were just being organized on a university basis and who were beginning to develop systematic research. It was a young crowd and was to be confined to the men who were active in clinical investigation rather than men who had become eminent in medical practice and teaching." This was part of the far-reaching reform movement in medicine going on at the time, which Robinson characterized as "the intrusion of science into clinical medicine."[28]

Significant components of the new outlook were the beliefs that clinical medicine was a science in its own right, that the investigation of disease was the legitimate concern of the "clinician," and that the work of clinic and laboratory, of physician and basic scientist, ought to be more closely integrated and, in fact, combined in the person of an essentially new type of medical worker—the clinical investigator or clinical scientist. The cultivation of a "research atmosphere" in medical schools and hospitals necessitated, first, professors of medicine able to devote full time to research and teaching without the distraction of an extensive private practice; second, students and staff members trained in the methods and imbued with the spirit of science; and third, adequate laboratory facilities available to clinicians for the systematic study of clinical problems. Reform in these areas became the rallying cry of the "Young Turks."[29]

What was taking place to dissipate the schism between the basic scientist and the practicing clinician is revealed in the following statement, by Dr. James H. Means, of the situation when he began his own medical training in 1907:

> The transition from the preclinical to the clinical years in medical school involved almost as great a change in direction as that from college to professional school. The teachers of the first and second year subjects and those of the third and fourth year subjects constituted two distinct groups with quite different viewpoints and there was limited communication between them. The clinicians brushed off the preclinical scientists as mere laboratory men who knew but little of medicine and the scientist looked upon the practice of medicine as largely unscientific guess work. The whole manner of life between these two groups was different. The preclinical scientists were in the mold of college teachers on the campus. They were full-time, salaried people. There were no full-time clinical teachers in those days or salaries either for that matter. Small token honoraria were given by the University but nothing by the teaching hospitals. These men taught and attended hospital patients for love or kudos or a mixture of the two and made their livelihood in private practice. Any degree of unanimity

in a faculty so constituted I am sure was hard to come by. This gap was later to be closed by the development of the middle estate in medicine, namely, the full-time, academic, salaried clinician.[30]

The essential difference between the old-type clinical teacher and what was called for here was the difference between the German and British schools of medicine. At the time the society was founded, the predominating medical influence in America was British and French,[31] as represented, for example, by Osler. Many of the members of the younger generation were then strongly influenced by the medical traditions of Germany. Some of them had been fortunate enough to have studied at German university clinics, where clinical medicine enjoyed a status equal to that of the other sciences and where its teachers devoted most of their time to instruction and investigation. It was in this direction that the reformers of American medical education hoped to move, and it was this tradition, with its emphasis on research in academic clinical medicine, that was the motivating factor in the society.

The training and accomplishments of those physicians who accepted an invitation to join the American Society for Clinical Investigation in 1908 give a picture of clinical science at that time. Twelve of them were interested in some aspect of infectious disease and immunology, including tropical medicine; four, in cardiovascular-renal disease; and four, in some aspect of metabolic disease. One was a pharmacologist, another a physiologist and pharmacologist. The primary interest of two was in neurology. The others were physicians who were interested in some aspect of clinical investigation, but are difficult to classify as to their specific field.

The age of these new members ranged from thirty-one to forty-four, with an average of thirty-five. Five received their M.D. degree from the Johns Hopkins University School of Medicine, five from Pennsylvania, four from Harvard, three from the College of Physicians and Surgeons, two from Michigan and Rush, and one each from Georgetown, George Washington, Maryland, Yale, New York University, and Northwestern. The average interval from graduation to election was eleven years, with a range of six to eighteen years. Twenty-one had an internship, whereas four entered the army immediately after medical school. Four trained in pathology laboratories, and one became a pharmacologist. Fifteen studied abroad, all but one in Germany. All continued to contribute significantly in research or education. Two became directors of a research institute, and two had army careers. All of the others maintained a faculty position in a medical school, twelve becoming chairman of a clinical department and two of a preclinical department. Eighteen achieved full professorial status. That the selection of these men was perceptive in terms of the future of clinical investigation is shown by their subsequent activities: twenty-four of them did research that involved the application of the experimental methods of the basic sciences to clinical problems.[32] For further biographical information about the society's charter members, see Appendix A.

## Program of the First Meeting

In his presidential address to the new society, Meltzer said:[33]

I feel sure that the efficiency of that practice will be best attained when the search for the knowledge which the practice has to use should be carried on in the same manner and by the same methods as are employed in the search for knowledge in the other branches of intellectual activity. In other words, clinical research should be raised to a department of clinical science and be theoretically and practically separated to a considerable degree from the mere practical interests, that is, separated so far as the various and variable conditions permit. It will be the practice not less than the science which will benefit by such a separation.

Meltzer, who felt that the efficiency of practice should be the supreme object in medicine, went on to say:

Each disease is an experiment which nature makes on the organism. The very large number and the great variations of these experiments of nature offer favorable opportunities for testing the theories made regarding the nature of these spontaneous experiments. Furthermore, clinical research should, indeed, be coupled with animal experimentation; any new point of view gained by observation in clinical medicine which cannot be verified on human beings should be tested by experiments on animals. By such a procedure not only clinical medicine but also physiology may learn a great deal for which the following facts from the recent history of medicine are classical illustrations: the recognition of myxedema as a special type of disease led to the understanding of the function of the thyroid gland, and the observations of the coincidence of pathologic processes of the pancreas with diabetes led to the discovery by clinical investigators of the glycolytic function of the pancreas.

Clinical science will not thrive through chance investigations by friendly neighbors from the adjoining practical and scientific domains. Such volunteer service which for the present is keeping up the cultivation of the unacclaimed region is almost certainly very welcome. But the acclimation, cultivation and maintenance of a field of pure science of clinical medicine cannot be accomplished by chance services by volunteers. For such a purpose we need the service of a standing army of regulars. The investigator in clinical science must devote the best part of his time and intellectual energies to the cultivation and elevation of this field just as the physiologist does in his domain ... without the development of such a department of clinical science the efficiency of the practice of internal medicine will lag behind no matter how progressive the allied sciences of medicine are and how great their efforts to be useful in medicine may be.

Meltzer's stirring presidential address, entitled "The Science of Clinical Medicine. What it ought to be and the Men to Uphold it," was followed by fourteen papers.[34]

## Advance of Clinical Investigation

The years 1910 to 1945 witnessed striking advances in the status of investigative medicine and a veritable revolution in American medical education. The presidential addresses delivered annually at the meetings of the society give a picture of the development of clinical science and the problems faced in its implementation and expansion. For example, the increasing tendency among investigators to adulate experimentation at the expense of the descriptive method received the frequent attention of critics. Many looked upon the descriptive method as being outdated, but, in his presidential address of 1931, Francis G. Blake stated that there were, of course, two methods—on the one hand, observation, analysis, and deduction, the so-called descriptive method, which was still held honorable by some because of its antiquity, if for no other reason; on the other hand, the inductive experimental method, held in higher esteem by most because of its relatively recent use and the vigor of its advocates. He called the argument concerning the relative superiority of either method a somewhat fruitless pastime. The important thing was that the investigator stopped to think about what it was he hoped to accomplish, regardless of which method he chose.[35]

The science of clinical investigation was greatly enriched by the growing array of instruments and techniques that enabled clinicians to transcend simple observation in their study of the mechanisms of disease. If clinical research activity boomed in the 1920s and 1930s, it exploded in the years following World War II. In the interval between 1945 and 1955 alone, the number of physicians trained in clinical investigation increased tenfold. The funds available for medical research likewise multiplied at a rapid rate, in large part due to the federal government's support of scientific activities on a massive scale. The stimulus provided by the work of the members of the American Society for Clinical Investigation played an important role in these developments.

## The *Journal of Clinical Investigation*

At the sixth annual meeting of the society (May 11, 1914), Meltzer moved that the president should appoint a committee to work out a mode of publication of the society's transactions.[36] The committee, composed of Meltzer, Christian, and Morris, presented the following proposition at the seventh annual meeting on May 10, 1915: "The Committee ... considers it as desirable that the ... Society shall ... publish a volume containing the transactions of each annual meeting, which would embody fuller information ... of the papers presented and the discussions which followed, a volume which should be accessible through libraries, etc." Meltzer voted in favor, but Christian and Morris were opposed. Because the majority of the committee was opposed to it, the chair ruled that "the publication of the Society's proceedings will continue as in the past."

There was no further reference to publication of the proceedings until 1919, when it was voted to ask the *Journal of the American Medical Association* to publish the proceedings.

George Canby Robinson appeared before the council on May 4, 1924, and reported the president's appointment, on September 15, 1923, of a committee on the formation of a new journal that at some future time could be affiliated with the society. The committee consisted of Drs. Austin, Rollin T. Woodyatt, Cole, Longcope, Cohn, Peabody, and Robinson (chairman). It had been directed to confer with the representatives of the Rockefeller Institute about the formation of the new journal.

Robinson read the following minutes of this committee's meeting, which was held October 12, 1923, at the HRI:

> The Committee unanimously recommends that the Council of the American Society for Clinical Investigation offer the following plan to the Society at its annual meeting. That there be established a journal to be called the *Journal of Clinical Investigation.* That there be an Editorial Committee consisting initially of the following 15 members of the American Society for Clinical Investigation: C. C. Bass, Francis G. Blake, Henry A. Christian, Eugene DuBois, A. W. Hewlett, C. P. Howard, John Howland, Edward B. Krumbhaar, William S. McCann, Franklin C. McLean, W. McKim Marriott, Edward H. Mason, L. H. Newburgh, Walter W. Palmer, and Leonard G. Rowntree.
>
> That there shall be an Editorial Board consisting of G. Canby Robinson, editor-in-chief, and of J. Harold Austin, Alfred E. Cohn, Rufus Cole, Warfield T. Longcope, Francis W. Peabody and Rollin T. Woodyatt. The editor-in-chief shall have direct responsibility and authority for the active editorial conduct of the Journal and shall have discretionary power in arranging the details as to the conduct of the Journal.

This plan for the establishment of the *Journal of Clinical Investigation* was presented tentatively by Robinson to the Board of Scientific Directors of the Rockefeller Institute, at their meeting on October 29, 1923, with the request that the institute give financial assistance sufficient to allow this project to be undertaken without expense to the society.

Robinson reported that the board, at its meeting on April 26, included in the preliminary draft of the budget for fiscal year 1924–25 an item of $3,000, to be paid as a grant to the Society for Clinical Investigation for the publication of a new journal, contingent upon the acceptance of the just-outlined plan by the society at its next meeting. It was proposed to provide that sum to the journal for a period not to exceed three years, by which time it was expected that it would be self-supporting.

On motion duly made and seconded, it was voted to approve the plan of organization for the new journal and to recommend to the society that it be accepted; and, furthermore, to recommend that the council be authorized to incorporate the society, in order that it might own the journal.

### The First Issue

The first issue of the *Journal of Clinical Investigation* appeared in October 1924. It contained a scholarly lead article entitled "Purposes in Medical Research," written by Alfred E. Cohn, who was on the staff of the HRI. After thoughtful consideration of the history of the research process, Cohn stated that

> medicine has significant tasks, tasks of great complexity. . . . We have begun to study these diseases which involve abnormal physiological processes as scientists always study, by whatever means natural science has to offer which promise success. We are engaged now in the struggle to fit ourselves for the work of overcoming the difficulties involved in mastering the methodology we must use—be it physics, physiology, nosology, or chemistry. These are, it need scarcely be pointed out, the methods employed likewise in biology; that the methods are the same is not surprising, in view of the fact that the living system which is studied in medicine does not differ from that which is the concern of biology in general, except that one has in medicine not always the advantage of adopting simple material to serve the purposes of one's experiments.
>
> This, then, is the task which academic medicine in the United States, now become self-conscious, has set itself; it is the task of clinical investigation. . . .
>
> To give substance to ideas like these is the purpose which lies behind the work of the new university clinics which are being founded in many parts of our country. They mean to take on new functions. . . . In addition to the traditional responsibility for teaching, they avow the desire to contribute to an increase of knowledge. They are drawing to themselves new men, trained in a new way; they are being supplied with new hospitals properly equipped with laboratories in which to pursue what Bernard called the *observation provoquée*. These activities testify to the development of a new spirit. This is the spirit which has called the American Society for Clinical Investigation into being. It is the spirit to which the *Journal of Clinical Investigation* desires to give expression.[37]

Over the five decades of its being, the journal, due to the distinguished work of its contributors and editors, has succeeded in full measure in serving this important function.

Isaac Starr, in his presidential address to the society, referred to the importance of the *Journal of Clinical Investigation* as follows: "a godsend to those of us who are considered to be clinicians by physiologists, biochemists and immunologists and considered to be physiologists, biochemists or immunologists by most clinicians." By serving as an organ for clinical research made by quantitative methods, the journal was: "in the forefront of that change from descriptive and qualitative methods to the more exact quantitative methods. . . . which has made possible the great advances of physics and chemistry and may well produce as great a revolution in medical practice."[38] What prophetic words these were.

When the subsidy from the Rockefeller Institute ceased, financial aid was given for several years by the Rockefeller Foundation. For the next few years, many departments of medicine accepted associate memberships in the society, as a form of subsidy for the journal. Beginning with volume eleven, in 1932, the Chemical Foundation began meeting all deficits in the costs of the journal and continued this until the growth of the subscription list placed it on a self-supporting basis.

The editorial staff for the first few years of the journal is not recorded in the bound files of the journal, for this information appeared only on those issues' cover pages, which were discarded in binding. The names have been recorded, however, in an historical note by James Harold Austin.[39]

After the inauguration of the journal, the proceedings of the meetings regularly appeared in abstract form, beginning with the seventeenth annual meeting, in May 1925. The most complete library collection of the early *Proceedings* is, according to the Union Serials List, at the New York Academy of Medicine Library.

## The Central Society for Clinical Research

Although the American Society for Clinical Investigation provided a forum and a journal for the presentation and publication of the results of clinical investigation in the East, it was difficult for a young investigator from the Midwest to present work before these existing organizations. Since World War I furnished a tremendous stimulus to clinical research, the problem grew more acute with each passing year, as the number of young men engaged in clinical research in the Midwest medical centers rapidly increased. The founding of the Central Society for Clinical Research helped to alleviate this problem. The early history of this society has been ably reviewed by Lawrence D. Thompson of St. Louis.[40]

In December 1919, a group of prominent physicians from the Midwest centers of Chicago, Iowa City, Minneapolis, Rochester (Minn.), and St. Louis decided to organize the Central Interurban Club.[41] The club was to be patterned after the Interurban Clinical Club, founded by Osler.

The original members of the Central Club were: Frank Billings, Joseph A. Capps, James B. Herrick, Ernest E. Irons, Joseph L. Miller, and Rollin T. Woodyatt (Chicago); Campbell P. Howard (Iowa City); S. Marx White (Minneapolis); Henry S. Plummer and Leonard G. Rowntree (Rochester); George Dock and George Canby Robinson (St. Louis).

The objectives of the club were: (1) the stimulation of investigation,

(2) the improvement of methods of teaching, (3) demonstrations of work in "borderline" subjects, (4) a better knowledge of the men, methods, and work of other clinics, and (5) the promotion of good fellowship among the members. Informal meetings were held twice a year, and various clinics were visited in rotation. Membership slowly increased, but it became obvious that gaining admission to the established societies for clinical investigation was still difficult for young men in the Midwest.

In November 1920, Billings discussed this matter before the club, and, in June 1923, he brought up the subject of "the organization of a new society." It was decided, in November 1924, to organize a club similar to the Central Club for the younger men of the schools represented.[42] Two young men from each of several Midwest cities were invited to meet with the Central Interurban Club in Rochester on December 5, 1925. These men were: from Chicago, Robert W. Keeton and W. H. Nadler; Iowa City, Lee C. Gatewood and Frank J. Rohner; Minneapolis, C. A. McKinley and Jay A. Myers; Rochester, George E. Brown and Frederick A. Willius; St. Louis, A. P. Briggs and Lawrence D. Thompson. The Central Clinical Research Club was formed, which was the first step in the plan for a larger society for clinical research.

The idea of a new society for clinical research was the major topic of discussion at the meetings of both clubs until the fall of 1926, when a joint committee was appointed to proceed with the plans for organization of a new society. Rowntree was instructed "to write a letter on behalf of the Central Interurban Clinical Club to the secretary of the American Society for Clinical Investigation stating the intention to further such a society in the middle west and that they would like to cooperate with the parent society [American Society for Clinical Investigation] in every way." Rowntree learned that the foundation of the new society had the best wishes of the American Society for Clinical Investigation, but that the latter did not wish to participate formally. It was then decided to have a joint meeting of the Central Interurban Club and the Central Clinical Research Club in the spring of 1928, and to invite to this meeting a number of representative men from the Midwest, so that plans for the formation of the new society could be formalized. The meeting took place in Rochester, Minnesota, on April 20–21, 1928. A constitution was officially adopted, and the name "Central Society for Clinical Research" was decided upon. Billings was elected the first president; Rowntree, vice-president; Thompson, secretary; and William S. Middleton, treasurer. Counsellors were Irons, Brown, and Roger S. Morris. At the first annual meeting of the Central Society for Clinical Research, held at the Albert Merritt Billings Hospital in Chicago, on November 23, 1928, twenty-two scientific papers were presented. The further growth and activities of the Central Society for Clinical Research are a matter of record. The abstracts of papers presented at the annual meetings were first published in the *Journal of Clinical Investigation* and then, for a number of years, in the *Journal of the American Medical Association*. In

1944 the society adopted the *Journal of Laboratory and Clinical Medicine* as its official publication, and since then all abstracts and many full manuscripts have been published in that journal.

## The American Federation for Clinical Research
### (The Young Men's Christian Association)

The number of clinical investigators in the United States expanded so rapidly that the American Society for Clinical Investigation, too, reached a stage at which it no longer provided an adequate forum for all of the young men, beginners in investigation, that needed an association in which they could participate and present their work. Another society to stimulate clinical investigation was successfully launched through the efforts of Henry A. Christian of Boston.

In November 1940, Christian sent a letter to a number of individuals in different parts of the country, designed to obtain their reaction about his proposal. The letter read as follows:

Dear Doctor: In May 1908 on the invitation of the late Samuel J. Meltzer, a small group of men met in Washington, D.C. to discuss the desirability of organizing a new society, whose chief aim was to stimulate investigation in the field of clinical and allied medical sciences and to make a place for young men, already having evinced an interest in investigation, to meet to discuss their problems. . . .

Similarly, on May 6, 1940, a small group of surviving charter members of this society met in Atlantic City . . . to discuss the desirability of forming again a new society to carry out, especially as concerns young men, the purposes which those who met in Washington in 1908 had in mind. The original Society having by now so progressed that no longer does it give a place to young men, beginners in investigation, and to men not connected with medical schools or research institutes, this group proposes the organization of a new society, not to compete with, but to supplement, the "American Society for Clinical Investigation," to stimulate among young men a persisting interest in investigation in clinical and allied medical sciences. A tentative constitution has been prepared as a basis for discussion at the first annual meeting of this new society. . . . A meeting for organization and discussion and adoption of a constitution probably will be held in Atlantic City in May 1941. . . .

Do you approve of such a new society? If so, please send us the names of young men (preferably under 35) in your clinic or department or city, who you consider eligible for membership in such an organization and probably interested in its purposes. Have you an activity, a research club, or other organization in which young men take an active part by presenting the results of their investigations and by discussing papers presented by others? Will this organization care to participate in such a national organization as is proposed in this letter? Please send the name of the presiding officer or secretary of this organization. Sincerely yours, Henry A. Christian[43]

Although Christian had retired as Hersey Professor at Harvard, his continuing interest in young investigators is evident. He received a favorable response to this letter, and the first meeting of the American Federation for Clinical Research took place in Chalfonte-Haddon Hall in Atlantic City, on the afternoon of May 5, 1941. There were approximately three hundred young men and women there, who exuded great enthusiasm about this new society and who unanimously approved the constitution and bylaws presented. Charles Janeway of Boston was elected temporary chairman. Each of the speakers, not one of whom was over thirty-five years of age, presented a ten-minute paper. Discussion of the papers was active and stimulating. Maurice A. Schnitker of Toledo, Ohio, was elected the first president, and the first annual meeting was held in Minneapolis, Minnesota, on April 20, 1942.

In contrast to the Association of American Physicians and the Society for Clinical Investigation, there were no numerical limitations to membership in the American Federation. The organization was open to any young man or woman conducting investigation in any branch of medical science or allied fields, including medicine, surgery, obstetrics, gynecology, pediatrics, pathology, bacteriology, chemistry, and so forth. Anyone qualified could become a member, but the vast majority of the active members were under thirty-five years of age. No one over the age of forty could hold an office, and, in line with the precedent set at the original meeting, no one over that age was to appear on the program or to raise a voice in discussion at a national meeting. Thus, this was to be a society for young investigators, and its affairs were to be conducted by young investigators. Provided one was in the proper age group, however, more was required than the simple expression of an interest in investigation. There had to be tangible evidence in the form of at least one completed piece of research. It was decided that a single interesting case report was not a sufficient prerequisite for entry. The work involved had to pose a question and present good quality work to answer it. The data involved could be in the form of a statistical analysis, an analysis of bedside or laboratory observations, or an original piece of experimental research. These criteria represented an attempt to place a premium on membership sufficiently high to make such membership valuable to the individual and to the organization as a whole. The requirements were not so stringent as to place membership beyond the reach of the majority. No letters of recommendation were required to obtain membership. Many of the members were in the practice of medicine, but this society provided a stimulus for them to contribute, in the limited time they had, to the growing body of new knowledge.

The activities of this group grew rapidly, and the society ultimately published a journal called *Clinical Research*. Since the American Federation for Clinical Research was meant to be a national organization, plans were made to put attendance at annual meetings within the reach of all.

The annual meetings were to be held in conjunction with the meeting of some other large society, but in a different part of the country each year. As it has worked out, the annual meetings have been held in conjunction with those of the American Society for Clinical Investigation and the Association of American Physicians. The society has persisted in the organization of local research clubs. These local clubs are not officially tied to the national organization. Members of such local research clubs may attain individual membership in the American Federation for Clinical Research, but local clubs as groups are not admitted. In these local clubs, encouragement is given to the presentation of work still in progress, thus giving the investigator opportunity for criticism and suggestion in the active phase of his study. Adequate time is always given for critical discussion.[44]

Although effective associations were formed for the promotion of clinical research, as time passed and the areas of research became more and more specialized, even these societies proved inadequate. First, groups such as the American Society for Clinical Investigation and the American Federation developed specialty groups within their own organizations and had, at their annual meeting, a general session and sessions for each of the specialty areas. This was necessary to take care of the large number of papers and the increasing number of papers in highly complex fields, which were only of interest to specialists in those fields. This proved insufficient, however, and other research organizations developed, which were supported by those interested in narrow fields of medical research. For example, in the East, a club known as the Pus Club was organized for specialists in infectious diseases, and a Gut Club was formed by the gastroenterologists. At the national level societies were organized in all of the various medical specialties. These organizations, such as the American Heart Association and the American Gastroenterological Association, are larger in scope and include clinical programs, as well as programs involving the latest investigations in the particular area concerned. Thus, there has occurred a striking tendency toward specialization in the scientific societies.

# Summary

The last quarter of the nineteenth century was highlighted by the professionalization of the basic sciences and by the creation of several laboratories of experimental medicine in which young people learned to apply the methods of laboratory research to clinical problems. It was also characterized by the introduction of the residency system of clinical training. These developments made it possible for young men and women to emerge from their training period skilled both in the methods of investigation in the basic sciences and in clinical medicine.

Franklin Paine Mall emphasized the importance of putting the clinical departments in the medical school on a university basis—a theme that was effectively articulated by Lewellys Franklin Barker. When Barker succeeded Osler as professor of medicine at Johns Hopkins in 1905, it was not possible for him to be on a full-time basis because of lack of sufficient funds, but he was able to create full-time research divisions. The importance of the research divisions established by Barker cannot be underestimated. Scientific investigation in clinical departments did not begin with the opening of these laboratories, but the institution of special facilities for this puspose started a movement that was to influence greatly the character of university clinics. Just as Barker did in medicine, William Stewart Halsted made many innovative moves in surgery with the establishment of special divisions in the surgical specialties, which had an obligation to advance the existing knowledge in these fields by research. Among the most productive was the division of neurosurgery under Harvey Williams Cushing.

In 1901 a key step in creating the facilities for clinical science was the incorporation of the Rockefeller Institute for Medical Research. In 1903 Simon Flexner began work there as director, and William Henry Welch was chairman of the Board of Scientific Advisors. The institute took over the *Journal of Experimental Medicine* in 1905 as an outlet for the publication of research. A few years later, John D. Rockefeller was persuaded to endow a research hospital that was to be connected with the institute. The greatest proponent of the hospital was Christian A. Herter, who was one of the first researchers to stress the importance of biochemistry for clinical science.

Rufus I. Cole was appointed director of the hospital in 1908, and his plan for the operation of the hospital—in which young men and women trained both in research and in clinical medicine would have the opportunity to select a specific disease and have both clinical and laboratory facilities for the pursuit of their research—was a major step forward in the evolution of clinical science in the United States. When the hospital opened in 1910, Cole implemented his plan to train the leaders of the new movement to develop so-called university departments of medicine, where a basic responsibility, in addition to teaching and patient care, would be the application of the knowledge of the basic sciences to the study of disease in man. The research areas chosen for work at the hospital represented the most common and most important medical problems of that day: pneumonia, syphilis, diabetes, cardiovascular disease, and poliomyelitis. The basic work of Avery and his colleagues on the antigens of pneumococci represented an important foundation of the modern sciences of immunochemistry and demonstrated how clinical investigation may lead to important discoveries of a basic nature. The importance of chemistry to medicine was emphasized by Van Slyke's studies of the acid-base relationships of the blood; respiratory gas exchange; the transport of oxygen and carbon dioxide in the blood stream; the distribution of the gases and electrolytes in the tissues; the physical chemistry of nephritis; and the clinical course of the different types of Bright's disease. His contributions have affected the thought of every physiologically minded physician. These are only a sample of the many important advances made in clinical science during the period of Cole's directorship. The HRI, under Cole, had a tremendous impact on the development of medical science, both by the specific discoveries made and by its influence on medical thought and practice through those trained there.

Thomas M. Rivers, the second director, not only carried on the important traditions begun by Cole but also established the hospital as a key center for virology; the hospital played an important role in the emergence of virology as an independent branch of science.

Thus, the development of scientific research into a separate profession at the clinical level brought about a considerable acceleration in the process of discovery. It was one of the developments that made it possible to turn science from an unpredictable process into a tool that could be used for practical purposes.

An important influence on clinical science was the development of appropriate societies that could establish standards and serve as forums for the discussion of new work, free of the distractions of political, economic, and social problems. A significant organization of this type was the Association of American Physicians, founded in 1885. Practicing physicians, as well as basic scientists, came together to exchange information and to promote high-quality research work relating to the problems of disease. Later, as the number of young clinical scientists increased, Samuel James Meltzer recognized the need for these scientists to have a separate organization where they could exchange ideas; this realization led to the founding of the American Society for Clinical Investigation in 1908. After a few decades, the numbers had swelled to such an extent that even this organization was unable to meet all the needs of young investigators. Henry A. Christian pioneered the establishment of another organization for these investigators, the American Federation for Clinical Research.

These professional clinical-research organizations have played an active part in influencing the academic and research policies of medical schools and have provided an efficient means of communication between practitioners and scientists. In Germany, the role of research and teaching was entirely separated from that of practice by the end of the nineteenth century. About this time, the differentiation of the roles of research and practice began in the United States. In Germany, this role differentiation led to the deprivation of the practitioners from all the facilities necessary for research and to a lowering of the status of the practitioners as compared with the basic scientists. Similar results did not follow the large-scale development of medical research in America. Practitioners have continued to have a role in teaching and research, and the effective role of the full-time clinical investigator in providing a bridge between practice and the basic sciences has led to better medical teaching and to elevation of the standards of medical practice.

# Part III

❧

# The Professionalization of Clinical Science:
## Full-time Professorships

⚜

# The Concept of Full-time Professorships in Clinical Departments: The Implementation of the Idea

In his presidential address to the Association of American Physicians in 1901, William Henry Welch predicted the establishment of professorships in clinical departments on a full-time basis. Welch noted that a preclinical scientist could "look forward with reasonable assurance to securing a desirable position as a teacher and a director of a laboratory of his special branch of science," but young physicians desiring corresponding careers in clinical medicine and surgery had to face the fact that, with few exceptions, American hospitals did not offer such opportunities for training; and, in addition, the prospect of securing a stable position to carry on their work in clinical science was poor.[1] Welch did not make specific recommendations as to how the organization in clinical departments should be altered. At that time, with the exception of Johns Hopkins, whose clinical professors had been chosen on the basis of merit alone, medical schools selected their professors from among the local practitioners. Would-be clinical scientists could obtain important academic positions only if resignation or death created a vacancy in a medical school in the city where they practiced. They had to be successful practitioners before they could anticipate any appointment at all. No one could obtain a clinical position through pursuit of the scientific side of medicine alone. The pay was so small in the clinical departments that the staff had to support themselves by private practice and could, therefore, give only a limited part of their time to medical school activities. Essentially all the research done by clinically trained individuals was done in the laboratories of the basic science departments. At the turn of the century, with the rapid advances in physiology, physiological chemistry, and pharmacology that had potential applications to disease in man,

it became increasingly clear that the organization of the clinical departments would have to change if medicine was to progress.

The story of Franklin Paine Mall's interest in the development of
clinical science and its influence on Lewellys Franklin Barker has already
been recounted. Barker's famous 1902 address, "Medicine and the Universities," made the question of full-time professorships a national issue
overnight. In his address, Barker stated that "like other university professors, clinical professors should give their whole time and energy to the
work of the university, to teaching and to investigating in the hospitals.
. . . They should be well paid by the university. They should not engage in private practice." Although Barker believed that the services of
part-time men were also necessary, he believed that the greatest need
was for full-time "physicians and surgeons trained in physiology and
pathology," who, after careful observation in the wards and over the
operating table, would submit the ideas there gleaned to experimental
tests "in laboratories adjacent to the wards."[2]

The *Journal of the American Medical Association* took notice of Barker's
talk, although only to criticize the plan as impractical. "It would be pro-
hibitively expensive," the journal said, "and furthermore professors
need the experience gained from daily private practice."[3] In 1902 John
M. Dobson, professor of pediatrics at Rush Medical College, supported
Barker's plea.[4] In the following year, Frank Billings urged, in his address
as president of the association, that professors of medicine, surgery, and
obstetrics "should give their whole time to the work of teaching and to
original work in the hospital." He also emphasized that other professors
who engaged in private practice would also be needed, for they would
"impart to the student a better idea of medicine as a whole" and coordinate and arrange the isolated facts of clinical and laboratory investigation.[5]

The idea was strongly attacked by Arthur Dean Bevan,[6] head of
surgery at the University of Chicago. But Abraham Flexner recalled that
"Frank Billings once stated in a speech that a resolution was adopted by
the faculty of Rush Medical College after it became affiliated with the
University of Chicago [in 1898], pledging the school to the establishment
of full-time clinical teaching whenever funds could be procured."[7]

Welch had, of course, joined the ranks on the side of Mall. In an
address at Harvard (1906) he stated the case as follows: "The most
urgent need in medical education at the present time in this country I
believe to be the organization of our clinics both for teaching and for
research in the spirit of this modern movement and with provision for
an intimate, prolonged, personal contact of the student with the subject
of study as he finds it in the laboratory."[8] Welch knew, however, that
implementation of the full-time concept would be so expensive that its
promotion would be useless as long as medical endowments remained
meager. Thus, he waited patiently in the wings for the proper time to
strike in the interest of full-time appointments. In 1907, in an address at

the University of Chicago, he took a cautious step forward when he said: "The heads of the principal clinical departments, particularly the medical and surgical, should devote their main energies and time to their hospital work and to teaching and investigating without the necessity of seeking their livelihood in a busy outside practice and without allowing such a practice to become their chief professional occupation."[9] A year later Welch played a major role in the establishment of the HRI, which was on a full-time plan.

William Henry Howell, then dean of the medical school at Johns Hopkins, publicly endorsed the full-time concept in 1909:

> The university school which shall first establish departments on this basis [full-time] may . . . secure both reputation and students as compared with schools organized on the present system. . . . Our country is in a peculiarly favorable position to make such an experiment. Our system of medical education has heretofore simply developed along lines laid down by the experience of foreign countries; perhaps in the direction suggested . . .we may have the opportunity to take the lead instead of trailing along in the rear.[10]

After several years of discussion, the reform of clinical teaching received wider acceptance. When many leading educators became convinced that the possibility of full-time clinical professorships was real, the debate became "sharp and personal." In 1911 Mall wrote the following letter to Charles S. Minot:

> We are also thinking of reform in medical education, but on the hospital side. The problem would be easy if the pork barrel were removed. Its removal would no doubt remove the exploiting medical professor and open the way for a real university professor of medicine. We are told that medical and surgical professors cannot take interest in medical problems and the sick unless they are paid for each move; that the sick man is not as conducive to real science as the dead or as a dog. It falls to us to demand of the last two years of medicine what they demanded of the first two and I think that the day of reckoning is near at hand.[11]

Barker's replacement of Osler as professor of medicine at Johns Hopkins in 1905, when Osler left for Oxford, had a definite bearing on the full-time plan of clinical teaching in American medical schools. Indeed, Barker's appointment was symbolic of changes that may be characterized as the intrusion of science into clinical medicine. The contrast between Osler and Barker was striking, although both were Canadians and students at the University of Toronto in 1870 and 1890, respectively. They belonged, however, to different "schools of medicine"— Osler, to the British school, Barker, to the German school.[12] Osler was, as Robinson pointed out, a great physician and a preeminent teacher, but he was not an investigator, in the present-day sense of the word. His primary interest, the direct study of patients, could be carried over directly into the practice of medicine outside the hospital, and, because of his experience, skill, and personality, he was constantly in demand by practicing physicians as a consultant.[13] Barker's concept of a professor of medicine was that of a teacher involved in research, whose primary interest would not be interrupted by medical practice outside his departmental activities. Barker was among the first to advocate full-time teachers, whereas Osler was definitely opposed to the plan when its adoption at Johns Hopkins was under discussion, some years after Osler's departure for Oxford. This opposition was strongly expressed in a letter to Ira Remsen, then president of the university.[14] Some twenty-five years later, when the same proposition was under consideration at Osler's Canadian university, McGill, Osler wrote supporting the idea of full-time clinical teachers.

In 1910 Clement von Pirquet, who had already spent time as a professor of pediatrics at Johns Hopkins, expressed a willingness to return there, if his appointment was placed on a full-time university basis. On November 22 of that year, Welch wrote to Flexner, stating that if an endowment of $200,000 could be obtained to place the professorship of pediatrics on a full-time basis, Pirquet would not only be an ideal candidate, but would also probably accept. There is no evidence that Welch presented the matter formally to the Rockefeller office at that time, but it seems unlikely that it would have had any appeal as an isolated undertaking.[15]

The next relevant communication was a letter, dated January 6, 1911, from F. T. Gates, adviser to John D. Rockefeller, Jr., to Welch.[16] Gates expressed his interest in getting cost estimates from Welch: first, to accommodate an entrance class of one hundred each year, with as good facilities as the institution could at that time offer to an entering class of fifty; and second, to conduct the institution in such a way ("I speak now of an ultimate ideal") that none of its professors would be permitted to make anything beyond a nominal charge for consultation or other services. Welch wrote back that the first item would present no difficulty, but that the support of clinical professors was a perplexing question because of the large sums of money involved. He hesitated to send Gates an estimate of what it would cost. Gates stated, in a second letter, that it was important to establish a cost estimate of the ideal arrangement so that there would be a plan to build toward.

Meanwhile, the contrast between the clinical and the preclinical departments was becoming increasingly evident as medical schools raised their standards. In 1910 Abraham Flexner, under the auspices of the Carnegie Foundation for the Advancement of Teaching, published his epoch-making investigation of medical schools in the United States and Canada. He showed that, out of the 155 institutions in existence, 50 (a little less than one-third) were integral parts of universities.[17] He was particularly critical of the quality of the clinical departments. His report touched off a great movement toward reform.

Flexner's report impressed Gates, because it was a subject near to his heart. Gates asked Flexner what he would do with $1 million to be used for medical education. Flexner's reply was: "I should give it to Dr. Welch." As a result, Flexner was sent to Baltimore to make a detailed study of what might be done there, and, at a dinner party (which included Welch, Flexner, Mall, and Halsted), Mall argued eloquently that all of the money that might be obtained should be spent to place the heads of the clinical departments on a full-time basis.[18] After his visit, Flexner made a report to Gates that presented several alternative plans, one of which was that the school should be endowed and reduced to 250 students (a cut in the enrollment for that year of 97), and the main clinical chairs placed on a university or full-time basis. On May 10, 1911, Welch wrote to Gates apologizing for the delay in the conclusion being reached by the faculty and trustees and pointing out that there was considerable difference of opinion on essential points. By June 11, Welch told Gates that "the opinion prevails in our medical faculty and among the trustees of the university" that the proposal to set up full-time clinical professorships, "if it could be carried out upon an adequate financial basis is the one which meets the most urgent needs and promises the largest benefits not to the Johns Hopkins school alone but to medical education in general."[19] Welch spoke of the main objections as follows:

> The alleged difficulty or impossibility of securing and holding the best men for the positions with such salaries as could be contemplated seemed to be the most serious although only temporarily so. It would be hazardous in the extreme to start the new arrangement with young men in the clinical chairs without considerable experience and without established reputations however promising they may seem to be. At present the field of choice is a very restricted one but one of the great benefits to be expected from the suggested plan is the wide extension of this field by the training of men for the higher clinical walks.[20]

Once the new system had been put into effect it would generate its own professors, who had not become used to living on the scale of successful practitioners. There were other objections, including the difficulty of keeping the public and the profession away from men with the reputations of these clinicians, and the loss to the community and medical practitioners by withdrawal of such men from outside practice. A further objection was the contention that limitation of practice within the hospital would deprive teachers of opportunities and experience valuable to their own development and in their training of students destined to become practitioners. Welch stated that such difficulties could be overcome if the salaried clinicians "should be permitted to have consultations at the hospital and to have patients in the private wards, but the professional fees from such patients should go to the hospital or university.... The number of these private patients should be limited and determined mainly by the scientific interest of the cases."[21] He pointed out that the new plan, of course, does not contemplate dispensing with the service of men engaged in practice who can give only a part of their time to teaching. . . . Among the practitioners are some who love to teach and are really excellent teachers, whose services it would be a detriment to the school to lose. . . . That the imposition of fixed rules and regulations upon the conduct and the use of the time of such men as would be entrusted with these clinical chairs would be harassing, improper and unnecessary.[22]

Welch also stated that once the proposal was put into action, established and rigid stipulations regarding the full-time service would no longer be needed: "While the principle must be safe-guarded contingencies may arise which might make proper and desirable an exception to the rule that the salaried, full-time professor should not receive a fee from professional services."[23] In Welch's view, the incumbents in these new chairs would not be attracted by salary, but by the facilities and opportunities for scientific work of high quality; thus they should not be overburdened with administration and patient care, and they should have a young, capable staff, acting as associate professors, associates, and assistants, who would themselves be in training for these higher positions in other schools. He emphasized that laboratories for clinical teaching and research should be provided and that there should be an ample budget for running expenses.

It was Welch's firm belief that the disadvantages of the plan were minimal in comparison with its advantages:

The establishment upon the clinical side of the medical school of academic ideals like those which prevail in other departments of the university would be a forward movement of far reaching significance. These ideals imply single minded devotion to the work belonging to the university chair. An absorbing outside practice is not a part of this work and is incompatible with such devotion to teaching, to investigating and to the duties of a hospital physician or surgeon which should characterize a university professor and which is required to obtain the best results and the activities which properly belong to his chair.

It is inspiring to contemplate the possibilities of a well supported and properly organized medical and surgical clinic upon a true university basis. It would introduce new opportunities and higher standards of teaching and of productive research. It would place before students and the profession higher ideals of the mission of the physician and of his relation to the community. It would advance both the science and the art of medicine by training investigators, by making better physicians, and by contributing to useful knowledge. . . . We who advocate this change believe that it will initiate a reform in medical education so far reaching as to constitute a new era.[24]

On August 2, 1911, John D. Rockefeller, Jr., wrote to his father that he was in accord with Murphy and Gates in recommending a gift of $1.2 million to Johns Hopkins for the establishment of full-time clinical chairs.[25] Gates believed that such a sum, utilized in this manner, would result in a revolution in American medical education, which would place medicine throughout the world on a scientific basis and would have immense value to mankind.

Nothing happened immediately as Welch was working behind the scenes, endeavoring in his own way to arrive at a general agreement that would "make it unnecessary to hurt feelings by the use of force." He felt that the spirit and atmosphere at Johns Hopkins was so valuable that it should not be damaged by unnecessary haste in such an important matter. On May 23, 1911, Osler wrote to Welch stating that he had not heard of the proposal in detail and thus found it difficult to express his opinion.[26] He was concerned, however, that the payment to clinicians of salaries on an academic scale would spell ruin for the hospital. He felt that one might get good men for a few years for such salaries, but that they would ultimately leave. On the other hand, if the trustees paid liberal salaries of $15,000 to $20,000, they could always command the best men, and Osler stated that, under such circumstances, he would be strongly in favor of it. He also stated that the hospital should not be converted into a sanitorium and a large part of the professor's time taken up with earning money for the hospital from private patients. Osler wrote to Dr. Henry M. Thomas, on April 18, that: "Personally, I feel that to cut off the heads of departments from a practice is a utopian scheme admirable on paper but the very men who would be most in favor of it would be the first to get the professors to break the rules. . . . It is an experiment I would like very much to see tried but not at the Johns Hopkins first. It might have been different if we had started so, but I do not believe there is any possibility of success at present."[27]

In March 1912, Welch attempted to interest Gates in providing support to bring von Pirquet back to Johns Hopkins as professor of pediatrics. Gates expressed no interest, however, in this pilot approach to the problem. On September 23, Welch wrote Osler: "We could not raise the money to put the children's department into the shape which would justify von Pirquet in leaving Vienna and we have secured Howland who begins in October."[28] Little did he know at that time that Howland would create the most successful full-time clinical department at Johns Hopkins.

While acting head of the university, Welch continued his negotiations with the Rockefeller Foundation and brought them to a successful conclusion. On October 21, 1913, he wrote to the General Education Board that "the faculty of the medical school are fully convinced of the wisdom and necessity of commanding the entire time and devotion of a staff of teachers in the main clinical branches," and that the trustees of the university and hospital had authorized him to ask for funds to place the departments of medicine, surgery, and pediatrics on this basis.[29]

Two days later the board took action:

Resolved, that the General Education Board hereby agrees to appropriate the funds necessary to carry out the full-time scheme described in Dr. Welch's letter under date of October 21, 1913, and empowers the Finance Committee to take the necessary step looking to the execution of this agreement.

Resolved, that in view of Dr. Welch's great services to the cause of medical education in America the fund appropriated as above be called "The William H. Welch Endowment for Clinical Education and Research."[30]

## The Debate over the Impact of the Full-time Plan on Education and Research

Initial reaction to the full-time plan at Johns Hopkins was mixed. The *Medical Record* referred to the plan as a "somewhat doubtful experiment" and went on to state that full-time would make clinical professors into laboratory workers and that laboratory workers had narrower experience than practitioners.[31] The *Journal of the American Medical Association* at first declared that a full-time system would "not only elevate the standards of clinical instruction, but also develop more extensive research along the lines of clinical medicine, leading to a wider application of new discoveries in the treatment of disease."[32] The next year, however, the editors changed their minds.[33] During 1914 a series of attacks on the Johns Hopkins plan were published, contending that first-class clinicians could not be expected to make the financial sacrifice of accepting university salaries. The Council on Medical Education of the AMA took a hostile attitude. Thus, full-time became a subject of heated debate over a period of years, a main contention being the payment of consultation fees to the university rather than to the physician. A committee of experienced clinicians appointed to study the matter made their report at the annual meeting of the council in Chicago in February 1915:

"Is some private practice by clinical teachers essential to keep medical education in sympathetic touch with the human side of medical practice?" they asked. "Will the placing of clinical chairs on a full-time basis result in a gradual separation of medical teachers from perhaps some of the most vital problems of active medical service? . . ."

The principle that the practice of clinical teachers should be restricted appears to have general acceptance. In determining to what extent that practice should be limited there are two extremes somewhere between which it is possible to construct a rational scheme. On the one side is the whole time experiment as adopted at Johns Hopkins, and on the other side is the condition in some medical schools where clinical teachers are so busy with their private practice that their teaching is badly neglected. Opinion is by no means unanimous that the whole time requirement is ideal.[34]

Others, including the famous surgeon Bevan, labeled the plan as "fee-splitting, dichotomy, unethical, immoral and wicked."[35] Those who were on the side of full-time were characterized as unable to understand this because they were laboratory men and not clinicians.

Mall knew, of course, that securing the endowment was only the start; the necessity was to make the plan work. Mall believed that a concession should be made to the greater earning power of the clinical men as the only practical method, and he advocated that they should be offered salaries twice those of other professors in the medical school. In the full-time plan, the principal issue was a constructive one—the advancement of medicine and the training of men who would contribute to that advance. There was no prohibition against practice, but only against taking fees. The plan was to release the head of the clinic from indiscriminate consultation and enable him to choose and limit his consultation to the cases related to his own area of research. The plan in Baltimore was meant to put the head of the clinic on a full-time basis and to make him the judge of the number of his assistants, who should also devote their entire time to the clinic. It was intended to include only the major clinical departments. The minor specialties were to be added only if they became fully organized departments and acquired an adequate endowment.

## The Start of Full-time Professorships at Johns Hopkins

In Baltimore, the plan went immediately into effect in surgery, because William Stewart Halsted had, in essence, been a full-time professor from the time he joined the faculty. The appointment of Howland as professor of pediatrics, in 1912, made the introduction of the full-time plan into that department very simple. In medicine, however, Barker had acquired a large private practice and, when offered the full-time chair, he declined. The chair was then offered to William Sydney Thayer, a clinical professor of medicine, who also declined. The advisory board finally turned to Theodore Caldwell Janeway, Bard Professor of Medicine at Columbia University. Despite the heavy pressure of teaching and practice, Janeway had carried on investigative work on diseases of the heart and circulation, particularly in the field of hypertension, on which subject he had published an important book. Janeway accepted on April 28, 1914.

On June 5, 1911, Barker gave an address, at the convocation exercises at McGill University, entitled "Some Tendencies in Medical Education in the United States."[36]

He stated that there were four functions of clinical departments:

1) the practice of medicine—the actual diagnosis and treatment of disease; 2) the teaching in the wards, in the dispensaries, and in the laboratories of a) undergraduate medical students, b) assistants and associates, and c) physicians taking postgraduate courses in the department; 3) the prosecution by professors, assistants and postgraduate students of original in-

quiries in internal medicine; the search for new methods of diagnosing and treating disease; the attempt to advance our knowledge of the subject beyond its present boundaries; and 4) the administrative duties including the arrangements for patients, relations of the clinic to housekeeping and nursing, the maintenance of records and statistics, the arrangements for publication, the superintendence of budgets and expenditures, the making of appointments and promotions, the attendance on departmental and interdepartmental conferences, the formulation of curricula, the organization, equipment and running of several clinical laboratories, the library, and the museum, the integration of departmental activities, the development of an esprit-de-corps.

Thus, he outlined a heavy responsibility for a professor of medicine, which could hardly be accomplished without full-time attention to his many duties.

Barker felt that the clinical activity would, to a great extent, be carried by students, house officers, and senior assistants; however, an associate professor or, in the larger institutions, a full professor could devote the major part of his time to it, leaving most of the teaching and experimental investigation to others.

He believed that the aim of the clinic was to make new applications of the facts of anatomy, physiology, pathology, and chemistry to diagnosis and therapy. "Clinicians are sure now and again to make certain contributions to pure physiology or pathology when trying to solve their problems in diagnosis and therapy. They will be glad when their work so contributes, but this should not be the main aim and purpose of that work; as soon as a man in the clinic finds it to be so, it is time that he left the clinic and transplanted himself to a laboratory of physiology or pathology."

He felt that "every university professor should himself be an investigator. A department of medicine in this setting would be not only a place for transmitting what is known to medical students but also a place in which the unknown is actively explored. . . . Thus introduced to the spirit and method of scientific inquiry, the students are protected from the dogmatism which so often accompanies mere traditional teaching."

Barker believed in creating two types of activity in the department: one supervised by a research professor and offering some research opportunities to the younger people on the staff and the postgraduate students; and another supervised by a professor whose primary responsibility would be the care of patients and the teaching of students. This view corresponded more to the plan Herter had for the HRI. Cole's belief was fundamentally different in that the professor was both a skilled physician and a talented investigator.

In conclusion, Barker stated: "We must find places for the different kinds of clinical men—practitioners, teachers, investigators." As his final recommendations he suggested the following: "Provide endowment for the maintenance in each clinic of a group of young scientists of proved ability, and relieve these men of most of the routine work, that they may have the leisure for investigative work in the wards and clinical laboratories." This is what Cole had initiated at the HRI.

Of course, the full-time movement was not limited to Baltimore; this plan was actively discussed in other medical schools across the country. Encouraged by the progress under the Johns Hopkins grant in obtaining distinguished professors, the General Education Board made grants of $750,000 to Washington University in St. Louis and $500,000 to the Yale University School of Medicine, with the understanding that they would reorganize their work in order to put their clinical teaching upon a full-time basis.

With all of the controversy over full-time, there was inadequate analysis of what the needs were in clinical departments in regard to teaching and research, and how they might be accomplished. One who did comment critically on this situation was Samuel James Meltzer.

Meltzer published an article in *Science*,[37] in 1914, in reply to the president and trustees of a well-known university who posed the following question: How important do you believe full-time positions in the clinical subjects are for a satisfactory connection between the school and hospital?

Meltzer stated that "the teaching of medicine is for nearly all the heads of clinical departments (in 1914) only a secondary occupation and in some instances it is not more than a legitimate business advertisement," and that "most of the present heads of departments do not possess sufficient familiarity with the modern medicine to be the instructors of present-day medicine to the coming physician."

He then presented his suggestion for improvement: heads of departments should be chosen from a class of physicians who, from the time of their medical school graduation, never ceased to be close students of their science and for whom the study of, and instruction in, a chosen clinical subject constituted their primary occupation.

> To the question, where can we get this class of physicians? My answer is: create it, or, more correctly expressed, accelerate its development, since a fairly good beginning has been made in the last few years.
>
> The Johns Hopkins plan remedies the evils.... The Johns Hopkins Medical School does not offer its new procedure as a general plan to be used in all other colleges. . . . It probably originated in the desire to put the teachers of clinical subjects on a university basis, and thus maintain a university atmosphere in the medical school, an atmosphere which is essential to the mode of life of the scientific men of that school, and which is readily disturbed by the mode of life of a head of a department "who in a very limited amount of time devoted to practice could obtain for his service much more than the amount of such a salary."
>
> The election to headship must be based upon evidence that for the past years the appointee has been continuously a close student of modern medicine and showed efficiency in teaching, as well as in research, in the scientific and practical fields of medicine. The work of the department should be conducted with the aid of scientific assistants. These shall be

elected from graduates who have given evidence of possessing higher abilities and ambitions, and who had one year service in a good hospital and one year laboratory work in the science of medicine.

Meltzer had no university medical school appointment. He was, however, a well-trained experimental physiologist and an experienced practitioner of medicine. He emerges as the scientific physician of his day who was, in most respects, in the best position to see this problem in perspective. He was convinced that medicine must become more scientific and that this could be done with the help of trained clinical scientists, without losing the important contributions of the practicing physicians to the educational program. In their solution to the problem, most schools have followed the general principles that he espoused in this essay.

Simon Flexner, in his presidential address before the Association of American Physicians in 1914, strongly endorsed full-time clinical professorships:

> The growth in medical knowledge and improvement in medical instruction are traceable in last analysis to the segregation of groups of men of scientific attainment and temper, who were thus enabled to work in a favorable environment; their sheltered situation protects them from the diversions and distractions of ordinary professional life, and encourages them to devote all available energies to the advancement of science and the teaching of students. . . .
>
> Established midway in the course of the development that I have sketched, the independent institution for medical research has within a decade begun to exercise a distinct influence on medical progress. The foundation of these institutes was impossible until improved medical schools furnished an adequate supply of students whose training approximated that of the older European countries.
>
> In turn, all these conditions have reacted more and more powerfully on clinical teaching . . . the amount of knowledge to be communicated and the difficulty of the techniques to be acquired, necessitate that more and more hours be spent in teaching in or adjacent to the hospital wards. It has thus become physically impossible for the teacher to remain in general practice and at the same time attend to his university duties. . . . The function of the clinical teacher has been newly defined within the past one or two decades, and a process of selection within the terms of this definition has been going forward. Hence we are confronted not so much by an experiment as by a development. The full-time clinical teacher is simply the consultant as developed in recent years, completely protected by his university status.[38]

## A Department of Research Medicine

One of the proposed alternatives to appointing full-time professors who would be responsible for research, teaching, and patient care was to have a separate department of research medicine. Such a venture was the John Herr Musser Department of Research Medicine at the University of Pennsylvania. In 1916 Richard M. Pearce presented a report of the department's first five years.[39]

The goals of the department, which was endowed in 1909, were set to a significant degree by the following conditions of the gift: (1) that the department concern itself especially with the study of chronic diseases, working in the laboratory and, when necessary, with patients in the university hospital; (2) that the professor of research medicine devote his entire time to the conduct of the department, his duties as a teacher being limited to no fewer than fifteen lectures or demonstrations on the work of the department, to be given to students of medicine; (3) that the facilities of the department be opened to members of other university departments and to students and practitioners who might be considered capable of conducting research work; and (4) that the income of the endowment be applicable to the purposes of the department of research medicine and to no other department of the university.

During the first five years, the principal lines of investigation were kidney diseases, and the spleen in relation to anemia and hemolytic jaundice.[40]

Pearce's department developed, with the department of medicine, a community of interest and a cooperative effort, which both departments regarded as a most important experiment in medical education. At the suggestion of Alfred Stengel, a professor of medicine, the two associates most intimately concerned with clinical teaching and patient care in the university hospital gave half of their time to investigations in the department of research medicine. As clinical teachers, there was abundant evidence that they found this experience of great value.

It should be pointed out that there was no lack of opportunity for laboratory research in the hospital. The university hospital had two spacious and well-equipped laboratories; one in the hospital proper for the usual routine examinations and the other, the William Pepper Laboratory of Clinical Medicine, in a separate building, with an independent endowment and a large staff engaged in various clinical research problems (see chapter 10).

The department of research medicine also offered special elective courses dealing with the experimental side of medicine. During the first year, a comprehensive series of demonstrations in experimental pathology was given for the second-year class in pathology. As far as possible, the gross and microscopic lesions of disease in man were correlated with experimental lesions, and the relations to clinical medicine were emphasized. Physiological methods of graphic registration were employed whenever possible, changes in urine and other secretions were demonstrated, and methods of chemical examination were shown.

A seminar for the discussion of various clinical problems was inaugurated. In this seminar the chairs of medicine (Alfred Stengel), pharmacology (A. N. Richards), physiological chemistry (A. E. Taylor), and research medicine (Richard M. Pearce) met with their respective staffs. These seminars proved a dismal failure, since very few students attended; they apparently lost interest because of the detailed discussions of opposing and often irreconcilable views, which led the disputants away from the fundamental basis of accepted facts. For the teaching and research staffs represented, the exchange of views was very profitable, and, despite the absence of students, the seminar was continued throughout the year.

Another important object of the department was to furnish the opportunity for investigation to properly trained students and practitioners in medicine. As far as students were concerned, this was not successful; the failure was due to the demands of an overcrowded, inflexible curriculum and an inadequate elective system. During the five-year period, however, about fifteen practitioners entered the department for the purpose of carrying out a definitive investigative study. In part, these researches had a close relation to clinical problems, but, in a number of instances, they were fundamental investigations in experimental pathology. The practitioners involved were usually younger men with their hospital internship behind them, who were starting the practice of medicine and wished to divide their free time between outpatient and research work or to devote it entirely to investigative work.

Pearce, in reviewing the five years, posed the question whether it would not be better to divide the endowment for research among existing clinical departments rather than to have a separate department of research medicine. His answer was that teaching and investigation should go hand in hand. If adequate endowment could be procured to establish teaching and research in every department of the medical school, there would be no need for a separate department of research.

## Report on Medical Research and Its Relation to Medical Schools

The Committee on Medical Research of the Association of American Medical Colleges published a report, in 1917, on the extent to which medical schools should encourage research. Should all schools undertake it; and, if undertaken, by whom should it be carried on? Should there be, within the schools, professorships or other positions devoted to research alone and distinct from teaching positions and departments of research distinct from teaching departments? What should the relation of medical schools be to research foundations?[41] The committee consisted of Frederic S. Lee, professor of physiology at Columbia; Walter B. Cannon, professor of physiology at Harvard; and Richard M. Pearce, head of the department of research medicine at the University of Pennsylvania and later medical director of the Rockefeller Foundation.

The committee members concluded that no faculty member was performing his full duty to the school unless he investigated. This idea was becoming generally recognized by the best schools in the so-called medical sciences, but it was as true of the clinical as of the preclinical departments. In this respect, the committee members pointed out that the evolution of clinicians, and of clinical departments from their traditional position as exclusively teaching branches of the schools, had been slower than that of the preclinical branches. Such a distinction, they said, was wholly artificial and was destined to pass away. The establishment of full-time chairs, already achieved in the preclinical branches, and greatly to be desired in the clinical ones, would help to break down this distinction.

The committee went on to discuss separate chairs in research departments, saying that, insofar as they supplement and work in cooperation with other research activities of the school, they are to be commended; but, insofar as they assume the sole research functions of the school and afford an excuse for other chairs or departments to refrain from such activities, they can offer only an imperfect, even harmful, substitute. Thus, the basic scientists were still in the forefront in stressing the need for clinical science.

## Later Evaluations of the Results of Establishing Full-time Clinical Chairs

An appraisal of the full-time system was presented, in 1922, by George Canby Robinson. Robinson, at that time an acting professor of medicine at Johns Hopkins, spoke as follows:

> We may say that the science of clinical medicine has recently come into being, and in some instances departments of clinical medicine have attained the scope and atmosphere of true university departments. . . . The quality and quantity of its research work, the attitude of the head of the department and all its members toward original investigation, the facilities for research and the publications issuing from it determine to what degree a department has attained a true university position.
>
> No one who has had any actual experience with the university plan now holds that clinical departments are to be manned exclusively by men who have no interests outside the medical school and who do not engage in private practice. Everyone recognizes the desirability of having the clinical departments composed both of men whose main interest is in the academic activities of teaching and research, and men to whom these activities are to a greater or lesser extent secondary to the practice of medicine within and without the confines of the medical school. There is one requirement, however, that must be insisted upon in the case of every member of a department who has any clinical responsibilities. He must have a fundamental interest in patients. . . . This interest must be sufficient to impel him to master the technic of clinical methods, and to awaken the humanitarian spirit without which the physician in the true sense of the word does not

exist. A man who lacks this interest, or who allows his desire to accomplish successful research to overshadow it belongs rather in the department of pathology or physiology. . . . If men whose chief interests are in the laboratory are put into positions of prominence in clinical departments, the university department will fall far short of meeting its basic obligations.

It is essential to have practitioners as an integral part of the department of medicine, not primarily because of their direct influence on the students, but because of their influence on the department as a whole, and especially on the men who have chosen to follow the academic career in clinical medicine. The two groups of men, one devoting part of its time to intensive study and research, and the other devoting the greater part of its time to private practice can be of the greatest mutual benefit to each other, and it is only when these two groups can be brought into a harmonious, united, contented whole, each with respect, esteem and a cooperative spirit toward the other, that the ideal department of medicine will exist.[42]

W. McKim Marriott of St. Louis contributed the following remarks in discussion of Robinson's talk:

What we need is more men who are prepared to apply the biological sciences to the solving of clinical problems. Since the establishment of full-time clinical teaching in some of our schools a considerable number of younger men have been preparing themselves to fill full-time positions. These younger men are thoroughly trained in the fundamental sciences as well as in clinical medicine. . . . Already as the result of this newer generation of scientific medical men . . . medicine has advanced more in a few years than it did during preceding generations.[43]

George Dock, professor of medicine at the Washington University School of Medicine, pointed out that the first essential toward filling full-time positions was an adequate university hospital—fully controlled by the medical school, with proper clinical material, well-equipped laboratories, library, and staffs—not only for teaching and research but also for the care of patients. The second essential was money to pay the full-time staffs and all others whose services seemed valuable to the institution. A large enough staff had to be provided, so that each member would have adequate time for study, research, writing, and study travel. Dock observed that these needs were disregarded almost wholly in many tentative plans. He emphasized that, in order to provide satisfactory facilities for the full-time faculty, it was essential that there be a fairly large technical staff. The full-time system was therefore costly, and Dock believed it would become costlier as medicine became more complex. He pointed out that the full-time staffs, which were to have led lives exempt from the cares and temptations of practice, were now expected by many universities to earn the income needed not only for their own salaries but also for their departments or even other departments. This income was to result from securing rich patients and charging them large fees or even by collecting small fees from a large clientele. He stated that this idea was enticingly set forth in an essay by Dean Hough in the *University of Virginia Alumni Bulletin* of January 1921. It was also put forward in an address by the then president of the University of Michigan in an address published in the *Journal of the Michigan State Medical Society* in February 1921.

It is clear that Robinson and Marriott, both of whom organized successful full-time departments—the former in medicine, the latter in pediatrics—appreciated the need to retain the valuable contributions of the part-time practicing physicians. Dock, who during his later years held important administrative posts, soon appreciated the problem created when the university depended on funds derived from the private patients of the full-time clinician for his salary support. Equally important, and a development that reached its peak much later, was the tendency of medical schools to choose men for full-time clinical posts who were not outstanding clinicians and whose major interest was in the laboratory. This problem became more serious as research done in clinical departments became more basically oriented and the use of patients for research more restricted. Research grants depended on productivity, and work in molecular biology was considered more scientifically elite· than clinical investigation.

## McCann on "Full-time" Professorships in Clinical Departments

William S. McCann, who was a full-time professor of medicine at the University of Rochester School of Medicine for many years, described his experiences in relation to the full-time system in his unpublished memoirs:

> The difference between the Hopkins and the Harvard systems lay in the disposition of fees earned by the incumbent "whole time" staff. At Harvard there was no set limit to the amount of fees which might be earned, other than the stipulation or gentlemen's agreement to limit the amount of time devoted to private practice so that it would not encroach on the time required for the proper administration and development of the department for which the professor was responsible. At Johns Hopkins the whole-time professor received a salary, supposedly adequate to relieve him of financial worries, and leaving him free to devote all his time and effort to the development of his department. There was no prohibition of private practice, only the stipulation that the fees be turned over to the university or to the department in which they were earned. This concept of "whole time" was the product of the mind of Abraham Flexner, and backed by the potent influence of the General Education Board of the Rockefeller Foundation. There were fallacies in both concepts of "whole time" as experience was to prove, but at the inception discussion was bound to be largely theoretical.
>
> As a young associate professor from 1921 to 1924 the Flexner plan worked well for me. I was in my early thirties, with a salary of $4,000 to $4,500 which was equivalent to $15,000 to $18,000 in present purchasing

power. I was in charge of one of the best teaching wards in the hospital, with a metabolism ward of four beds attached. I had an excellent associate in Robert Hannon, who assisted me in our research laboratory, and in addition we were responsible for the clinical biochemical laboratory serving the whole hospital, and presided over by my associate William A. Perlzweig, who later became professor of biochemistry at Duke University. We had thus an unrivalled opportunity to study a very wide range of clinical conditions. The daily teaching rounds with the fine students enabled us to develop diagnostic acumen at the bedside and at the same time explore the meaning of clinical phenomena by laboratory studies of our own and those of my colleagues in charge of special laboratory services in hematology, cardiology, and in infectious diseases. Freely available were the finest consulting specialists in the surgical and neurological fields, in otology, ophthalmology, urology, and gynecology. To have the opportunity to integrate these special fields into a diagnosis, and from it to formulate a plan of treatment for each patient gave me the best possible preparation for taking charge of the development of a clinic of my own. There was only one special ingredient lacking and that was the fact that we did not see the patients in their own environment; we had to learn in taking the history, or through the observations of social workers who did go into the homes, and the rest we had to draw from our own life experiences. Not infrequently there were excellent letters from the referring physicians, but in many cases these were lacking. However, we should realize that the whole focus of interest in clinical medicine of that period was directed toward the mechanisms for maintaining homeostatic equilibrium in the internal environment. The summer of 1923 was long and hot in Baltimore. . . . I was beginning to be asked by local medical societies over the state to come and discourse on the newer treatment of diabetes. I recall one such trip to Port Tobacco on the Potomac River. The meeting was held in a grove in a picnic setting, with an abundance of Maryland fried chicken. The rural physicians were attentive but asked few questions as I told them that the wonderful gift of insulin would be of little use unless the patients were well controlled in the matter of diet. To most of the older among my listeners the discussion of the pathological physiology of diabetes mellitus might just as well have been given in Greek. Except those who had received their training in a few top schools, medical education of the period had given them very little of biochemistry or of the physiology of the metabolism.

To me the experience of meeting these practitioners was invaluable. They were dealing with environmental factors in the management of patients of which we in Academe did not often think about, since our whole effort was devoted to understanding the adaptive forces at work within the internal environment of diabetic patients. This situation was very typical of the early movement toward the development of whole time clinical teachers. The situation would have been worse had there not been men in the great medical centers, such as Elliott Joslin, who were long experienced in the management of the external environmental factors and at the same time able to participate in the scientific investigation of the internal environment. Thus I was convinced at an early date that a balanced medical education could not be given by an unbalanced whole-time faculty. It was precisely this balance in the faculty of the Johns Hopkins Medical School that made it so outstanding at that time.[44]

By 1960, the newly emerging problems of full-time departments of medicine drew the attention of one of the most outstanding American clinical scientists, William B. Castle.[45] Castle noted that, in 1960, stresses were clearly set up within university hospital medical units by the progressive compartmentation of clinical knowledge, the increase in the length of the training period within the hospital, and the vast expansion of hospital-based research. Because the appraisal of many clinical problems had passed, with the proximal identification of the nature of the disease process, from the stage of patient-study to its replication in laboratory animals or to studies of tissues, cells, and biochemical systems in vitro, the clinical investigator went less often to the bedside and spent more time at the laboratory bench. Hence Castle's chief concern: the possible effect, upon full-time teachers of medicine and their students, of the increasing preoccupation with research that does not frequently renew its purpose with studies of patients or their diseases.

To Castle, it seemed inappropriate to the functions of a university hospital—and unwise for progress in medicine—for clinical investigators to pursue too far problems that had become possible of solution by preclinical as well as by other basic scientists:

> Admiration for the penetrating character of fundamental experiments in biological science should not lead us as physicians to depreciate the unique opportunity and responsibility of the clinical investigator. . . . I believe that he should keep the problems of disease at least in the back of his mind and as often as possible in the front, for the record of his accomplishment provides many examples of matters now under intensive scrutiny by basic scientists that became apparent originally from the bedside study of disease. Indeed, F. M. Burnet has recently pointed out, "It is only when things go wrong that it becomes possible to perceive that there is something in normal function which requires understanding. . . ."[46] As I see it, the all-important task of the clinical investigator is to take the essential first step away from the bedside toward the laboratory. This may be an achievement requiring new scientific insight, the invention of a method never before used or even a wild surmise. However, once his discovery is in the laboratory, it has become available, or today soon will be, to all biological workers. To proceed much beyond this point within the university hospital's walls then runs the risk of attempting something that others are better suited to accomplish or for which they must be introduced into the hospital, there possibly to become persons displaced from their native departmental environments. Surely, at that point, it is better for the clinical investigator to begin again with a study of some new facet of disease. . . .
>
> There is, of course, no universal formula for success as a clinical investigator other than perhaps to be lucky and, according to Fuller Albright, to apply one's mind, whether a "one story, two story or three story intellect with skylights" to appropriate problems.[47] For outstanding achievement, many are called but few are chosen. It is therefore well that throughout his

career, the full-time physician-teacher-investigator keep in mind, despite inevitable compromises, his responsibilities to this familiar triad of activities as the guiding principles of his academic life. By no man can all be fulfilled, much less at one time. Youth is surely the time for high adventure and for experiment, and with maturity some will gladly teach and some more wisely tend the sick.[48]

# 8

## ∝∮∾

# Implementation of the
# Full-time Plan at Johns Hopkins

### The First Full-time Professor of Medicine:
### Theodore Caldwell Janeway

Theodore Caldwell Janeway, born in New York City on November 2, 1872, was the son of Edward G. Janeway, one of the foremost physicians of his day. His association with his father furnished a wonderful training, because he knew more medicine than could be derived from any of the then current textbooks.

The younger Janeway came under the influence of Chittenden at the Sheffield Scientific School of Yale University, from which he graduated in 1892. Three years later he received the M.D. degree from Columbia's College of Physicians and Surgeons and then interned at St. Luke's Hospital in New York City. From 1898 to 1905 he was instructor in medical diagnosis at New York University and Bellevue Hospital Medical College and, from 1902 to 1911, visiting physician to New York Hospital.

Janeway emphasized the rational interpretation of symptoms and the importance of pathological physiology to his students. His inspiration in this effort was Graham Lusk. This was a forward step from the method of parrot-like response to which medical students had, for the most part, been trained previously. His expertise in teaching and his work with hypertension led to his appointment as Bard Professor of Medicine at the College of Physicians and Surgeons in 1909. Janeway became the leader of a younger group of "physiological clinicians" who quietly but surely transformed American medicine.

In 1911 he succeeded Christian Archibald Herter on the Board of Scientific Directors of the Rockefeller Institute for Medical Research. He represented scientific internal medicine on the board, and his service in planning the activities of the Institute was important.[1]

Janeway's greatest contribution to clinical science was his work on blood pressure.[2] His treatise on this subject was published in 1904. Its subtitle, "A Guide to the Use of the Sphygmomanometer in Medical, Surgical and Obstetrical Practice, with a Summary of the Experimental and Clinical Facts Relating to the Blood Pressure in Health and Disease," is revealing of its contents. Thus, Janeway was among the first American students of hypertension and its relation to the heart and kidneys from a clinical and experimental point of view.

In 1908 Janeway emphasized that for minor grades of cardiac insufficiency the continued use of small doses of digitalis was advantageous. In 1914, at least five years before any one else mentioned the subject, Janeway wrote as follows: "In certain cases with normal rhythm, I have seen digitialis followed by speedy relief of symptoms as in fibrillating cases. This has been particularly true in patients with cardiac insufficiency secondary to prolonged high blood pressure." Another important point related to the toxic arrhythmias induced by digitalis: "In all these hearts with regular rhythm I believe that dosage should be more cautious than in the fibrillating heart. The onset of abnormal rhythm is one guide to toxic effects."[3]

After he became professor of medicine at Columbia, Janeway found little time for experimental work. He was invited, in 1914, to become the first full-time professor of medicine at the Johns Hopkins University School of Medicine. Janeway found there a medical clinic organized largely in accord with his ideals for patient care, laboratory work, teaching, and investigation; this clinic existed alongside others similarly developed and associated with strong departments in the preclinical sciences. He maintained the research divisions that Barker had organized and brought with him Herman O. Mosenthal, who was interested in metabolic studies, as an associate professor in charge of the chemical division.[4] Janeway retained, either on his "whole-time" staff or on an associated "part-time" staff, nearly all of the workers already in the department and quickly made the readjustments necessitated by reorganization on the "whole-time" basis.

Leonard G. Rowntree, who had been working with John J. Abel in the department of pharmacology, joined the department of medicine.[5] In September 1916, Clyde G. Guthrie assumed directorship of the clinical laboratory, a post he was to hold until September 1922. Paul W. Clough joined the biological division in 1916, after finishing his duties as a resident physician.[6] A. L. Bloomfield, also a member of this division, was very active in research.[7] Charles R. Austrian was an assistant physician from October 1914 to June 1915.[8] Allen K. Krause, whose special interest was tuberculosis, joined the department in 1916.[9]

References to research in the department of medicine during Janeway's tenure show the tremendous increase in clinical investigation resulting from the recruitment of a full-time staff.[10] In spite of the progress made, Janeway was not happy in his transformation from active New York consultant and teacher to full-time university professor. In 1917 he resigned his professorship with the idea of returning to New York, partly because his restrictions from practice created a financial hardship and partly because he was no longer entirely in sympathy with the full-time plan. After Janeway's tragic death in December 1917, Mosenthal assumed temporary chairmanship of the department.

In his brief period at Johns Hopkins, Janeway made a deep impression, winning the respect and esteem of his colleagues. He helped to plan a new building for the Hunterian Laboratory for Experimental Surgery and Medicine, improved the facilities for metabolic studies, fostered researches in the heart station, and secured a substantial increase in the endowment for studies in tuberculosis known as the Kenneth Dow Fund.[11] According to Mosenthal, Janeway accomplished a great deal.[12] The medical department and medical division of the hospital, which had wards, laboratories, dispensaries, and classrooms, constituted an administrative problem of considerable magnitude, which was largely solved by Janeway.

As one reviews the names of those who served on the resident staff or as fellows under Janeway, the importance of Johns Hopkins during this period as a training center for scientifically based clinicians who later occupied positions of importance in other medical schools becomes evident. For the years 1914 to 1917, the following were assistant resident physicians: A. L. Bloomfield, who became a professor of medicine at Stanford; Robert L. Levy,[13] who became a distinguished cardiologist and a member of the staff at the College of Physicians and Surgeons; Dana Atchley, who became a professor of medicine at Columbia; R. L. Haden, who became the medical director of the Cleveland Clinic; Verne R. Mason, who became a clinical professor of medicine at the University of Southern California; Thomas M. Rivers, who became the second director of the HRI; and V.P.W. Sydenstricker, who became a professor of medicine at the Medical College of Georgia. Norman M. Keith, an assistant in medicine, became a distinguished member of the staff of the Mayo Clinic. Henry Barber Richardson, who later served on the staff at the Cornell Medical College–New York Hospital medical center, was a fellow for two years.[14] George R. Minot was an assistant resident physician and then a fellow under William Henry Howell, at which time he developed his interest in hematology.[15] Frank A. Evans served as an instructor in medicine from 1916 to 1921 and, with Thomas P. Sprunt, gave the first complete description of infectious mononucleosis, pointing out that it occurred in adults as well as in children. Evans later became a professor of medicine at the University of Pittsburgh.[16] Many of the others who served under Janeway established themselves as leading practitioners of medicine in various parts of the country, and most of them had part-time teaching positions in local medical schools.[17] Meanwhile, the spirit of research had been constantly fostered and teaching put on a high plane. Janeway felt that the experiment of full-time medicine had justified itself and that he had brought about more adequate teaching, research, and administration than had been possible under the "part-time" system.

The events that took place during Janeway's tenure were commented on by Dana Atchley, who was at that time a student of medicine:[18]

> I remember the [effect of the] change on students and faculty with great vividness. Dr. Theodore C. Janeway came as professor of medicine, supplanting Dr. Lewellys Barker, and Dr. William S. Halsted was made professor of surgery and Dr. Howland professor of pediatrics, all on full-time. Each had his own laboratory. They were given these laboratories, a budget for their laboratory work, and an associate professor apiece, also full-time, to work with them.
>
> Janeway, a man of great prestige in New York, arrived in Baltimore and became professor of medicine. . . . He brought in an entirely new point of view. Whereas Barker was a tall, handsome articulate charmer, Janeway was short, homely and inarticulate; but he was a highly intelligent man and a dedicated person. He gave up a huge practice to come down at $10,000 a year.
>
> I immediately established a rapport with him.

As a student, Atchley conceived a research project for himself that involved some chemical tests. When he found a suitable case for his experiment, he went to Janeway, who turned him over to his chemical associate and gave him a place in the laboratory. Atchley's experiment worked out satisfactorily, and Janeway was quite pleased with this original student work.[19] After spending a year in New York, Atchley returned to Johns Hopkins as an intern, taking care of Janeway's private patients. Janeway had a number of private patients, but his fees were allocated to the research fund. Atchley described his internship in the following fashion:

> My internship under Janeway was similar to the work an intern would do nowadays. I think that Janeway did with me just what I do with the interns that are assigned to the private pavilion. . . . We would go over the cases. I did histories and did physical examinations on the cases just as the boys do for me here [the College of Physicians and Surgeons]. Every morning at 8:30 I spent an hour with him going over the cases and discussing them.

Atchley spoke further of Janeway's period at Hopkins in an address entitled "The Uses of Elegance":[20]

> I arrived at the Johns Hopkins Medical School in 1911, during the heyday of physical diagnosis. At a time when biochemistry was discussing the structure of nucleic acid, clinical medicine was presenting physical diagnosis as an independent subject which had made little sophisticated progress in the many years since Auenbrugger and Laennec. Physical signs

were collected with less interest in their relevancy than in the virtuosity by which they were obtained. Elegance was the keynote of percussion; in vain did I try to develop the graceful wrist action that would have been more appropriate to Paderewski's piano playing. It was not sporting to look at a chest x-ray until the patient had been worn out by a tiresome period of physical diagnosis, and much time was spent on estimating the blood pressure by palpation before the sphygmomanometer was applied, although the inaccuracy of palpation had long since been proved. As I look back, I realize that it was a misuse of elegance to draw a cleft and place the heart murmurs on it in absolute pitch. . . .

Into this atmosphere with emphasis on clinical minutiae there came in 1914 the new full-time professor Theodore C. Janeway. He was one of the first modern internists to think in terms of the natural history of a disease and its dynamics.

Graham Lusk[21] recognized that Janeway was the first instructor in medicine in New York City who attempted to teach his subject from "the standpoint of disease being a deviation from the physiological normal" and observed further that he was the first man to take routine blood pressures in his office. . . . Janeway wrote that medicine is "now consciously an experimental science" and he spoke accusingly of the "intensely practical men" who "discourage all attempts at systematic thinking who decry laboratory studies and hold that a true knowledge of disease can be acquired only at the bedside." To quote further from the same essay: "When we have comprehended a disease . . . we see it not as an entity, not static, but as something dynamic, a process . . . all treatment of disease is a therapeutic experiment based on a theory. This theory we call a diagnosis. . . . The science of disease [is] the only sure basis for the successful practice of the art of medicine." I can testify from sad memory that this precociously enlightened attitude toward clinical medicine was considered by most of my associates as little short of heresy, and silly heresy at that.

Introduction of the academic full-time policy, with its corollary that research laboratories should be an integral part of the clinical equipment, was the turning point of medical education in this country and thus of medicine itself. The forty-five years since Janeway went to Johns Hopkins have seen a greater advance in the understanding and management of disease than had the previous 500 years. Much of the new knowledge and most of its critical application to patient care are the result of freeing the clinical teacher from the distractions of private practice and offering him both the time and the facilities for his own research. With investigative experience the academic physician became a better teacher, a sounder critic of new scientific contributions and a more competent clinician, for modern medicine depends more on logical thinking than on encyclopedic knowledge.

Janeway felt, as a result of his experience, that the strict limitations placed on the full-time system needed modification. In 1915 he commented on the full-time plan at Johns Hopkins.[22] He outlined a modification, based on his brief experience, that contained five essential points:

1. Clinical teachers should be chosen because of their possession of the same qualities that govern choice for other university positions. Such selections should be absolutely without geographical limitation.
2. There should be provision of adequate facilities for laboratory investigation, hand in hand with clinical training for every member of the department staff.
3. Salaries should be sufficiently ample to make outside practice unnecessary, especially for the younger men who show ability as investigators. Salaries should be proportional to the time given to teaching and research.
4. There should be full freedom for every member of the staff to develop into practitioner, consultant, teacher, or investigator, as best suited the individual talents of each; but original appointment, reappointment, and promotion alike to be for true university accomplishment.
5. All appointments of clinical teachers should be term appointments; not even professors should hold lifetime chairs.

Janeway suggested this deviation from ordinary university practice, because he viewed the hospital clinic as a monopoly, put into the hands of the professor, that contained the potential of exploitation for private gain. The reason for life tenure for the university professor, he pointed out, is that the older he grows in the university service and the more valuable in his devotion to his subject, the less capable he becomes of earning his living in any other way. "The professor of medicine . . . on the other hand by virtue of his very position acquires an increasing money value. The more illustrious he becomes, as the university should wish him to become, the greater is his potential earning power."

In conclusion, Janeway stated that he had been an unpaid instructor, a professor giving part of his time to consulting practice, and a well-paid full-time teacher. He could therefore speak from personal experience:

> I know that the conduct of a large clinical department along university lines requires a man's best thought and effort. Only a small fraction of his time can he spare for outside engagements. . . . He must give . . . more time than any of his colleagues in the university devoted to routine duties, and he must keep up with an enormous literature and do research work. To earn any considerable part of his own living is manifestly impossible. But as well say that he must not be a good musician, or a devotee of chess, as to insist that he must never sharpen his wits on a case that has puzzled some physician outside the hospital who wishes his help. If he is to do this, it is unnatural and repugnant to the patient's sense of judgment that he should not receive the usual fee for such service. . . .
>
> For the rest, one man may be valuable to the clinic because of his ability to train students in methods, another for his encyclopedic knowledge, a third for his suggestiveness. Specialists are vital to progress, but all around men are indispensable to sane teaching. The widest variety of interests will create the strongest department and men of varied interest cannot be

produced by any single type of training. For this reason I am of the opinion that, if the liberal support for research provided by the whole-time plan could be secured without its limitations, the ends of medical education would be best served.

I would conclude, therefore, that outside professional engagements may be desirable for most members of medical faculties at some period of their careers, and that clinical teachers who engage in some outside practice are necessary in any scheme of medical education. Uniformity of environment is not the distinctive feature of the university, but unity of purpose.

Thus, although Janeway felt that much more flexibility was desirable, he still was completely in keeping with the spirit of the development of new knowledge as an essential feature of a university clinical department and the belief that there should be men fully engaged in such work.

## The First Full-time Department to Win Complete Success: Pediatrics under John F. Howland

In September 1912, John F. Howland became the first full-time head of the pediatric department at Johns Hopkins.[23] In the next fifteen years, pediatric biochemistry flowered under Howland and the remarkable group of young men associated with him.

Howland entered Yale in 1894 and then attended the New York University School of Medicine. After graduation, Howland was a house officer at Presbyterian Hospital. Two years later, he interned at the New York Foundling Hospital. Howland's contact there with L. Emmett Holt, a dynamic personality, was responsible for his choice of pediatrics.

After this internship, Howland studied in Europe, first in Berlin and then in Vienna. It was this trip that kindled his interest in research. On his return to America, in 1902, Howland became an assistant to Holt.

Holt actually laid the foundation of biochemical investigation in pediatrics. He had trained as a resident under William Henry Welch at Bellevue Hospital. He chose pediatrics as a career and, when the *Archives of Pediatrics* was first published, in January 1884, was a member of the editorial board. Holt's marriage brought him into intimate contact with one person who became a particularly stimulating influence upon him along scientific lines—Herter,[24] who had married a relative of Mrs. Holt's. Herter, who had fallen under the spell of Welch, followed him to Baltimore to work in pathology and bacteriology. He returned to New York and, in 1889, joined the staff of the Babies' Hospital. Herter performed autopsies (and did bacteriological work), but there were few, if any, autopsies at which Holt was not present. Using postmortem specimens, Holt measured the stomach's capacity at various ages, to determine how much a baby should receive at a single feeding.[25]

The Rockefeller Institute for Medical Research, which Holt had been instrumental in founding (chapter 5), gave him the means of fulfilling his ambition to establish laboratory facilities for research in pediatrics. One of the first grants the institute made was to aid bacteriological and pathological studies at Babies' Hospital. Studies were conducted on the bacteriology of milk; on the bacteriology of meningitis and of infant diarrhea; on calcium and fat metabolism. In 1911 the institute supplied two chemists (Francis McCrudden and Helen L. Fales) and a chemical laboratory, which maintained an interest in metabolism and nutrition for another decade.[26]

> Holt's pupil, John Howland, played a major role in launching the chemical era in American pediatrics, and perhaps he did as much as any one to turn his former chief in that direction. Holt's task was that of planning the work, interpreting the data and writing the papers; the actual determinations were done by the others. The problems were usually discussed with Levene or Van Slyke of the Rockefeller Institute, who collaborated in some of them. Their counsel was invaluable, but the guiding hand was that of Holt.
>
> From 1911 to 1923 the chemical laboratories of the hospital turned out a series of balance studies—the intake and output of nearly every chemical substance for which an analytical method was available were measured in health and in disease. . . .
>
> Holt and Howland remained in close touch with each other even after Howland left New York.[27]

As a result of his investigative work under Holt, Howland became a professor of pediatrics in the reorganized full-time medical school at Washington University in 1910. In preparation for this appointment, he studied under Adalbert Czerny in Strasbourg, where he developed his interest in nutritional disorders of children. Most important, he saw a great German clinic in which the advancement of knowledge was a major interest. He returned in 1911 and, six months later, was invited to succeed von Pirquet as head of pediatrics at Johns Hopkins.

When Howland arrived at Johns Hopkins, there was no separate pediatric department—pediatrics was part of internal medicine. Although von Pirquet had been a professor since 1910, there was no inpatient service in pediatrics. Von Pirquet worked in two small rooms in the medical dispensary, and it was he who designed the pediatric inpatient building, on the basis of some preexisting plans.

Howland also found no pediatric staff. He selected his own group, and, as stated in Genesis, "there were giants on the earth in those days and they became mighty men—men of renown." Almost every one of Howland's original staff later became the head of a pediatric department in a medical school.[28] Edwards A. Park joined him as chief of the outpatient service.[29] Park became interested in rickets while at the New York Foundling Hospital and went to Marburg, Germany, in the summer of 1912, to study the pathology of that disease under Professor M. B. Schmidt. While there, he received his offer from Howland. Kenneth

Blackfan, who had been Howland's chief resident in St. Louis, was appointed chief resident of the inpatient service.[30] Grover Powers, later head of the pediatric department at Yale University, joined the group in 1913; W. McKim Marriott in 1914; and James L. Gamble in 1915. In 1916 Marriott left to become head of pediatrics at Washington University in St. Louis, and, the following year, Benjamin Kramer took his place at Johns Hopkins.

The members of the research staff were allowed to work in the outpatient department, but were not given any ward privileges. Howland, along with his resident staff, took sole care of the children on the wards, and he personally had charge of all private patients. Marriott was so essential to Howland in the laboratory that he had the greatest difficulty in obtaining consent even to work in the dispensary. Howland would not allow any special clinics (with the exception of one for the treatment of congenital syphilis) to be organized. His policy was to keep the department completely under his immediate control, and his system was certainly conducive to successful research.

As an investigator, Howland was an opportunist. He generally chose subjects for his studies in which, from the beginning, he could see the end. After he became interested in rickets, his investigations had a continuity, but his earlier studies seemed to involve what chance offered. In his studies with the calorimeter, Howland worked alone, but, in almost all other cases, he worked in collaboration with someone else. The collaborator might be chosen because his problem appealed particularly to Howland, but more often because he possessed some special knowledge or ability that Howland himself lacked. His coworkers were unusual men—for example, A. N. Richards was an early colleague, and later work was done chiefly with Marriott and Kramer. Howland apparently did not have a very imaginative or creative mind, but he did possess unerring judgment.

Howland did not provide technicians in the chemical laboratories. He insisted that investigators must gain, through experience, resourcefulness in the use of the required methodology, in order to have full faith in their results. Although Howland himself had little knowledge of theoretical chemistry, he was remarkably skillful in technical procedures.

Edwards A. Park vividly described Howland and the stimulating environment he created in the Harriet Lane Home:

> What a joyous place the Harriet Lane was in those early days under this virile man. We were all young, our chief not much older than we, certainly not older in spirit, a happy family in which each had his duty. There was not a discordant soul amongst us—all the fresh, hard work was a delight and each day brought the new experiences and excitement of creative work. It must be remembered that this pediatric oasis was set in the larger oasis of Johns Hopkins, then still in its early glory, filled with interesting and distinguished men, engaged in important work and having wide outlooks. . . . In pediatrics he [Howland] had become a world figure as the

result of his investigative work ... Abraham Jacobi was the pioneer in pediatrics. Holt established pediatrics in this country as a special branch of medicine. ... John Howland, on the other hand, modernized pediatrics. He changed the course of pediatrics by substituting for bedside observation and conjecture, the study of disease through laboratory methods and experiments. ... He did this by example—by the development of a model clinic; model from the point of view of administration, medical care, teaching, research and spirit. ... He created and sent out missionaries, his pupils, filled with his ideas and his spirit. A new era in medicine founded on the application of scientific methods to the study of clinical problems was coming anyway ... but Howland started the movement in pediatrics ... and the Harriet Lane Home under his guidance was the first full-time university clinic to win complete success.[31]

Howland's first great accomplishment in Baltimore was proving that an acidosis existed in children with diarrhea. The selection of the problem was Howland's; the development of a better method for the recognition of the acidosis was Marriott's contribution. They demonstrated marked increase of urinary ammonia, severe reduction of carbon dioxide tension in the alveolar air, increase in the hydrogen ion concentration of the blood, and increase of three to five times in the amount of sodium bicarbonate required to alkalinize the urine, which was always highly acid. They noted, but without pursuing the matter further at that time, "the continual drain of water from the tissues." They knew, however, that the "acidosis may be entirely overcome, and yet death ensue as a result of it; it probably initiates many abnormal processes that we do not understand and that we have no way of overcoming."[32]

Howland and his associates made important advances in replacement therapy. Thomas Latta, a physician in the town of Leith, near Edinburgh, was the first to inject intravenously a solution containing sodium chloride and sodium bicarbonate, to treat a patient severely ill with cholera. The outcome was dramatic, but, after Latta's magnificent experiment, nothing more was done about replacement therapy until almost one hundred years later. Indeed, it was not until Marriott and K. Utheim[33] directly measured the large reduction of the volume of blood in dehydrated infants that circulatory failure was recognized as the immediately dangerous event in infant diarrhea and it became clear that volume was the critical dimension of effective replacement therapy. Blackfan, Howland's perennial resident, who later became director of the Children's Hospital in Boston and a professor of pediatrics at Harvard, became convinced earlier, on clinical grounds, that infants dehydrated by diarrheal disease needed more salt solution than could be provided by subcutaneous infusions. He successfully argued his case with Howland and was permitted to try more vigorous therapy. This is an example of an important advance in medical science made at the bedside by an observant physician.[34]

In 1914 Marriott and Howland began to study what prevented the deposition of calcium salts into the bone and bone-forming cartilage in patients with rickets.[35] Marriott, Haessler, and Howland had to devise suitable methods for the detection of calcium and phosphorus in small amounts of blood.[36] Marriott and Howland showed that, in the active phase of so-called idiopathic tetany of infancy, the serum calcium was 5 to 7 mg/dl, as opposed to a normal concentration of 10 to 11 mg/dl.[37] In 1916 Marriott and Howland found the serum calcium concentration in rickets without tetany to be normal or only slightly reduced.[38]

In 1919 Kramer and Howland began a systematic study of rickets.[39] They found that even in severe rickets with marked deformities the serum calcium was only slightly changed, but the concentration of serum inorganic phosphorus in uncomplicated rickets was always lower than normal. Kramer successfully developed even better micromethods for analysis of inorganic ions in serum, particularly calcium and magnesium, which were useful as diagnostic and research tools.

## The Discovery of Vitamin D

In 1917 E. V. McCollum set up a rat colony in the new School of Hygiene and Public Health at Johns Hopkins. Howland learned in the autumn of 1918 that Simmonds, a colleague of McCollum's, had produced a condition in young rats that the two researchers thought might be rickets. Howland confirmed that the gross appearance of the thorax in these rats was similar to that seen in severe rickets in children. An experimental team was organized to study this disease, with Park in charge of the bone pathology, McCollum and Nina Simmonds doing the experimental work with the rats, and Howland and his group working with the microchemical determinations.

By 1921 they had completed studies of three hundred experimental diets on hundreds of rats.[40] The most significant factors for safeguarding normal bone growth were the ratio between the calcium and the phosphorus in the blood and the kind of fat supplied. Low calcium and high phosphorus—or low phosphorus and high calcium—were disturbing to bone growth. The former relationship caused rickets complicated by tetany. Kramer showed that the blood phosphate was low in the animals with rachitic lesions. The unfavorable ratios between calcium and phosphorus seen in rickets were prevented by a small amount of cod liver oil or a large amount of butter fat. They discovered a second fat-soluble vitamin, an antirachitic substance that they named vitamin D. These and other experiments clarified the pathogenesis of this crippling disease of children and led to its eradication.

## James L. Gamble and "Gamblegrams"

James L. Gamble[41] graduated from the Harvard Medical School in 1910 and interned at the MGH. After spending six months in 1913 at

Children's Hospital in Boston, he visited various European clinics and became interested in the study of disease in man by the quantitative methods of biochemistry. Gamble worked for a period with Otto Folin and then returned to the MGH, under Fritz Talbot. While there, Lawrence J. Henderson's physicochemical approach to physiologic processes made a deep impression on him.[42] In 1915 Gamble joined the full-time staff, under Howland. He remained until 1922, when he joined Oscar Schloss to establish a full-time staff in pediatrics at Harvard. Schloss left Boston within a year, but Blackfan succeeded him as head of the department. Gamble remained at Children's Hospital until his death on May 28, 1959.

In 1919 Gamble studied the ketosis of starvation with Graham Ross and F. F. Tisdall. Rarely have data been subjected to more original deductive reasoning than they were in these classic metabolic experiments.[43] The results are best summarized in Gamble's own words:

> One, the data display, in operation, the two adjustable components of the acid-base construction of urine (titrable acidity and ammonia production) which Henderson and Palmer described and which permit the removal of anion excess within the prescribed limits for urine acidity without expenditure of fixed base beyond the quantity which probably presents for removal. Two, they show the determining role of fixed base in sustaining the osmolar value of the body fluids because of the adjustability of the total cation-anion equality. Three, they show the relation of volume of the body fluids to fixed base content on the premise of preservation of the normal osmolar value with the corollary that, so long as the kidney is operating accurately, loss (or gain) of water and electrolytes will be parallel. On this basis the data were used to allocate losses of water from the body fluid compartments from measurements of outgo of intracellular and of extracellular base.[44]

These experiments were an important milestone in clinical investigation.[45] At a time when most clinical investigation consisted of the recording of endless observations made using some new method, Gamble planned a crucial experiment to elucidate basic problems of function and applied chemical means to this end. In the words of Robert F. Loeb: "These experiments constituted a pioneer approach to the interpretation of quantitative description in terms of the mechanisms involved. Meaning received the primary emphasis. The general design of the experiments devised by Gamble continues to be the pattern for most studies dealing with electrolyte and water metabolism today. Even the expression of data by simple graphic means, now known as 'Gambelian diagrams' or 'Gamblegrams,' has been generally adopted."[46]

Gamble emphasized that his work would not have been possible without the methods of measuring sodium, potassium, calcium, and magnesium that Kramer provided.[47]

The principal feature of Gamble's investigations was the remarkably clear demonstration that the total electrolyte concentration of the body fluids remained constant in the face of a great variety of drastic attacks; a constancy he showed to be closely dependent upon the acid-base construction of the urine. From these observations, he deduced the fundamental role of the concentration of electrolytes in extracellular fluid for determining the distribution of water among the body-fluid compartments.[48]

In 1931 Peters and Van Slyke epitomized these investigations as follows:

> A corollary of the generalization [Gamble's], that the total base concentration per unit of water in all tissues of the organism remains constant is that changes in the base and water content of the organism parallel one another. Gamble and his co-workers have demonstrated that measures which reduce the water content of the organism lead to the excretion of an equivalent amount of base and, conversely, measures which deplete base are attended by equivalent losses of water. Retention of base entails retention of water and accumulation of water is associated with storage of base. When the water changes affect chiefly the extracellular fluid, the base simultaneously retained or lost is chiefly sodium; when the cellular fluids are involved the base which accompanies them is chiefly potassium.[49]

These ideas of Gamble's form the basis for our understanding of dehydration and edema and for rational techniques of therapy.

At Harvard, Gamble studied the effect of various lesions of the gastrointestinal tract upon the volume and composition of body fluids. In 1933, with Allan M. Butler and Charles F. McKhann, he pointed out the potassium deficits in diarrheal disease, which Daniel C. Darrow and Gamble's pupil, Edward Pratt, reinforced the importance of a decade later. By 1939 Gamble had assembled his observations and experiments in a looseleaf syllabus, first privately printed and subsequently published by Harvard University Press, entitled "Chemical Anatomy, Physiology and Pathology of Extracellular Fluid." This medical classic had enormous impact upon a whole generation of medical students and physicians.[50]

In accepting the Kober Medal of the Association of American Physicians, Gamble spoke of his career as follows:

> In 1913 the gentle and kindly Folin gave me headspace . . . and I found it an exciting experience to learn these new techniques which made quantitative information so easy to come by . . . I had a great affection for Van Slyke's first $CO_2$ burette. It was not the larger machine of nowadays with the noisy mechanical shaker. One rocked it gently by hand as a little girl does her doll. . . .
>
> On leaving Folin's laboratory my luck continued. In a small chemistry laboratory at the MGH my classmate Bill Palmer was measuring pH in the urine for the first time and carrying out under Lawrence Henderson's guidance their classic description of the process of acid excretion . . . Henderson appeared about twice a week to see how Bill was getting on. It was evident that he did not like the clatter that I made dashing about the

laboratory tending my various analyses and one day he came over, placed his hand on my shoulder, and said: "Young man, you will never get anywhere in this game until you learn an attitude of leisure. . . ." I learned from him [Henderson] to admire the beauty of the physico-chemical systems which sustain the body fluids, the marvel of their automaticity and their remarkable resiliency in the presence of obstacles imposed by disease, and ever since I have been content to work in this field as an humble artisan applying the simple tool of quantitative description to the pattern provided by this great architect of concept.[51]

## William Sydney Thayer[52] as Professor of Medicine at Johns Hopkins

William Sydney Thayer refused the chairmanship of the department when Barker resigned in 1914. After Janeway's death in 1917, Mosenthal served as temporary chairman for a few months, and Thayer, when again offered the professorship, accepted. Before assuming his position, however, he went to Poland to investigate typhus fever. He then served as the chief medical consultant of the American Expeditionary Forces in France and did not assume his duties as professor until 1919. During the war, the full-time plan was temporarily in abeyance, and the medical department was ably directed by a part-time physician, Louis Hamman.[53]

Thayer received his M.D. degree from Harvard in 1889, after which he served as a house officer at the MGH. He then spent time abroad before coming to Johns Hopkins as an assistant resident physician in November 1890. In September 1891, he was appointed resident physician, a post he held for seven years.[54]

While abroad, Thayer acquired expertise in Ehrlich's new blood-staining technique. Thayer's experience with this new method attracted many physicians to the clinical laboratory to study under him.

In the 1890s, two infectious diseases—malaria and typhoid fever—were rampant in Baltimore. Thayer's studies were directed toward malaria.[55] The discovery of the malarial parasite by Alphonse Laveran, ten years earlier, had already been confirmed in America by Councilman and Osler. Thayer's investigations with John Hewetson enlarged this expanding subject, and Thayer's *Lectures on Malarial Fever*,[56] published in 1897, carried the new knowledge throughout the English-speaking world.

Thayer's studies of the physiological third heart sound, an auscultatory event he discovered with Hirschfelder about the same time as did Gibson of Edinburgh, and some two years after Obrastzow of Kiev, were exemplary. He thought that this sound was due to "the sudden tensing of the mitral leaflet and perhaps the tricuspid valve at the time of the first and most rapid phase of diastole.[57]

Thayer also introduced the term *opening snap* for the characteristic
sound heard in mitral stenosis. He was among the first to describe an
epigastric venous hum with hepatic cirrhosis.[58] With William G. MacCallum, he studied the effects of anemia in dogs upon the auscultatory
findings in the heart.[59] Thayer was one of the early clinicians to employ
blood cultures in the study of patients with fever and heart murmurs.
The first definitive proof of the existence of a gonococcal septicemia, as
well as of an ulcerative endocarditis due to the gonococcus, was reported
by Thayer and George Blumer in 1896.[60]

Thayer rapidly became a vital force in medicine in the United States.
In his delightful essay, "The Medical Education of Jones,"[61] he stated:
"Twenty-five years have passed by. Great changes have taken place in
medicine through the introduction of new procedures, both diagnostic
and therapeutic. Based on the application of the fundamental sciences,
remarkable advances have been made in the art and science of medicine.
Researches in no way inferior to those carried on in the laboratories of
the fundamental sciences are being pursued by members of the clinical
staff." With this advance, Thayer detected a "regrettable tendency"
against which he warned: "A sound basis in the fundamental sciences so
desirable for the trained and scholarly physician, is in no way a shortcut
to experience, practical and human, which always has been and always
will be necessary to make a good diagnostician, a good doctor and a good
clinical teacher." He insisted that interest in bacteriological, serological,
and chemical tests was indispensible, but that "the newer physical
methods of exploration should not lead us to forget the necessity of
prolonged and systematic training in ward and outpatient departments,
in pathological anatomy and in physical diagnosis." Thus, Thayer represented a transition between the old school and the modern school of
"physiological medicine."

A year before accepting the full-time professorship, Thayer gave an
address (May 9, 1916) in which he stated his views on a modern department of medicine.[62] Thayer believed that a department of medicine
should be a well-organized unit under the control of a single director
and a corps of associates and assistants. None of the directors of the
subdepartments should be expected to give any essential part of their
time to the practice of medicine. In the ideally arranged department of
medicine, however, all of these directors should have clinical duties and
responsibilities. Thayer felt it would be impossible for any man with a
consulting practice to organize and direct a medical clinic such as he
outlined. He came to the conclusion that there was a new class of consulting physicians. Long-continued service in institutions in which proper
opportunities for study and research were offered was creating men,
who, well-trained in modern methods of diagnosis and treatment, had
accumulated, at a relatively early stage, a store of actual clinical experience, such as is acquired in independent practice only after a much
greater time. It was from this class of men, in his opinion, that professor-

ships of medicine were more and more likely to be filled. In order to provide opportunities for students with scientific aspirations, there should be a considerable number of assistantships commanding salaries. Such salaries should be adequate to enable these men to continue their work for many years, should they prove themselves of suitable character and ability.

In Thayer's view, training that best fitted a man for professorship differed in no way from that which best qualified him for a career as a practitioner or a consultant. Some of the men who started their careers in modern departments of medicine would remain connected with these departments in one capacity or another for ten to fifteen years, or even more, until positions as professors at other large clinics were offered to them. As Thayer pointed out, however, many men, after eight to ten years' experience, would find themselves well fitted to enter the practice of medicine or surgery as consultants. Thayer concluded his discussion as follows: "No effort can be too great; no sacrifice too costly that may afford to the student of the medical sciences the most active stimuli, the best opportunities for training and for research."

## The Structure of the Department under Thayer

Thayer maintained the same departmental organization that Barker had instituted and recruited a promising group of young men.[63] Allen K. Krause, a leader in tuberculosis research, had been an assistant physician since September 1916. Edward Perkins Carter was placed in charge of the physiological research division (the heart station).

Carter[64] received his M.D. degree from the University of Pennsylvania in 1894. He became a resident house officer at the Johns Hopkins Hospital and, two years later, a fellow in pathology. In 1898 he was the first resident physician in the newly opened Lakeside Hospital in Cleveland. From 1912 to 1914 he worked with Sir Thomas Lewis. When the Cleveland City Hospital became affiliated with Western Reserve Medical School, in 1914, Carter became full-time chief of medicine there. His interest in research and the field of cardiovascular disease began early in his career. While still in practice, Carter acquired a Mackenzie polygraph, with which he obtained records of the heartbeat and pulse of patients in their homes. At Cleveland City Hospital, he had the first electocardiograph machine in his area. His study of bundle branch block is a classic. He was among the first to recognize the high alveolar $CO_2$ content and the unusual $CO_2$ tolerance of patients with emphysema. An important study on determination of the direction of the electrical axis of the heart was published, in 1919, with C. P. Richter and C. H. Greene. Francis Dieuaide[65] joined Carter soon after his arrival in Baltimore, and they carried out further studies in the same field.

From New York, Thayer recruited W. W. Palmer[66] as chief of the chemical division. After graduation from the Harvard Medical School in 1910, Palmer served two years as house officer at the MGH and was then appointed its first chief resident physician. During this residency, he worked under Lawrence J. Henderson, producing five important papers on the acid-base equilibrium of the blood. His work continued with Donald D. Van Slyke at the HRI, where Palmer was an assistant resident physician from 1915 to 1917. In 1917 Palmer served as acting director of the medical service of the Presbyterian Hospital.

Dana Atchley, a graduate of Johns Hopkins, returned to Baltimore from New York as Palmer's assistant, and Robert F. Loeb came from the MGH to be the assistant resident physician who would serve as Atchley's contact with the clinical service.

Alphonse Raymond Dochez, recruited as director of the biological division, was a 1907 graduate of the Johns Hopkins University School of Medicine. He had been an important member of Rufus I. Cole's pneumonia research group at the HRI for a number of years (see chapter 5). While in Baltimore, Dochez undertook his important investigations of the etiology of scarlet fever.[67] Prior to Dochez's arrival, Paul W. Clough[68] was in charge of the biological division.

There were a number of other talented younger scientists in the department, including A. L. Bloomfield, who worked in the biological research division (bacteriology) and who later became a professor of medicine at Leland Stanford University School of Medicine; William S. Ladd,[69] from New York, who later became dean at Cornell; Hugh J. Morgan, who became a professor of medicine at Vanderbilt University School of Medicine; George A. Harrop, Jr., later an associate professor in charge of the chemical division; Henry S. Willis, an associate of Krause's in the tuberculosis division; William S. Tillett, later a professor of medicine at the New York University School of Medicine; Henry Jackson, Jr., who had a distinguished career at the Boston City Hospital; and Henry M. Thomas, Jr., who became an associate professor at Johns Hopkins.[70] Verne R. Mason[71] was a resident in medicine at that time and, as such, was in a position of great power. He had been a classmate of Atchley's at the Johns Hopkins University School of Medicine.

The clinicians who had a great interest in demonstrating their skills in physical examination and who, for the most part, were strongly opposed to the full-time system, held sway during Thayer's regime. Their hostility to the full-time system was directed at the new arrivals, including Palmer, Dochez, Atchley, and Loeb, and not against the professor himself.

In 1921 Palmer received offers to be the head of the department of medicine at Yale, Michigan, and Harvard. Palmer was ultimately offered the position at Columbia. In Atchley's words: "When Hopkins saw that they were going to lose Palmer, Thayer resigned and they offered Palmer the headship of the department of medicine. Thus, he had some five top schools to choose from. . . . All the time he knew well that he wanted to go back to Columbia but he was cagey and investigated all the offers carefully which is what you should do."[72]

George Canby Robinson was asked to serve, during the year beginning July 1, 1921, as acting professor of medicine and physician-in-chief of the Johns Hopkins Hospital.[73] Vanderbilt University granted him a leave of absence; its administrators realized that the position would be an excellent preparation for his duties as dean and professor of medicine in Nashville.

## Professor Pro-Tempore: George Canby Robinson

During Robinson's year as professor, Bloomfield remained the associate professor in charge of the biological division;[74] Allen K. Krause continued as head of tuberculosis research, Clyde G. Guthrie[75] as head of the clinical laboratories, and Edward Perkins Carter as director of the physiological division. Krause was assisted by Henry S. Willis, who was an instructor, as was John G. Huck. In 1923 Huck[76] presented evidence that strongly indicated that the sickling phenomenon was a property of the red cell itself, inherited according to the Mendelian Law. Among the fellows were Harold J. Stewart,[77] who was to have a distinguished career in cardiology at the HRI and at Cornell; and John B. Youmans,[78] whose magnificent career in the field of nutrition began at Michigan and continued at Vanderbilt.

Robinson's first problem was to fill up the ranks of the department. Alan M. Chesney was recruited from Washington University, and William S. McCann from Cornell Medical College. Chesney, a Johns Hopkins graduate and former member of the Johns Hopkins Hospital house staff, had a thorough training in bacteriology at the HRI. He joined the faculty of Washington University just before the United States entered World War I and served in France at its base hospital. Chesney was assigned to direct the experimental research laboratory of the syphilis division of the medical clinic. His major research contributions were related to the study of immunity in syphilis.[79] McCann, who had trained under Eugene F. DuBois and Graham Lusk at Cornell, was director of the metabolic research division of the medical clinic until called to be a professor of medicine at the new medical school at the University of Rochester.

Robinson's task of selecting a resident physician proved most difficult. There was no one in Baltimore suitable for such a responsible post, and no one had ever been brought in from the outside to fill this position. On the recommendation of Roger I. Lee and Paul Dudley White of Harvard, the position was offered to C. Sidney Burwell.[80]

McCann described the department of medicine at Johns Hopkins in his unpublished memoirs:[81]

In the autumn of 1921 the medical clinic of the Johns Hopkins Hospital was in a state of flux. . . . As Canby Robinson reorganized the department he had several associate professors, each heading a division of the clinic. I was given charge of the metabolic or chemical division of the clinic. Each division had its own appropriate laboratory and also a ward of general medical patients on which he was to make the teaching rounds. Each division chief had an assistant resident physician attached to his ward for the entire year, and under him were the interns and the clinical clerks assigned to it.

Dr. Carter had two wards and two assistants, Dr. Francis Dieuaide and Dr. E. Cowles Andrus. The two wards were for colored patients, male and female. Before leaving New York I had sought the advice of Dr. W. W. Palmer, who counselled me to ask for the white men's ward "F," which could always be relied upon for a rich variety of clinical "material." When I arrived the daily ward rounds were being made by Dr. Louis Hamman, one of the senior physicians to the hospital, a man of great experience who was much sought after as a consultant and immensely popular with the fourth year students assigned to him as clinical clerks. . . .

The assistant resident physician on my ward was Dr. Roger Hannon, who was ultimately to become chief resident physician, and later to come to Rochester as an associate professor. He associated himself with my own research in the laboratory of the chemical division, and the metabolism ward.[82]

At this time there was great excitement over Banting's discovery of insulin. We were able to secure some of the earliest product of the Eli Lilly Company. . . . Soon we had a large number of patients in the hospital with severe diabetes, and at times Dr. Hannon and I were following 80 patients with this dreaded disease. . . . In order to make the insulin go as far as possible I felt that we needed more than ever to bring patients under the closest dietary control. . . .

About this time Hannon and I were studying in the metabolism ward some patients with severe diabetic acidosis. We were testing the ideas of Dr. Rollin T. Woodyatt in trying to balance the ketogenic and antiketogenic substances in the metabolism at the threshold at which acetone and diacetic acid would appear in the urine. . . .

Woodyatt had calculated that the glycerol derived from the fat was antiketogenic. This led us to add glycerol to the diet of acidotic patients, and we found this to be a ready method of bringing acidosis under control, and one which could still be used as a temporary measure when a supply of insulin was not available. . . .

Dr. Halsted, who was still surgeon-in-chief at this time, asked me to see one of his patients who was in severe tetany. This patient had a large diaphragmatic hernia within which was what the newspapers called an "upside down stomach." When I saw her she was in severe tetany with spasmodic contractures of both hands and feet. She had had a prolonged period of vomiting, so that I felt sure we were dealing with the same sort of situation which I had produced in dogs when I was in Boston with Harvey Cushing. Quickly we drew blood for determination of the carbon dioxide combining power and found it to be very high. . . . I dissolved 5 grams of ammonium chloride in water and introduced it into the rectum of the patient by means of a small catheter, in the belief that the neutral salt $NH_4Cl$ would be absorbed into the portal blood stream, and that on arrival at the liver the ammonium ions would be converted into urea leaving the chloride ions to replace those lost by the patient in her prolonged vomiting. We were rewarded by seeing the spasms relax as the tetany was relieved. Another blood sample drawn revealed a pronounced drop in the $CO_2$ combining power to normal levels.... This simple demonstration of the bedside application of biochemical knowledge made a deep impression on the students who took an increased interest in what was going on in our "metabolic" division of the medical clinic.

## Warfield Theobald Longcope as Professor

Warfield Theobald Longcope[83] was appointed professor, in March 1922, and assumed office in July of that year. He had received his A.B. degree (1897) and his M.D. degree (1901) from Johns Hopkins. Although he had no way of anticipating his ultimate appointment as the third full-time professor of medicine at Johns Hopkins, Longcope's training prepared him admirably for this post. As Tillett pointed out:

> It is very informative to follow Dr. Longcope's career after graduation since his growth reflects what was taking place in relation to medical education and the preparation for academic medicine during that period. During his four years in medical school he had close contacts with Welch, Halsted, Osler, Mall, Howell and Kelly. It was Mall in particular who opened a door that let him see both the rewards and difficulties of medical research. From Johns Hopkins, Longcope went to the Pennsylvania Hospital in Philadelphia as resident pathologist. It seems paradoxical that this great American clinician took no medical internship. At the time Longcope went to Philadelphia, experimentation in clinical medicine was almost unheard of. Observations made at the bedside were with very simple forms of apparatus, inquiries into the etiology of disease were carried out with rather crude bacteriological techniques, and pathological examinations of material obtained at autopsy formed the major basis for clinical studies. Venapuncture for bacteriological culture was such an innovation that he recalled "as a daring novice trembling with apprehension I made the first blood cultures ever performed at the Pennsylvania Hospital."[84]

While working at the Ayer Laboratory under the direction of Simon Flexner, Longcope began his studies in immunology. His activities there included work in pathology, biochemistry, bacteriology, and serology. He also visited the wards frequently and gave advice about the diagnosis and treatment of patients. In 1909 he received an additional appointment, as an assistant professor of applied clinical medicine at the University of Pennsylvania. When he finished his term of service at the Pennsylvania Hospital, he was a uniquely trained academician who set a new standard of learning in several scientific disciplines, all of which merged in a broader approach to the problems of disease and an under-standing of its nature, both etiologically and pathologically. In 1911 he was appointed an associate professor of medicine at Columbia's College of Physicians and Surgeons. When Janeway left for Baltimore, Longcope, aged thirty-seven, succeeded him as Bard Professor. He re-signed this position one year before he assumed the professorship of medicine in Baltimore in 1922.

Longcope saw the superficial analogies between serum disease and acute Bright's disease. Although his studies did not throw much direct light upon the origin of acute nephritis, they did arouse an interest in the general subject of anaphylaxis and allergy; Longcope became one of the pioneers in this area.[85] Crude experiments made at that time showed that inflammatory reactions occurred in the kidneys, involving par-ticularly the glomeruli, when animals sensitized to a specific protein were reinjected with the same antigen or, indeed, in some animals within three weeks after the injection of a single large dose of antigen. Later, the realization that acute infections such as tonsillitis and scarlet fever frequently preceded the onset of acute glomerular nephritis induced Longcope to concentrate attention on this association. Dochez's démon-stration that scarlet fever was the result of an infection with hemolytic streptococci, combined with Bela Schick's suggestion that many of the complications of scarlet fever could be interpreted as allergic reactions, formed further incentives for Longcope's work along these lines. His studies on nephritis were continued in Baltimore with the aid of Drs. D. P. O'Brien, O. Hansen, W. A. Winkenwerder, James Bordley III, Robert H. Williams, Charles Janeway, Francis Lukens, Calvin· F. Kay, and others.

Longcope's classic paper, "Clinical Features of the Contracted Kidney Due to Pyelonephritis," written in collaboration with Winkenwerder, was published in the *Johns Hopkins Hospital Bulletin.* [86] Here, for the first time, the fully developed clinical picture of chronic nephritis due to bilateral pyelonephritis with shrunken kidneys was clearly described and its im-portance emphasized. A notable contribution was Longcope's excellent study, with British Anti-Lewisite (BAL) during World War II, for use in the treatment of metallic poisoning by such substances as arsenic and mercury. Other examples of his brilliance at clinical observation were his description of the syndrome of sarcoidosis (1937)[87] and his early report on mycoplasma pneumonia (1940).[88] Of greater diagnostic value than the streptococcus m.g. agglutination in this disease is the appearance, late in the illness, of cold agglutinins for human type "O" red cells, a phenomenon first described in 1918 by two members of the house staff in medicine at the Johns Hopkins Hospital—Ina Richter and Mildred Clough.[89]

Longcope not only stimulated research activity in clinical fields during his tenure at Columbia and at Johns Hopkins, but he also served as a bridge between the old-time clinician and the modern clinical investigator. Upon being awarded the George M. Kober Medal of the Association of American Physicians, Longcope spoke as follows:

> But all of us who have spent much time in the wards of a hospital are subject to the irresistible temptation of describing rare forms of disease, or of recounting the clinical features presented by a group of patients suffering from a malady that has not previously been clearly defined. Though information gained from this simple type of observation, in which I must confess to have indulged, still has some place in clinical medicine, we all know that the most fertile field of work lies in the investigation of the fundamental processes that form the basis of disease in man.[90]

Thus, Longcope was one of that generation of Renaissance physicians who had the ability to perform skillfully both in the clinic and in the laboratory, an ability that is still important if one is to maintain leadership in the training of young physicians who may ultimately find their career pattern in clinical science.[91]

## Organization of the New Osler Clinic

In 1928 Longcope had the opportunity to redesign the medical clinic of the Johns Hopkins Hospital.[92] This new clinic was planned as a complete unit containing wards, dispensaries, laboratories for students, laboratories for routine work and for investigation, and rooms and small amphitheatres for teaching. The facilities for research were organized along essentially the same lines that Barker had started in 1905. There was a chemical division, a physiological division, and a biological division. The chemical suite consisted of a small laboratory for an individual worker, a large research laboratory, a balance room, a darkroom, iceboxes, a routine chemical laboratory, a laboratory planned for work in physical chemistry, a laboratory for gas analysis, a room designed for metabolic determinations, and two offices. The physiological suite consisted of one large laboratory for general physiological work, an experimental laboratory with operating tables, a galvanometer room, a darkroom, an office, and a technician's room. The Kenneth Dows Tuberculosis Research Laboratories[93] occupied floor space of 56 by 45 feet. There were two large and two small laboratories, an office, a room for a secretary, a darkroom, a preparation room, an incubator room, a technician's room, and a storeroom. The suite of laboratories for research and routine work in bacteriology and serology extended 125 feet. There was a moderate-sized room for general diagnostic work in bacteriology and serology, a large laboratory for student research work, five rooms for individual workers, two offices, a room for a secretary, a large thermostat room, cold rooms, and a room for transplanting cultures.

In 1930 the new Osler medical clinic opened. The fifth floor was devoted to a metabolism ward for clinical investigation. This grew out of an earlier unit created in 1916, when the trustees of the hospital authorized a metabolism ward, where patients whose illnesses required special dietetic measures could be studied. The ward, which consisted of four beds, was adjoined by a diet kitchen.

On the medical staff were those who devoted their entire time to the department and those who were in practice and devoted only part time. There were five full-time associate professors, each responsible for a clinical service. In addition to their ward responsibilities, one associate professor directed the routine biological laboratories, another directed the routine physiological laboratories, while a third had charge of the clinical chemical laboratories. One associate professor was director of the Kenneth Dows Tuberculosis Research Laboratories, and another was in charge of the syphilis laboratories and of the student course in clinical microscopy. Aside from the technical assistance in the laboratories, each associate professor had one or more instructors or fellows as assistants. The resident and, as a rule, one assistant resident were especially associated in their work with the professor, whereas each of the other assistant residents conducted his work under the supervision of the associate professor to whose ward he was assigned. This system gave the resident and each assistant resident considerable responsibility on the medical wards but, at the same time, gave them an opportunity to carry on some clinical investigation under the direction of a more experienced physician.[94]

## The Scientific Family of Warfield Theobald Longcope

During his tenure of almost a quarter of a century as chairman of the department of medicine at Johns Hopkins, Longcope had an important influence on a large number of young students in medicine who later went on to have distinguished careers in medical science. A productive group of clinical scientists under his guidance populated the research divisions of the department.[95]

### The Chemical Division

When William S. McCann moved to the University of Rochester School of Medicine as departmental chairman, in 1924, George A. Harrop, Jr., returned to head the chemical division. Harrop made important studies of the adrenal cortex and various metabolic problems before leaving, in 1936, to become director of the research laboratories at E. R. Squibb and Son.[96] It was Harrop who first had a definite concept of the  mineralocorticoid action of the adrenal cortex. Harrop (M.D., Johns Hopkins, 1916) began his career as a house officer on the medical service of the Johns Hopkins Hospital. From there he went to the Presbyterian Hospital in New York City, serving as chief resident under Palmer. From 1923 to 1924, he was an associate professor of medicine in Peking Union Medical College, and it was from that institution that he returned to Baltimore.

In the academic year 1929–30, William A. Perlzweig, the chemist to the medical clinic who came from New York with McCann in 1924, left to occupy the chair of biochemistry at the newly organized Duke University School of Medicine. Perlzweig was a graduate of Columbia. While at Johns Hopkins, his investigations concerned certain aspects of immunology, the properties of semipermeable membranes, and, later, the development of improved methods for the quantitative determination of bile derivatives in the blood.

Read McLane Ellsworth (M.D., Johns Hopkins, 1924) served for two years as a house officer at the MGH. On returning to Baltimore, in 1926, he was an assistant resident for two years and then a resident physician. He remained on the staff as a full-time member of the chemical division, where he pursued his interest in the pathological physiology of the parathyroid gland.[97] He also collaborated with Harrop in his studies of mineralocorticoid control by the adrenal cortex. Shortly thereafter, he developed tuberculosis, which led to his death in 1936.

In 1930 John Eager Howard (M.D., Johns Hopkins, 1928) became an assistant in medicine. After two years as a house officer at the MGH, he returned to Johns Hopkins to complete his residency training. He was a fellow in medicine (1932–35) and then joined the chemical division, under Harrop.

Howard's research contributions illustrate the meaning of serendipity, as well as creative talent and ingenuity. In 1937 Barker and Howard analyzed the clinical syndrome in individuals with pheochromocytoma.[98] Because of this work, they were asked to see a patient who recently had a normal appendix removed. Hypertension developed abruptly after the operation. Because of the suspicion, from x-ray findings, of an adrenal tumor, the patient was explored, but no tumor was found. The surgeon removed the kidney, however, in the mistaken belief that it was cancerous. The patient's blood pressure promptly became normal. The lesion proved to be an infarcted area to which the blood flow had been abruptly diminished. Thus, an extraordinary series of circumstances and "errors of both head and hand" led to the patient's cure.

Some fifteen years later, this unique clinical event yielded fruit of wider scientific moment. A patient had a normal appendix removed and then developed severe hypertension. After exhaustive tests, his physician concluded that he had hemorrhagic nephritis. Howard remembered the previous experience. As in the first patient, an operation was performed, with similar findings; the blood pressure returned to normal after removal of the kidney. Thus, Howard opened up the area of unilateral renal hypertension and then greatly advanced our knowledge concerning its recognition and management.

Howard did significant work on kidney stones, demonstrating that in uremic serum there is a factor preventing deposition of calcium phosphate crystals in rat cartilage. In the search for a possible inhibiting factor, Howard and William C. Thomas put rachitic cartilages in normal urine. Despite an enormous concentration of calcium and phosphorus in the urine, the cartilage failed to calcify. Urine from the first four patients who suffered from kidney stones did, however, calcify the cartilage, although the calcium and phosphorus content of their urine was no higher than normal. Howard and Thomas soon found that an inhibitor to calcification is normally present in urine and in blood.[99]

Other investigators at Johns Hopkins have contributed importantly to our knowledge of the adrenal glands, beginning with William Osler, who studied six cases of Addison's disease, with report of a case greatly benefited by the use of the suprarenal extract.[100] Osler emphasized the need of preparing the extract from fresh glands that are kept cold. He used hog adrenals, and, years later, it was demonstrated that hogs have a much higher concentration of corticoids in their adrenals than do grazing animals. Furthermore, Osler recommended extracting the glands with glycerin; this was also shown by Arthur Grollman, another Johns Hopkins contributor, to be a particularly effective solvent for adrenal steroids.

George W. Thorn was also a major Johns Hopkins contributor to this field. In November 1930, Hartman and Thorn described a standard assay for adrenal cortical extracts, based on maintenance of the normal growth curve in adrenalectomized rats. In 1931 they demonstrated that their extract could maintain patients with Addison's disease for a prolonged period. By 1936, while at Ohio State University as an assistant professor of physiology, Thorn demonstrated that the administration of a potent adrenal cortical extract could modify the renal excretion of electrolytes in normal subjects. In that year Thorn joined George A. Harrop, Jr., in Baltimore.[101] Harrop had developed an excellent technique for carrying out mineral balance studies on dogs. The standardization of the metabolic cages for the experimental animals, the technique for repeated bladder catheterizations, the well-controlled diets, and, above all, the skill of Harrop's laboratory associate, Harry Eisenberg, were important in laying the groundwork for future explorations in this field of medical research.

In 1937, when Harrop accepted the post of medical director of Squibb, Longcope asked Thorn to head the chemical division. Thorn invited Lewis Engel, a young steroid chemist who was at that time studying in Zurich, to join him. Thorn and his collaborators made outstanding contributions to our knowledge of adrenal physiology and Addison's disease.[102] The first instance of desoxycorticosterone acetate (DCA)–induced hypokalemic paralysis was reported in 1940 by Thorn and Warfield M. Firor. Severe paralysis occurred in a patient with Addison's disease who was given large quantities of DCA and supplementary saline and glucose solution. There was complete recovery following reduction in DCA dosage and supplementary feeding of foods high in potassium.

Thorn gives the following account of the early use of the special clinical research facility (Osler 5) during his period at Johns Hopkins:

When George Harrop, Jr. left in 1937 I was responsible for the operation of Osler V, the routine biochemistry laboratory (supervised by Mary Buell) and the research laboratories of the chemical division.

The hospital did not charge the patients. It was my responsibility to recruit the nurses. George Koepf joined me as a research fellow. His wife was a graduate nurse and she recruited from her friends at the Buffalo General Hospital who enjoyed a year in Baltimore.

Dr. Longcope made regular rounds on Osler V and we had some of Dr. Taussig's polycythemic cardiac patients who received DCA to reduce their hematocrit. . . .

Palmer Howard was one of our first fellows and Kendall Emerson was one of the early residents.

In summary, this was an extremely efficient and effective research unit, combining patient care, clinical investigation, student and house staff teaching, and basic research in the biochemical laboratories, economically operated by having a joint relationship with the routine laboratory under Mary Buell.[103]

In 1942 Thorn became Hersey Professor of the Theory and Practice of Physic at the Harvard Medical School, as well as physician-in-chief at the Peter Bent Brigham Hospital. His career since leaving Johns Hopkins included not only the continuance of his productive work in the study of the adrenal gland and its diseases, but also many other important endeavors in the field of endocrinology and renal disease.[104]

## The Physiological Division

In 1927 E. Cowles Andrus[105] joined Carter in the physiological division. Andrus (M.D., Johns Hopkins, 1921) was a house officer (1921–22) and an assistant resident physician (1922–23) in medicine at the Johns Hopkins Hospital. He received a fellowship from the National Research Council and studied in London and Vienna from 1923 to 1925, returning to Baltimore as chief medical resident (1925–27). Andrus's research interests were always related to the heart. Between 1921 and 1936 he and Carter reported a number of studies on the mechanism of cardiac rhythm. In 1921 they demonstrated that increase in the pH of the perfusate of the amphibian heart increased heart rate and accelerated conduction, and vice versa. They advanced the theory that the rhythmic polarization and depolarization of the cell membrane and, therewith, the potential difference so developed and discharged, was because of the gradient in hydrogen ion concentration across the cell boundary. They later extended this concept to explain ectopic arrhythmias, assuming that local changes in hydrogen ion gradient increased local excitability. In 1937 Andrus produced anaphylaxis in the isolated perfused hearts of guinea pigs sensitized to horse serum. The reactions, which included tachycardia and decreased coronary flow, were mimicked by the injection of small amounts of histamine. In 1940, with Philip Hill, Andrus showed that angiotensin provoked constriction of the coronary arteries in a perfused heart and also conspicuously increased cardiac output in the heart-lung preparation. This finding was overlooked until 1960, when it was confirmed by Jan Koch-Weser and others.

Among the fellows who worked under Carter and Andrus, many later had distinguished careers in academic medicine. Perhaps the most important, in terms of the significance of his research, was W. H. Craib, a South African who later became professor of medicine at the University of Witwaterstrand in Johannesburg. As a novice in research, Craib took a critical view of J. Bernstein's "membrane theory" and conceived the hypothesis that the excitatory process is due to the formation of electrical dipoles or doublets. Despite the storm raised over his revolutionary ideas, Craib's conclusions have been abundantly confirmed and form the basis of our present understanding of electrocardiography and vector-cardiography.[106]

Another fellow, Donald McEachern, became professor of neurology at the Montreal Neurological Institute.[107] John K. Lewis, who worked with him, became a member of the faculty at Stanford, under Hewlett and, later, Bloomfield.

Three important fellows who remained at Johns Hopkins were Benjamin M. Baker, Caroline Bedell Thomas, and Helen Taussig.[108]

## Hematology

Alan M. Chesney continued his productive studies of immunity in syphilis and, in addition, was responsible for the clinical microscopy laboratory, which included hematology.

In 1929 Maxwell M. Wintrobe[109] became a member of the department of medicine. Wintrobe's graduation from the University of Manitoba medical school in 1926 coincided with Minot's discovery of liver therapy for pernicious anemia. As a research fellow, Wintrobe's goal was to reproduce pernicious anemia experimentally. In 1927 he went to Tulane University, where his attention was drawn to the virtually nonexistent knowledge of normal blood standards and the gross inaccuracy of the methods used for estimating hemoglobin content and red blood cell numbers. He began work on this problem, and the Wintrobe hematocrit tube was soon devised. Out of this invention grew the idea of the calculation of the indices of the red cells, which became a basic technique in modern hematology. These developments made it possible, for the first time, to propose a sound morphological classification of the anemias. John Musser, Jr., Wintrobe's chief at Tulane, asked him to assist in the writing of the hematology section in Tice's *System of Medicine*. The result was a classic monograph on hematology, based largely on Wintrobe's own work, which ultimately led to Wintrobe's famous book, entitled *Clinical Hematology*.

Wintrobe wrote an article, "The Erythrocyte in Man," that was published in *Medicine* in 1930. Alan M. Chesney, editor of the journal, recognized the talent of this young physician, who was highly recommended by Raymond Pearl, of the School of Hygiene and Public Health, whom Wintrobe had consulted about the statistics involved in his (Wintrobe's) studies on normal blood values. Chesney invited him to join the staff at Johns Hopkins, as his assistant in clinical microscopy. At Johns Hopkins, Wintrobe continued to study the pathogenesis of pernicious anemia. Knowing that Ehrlich had described the early blood cells of the embryo and fetus as megaloblastic, Wintrobe decided to study the blood of the embryo and fetus in man whenever possible, but, more importantly, in animals. The most dramatic finding was that the younger the fetus, the more striking the macrocytosis. In his effort to reproduce pernicious anemia, Wintrobe then studied the newborn pig during the growth phase while the pig was on a diet lacking an extrinsic factor. From these studies came observations concerning the role played by various vitamins in blood formation, and the effect of a deficiency of these vitamins on the blood and on the nervous system.

Wintrobe reported the first case of cryoglobulinemia and described thalessemia minor. In 1943 he was invited to head the department of medicine in the new medical school of the University of Utah.

## The Biological Division

When Longcope assumed chairmanship of the department in 1922, A. L. Bloomfield was the director of the biological division. In 1926 Bloomfield,[110] who had done outstanding work in the field of infectious diseases and in the study of gastric secretion, succeeded Albion W. Hewlett, a Johns Hopkins graduate, as professor of medicine at Stanford. Allen K. Krause and Henry S. Willis continued their outstanding work on experimental tuberculosis.[111]

Longcope recruited Harold L. Amoss to direct the biological laboratory. After obtaining his B.S. degree in 1905, from the University of Kentucky, Amoss worked for two years as a chemist for the Kentucky Agricultural Experiment Station and the Hygienic Laboratory of the U.S. Public Health Service. During this time, he obtained his M.S. degree from Kentucky. Four years later, he graduated from the Harvard Medical School and, one year after that, received the degree of Doctor of Public Health from Harvard. In 1912 he went to the Rockefeller Institute for Medical Research, where he was associated with Simon Flexner. He worked with meningococcus infections and participated actively in the development of antimeningococcus serum. During his eight years at Johns Hopkins, he was active in teaching and in research in infectious diseases. In 1930 he became professor of medicine at Duke University, where he was one of the original faculty members. Three years later he moved to Greenwich, Connecticut, where he developed a large practice.[112]

In 1929 William S. Tillett assumed charge of the biological division.

Tillett received his A.B. degree, in 1913, from the University of North Carolina and his M.D. degree from Johns Hopkins four years later. After World War I, he returned to Johns Hopkins, for an internship and an assistant residency in medicine. In 1922 he worked in the laboratory of Oswald T. Avery at the HRI and also participated in Rivers's studies on vaccinia. Tillett's research focused on the biology of the pneumococcus and the streptococcus, as well as on the role of immunity in infectious diseases. At Johns Hopkins, he explored a chance observation on the lysis of blood clots by streptococcal cultures that occurred in tubes that had been left standing. This original observation led to a series of classical studies that resulted in the discovery of streptokinase and streptodornase. In 1937 Tillett accepted the chairmanship of the department of bacteriology at New York University School of Medicine. The following year, he became director of the department of medicine at New York University and moved to Bellevue Hospital. Work done there in association with Sol Sherry culminated in the isolation, identification, and partial purification of streptokinase and streptodornase from streptococcal filtrates. Tillett and his associates pioneered the principles of enzymatic dissolution of thromboemboli and the enzymatic debridement of purulent exudates. Tillett also carried out some of the early clinical studies on penicillin in the treatment of pneumococcal infections.[113] He combined enzymatic therapy with penicillin to reduce the need for surgery in empyema. The high standards of excellence set by Tillett in his research inspired a series of young investigators, whose work led to the development of a distinguished department of medicine at New York University.

In 1929, with Tillett's departure for New York, Perrin Hamilton Long became director of the biological division. Long and Eleanor A. Bliss were the pioneer American workers in sulfonamide therapy.[114] They had previously been developing specific antisera for the treatment of streptococcal infections. Their work was well advanced when, in early 1936, after reading reports about prontosil in the German literature, they became interested in the sulfonamide compounds. Obtaining supplies of the material, they studied experimental hemolytic streptococcal infections in mice, with what appeared to be miraculous results. They then began their monumental study of this drug and, later, of sulfanilamide in streptococcal and other infections in man. By November 1936, they had accumulated enough data to warrant a report before the Baltimore meeting of the Southern Medical Association. Their first report was published in the *Journal of the American Medical Association* on January 2, 1937. Later they teamed up with E. Kennerly Marshall, Jr., whose development of a method of estimating the concentration of these drugs in serum led to observations that laid the foundation for the science of chemotherapy.

Perrin Hamilton Long[115] attended the University of Michigan and, after service in World War I, obtained his M.D. degree there. In 1924 he went to Boston for three years, first as a fellow in the Thorndike Laboratory, and then as an intern and resident in the fourth medical service of the Boston City Hospital. His chief was Francis W. Peabody. After this, he spent several months at the Hygienic Institute in Freiburg, Germany, and, in 1927, joined the staff of the Rockefeller Institute. Here, under the guidance of Simon Flexner and Peter Olitsky, he began his work in the field of infectious disease, concentrating on problems in virology.

Eleanor A. Bliss received her Doctor of Science degree from the Johns Hopkins University School of Hygiene and Public Health in 1925. As a fellow in the department of medicine, she worked with Amoss on recurrent erysipelas, showing that it could be prevented by immunization with hemolytic streptococcal toxin. In 1930 she joined in Long's study of the common cold and was delegated to make friends with fourteen chimpanzees. After this project was terminated, Bliss continued to work with Long, and, in 1931, they identified the "minute" hemolytic streptococci, which seemed to be particularly prevalent in the throats of patients with nephritis and rheumatic fever. They were attempting to produce type-specific streptococcal antisera in some forty rabbits, housed in the chimpanzee quarters atop the old physiology building, when the sulfonamide era arrived.[116]

## Other Members of Longcope's Department

Among those who served on the faculty, on the resident staff, or in fellowship positions during Longcope's tenure were C. Sidney Burwell, later to become professor of medicine at Vanderbilt and then at Harvard, where he was also dean; Chester A. Keefer,[117] who was later to become an important member of the Thorndike Laboratory in Boston and professor of medicine at Boston University; Bruce Webster, who worked with Chesney on the goitrogenic substance in cabbage and later became clinical professor of medicine at Cornell; Tinsley R. Harrison, who became professor of medicine at Vanderbilt and later at Winston-Salem, Southwestern, and, finally, Alabama; E. G. Guzman-Barron, who became professor of biochemistry at the University of Chicago; Fuller Albright, who was to make his name in clinical endocrinology at the MGH; George P. Berry, who became professor of bacteriology at Rochester and later dean of the Harvard Medical School; James Bordley III, who, after serving with A. N. Richards in Philadelphia, returned to Longcope's faculty and, ultimately, became professor of medicine at Columbia and director of the Mary Imogene Bassett Hospital in Cooperstown, New York; F. D. W. Lukens, who became professor of medicine at Pennsylvania and director of the Cox Laboratory for Research in Diabetes; R. L. Waterfield, who returned to Guy's Hospital, London, as director of hematology; Harry S. Eagle, who became professor of microbiology at the Albert Einstein School of Medicine; Hugh Levell, who became professor of public health at Harvard; Thomas

MacPhearson Brown, who became professor of medicine at George Washington; Alan Bernstein, who became a distinguished Baltimore internist; Charles Janeway, who became professor of pediatrics at Harvard; A. McGehee Harvey, who succeeded Longcope as professor of medicine at Johns Hopkins; Joseph L. Lilienthal, Jr., who became professor of environmental medicine in the Johns Hopkins University School of Hygiene and Public Health; W. Barry Wood, who became professor of medicine at Washington University and later professor of microbiology at Johns Hopkins; Ludwig W. Eichna, who became professor of medicine at the Long Island School of Medicine in Brooklyn; Robert W. Wilkins, who became professor of medicine at Boston University; and Charles Ragan, who became professor of medicine at Columbia.[118]

# Summary

No single event has had a more profound effect on medical education and medical practice than the movement to full-time positions in clinical departments. Out of this emerged the clinical scientist, versed in the bedside practice of medicine and capable of applying the knowledge and techniques of the basic sciences to the study of human disease. He occupied the position of middle man in the medical world—a compleat clinician who served to bridge the gap between the practicing physician and the laboratory-based scientist.

The senior clinicians of the last part of the nineteenth century did not have, for the most part, sufficient background to appreciate what physiology and biochemistry had to offer to future developments in medical practice. There were few among them like James B. Herrick, who, upon finding himself unable to understand articles involving biochemical studies, took time from his practice to study chemistry both at home and abroad. It was the basic scientists, including Ludwig, Mall, Welch, Bowditch, and Newell Martin, who understood the need to make the clinical branches true university departments. This need became more evident with each passing year, and, by the time of the Flexner Report (1910), it was the overriding concern about the medical schools' structure and their ability to advance knowledge and accelerate the creation of a scientific base for medical practice. At the time of the Flexner Report, changes in the professionalization of the basic sciences were already well under way. Flexner's main target was to stimulate improvement in the organization of the clinical departments.

The implementation of full-time professorships took place over a number of years, during which ideas changed on the basis of experience, leading to various modifications. It seems reasonable to assume from the available evidence that the rigid "all or none" approach taken in the beginning stemmed from the opposition met as the idea germinated and took shape. There was a storm of protest following Barker's famous address, and, as the implementation of full-time reached fruition, the exchanges became more bitter and more personal. The feeling that role models had to be created, and that halfway measures would be circumvented by the part-time professors chosen for such posts, probably accounts for the firm stand against the receiving of any fees by the full-time professor.

Although Barker was a strong advocate of full-time clinical professorships, he could not be provided with one when he succeeded Osler at Johns Hopkins, because there was not sufficient endowment to support it. Barker had a large private practice within a short time, and, when offered a full-time professorship, in 1914, he refused it. This undoubtedly helped reinforce the strict full-time salary arrangement insisted on by Gates and supported by Welch.

This demand for total dedication in an environment charged with emotion set off a controversy, which continued in many centers for decades and has still not ended. Some clinicians were quick to perceive that it was the basic scientists who gave the major impetus to the development of full-time clinical positions. They derided the idea as an impractical scheme formulated by a group who had no knowledge about clinical medicine and its teaching. Negative reaction stemmed from a number of factors. These included pride; insecurity of part-time incumbents in terms of loss of prestige (for it was prestige that generated patient flow); competition with full-time faculty for hospital beds for private patients; and competition in terms of lower pay scales, if charges were made by full-time practitioners who generated money for the hospital or school and, in turn, received a salary. The idea of turning over a fee to a third party (which Bevan called fee-splitting) was repugnant to Janeway. In large measure, the outcome was determined by the attitude and the power of the local practitioners. In the department of medicine at Johns Hopkins, the senior part-time faculty, many of whom were protégés of Osler, formed a determined opposition, and the controversy was bitter. The same situation existed at Cornell. Most of these factors did not enter the picture in pediatrics, and Howland's department at Johns Hopkins was the first truly successful full-time university department, as envisioned by Mall.

In the setting of vocal opposition by the part-time professors who were, at the same time, the leading practitioners in the community, young men with the potential for a successful academic career on a full-time basis were slow to choose such a career. There were a number of reasons for this reluctance; there were only meager facilities for clinical research, there were no role models to stimulate them, and the number of potential career positions was minimal. Most of the hospital beds were still in control of the local practitioners, because—with few exceptions—the medical schools did not have their own hospitals, or affiliations with appropriate institutions that gave them control over beds, staff appointments, and 'the making of general policy. Since Johns Hopkins had its own hospital, it was able to find the best man for each position. Such control of a hospital service was not available at Harvard until 1912, when David Linn Edsall became a professor at the MGH, and, a little later, Christian and Cushing had the necessary authority at the Peter Bent Brigham Hospital. Arthur Ellis remarked that it was an act of faith on the part of all of the residents at the HRI that, under the leadership of Rufus I. Cole, they were preparing themselves for full-time professorships, which did not exist.

There were a few clinicians who were ahead of their time and were so highly motivated to do clinical research that they were virtually "full-time" before such positions were formally established at Johns Hopkins. A notable example in medicine is Edsall, who discouraged patient referrals in order to conserve his time for investigation. In the field of surgery, William Stewart Halsted provides another specific example. There were undoubtedly others, particularly those who had an independent source of income. As soon as there were facilities and role models to provide the proper incentive, recruitment was no problem. Barker's full-time research divisions were populated with young men eager to engage in clinical investigation, and Cole had no difficulty in recruiting outstanding young men for residency positions at the HRI.

It should be emphasized that Welch did not feel that full-time professors should not see private patients. The key point was the method of payment. This appears to have been a stipulation of the granting agency—the General Education Board. At Columbia, withdrawal of Rockefeller support was threatened when there was a move to relax the strict full-time status and to allow limited collection of fees by the full-time staff. At Harvard, Edsall did not receive Rockefeller support, because he felt that, although private practice should be limited, fees should go to the responsible physician. The attitude of Gates and his colleagues at the General Education Board is understandable. In the private sector, corporations paid full salaries to their employees, in return for full-time attention to their duties within the corporation, and the board looked upon the university–clinical professor relationship as analogous.

In the long run, the issue of full-time was not a matter of how the books were kept; it was a matter of motivation. In the early years at least, most of the men who assumed full-time positions were more concerned with the facilities and support that would enable them to do their research. They did not expect to receive in salary what their practicing colleagues received in patient fees. Mall was, of course, so motivated to see full-time clinical chairs established at Johns Hopkins that he advocated salary levels at twice those of the full-time basic scientists.

Perhaps progress would have been smoother if the opposing forces in the battle over full-time could have made an effective compromise at the beginning. There is reason to believe, however, that the idea would never have come to fruition without the strong approach that was taken. Joseph T. Wearn, who became professor of medicine and dean at Case Western Reserve University School of Medicine, emphasized this in terms of his experience at the University of Pennsylvania, where Stengal insisted that everyone in the department of medicine must earn his living through practice. This delayed the latter university's achievement of an outstanding position in clinical science.

Implementation of the full-time plan in the clinical departments at Johns Hopkins met with variable success. In surgery, implementation was no problem; Halsted had been on a quasi-full-time status in that, because of his deep interest in clinical investigation and the physical limitations imposed by his cocaine addiction, he engaged in little private practice.

In pediatrics, the plan was outstandingly successful. The private patients in the hospital were taken care of exclusively by John F. Howland, the professor, with the able assistance of his perennial resident pediatrician, Kenneth Blackfan, who later had a distinguished career as professor of pediatrics at Harvard.

Howland, and the outstanding staff of clinical scientists he assembled, presided over the flowering of biochemistry as a research tool, leading to advances that were largely responsible for the emergence of scientifically based pediatric practice. The full-time movement in the pediatric department was enthusiastically entered into from the start and served as a model of what the full-time principles could contribute in terms of improvement in medical education and medical practice.

In medicine, the course was more difficult. Janeway recruited a full-time staff and encouraged clinical science. The opposition of the part-time staff, however, and Janeway's belief, on the basis of his experience, that continuing contact with private patients was essential and that fees should go to physicians, impaired progress. It seems reasonable to assume that Janeway might have resigned for these and other reasons, if the war and his untimely death from pneumococcal pneumonia had not intervened. The interim period at Johns Hopkins was one of decline in achieving established goals. Thayer recruited an outstanding group of young men for the full-time staff, but the clique that was opposed to the full-time principle created a difficult environment in which to develop the plan. As a result, when W. W. Palmer received multiple offers to go elsewhere, he returned to Columbia, taking the key members of the full-time staff with him. George Canby Robinson made an outstanding contribution as an acting professor of medicine for one year, during which time he restored morale, recruited new full-time faculty to head the clinical research divisions, and paved the way for the next full-time professor, Warfield Theobald Longcope. Longcope's success in establishing an outstanding full-time academic department of medicine is described in detail in chapter 8.

# Part IV

**The Pattern of Development
in Selected Medical Centers**

# 9

⚜

## Columbia's College of Physicians
## and Surgeons and the Presbyterian Hospital

In October 1872, James Lenox presided at the opening of the Presbyterian Hospital at Seventieth Street and Park Avenue. Some thirty-six beds were ready for ward patients. A staff of twenty-one physicians and surgeons were to provide the best of medical care "for the poor of New York, without regard to race, creed, or color."[1]

Among the consulting physicians was Alonzo Clark (M.D., College of Physicians and Surgeons [P & S], 1835), who had studied under Louis in Paris. With G. P. Cammann, the inventor of the modern stethoscope, he made important additions to the principles of percussion. At P & S he held the chair of physiology and pathology (1845–55) and that of the theory and practice of medicine (1855–85). In 1885 William H. Draper, professor of clinical medicine at P & S, became president of the medical board. Among the consulting physicians was Edward G. Janeway, the father of Theodore Caldwell Janeway.

After a disastrous fire in 1889, new pavilions opened in 1892. The medical board was increased from ten to twenty-one members. Among those added were Walter Belknap James (a charter member of Osler's Interurban Clinical Club), James S. Thatcher, Francis B. Kinnicutt, and William P. Northrup. Each of these men served as professors of clinical medicine at both the Presbyterian Hospital and P & S.

James, who had studied for one year under Henry Newell Martin in Baltimore, had one of the earliest polygraphs.[2] The tracings were made by needles attached to rubber tubes connected with appropriately placed tambours. The record was made on a revolving drum with smoked paper. In 1909 James imported, from Germany, an Edelmann electrocardiograph machine, the first to be used in New York City.

In 1908 John Kennedy gave the Presbyterian Hospital $1 million to construct an administration building and to make other needed changes. During the study of a projected new hospital, two important questions arose: first, the future expansion of the hospital's education and scientific work, and the advisability of affiliation with a medical school; and second, a source of funds sufficient to erect and maintain an ideal hospital. The cost of operation would be increased by providing for research in bacteriology, pathology, biological chemistry, and other fields essential to modern medical and surgical practice. The hospital board preferred affiliation with P & S. In 1910 Harkness submitted to the hospital trustees a plan for an affiliation with P & S, in which he agreed to erect a surgical pavilion and a complete laboratory for advanced clinical work, in addition to providing an endowment valued at $1.3 million. Harkness visualized the medical needs of the future, and, through his influence, the Columbia-Presbyterian Medical Center was ultimately built. In December 1910, when the affiliation with Columbia appeared imminent, W. Gilman Thompson, president of the medical board and a visiting physician since 1887, resigned. Thompson wanted to retain his position as professor of medicine at Cornell Medical College. He was succeeded by James as president of the Medical Board.[3]

## Janeway and Longcope

Theodore Caldwell Janeway[4] was appointed to succeed Thompson as attending physician and became, in effect, head of the medical department. In 1912 Longcope became Janeway's first assistant. Janeway and Longcope (see chapter 8) devoted more of their time to hospital and medical school affairs than their predecessors.

The staff was divided into a surgical service, a medical service, and a pathological service.[5] The managers were to appoint annually a director for each service; these directors constituted the medical board. The provisions, which became effective on July 1, 1914, placed the hospital mainly on a university basis, but not requiring full-time service for all staff members. The resignations of several doctors followed, among them James. Janeway resigned in April, when he accepted the full-time professorship of medicine at Johns Hopkins.

The interest in the application of scientific methods to the study of disease problems during Janeway's tenure is well illustrated by the report of a case of an unusual paroxysmal syndrome, probably allied to recurrent vomiting, with a study of the nitrogen metabolism, by Janeway and Herman O. Mosenthal. At P & S, Mosenthal[6] worked in the laboratory of biological chemistry, which had been organized by Russell H. Chittenden. Janeway and Mosenthal made a study of urinary nitrogen during two periods of observation in the hospital. From the clinical description, it is evident that the subject of the case, a sixteen-year-old

Jewish schoolgirl, had familial Mediterranean fever.[7] They pointed out that the only careful study of the metabolism during recurrent vomiting that had appeared up to that time was that of John F. Howland and A. N. Richards.[8] Howland and Richards's findings for uric acid corresponded with those of Janeway and Mosenthal: a marked rise following the attack, with subsequent fall to normal. Howland and Richards interpreted their results as evidence of diminished oxidation of uric acid and provided figures for the sulfur metabolism in support of this. In the discussion of this paper, Joslin, James, and Edsall described similar cases.

On June 9, 1914, the managers appointed Longcope as director of the medical service.[9] He had just been made Bard Professor of the Practice of Medicine at P & S. In his first annual report, Longcope outlined the organization of the medical service. Each of the four wards was under the immediate charge of one of the attending physicians: David O. Bovaird, T. Stuart Hart,[10] Homer Fordyce Swift,[11] and George A. Tuddle. Appointed as an associate professor of medicine, in October 1914, Swift devoted his time exclusively to the hospital, where three beds were assigned to him for his studies of central-nervous-system syphilis.

In 1915 a division of metabolism was organized under the direction of H. Rawle Geyelin. He was soon joined by John P. Peters and Eugene F. DuBois, and, later, by William C. Stadie. After his internship, Geyelin studied in Europe, where his interest in medical research along chemical lines was stimulated. Geyelin had had little training in physics and chemistry. There were few men in New York who knew enough to be helpful, thus he had to rely mainly on his own resources. His initial interest was the study of carbohydrate metabolism in thyroid disease, but he soon shifted his attention to diabetes.[12] Only cumbersome and laborious methods were available for urine analysis. The Bertrand method was standard for blood sugar determinations. It required the withdrawal of 50 cc of blood, which was defibrinated by stirring it in an evaporating dish as it was drawn from the vein. The blood was heated and a deproteinized filtrate prepared. Then followed the preparation of a cuprous oxide precipitate, which had to be washed and weighed. Soon, however, Benedict, Folin, Kramer, and Van Slyke, among others, developed new microchemical tools for the determination of various constituents of blood. Geyelin established an efficiently functioning metabolic service, and his enthusiasm for clinical investigation spread to the resident staff and the students.

Much of Geyelin's early work in diabetes preceded the use of insulin. His best-known studies were on the famous C. K., who was considered to be totally diabetic. Geyelin studied him for many years, after which the patient went to the Russell Sage Institute of Pathology, where methods for the determination of total metabolism were available. In 1922 Geyelin published a carefully documented study of nine juvenile diabetics. He succeeded in arresting the downward course of the disease, achieving in each case a total food intake appropriate to the age requirement in calories. Thus, Geyelin was engaged in a full-time academic career before most medical schools recognized such specialization.

## The Merger of P & S and the Presbyterian Hospital

In 1917 it was decided that the Presbyterian Hospital and the medical school of Columbia should be rebuilt on a single site and that Presbyterian should function as a university hospital. The clinical staff was to be reconstructed on the full-time principle that was being followed at Johns Hopkins.

In 1920 a new agreement was made between the hospital and the university, and Edward Harkness gave the hospital and university a twenty-two acre site on Washington Heights.

Before Swift left for France with the Presbyterian Hospital unit in World War I, he tendered his resignation, to take a position at the Cornell Medical College. W. W. Palmer, then at the HRI, took his place at P & S. When Longcope was called to the surgeon-general's office in Washington, D.C., on July 15, 1917, Palmer took over as acting director of the medical service. In February 1919, Longcope resumed his duties as director of the medical service. Palmer became an associate professor of medicine at Johns Hopkins; Albert R. Lamb became Longcope's executive assistant. In 1921 Longcope resigned. For a short time he engaged in private practice; then came the call to be professor of medicine at Johns Hopkins.

## Other Faculty Members at Columbia during the Tenures of Janeway and Longcope

During the tenure of Janeway and Longcope, there were many distinguished physicians on the faculty: Francis Carter Wood,[13] later to head research in cancer at Columbia, was a professor of clinical pathology; Samuel W. Lambert,[14] a professor of applied therapeutics; and James,[15] a professor of clinical medicine. Other professors of clinical medicine whose names are well known for their clinical research contributions include Nathan E. Brill,[16] who described a peculiar form of typhus fever; Emanuel Libman,[17] who was a pioneer in the use of blood cultures and contributed much to our knowledge of infective endocarditis; and James Alexander Miller,[18] skilled as a chest physician, who was an assistant professor of clinical medicine. Edwards A. Park, who became a professor of pediatrics at Yale and then at Johns Hopkins, was an assistant in medicine, working in the laboratory with Janeway.

Others who joined the faculty during this period include Charles N. B. Camac,[19] as an assistant professor of clinical medicine; Haven Emerson,[20] widely known for his work in public health, as an associate in physiology and an instructor in medicine; Willard B. Soper,[21] later to do important work in the field of tuberculosis at Yale and elsewhere, as an assistant in pathology; Russell L. Cecil, known for his work in pneumonia, arthritis, and as the author of a new textbook of medicine, as an instructor in clinical medicine; George H. Draper, from the HRI; Harold E. B. Pardee,[22] a well-known cardiologist, as an instructor in physiology; and William A. Perlzweig, who later went to Baltimore in charge of clinical chemistry under McCann and then became a professor of biologic chemistry at the new Duke Medical School, as an assistant in biological chemistry.

After Janeway's departure the additions continued with Bernard Sutro Oppenheimer,[23] who later became a prominent cardiologist, as an assistant professor of clinical medicine; Sir Francis Fraser as an instructor in clinical medicine; George M. Mackenzie[24] as an instructor in pathology; Ralph A. Kinsella,[25] as an instructor in clinical medicine, who became a professor of medicine at St. Louis University; and John P. Peters, as an instructor in clinical medicine, who became a professor of medicine at Yale.

In 1919 Henry T. Chickering became an instructor of medicine, as did Kenneth McAlpin and Henry Barber Richardson.

## Walter W. Palmer and the Creation of Full-time Medicine at P & S

In 1917, when Longcope was called to Washington, Palmer agreed to serve as acting director of the medical service of the Presbyterian Hospital, assuming teaching responsibilities as an associate professor of medicine at Columbia.[26] At the end of World War I, he accepted Thayer's invitation to head the full-time chemical research division of the department of medicine at Johns Hopkins. In 1921 Columbia University appointed him as a full-time professor of medicine at the Presbyterian Hospital.

When P & S and the Presbyterian Hospital affiliated and established a joint medical center, in 1920, the medical and surgical services were placed on a full-time basis. Palmer brought Alphonse Raymond Dochez,[27] Dana Atchley, William S. Ladd, Robert F. Loeb, and George A. Harrop, Jr.,[28] from Baltimore. He also recruited Ethel Benedict (who later became Mrs. Alexander Gutman) to supervise the laboratory of the medical service. Mackenzie was already at the Presbyterian Hospital. In 1922 Randolph West[29] returned, from a year's work in chemistry at Chicago, to become an assistant physician, Alvan L. Barach received a similar appointment. In 1924 Loeb and Gerald Shibley were appointed as assistant physicians, and Franklin M. Hanger as a medical resident.

The resident system, which was not well developed in New York City, was strengthened and extended. Harrop, the first resident physician under Palmer, was followed, in succession, by Loeb, Hanger, Dickinson W. Richards, Jr., Alvin F. Coburn,[30] David Seegal,[31] Charles A. Flood, and many other distinguished physicians.

There were also appointments of basic scientists to the department staff. One of the most successful was that of Michael Heidelberger,[32] who became an international leader in immunochemistry. Working with Heidelberger over the years were many who became outstanding medical scientists, including Seegal; Forrest E. Kendall; Henry P. Treffers, who became a professor of microbiology at Yale; Manfred Mayer, who became a professor of immunology at Johns Hopkins; and E. A. Kabat.

The introduction of full-time clinical departments met with opposition from many leading physicians. In Palmer's view, no single scheme was free from criticism; a good quota of full-time men, combined with cooperative men in practice, appeared to be the best solution. In Palmer's arrangement, the so-called "geographic full-time" physicians, practicing solely in the hospital, contributed greatly in all fields, including research, and were an essential protection to the strictly full-time men. Doctors with downtown offices helped with the teaching and clinic work, but they too were free to do research, and a number of them did so successfully. Palmer's success was to a great degree dependent upon this flexibility of organization, together with a constant regard for the interest of the individual.

Just as in other medical centers, there were problems with the full-time plan, as pointed out by Dana Atchley:

All during the 20s . . . we ran into a great deal of antagonism among the practitioners working in the hospital. They were a good quality of men but . . . were embarrassed by their lack of fundamental knowledge. . . . They took the attitude that if you worked in a laboratory you couldn't possibly make a diagnosis. . . . We were trying to teach and study the mechanisms of disease, and to make the diagnosis by analysis of the mechanisms, rather than just an attempt to classify with one word. But we were criticized.

I'll never forget when I asked what the chloride content of the blood was in an obscure case. One of our most brilliant men burst out and said: "You're just interested in a lot of laboratory data. You don't really care anything about the patient"; which of course was not so because we had always felt that the patient was important. We just felt that we ought to know something about the patient. I had the pleasure of having him say to me many years afterwards: "Oh, I would give anything to have gone into chemistry when I got through and to have done what you did. . . ."

I would like to say just a few words about the full-time business. Medicine was run entirely by the big diagnosticians with successful practices who gave a little spare time to teaching. They had the kudos of it without doing much of the work. There was no research done; the professor and all the staff spent their entire time walking around listening to murmurs and doing physical examinations. There was this huge gap between the fundamental scientists who looked down their noses at the clinicians because they knew they were unscientific and the clinicians who looked down their noses at the fundamental scientists and said: "Well you don't know what patients are. You are not practical." It wasn't until the full-time professorships were started at Johns Hopkins by the Rockefeller Foundation, that we really began to have a department of medicine assume a role in the school that was scientifically and critically the equivalent of the department of biochemistry or physiology. At Johns Hopkins they made the serious mistake of not integrating the part-time men in it because you really need them. That was partly due to the fact that they were pioneering and partly due to the fact that that group was so uncooperative.

But Palmer immediately realized, in organizing his department, that you had to have three groups. . . . Dr. Palmer's third group was the part-time people who had offices in the city but who came to work in the clinic to do certain teaching. . . . The difference between what the practitioner could do for us in the 20s and what he can do in the 50s is because they are all now trained. We don't have anybody who isn't familiar with electrolytes and with all the basic fundamentals of disease.[33]

When Palmer arrived in New York, he made only two requests of the hospital—lunch facilities for the staff and increased laboratory space. A second story, built on the isolation pavilion, provided much needed laboratory space while the new center was being built. It was in these small laboratories that Dochez completed his work on hemolytic streptococcus  as the cause of scarlet fever; Loeb and Atchley started their studies on electrolyte balance in the blood and body fluids; West began his search for the active principle in liver that controls pernicious anemia; Hanger began his work on allergic phenomena and protein abnormalities in liver disease;[34] Richards became interested in the abnormal physiology of the cardiopulmonary system; Coburn began his study of the relation of hemolytic streptococcus to rheumatic fever; Draper organized the constitution clinic; and Barach developed the first portable oxygen room.

In 1925 the full-time program was modified, and there was a threat that the Rockefeller grants supporting the department would be withdrawn. Palmer made it clear that, in view of budget limitations, all physicians who would prefer to work on a full-time basis would not be able to do so. Palmer, Mackenzie, Atchley, and Ladd accepted the privilege of supplementing their salaries by limited private practice in the hospital. Dochez, Shibley, West, Loeb, and Ross Golden remained on strict full-time. The memorandum proposed some salary increase for these doctors and provided salaries for four new full-time men. The full-time physicians retained the privilege of seeing private patients of interest to them. The fees for such services were placed in a fund used to support research. Since the full-time position was not being abandoned, the General Education Board decided to honor its commitments.

In 1927 Loeb received a grant from the Rockefeller Foundation to study in Germany, and Richards, through the Proudfit fellowship, worked with Sir Henry Dale in London. In the same year, Mackenzie became director of the Mary Imogene Bassett Hospital.

In March 1928, the move was made to the new center. The shift was done so expeditiously that the director of the medical service opened his mail at nine o'clock one morning in the old hospital and at noon dictated replies in his new office at 168th Street.

## The Arthritis Clinic

Ralph H. Boots[35] received his M.D. degree from the University of Pittsburgh in 1914. In 1916 he joined the British Army Medical Corps, later transferring to the American army, where he was in the group that studied the influenza epidemic and its sequelae. He worked on rheumatic fever with Swift at the HRI. His research experiences there nurtured his lifelong interest in rheumatoid arthritis and his early suspicion that an infectious agent might play a role in pathogenesis.

In 1929 he founded the Faulkner Clinic at the Presbyterian Hospital with Fordyce B. St. John. Boots recruited Martin Henry Dawson,[36] from the Rockefeller Institute, to head the research unit of the clinic. Boots was closely involved with the introduction of the erythrocyte sedimentation rate into clinical medicine in this country, the study of rheumatoid factor, streptococcal agglutination through the sensitized sheep cell, the role of chrysotherapy and glucocorticoid in the treatment of rheumatoid arthritis, and many other projects. He was also a founder and president (1940) of the American Rheumatism Association.

## Other Clinical Resources

In 1936 Seegal and Kendall established the research division of the Goldwater Memorial Hospital on Welfare Island, which was associated with P & S. This was the first division of medicine devoted solely to the care of the chronically ill.

In 1937 an integration between the Neurological Institute and the Presbyterian Hospital was made. Palmer, medical director of Presbyterian Hospital, became professional director of the institute, and Loeb was appointed assistant director. As part of the agreement, a full-time program of research and education was undertaken, at a cost of $98,000 a year.

The first division of Bellevue Hospital was under the supervision of the College of Physicians and Surgeons for almost one hundred years. Earlier, Van Horne Norrie was director of the medical service; succeeding him was I. O. Woodruff, and, on Woodruff's retirement in 1945, Richards became director.

## Research

During 1921–22, the first year of the new full-time service, six full-time and three part-time medical faculty members were engaged in research. By 1946–47, at Presbyterian Hospital, there were twenty-four full-time and eight part-time; at Bellevue Hospital, four full-time and three part-time, and, at Goldwater Memorial Hospital, three full-time and four part-time, making a total of thirty-one full-time and fifteen part-time staff members.

It is not possible to give more than a brief outline of the men and the major research areas.

### Infectious Disease

While in Baltimore, Dochez and Walter Bliss had demonstrated the probability that the cause of scarlet fever was the hemolytic streptococcus. Later, in New York, this was established beyond any doubt; a discovery of great significance, since it led to improved methods of prevention and treatment. After returning to New York, Dochez began the investigation of the common cold, demonstrating, in collaboration with Shibley, Hanger, Yale Kneeland, and Harry Rose, that bacteria were not the primary cause of colds. This discovery led to a study of the tissue-culture method of cultivating viruses and, subsequently, the use of the developing chick embryo for this purpose. Of great importance was the transmission of the common cold to chimpanzees and, later, to man, by means of bacteria-free filtrates.[37] Dochez was later interested in the etiology of influenza.[38] He was an associate professor until 1925 and then a full professor until his retirement in 1947.

Hanger described, simultaneously with Gregory Shwartzman, the skin reaction known as the *Shwartzman phenomenon* and called attention to its nonspecificity. Later, he introduced the cephalin flocculation test, which was used for many years as an indicator of liver damage. With A. B. Gutman,[39] Hanger called attention to the cholangitic type of arsphenamine jaundice.

A significant contribution was made by Alvin F. Coburn, who demonstrated the relation between hemolytic streptococcal infections—chiefly upper respiratory—and the precipitation of attacks of acute rheumatic fever.[40]

Dawson was one of the pioneers, along with Gladys Hobby, in the use of penicillin in the treatment of infections. Together with Thomas Hunter, they were the first to show that large doses were necessary to cure patients with subacute infective endocarditis.

Important work on the relation of hemolytic streptococci to acute glomerulonephritis was done by a group that included Seegal, Emily M. Loeb, Walter Bloom, and David P. Earle.

### Physiology

Loeb and Atchley[41] made an excellent team and soon were responsible for guiding many young men in clinical research, one of their important pupils being Richards.

The activity of this group has been described by Atchley:[42]

Loeb and I saw eye to eye all the time. . . . If he had a good idea I leaped on it and if I had one he leaped on it. If he didn't like my idea, he would attack it thoroughly and without the slightest bit of antagonism and I would do the same with his. That same thing was true in our joint research. . . . One of the best papers we ever did was in 1933. It turned out to be a classic and concerned the mechanism of diabetic acidosis, a paper that is quoted regularly even today.

That work involved studying what happened to the electrolytes in acidosis. We knew from the people who were brought in terribly sick what state they were in but how they got that way we didn't know. I suggested—and this was one of the few things that was my idea—that we get a diabetic in and take away his insulin after having studied him very carefully and established a baseline, and see hour by hour what happens. In those days of unemployment we could hire a man for almost nothing so we hired three diabetics. We were very fortunate because just by chance with these three cases, it didn't do anything to one if we took the insulin away—he was so mild, the second was a little more severe, and the third was violent. We had to do rescue work on him a few hours after we had taken his insulin away. But we did a very elaborate experiment, and found that the loss of body water and potassium and sodium had definite results. . . . We were able, because we had done such accurate work, to figure out quantitatively where this had all come from, whether this was intracellular or extracellular, because, for example, it had to be intracellular water that was lost if potassium were lost. We could prove that there was potassium loss, you see. It was really quite a tour-de-force; there was tremendous luck in it but we had planned a very good experiment because we analyzed every bit of food and had duplicate meals right straight along. We went to elaborate lengths to have a perfect balance of every milligram in and every milligram out. And it turned out very well.[43]

At that time, fifty percent of uncontrolled diabetics succumbed in acidotic coma. From these experiments, Atchley and Loeb were able to devise a rational form of fluid and electrolyte therapy.

Loeb's chief research interest was in electrolyte physiology,[44] an interest that began with a study, at the Marine Biological Laboratory, of the replacement of potassium by rubidium and caesium in biological systems.[45] It was this preoccupation with electrolytes that took him first to Palmer's laboratory. His work there led to the publication of several papers, which were written with Atchley.[46] Later, Loeb observed that patients with advanced Addison's disease presented a picture of medical shock similar to that seen in salt depletion and dehydration; thus, he began a series of electrolyte studies in this disease. His discovery of the loss of sodium by way of the kidneys led him to suggest sodium chloride treatment.[47]

Loeb was the first to study the physiological consequences of mineralocorticoid excess, demonstrating that the administration of large doses of desoxycorticosterone acetate in the dog resulted not only in hypertension, hypernatremia, hypokalemia, and profound muscle weakness, but also in a diabetes insipidus–like syndrome unresponsive to the administration of pitressin.[48] These findings anticipated by more than a decade the description of the syndrome of excessive aldosterone secretion.

Loeb was an effective teacher, and his clinical erudition was skillfully integrated with the basic sciences, which he also knew well. Loeb predicted what lay ahead for medicine and medical research in his acceptance of the Kober Medal of the Association of American Physicians for 1959:

> In the years that lie ahead we who are concerned with the advance of medical science, medical education and patient care are going to have to be extraordinarily competent if we are to fulfill our responsibility in meeting the challenge—not of the Russians—but the challenge presented by the advance of the basic sciences if we are to capitalize on the products of this progress in the investigation of normal and pathological mechanisms. The opportunities are infinite and can be discerned and grasped only by the prepared mind. . . . It is inescapable . . . that in the future the student of medicine whether in practice or in the laboratory will have to have at his command an ever expanding body of knowledge of natural science if he is to exploit to the fullest extent the potentialities for the advancement of science provided by the enormous achievements of our colleagues in physics and chemistry. . . . The turning point of medicine in this country which has given rise to our leadership stems beyond question from the introduction of the full-time principle first in the basic sciences and then in the clinical departments yet the straining of the finances of medical schools by the inevitable growth of medical faculties and the mounting cost of research has resulted in an alarming distortion of the principle of full-time. Full-time is retained in a number of institutions in name but in many of these it is retained in name alone. In many institutions the so-called full-time man devotes a highly significant portion of his working hours to the care of private patients either for the purpose of earning a large part of his own salary or, yet more dangerously, to amass funds to help pay salaries and defray costs even in the preclinical departments. If it is granted that the purpose of the full-time is to afford a substantial corps of those with motivation, capacity and flare for research, as well as for teaching, freedom from the legitimate intrusions upon their time and thought by patients who pay for their services and for whom they should accept full and undivided responsibility, then it becomes apparent that the insidious trends now gaining momentum can only lead to a deterioration of the priceless standards which have been established.[49]

In 1926 Barach devised an ingenious apparatus for the administration of oxygen; it was he who introduced the use of helium and positive-pressure breathing, the latter being especially helpful in the treatment of asthma, dyspnea, and pulmonary edema due to obstruction.[50]

Richards[51] and André Cournand received the Nobel Prize for their cardiorespiratory studies.[52] Richards received his M.S. degree in physiology in 1922 and his M.D. degree in 1923 at P & S. He took his residency training at the Presbyterian Hospital, where he became a full professor in 1945. He was the first full-time director of the first (Columbia University) medical division at Bellevue Hospital. Cournand, in presenting the Kober Medal of the Association of American Physicians to Richards, made the following comment:

> Vivid in my mind are: his display of technical skill and efficiency; his care and caution in studying human subjects; his implementation of self-experiment in the true tradition of the British and Scandinavian respiratory physiologists; his foresight in planning which included taking advantage of the unexpected and stressing methodological innovations; and his thorough knowledge of medical literature, current and classical....
>
> In one of our early planning sessions, during which we were discussing methods for securing mixed venous blood for direct analysis of $O_2$ and $CO_2$ as an alternative to the rebreathing method, he produced an issue of the 1929 *Klinische Wochenschrift* describing Forssmann's self-experiment. The ultimate development which followed is well known to all, as this was the initial step in the development of cardiac catheterization and all that it has meant for clinical medicine and cardiovascular surgery.[53]

In his acceptance of the medal, Richards referred to three men who were responsible for molding his research career:

> "The archangel loved heights." With these words, Henry Adams begins his book, *Mont St. Michel and Chartres*. L. J. Henderson would be amused to find himself likened to an archangel, and perhaps equally, to be linked with Henry Adams. But he loved heights all the same. As a biochemist, he established as a young man the principles of acid-base equilibrium and explored the full significance of this, in nature and natural philosophy.... The Fatigue Laboratory at Harvard was his creation ... his was the stimulus for countless new ideas, experimental formulations, new modes of thought in many fields. He sought always the meaning beyond and above phenomena, and this could be true from the most casual topic of conversation, on to the hard business of research. To be with L. J. Henderson was an inspiration; he could lift a man out of himself.
>
> Sir Henry Dale could theorize, too, but his way was different. Dale was primarily an experimenter ... Walter Bauer and I worked in his laboratory in London in 1927–28. On a day when an experiment was planned, Collison, the head technician, would start at some time in the dark British pre-dawn; Walter and I would arrive at about nine—we were working on the dog's hepatic circulation. Just as we reached the key point of cannulating the blood vessels and bile duct, the laboratory door would fling open, and Sir Henry would come charging in, often in morning coat and striped trousers, grab a lab coat off the hook, and be with us in seconds. What is more, he would stay until the experiment was finished, whether at tea time, dinner time, or later.
>
> As it happened, it was in the spring of 1928 that the concept of the chemical transmission of the nervous impulse was born. Our job in this was the simplest, to test in cats the vasodilator principle—supposedly histamine—in extracts of horse's spleen. I recall one afternoon when the testing was finished, I had some extract left over, and I went on to acidify

and then alkalinize samples of it and test them again, to find, surprisingly, that on the alkaline side of neutrality all vasodilator activity disappeared. This would not occur with histamine, but would with acetylcholine. I reported this to Dr. Dale at tea that day, and he said, "Hmm," no more. But this was clearly one small addition to many things he had been thinking about, because only a few days later he began to construct for us the possibilities of acetylcholine as a biological agent. The generation of a great idea, in a first class research mind, over months and years, is a remarkable thing.

Alfred Newton Richards I came to know during World War II, when he was in charge of medical research in Washington . . . but I did not know him well until after the war . . . through our joint association with the firm of Merck and Co., and its research institute, he as Chairman of its Board of Scientific Advisers, and I as a member . . . Richards had long since given up his own research, but there was all of his careful and responsible study of everything that came before him, all of his warmth and enthusiasm, and his overflowing and irresistible sense of humor. And yet the goodness of his heart never dulled the keenness of his judgment. A special quality of mind and character, I think, was his passion for order; orderliness in ideas, manners, performance, even little things. One recalls how he would not even sit at an after-dinner discussion without clearing away the crumbs and ashes in front of him, and if the waiter did not take away the dishes, he would do it himself. As for listening to a sloppy scientific paper, we can all see him, sitting in the front row, shaking his head, grunting and muttering and tossing about, while the unfortunate speaker, sweating it out on the platform, looking down on this scene of agony, sinks even further into vacuous non-sequiturs. I cannot leave these three men without one word that characterizes all of them; this is what Walter Cannon, writing about Henderson, described as his "pervasive kindness" toward the younger men around him.[54]

As head of the first medical division at Bellevue Hospital, Richards demonstrated his qualities as a leader in clinical medicine. The words of one of his former residents show clearly that men of such stature are most important in the evolution of clinical investigation:

Members of the Bellevue Hospital House Staff who made rounds with Dr. Richards saw him as a multifaceted man—clinician, teacher-scientist, and chief-of-service. His impact on physicians in training can be fully appreciated only in his meld of these three roles. As a gentle clinician—concerned in the utmost for the comfort of his patient, but, above all, the master of clinical judgment—able to discern the proper course in a labyrinth of clinical and laboratory data though never reluctant to seek consultative advice. As a teacher-scientist—applying principles and results of research to interpretation of clinical phenomena and toward improved medical treatment, and awakening investigative potential in residents and interns through his attitude of constant inquiry. And finally as chief-of-service—always available to members of his house staff, fostering an atmosphere conducive to the happy blend of excellent patient care and fruitful clinical investigation, and willing (and able) to do combat with the administrative structure of a municipal hospital system.[55]

There were many excellent clinical investigators associated with Richards and Cournand during their thirty years of collaboration at Bellevue, including Eleanor Baldwin, Richard L. Riley, Robert C. Darling, Alice Lowell, and David G. Green.

Another important member of Palmer's team was Robert L. Levy,[56] whose main interest was in disease of the coronary arteries.[57] In Levy's group there were also a number of distinguished collaborators, including Kenneth B. Turner,[58] John M. Baldwin, Barach, Howard G. Bruenn, Francis Chamberline, and Rene Wégria.

At the Goldwater Memorial Hospital on Welfare Island, Arthur J. Patek, Jr., was joined, in his important studies of nutritional deficiency in the pathogenesis of cirrhosis of the liver, by such outstanding associates as Oscar D. Ratnoff, J. Post, C. Haig, R. Hillman, and many others.

George H. Draper[59] and his associates studied the constitution of individuals in relation to susceptibility to and behavior in disease throughout most of the years of Palmer's chairmanship. One of the first assistant residents at the HRI, Draper had had a long-time interest in poliomyelitis and in the type of individual most apt to contract the disease, and he extended such studies to other areas.

Psychosomatic medicine also evolved, to a significant degree, out of the activity in Palmer's department. This development was initiated by Thomas Salmon,[60] who assigned this task to Robert M. McGraw, a psychiatrist associated with the clinical services in the beginning. H. Flanders Dunbar Sproul began, after the move to the new medical center, a series of studies in an attempt to discover types of reaction among several diseases. Dana Atchley and others also took a deep interest, of course, in this area of medicine.

Reference has already been made to the research groups in chemistry, organized by Heidelberger and Green. Heidelberger's group studied the mechanisms of immunity, including the separation and isolation of various antigenic components of hemolytic streptococci and tubercle bacilli and their role in antibody formation and immunity. Kendall demonstrated, utilizing immunochemical methods, the presence of five different globulins, and at least two albumins, in normal human serum and crystallized human serum albumin. Green and his collaborators, among whom were W. Eugene Knox, John Taggart, Allan L. Grafflin, and Luis F. LeLoir, made important studies in the field of enzyme chemistry.

An important innovation was the development of an Isotope Committee, organized by the departments of chemistry and medicine in order to facilitate cooperation on problems of interest to the two groups and on the application of isotope techniques to clinical investigation. David Rittenberg and David Shemin, from biochemistry, and West and Irving M. London, from medicine, studied human red blood cell formation and found that the average life span was 127 and 128 days in two normal males and 133 days in an individual with polycythemia. The findings indicated that a mechanism for persistent overproduction of red blood cells, rather than a significant diminution in destruction, exists in that disease.

In his efforts to discover the liver's active principle, which is so spectacular in bringing about remission in pernicious anemia, West, in association with H. D. Dakin, was able to purify liver substance so that a single 10 mg dose was effective.[61] A. B. Gutman[62] and Ethel Gutman discovered, in 1936, that serum acid phosphatase is increased in carcinoma of the prostate. Utilizing newly developed immunochemical and electrophoretic techniques, the Gutmans identified Bence-Jone protein, as well as "M" protein, in multiple myeloma serum; discoveries that antedated the intense investigation of recent years in this area. Their observation that hyperproteinemia occurs in lymphogranuloma venerum and multiple myeloma was also a valuable new diagnostic approach in these conditions.

One of the most important by-products of this research, in one of the first successful full-time departments of medicine, was its beneficial effect on the quality of the clinical work. This can scarcely be overestimated, since it is true of all clinics that are organized to foster clinical investigation. One easily observable result is an increase in the accuracy of diagnosis; a change in part due to the introduction of laboratory aids developed by the research program. Another contributing factor is the improved clinical diagnostic skill that results from training in the scientific method. In the previous generation, even in the better hospitals, the clinical, when compared to the pathological diagnoses, were correct in only twenty to thirty percent of the cases. At the Presbyterian Hospital, Seegal and Turner reviewed a thousand consecutive records of patients who had pathological diagnoses; eighty-four percent of the clinical diagnoses were correct. Thus, the full-time program, including the emphasis on clinical investigation, clearly has had a very substantial effect on the quality of medical practice.

# 10

# The Development of Clinical Investigation
# at the University of Pennsylvania

At the University of Pennyslvania School of Medicine the basic approach in the developmental period of clinical research differed from that at Johns Hopkins. Johns Hopkins adopted the German method—that is, the professor did research and, it was hoped, inspired his students to emulate him. At Pennsylvania there was doubt that any practitioner of medicine would have time for effective research, so that endowed chairs were sought in which the incumbent, freed from the restraints of practice and routine teaching responsibilities, could give his full time and effort to investigation.

## The William Pepper Laboratory of Clinical Medicine

William Pepper (1843-98) was an important contributor to the development of clinical research at Pennsylvania. He had a successful private practice, yet found time to be a professor of medicine and provost; to found the university hospital (the first university-owned hospital in the country); and to establish a laboratory to promote clinical research. The William Pepper Laboratory of Clinical Medicine was named in memory of the provost's father, who also had been a professor of medicine. The laboratory was to be devoted to research and post-graduate teaching. "It is the first laboratory of its kind provided with its own building and amply equipped for research in this country," said Welch in his dedicatory address in 1895,[1] "and it is not surpassed in these respects in any foreign countries." Opened in December 1895, the laboratory provided facilities for study of the physiological, chemical, bacteriological, and pathological problems of human disease.

On October 17, 1894, William Pepper became the first director of the laboratory,[2] and, on October 1, 1895, Alfred Stengel[3] was appointed the assistant director. After Roentgen discovered x-rays in December 1895, Charles Lester Leonard purchased an x-ray tube and assembled his electrical equipment in the Pepper Laboratory. This was the beginning of fruitful laboratory investigations under the guidance of Stengel, who was, for all practical purposes, leader of the laboratory personnel.[4] Stengel (M.D., Pennsylvania, 1889) began his career at the university in embryology and pathology and as a clinical clerk to Pepper. After Pepper's death, Stengel became director of the laboratory, a position he held until 1911.

In 1903 William G. Spiller was appointed to a special professorship of neuropathology. After his graduation in medicine from Pennsylvania, he spent four years in Europe studying neurology. On his return, he joined the Pepper Laboratory, where he and Charles H. Frazier, a surgeon, conducted their studies on division of the sensory route of the trigeminus for the relief of tic douloureux.

The division of physiological chemistry was organized under Casper W. Miller, David Linn Edsall, George Woodward, and A. E. Taylor. The division of serology was also started in 1905 by Ravenel, Kness, and Evans and continued by John L. Laird and Frank B. Lynch, Jr. The division of clinical microscopy was established by C. Y. White and continued by William Pepper III, T. A. Cope, and Thomas Fitz-Hugh, Jr.

## David Linn Edsall

The most important individual to spend his early period in research in the Pepper Laboratory, in terms of the future development of clinical investigation, was David Linn Edsall.

Edsall received his M.D. degree from Pennsylvania in 1893. Following his internship, he studied in London, Vienna, and Graz.

Edsall became an associate in clinical medicine in the Pepper Laboratory during 1895. Edsall was interested in the chemical aspects of disease. He described what happened when he tried to go further with chemistry while at Princeton:

> I had a strong desire to know more about the subject and a rather vague but insistent idea that it might help me understand medicine better and perhaps aid me if I wished to attempt investigation in the vast area of the unknown in medicine. With the consent of the Dean I took the then radical step of asking the professor of chemistry ... to allow me to take the elementary laboratory course. He asked me what I was heading for and I said medicine. He replied with entire disapproval: "A doctor does not need to know any chemistry. You would be wasting your time" and looked at the door. I left with the feeling that I had been very stupid and impractical.[5]

Until very recently, speaking in the usual historical sense, serious devotion to research in medicine was looked at with askance by many of the medical profession itself. S. Weir Mitchell told a group of us once that after he had graduated in medicine and had a service in a hospital his father, then a prominent professor of medicine, asked him what he intended to do next, and he said that he thought he would spend a few years in research in an intensive way. His father threw up his hands in astonishment and almost anger and replied: "Weir, if you do that, people will look upon you as they would if you joined the circus."[6]

Edsall published over seventy papers between 1897 and his departure from Philadelphia in 1910. His chemical studies concerned, to a large extent, estimation of various substances in the urine. A good example of this interest is his work, with John K. Mitchell and Simon Flexner, on family periodic paralysis.[7] Edsall was responsible for the chemical studies. The study focused attention on the metabolism of potassium, the paralytic attacks having been shortened by large quantities of potassium given orally. Edsall and Miller demonstrated a retention of phosphorus and nitrogen in two children with acromegaly with a less marked retention of calcium, leading them to the view "that there is a growth of abnormal bone rather than a mere abnormal growth of bone and that there are very marked abnormalities in the solid tissues as well as in the bone."[8] Edsall delivered a Harvey Lecture, in November 1907, on the bearing of metabolism studies on clinical medicine.

In 1905, when Edsall's paper with John Herr Musser on the effects of x-rays on body function appeared, the profession was aware of the dangers of skin burns, but not of the more general reactions. Edsall checked the intake and excretion of nitrogen, phosphorus, and uric acid in the urine in two patients with leukemia. He discovered that a single mild exposure could have a profound influence on metabolism for days afterward.

Edsall, the "father of industrial medicine" in this country, published a paper in 1904 on heat cramps. He recognized that "it is, of course, a different disorder from heat stroke and clearly quite different from heat prostration. It appears also clinically to be different from any other recognized form of muscle spasms."[9] In 1909 he stated that the navy had reported good results by using enemas of salt solution.[10] Thus, he had the coil in his hands but it took some decades to unravel it. In the 1920s J. S. Haldane ascribed the cramps to salt depletion and prevented them by giving salt solution.

William Osler asked Edsall to write on the industrial aspects of medicine for *Modern Medicine;* the research for his paper taught him that a factory is a "genial garden to the lover of etiology, with much fruit on many a tree."[11] By 1910 he had such a reputation in the field that Professor Henry W. Farnam of Yale, the president of the American Association for Labor Legislation, appointed Edsall to a five-man committee that was to acquaint the president of the United States with these problems.

In December 1909, Edsall was invited to St. Louis, when the reorganizing Washington University School of Medicine was searching for a professor of medicine whose training was thoroughly scientific. After his visit, Edsall wrote a remarkable letter outlining in detail the plans for "a Johns Hopkins of the Southwest," in terms of faculty, financial support, and physical facilities.[12] When Edsall was offered this position, Pennsylvania took steps to make him a professor of medicine and he decided to remain there.

One of Edsall's greatest frustrations was that Stengel, the head of the Pepper Laboratory, did not fully cooperate with him. In developing his new department of medicine, Edsall wanted to have additional space in the laboratory. Stengel agreed, provided that Edsall could get an extra $5,000 from the trustees to cover the expense of the changes. The trustees declined to provide these funds, which was a great disappointment to Edsall. John F. Howland, who had recently been appointed a professor of pediatrics at Washington University, learned of Edsall's disappointments in Philadelphia and moved quickly to see that Edsall might again be offered a position in St. Louis, and this time find it more attractive.

The second offer from Washington University did come and Edsall accepted. He was given a year's leave of absence before taking up his new position. He used this time for study and research in metabolism at the Carnegie Nutrition Laboratory in Boston. While in Boston, he was asked to address the Aesculapian Club, one of the city's influential medical groups. His remarks show the stresses within academic medicine at the time of the Flexner Report, as well as the discussions concerning full-time clinical chairs:

> The life of the clinical teacher is and always will be more difficult than that of his academic colleagues. It is necessarily more complex, for under any circumstances he must have equal academic responsibility, the personnel of his department must always be more elaborate, and also he must carry the very serious responsibility of the lives and health of the hospital patients under his care. Further than this, entirely aside from the financial aspects of the matter, it is certainly questionable whether he can ever, without greatly endangering his usefulness, relinquish, as is being suggested, the added responsibility and complexity that comes with outside consulting work. . . . Aside from the fact that in the broad sense of the word research alone advances any subject, it is especially important that clinicians be trained into the judicial and inquiring spirit, and especially into the critical spirit that a little experience in research gives; for no one is more constantly an investigator than any thoughtful practicing physician and no one has more important or more complex problems to solve, and his mind must be trained to meet these. By training in research I do not mean simply training in discovering new things. Valuable as the results of research are, there is a more essential influence upon the clinician as an individual. His work is such that he must frequently act empirically and I think all thoughtful clinicians will agree with me that his greatest struggle is in avoiding the danger of falling into the habit of deciding all things upon

an empirical basis. While a hypercritical attitude makes a man ineffective, there is nothing more dangerous perhaps in practical medicine than an uncritical attitude. . . .

With a suitable combination of the German academic system and something approaching the English ward clerk system, the best results now possible for both students and medicine seem attainable. . . . It is quite apparent how essential it is that in carrying out this plan there be entire freedom in the academic use of large hospital facilities; that appointments to these hospitals be made by the medical school and hospital authorities together, but on a purely academic basis, and that medical school and hospital work in entire unison. . . .

It is not simply the important fact that these changes will provide men of higher training for the hospitals from the interns to the chiefs, and will imply that the attendants give more time and thought to their hospital work. It is not merely that they will increase the usefulness of the individual medical school affected in each instance. It is chiefly that they will change the work of the hospitals from simple ministration to the sick of the period to ministration to the sick of the future as well as the present, through providing advanced training as well as new information for the future.[13]

Edsall always had a broad concept of research—what it consisted of and what it meant in clinical medicine. He advocated broad fundamental training that would be focused on clinical problems in an effort to clarify the causes of disease and to provide more logical treatment. Clinical research had begun the modern surge in physiologic understanding of human disease, and Edsall was one of those who understood its importance to practical clinical medicine and to the future of medicine as a scientifically based profession.

Edsall constantly emphasized the importance of clinical investigation: "I do not feel the slightest sympathy with the frequently expressed fear that the tendency at present is to train investigators rather than clinicians, my reason being the very definite one that, to my mind, a sound clinician is essentially an investigator, whether he works in a laboratory with all possible facilities or in hard country practice; whether he conducts extensive studies of special questions or simply attempts to learn as precisely as possible what needs to be done for each separate patient."[14]

As the year 1911 drew to an end, Edsall found that things were not going well in St. Louis. The new department heads were younger than many of the distinguished clinicians on their staffs and did not have a well-organized tradition. Under such circumstances, it was difficult to break down the long-standing beliefs that established practice as the only worthwhile goal and provided no basis for understanding the need for research. Soon Edsall was called to Harvard, which was destined to reap the benefits of his hard-earned knowledge and experience relating to the proper development of clinical science.

Of Edsall's influence in Philadelphia, Isaac Starr spoke as follows:

Rated as the leader of the progressives in Philadelphia, Edsall was instrumental in attracting a group of new faculty members to the University of

Pennsylvania Medical School. The conservatives reacted vigorously and a bitter struggle for power resulted during which Edsall resigned. A. N. Richards, one of the new faculty, thought that Edsall had fled at the first sign of opposition and he never had any use for him after that. But Richards always saw people as either black or white and Edsall's later success in changing Harvard Medical School from a Boston based institution to a national one indicates that he might well have done the same in Philadelphia. From my contact with him at the MGH I would rate Edsall as a very dull teacher and this must have contrasted with the oratorical brilliance of the Peppers during his Philadelphia days. The Harvard experience showed clearly that he had great talent for organization and for finding and pushing talented men. I should judge that the fracas which caused Edsall to leave Philadelphia set back the development of the University of Pennyslvania Medical School about 10 years; many thought that had he stayed and fought it out he would have won.[15]

## Alfred Stengel as Professor

In 1910 Alfred Stengel, William Pepper's son-in-law, was made professor of medicine at the age of forty-three. Like Osler, he had had experience as a gross pathologist and, with Herbert Fox, had written a textbook of pathology. Both Osler and Stengel had a great ineterest in predicting during a patient's life the lesions to be found at necropsy. Stengel had more confidence in the drug therapy of that era than did Osler, however, and "some of the mixtures prescribed on his service at the University Hospital would cause the hair of a modern skeptic to stand up."[16]

Stengel's problem was to run a department of medicine with almost no money. The members of his department worked at the university hospital all morning without pay; their living was made by seeing patients in their offices all afternoon. Their "university pay" consisted of the privilege of admitting their patients to the hospital, and the intellectual rewards of discussing the patients with their peers. Stengel did little research himself and did not insist that his staff do any; however, if they wanted to, he did everything he could to help. He attracted no one to the University of Pennsylvania by his ideas and insisted that everyone in the department earn his living by the practice of medicine.[17] As Osler said of the University of Pennsylvania faculty in his essay "Equanimitas," "you let me alone, what more could you have done." One often forgets how very recent is the concept that a professor should do research.

## Alfred Newton Richards

Of the professors that Edsall was responsible for bringing to Philadelphia, Richards[18] had the greatest influence on the development of clinical science. Richards graduated from Yale, in June 1897, with honors in chemistry. He was greatly influenced by an elective given by Russell H. Chittenden; the course was designed for those who intended to study medicine; Richards at that time regarded himself as a member of that group. When Richards could not pursue his goal after graduation, because of financial stringencies, Chittenden offered him a fellowship for a year of graduate study at Yale. With Chittenden, he studied the starch-splitting power of saliva; their research led to a joint publication in the first volume of the *American Journal of Physiology*. When Chittenden agreed to modernize the department of chemistry at P & S in 1898, he invited Richards to participate. Richards was made an assistant in physiological chemistry and was allowed to work toward a Ph.D. degree, which he received in 1901, the first such degree awarded from Columbia's department of physiological chemistry. His thesis on the composition of yellow elastic connective tissue provided valuable experience for his later work. Philip Hansen Hiss, the professor of bacteriology who was interested in the development of differential culture media, asked young Richards to provide him with glycogen, which Richards soon isolated from scallops. Then Hiss called for a carbohydrate that would yield only levulose, and Richards found such a substance—inulin—in dahlia bulbs. This episode came back to Richards thirty years later when he was searching for a diffusible polysaccharide that would not be digested in the blood or urine of the frog's kidney. It led him (with B. B. Westfall and P. A. Bott) to study the renal clearance of inulin in dogs at least a year before it was utilized elsewhere.

Richard's accomplishments impressed Hiss, who spoke to Christian A. Herter, then a member of the Columbia faculty, who had just been named a trustee of the new Rockefeller Institute. Richards received the first scholarship ever granted by the institute, which enabled him to spend the next year working with Herter.

In 1904 Richards began a study of the influence of cyanide, chloroform, and other oxidation inhibitors on the ability of the liver to detoxify indole. This program was generated when Richards was asked to provide chemical assistance for Howland, who, as a young assistant to L. Emmett Holt, was trying to improve the treatment of a child suffering from cyclical vomiting. The studies of Howland and Holt led to a report in 1904 on chronic poisoning by indole.

After two years of effort to establish pharmacology at the Northwestern Medical School in Chicago (1908–10), Richards was invited by Edsall, then professor of therapeutics at the University of Pennsylvania, to reorganize the department of pharmacology.

Richards immediately attracted excellent young men into his laboratory, many of whom made distinguished contributions to clinical research. In June 1913, Cecil Kent Drinker, a member of the graduating class in medicine at Pennsylvania, worked with Richards while waiting to study under Howell at Johns Hopkins. The two designed a perfusion pump, which Richards and Plant used later to perfuse the kidney in their studies on the mechanism of the diuretic action of xanthines. After World War I, he and Plant resumed the kidney perfusion experiments, in an attempt to test the effects of raising perfusion pressure on urine flow while maintaining the quantity and quality of blood flowing through the kidney constant. This interest developed out of the work of Richards and Dale on histamine, which suggested the possibility of a rise in glomerular filtration pressure, along with a fall in renal arterial pressure. Out of these experiments came evidence that Richards regarded as support for the Ludwig filtration-reabsorption concept of urine formation.

In 1919 Richards conceived the idea that the effect of adrenalin on  perfusion pressure was due to relatively greater constriction of efferent rather than afferent glomerular arterioles—a totally new concept, which became an essential part of modern nephrology. Richards's next step was to search for direct experimental proof of his hypothesis. A report was found in which Ghiron claimed to have followed, under the microscope, the course of intravenously injected dye through the kidney of a living mouse. It was soon found that this was possible in the frog kidney; with this observation the experimental approach that brought fame to Richards and to his department originated.

Joseph T. Wearn, while a fellow in Richards's laboratory, improved the technique for microscopy of the living frog kidney and was responsible for the start of definitive chemical studies on glomerular, tubular, and bladder fluid. Richards, of course, had not forgotten the adrenalin hypothesis; when he saw a demonstration of Robert Chambers's new capillary pipette in 1921, Richards realized that this device would enable him to inject adrenalin directly into a glomerulus. Wearn later recognized that it should be equally possible to withdraw fluid from the glomerular space for chemical comparison with bladder urine. Thus was born the technique of micropuncture of the kidney. One cannot describe here all of the studies by Richards and his pupils, but the introduction of micropuncture has been such an important advance that it is worth recording in Richards's own words how it came about. The following quotation is from a letter to Paul Weiss, president of the Harvey Society, written in December 1962:

> Warfield Longcope was president of the Harvey Society during the year 1919–1920. He invited me to give one of the lectures.... Having done some perfusion experiments on the rabbit ... which led to the belief that the efferent arteriole was a contractile structure and could take part in the regulation of glomerular capillary pressure I thought that a description of these experiments might serve as the nucleus of a Harvey Lecture....
>
> During the months preceding the ... lecture I read August Krogh's work on the capillaries of the frog's tongue, and the thought occurred, if Krogh could see the minute vessels in the tongue perhaps if I tried I could see the small vessels in the frog's kidneys. Carl Schmidt and I tried and found that vessels of that kidney could quite easily be visualized....

In April of that year [1921] I saw Robert Chambers puncture erythro-cytes and imagined that I might with one of his pipettes, apply a little adrenalin to an exposed efferent vessel. In September of that year Joseph T. Wearn[19] came to work in my laboratory. After he had learned how to expose a living frog's kidney for direct microscopic study and come to realize its possibilities, I suggested that we make capillary pipettes and try to apply adrenalin to an efferent vessel. . . . He countered with the sugges-tion, why not puncture a glomerular capsule with the pipette, catch some glomerular fluid and find out what was in it. He went to work, succeeded, and this experiment gave the first direct proof of reabsorption of glucose and chloride from the tubule and pointed to the identity of glomerular fluid with the protein-free plasma.[20]

The initial publication with the description of methods and presenta-tion of results appeared in the December 1924 issue of the *American Journal of Physiology.*

## The Pupils of Alfred Newton Richards

Of interest are the subsequent careers of the young men who came to Richards, either as medical undergraduates or just after internship, at-tracted by the excitement of his work and by the personality of the man himself.[21]

Cecil Kent Drinker came in 1912 as a medical undergraduate. Drinker later became professor of physiology and dean of the Harvard School of Public Health. Francis Heed Adler worked with Richards for one summer in 1917 on the colorimetric analysis of urine for urea. Adler later was professor of ophthalmology at Pennsylvania. Carl F. Schmidt was the third young medical man to join Richards, doing so in 1919 after his internship at the University of Pennsylvania Hospital. Schmidt be-came a famous physiologist and pharmacologist with an interest in the brain and respiration and, in turn, was responsible for the research careers of such well-known scientists as Julius H. Comroe, George Koelle, and Robert Dripps. Schmidt succeeded Richards as the chairman of the department of pharmacology at Pennsylvania.

Joseph T. Wearn, after completing his internship at the Peter Bent Brigham Hospital, came in 1921 as the fourth of the young medical men to join Richards's research program. Wearn, after several years with Peabody at Harvard, eventually became dean, vice-president for medical affairs, and professor of medicine at Western Reserve University. In his Kober Medal acceptance speech at an Association of American Physi-cians meeting in 1965, he vividly described his work in Richards's labora-tory.[22]

Isaac Starr studied with Richards as an undergraduate and returned to his department after his internship at the MGH. After working on the mammalian kidney, Starr developed an interest in clinical pharmacology and the pharmacology of the circulation. He remained in Richards's department for ten years and then became professor and chairman of the department of therapeutic research at Pennsylvania. He was president of the American Society for Clinical Investigation in 1939. He received the Lasker Award in 1957 and the Kober Medal of the Association of American Physicians in 1967 for his cardiovascular research.

Joseph Marchand Hayman, Jr., was with Richards from 1923 to 1929, starting directly after internship at the Pennsylvania Hospital. He worked there on kidney problems until he went to Western Reserve with Wearn, eventually becoming a professor of medicine there. He was later dean and professor of medicine at Tufts University.

John Blair Barnwell joined Richards in 1923, after his internship at the Pennsylvania Hospital. He developed pulmonary tuberculosis and left in 1926. On recovering from this disease, he directed the tuberculosis service of the Veteran's Administration and initiated the well-known cooperative studies of chemotherapy in tuberculosis, for which he received the Trudeau Medal in 1950.

Howard Walter Florey came to the United States in 1925, sponsored by a Rockefeller Traveling Fellowship, to work in Richards's laboratory. Florey, who later was professor of pathology at Oxford, received the Nobel Prize in 1945 for his development of penicillin.

Eugene M. Landis,[23] after starting research in Bazett's laboratory as an undergraduate and later working with August Krogh and Sir Thomas Lewis, joined Richards's deparment to develop the clinical side of the kidney program. He became professor of medicine at Virginia and later professor of physiology at Harvard, succeeding Walter B. Cannon. His research on capillary pressure and other aspects of the circulation is well known.

William Osler Abbott[24] worked on choline derivatives in Richards's laboratory from 1932 to 1937. He was a pioneer in gastroenterology research, developing intubation methods for the study of the physiology and pharmacology of the intestinal tract and for diagnostic purposes.

Julius H. Comroe worked in Richards's department from 1936 to 1957, beginning there as a medical student and continuing after internship at the university hospital. After being professor of physiology at the University of Pennsylvania Graduate School, Comroe became director of the Cardiovascular Research Institute at the University of California Medical Center. He was largely instrumental in the development of modern clinical respiratory physiology.

There were many others among Richards's pupils, including Arthur Meeker Walker, Leonard Bayliss, Kendall Adams Elsom, James Bordley III,[25] André Simonart, Rudolph Theodore Kempton, James Paisley Hendrix, Charles L. Hudson, Thomas Findley, and Hugh Montgomery. A number of the young physicians who worked with Richards returned to clinical careers.

## The Department of Research Medicine[26]

Richard M. Pearce[27] was brought back to Pennsylvania, where he had received his early training under Simon Flexner, to head the department of research medicine. In 1909 Harriet C. Prevost (a patient of Pearce's father-in-law, John Herr Musser, one of the two professors of clinical medicine at Pennsylvania) offered funds to found a department of research medicine (see chapter 7). Musser was to be the director of the department and would have power to name a professor of research medicine. After Musser's death in 1912, the university obtained a revision of the deed of the gift, and from then on the department was known as the John H. Musser Department of Research Medicine.

Pearce soon left Pennsylvania to do executive work at the Rockefeller Foundation. He was succeeded by James Harold Austin, who had received his M.D. degree from Pennsylvania in 1908.[28] Austin interned at the university hospital (1908–10) after graduation. In 1911 he was appointed an assistant to the head physician of Philadelphia General Hospital and was an associate in research medicine from 1911 to 1914. After World War I, he became an assistant resident physician at the HRI, working with Van Slyke on gas transport by the blood. After returning to Philadelphia as John Herr Musser Professor of Research Medicine, he studied problems of a chemical nature having a clinical bearing.

Although his research achievements were not numerous, Austin made an important contribution to clinical science. He came across Fisher's book on biomathematics shortly after its publication and had the mathematical background to appreciate it. He introduced statistics into the university hospital, and for years every clinician writing a paper consulted him in this area. He also served with distinction as editor of the *Journal of Clinical Investigation*. Recognizing Austin's special talents, Richards appointed him director of the routine laboratories of the hospital. Austin's associate, Stadie, succeeded him as professor of research medicine.

Stadie[29] was a competent investigator, as evidenced by his research at the HRI (see chapter 5). He graduated in 1916 from Columbia and interned at the Presbyterian Hospital. In 1922 he became an assistant professor of medicine at Yale. He joined the staff at Pennsylvania as an associate professor of research medicine in 1925 and succeeded Austin in 1941.

Most of Stadie's important contributions can be classified into three broad fields: the blood gases, the metabolism of fats, and the metabolism of carbohydrates. In each of these areas, Stadie's work covered both the physiological and pathological conditions. His approach was characterized by a rare combination of scholarly study of the known facts and concepts, a plan of attack in breadth and depth that, coupled with research skill, made certain that significant advances would emerge.[30]

Isaac Starr spoke of Stadie's accomplishments at Pennsylvania in the following fashion:

> More mathematically minded than most clinical investigators he gradually became aware that the amount of $CO_2$, added to exhaled air by the pulmonary blood flow, far exceeded that which could be accounted for by current theory. Seeking an explanation he was led into a new field, that of enzymes, which occupied him for the remainder of his life. His studies led to a revolution in our thinking about the chemical abnormalities of diabetes mellitus and they are still, 17 years after his death, the last word on certain features of that disease. With the exception of his pioneering work during the influenza epidemic, Stadie could not be called a clinical investigator. Though interested in the enzyme changes in many diseases he worked all of his time in Philadelphia on animal preparations and muscle strips. However, he influenced the thinking and provided the stimulus for many at the University of Pennsylvania Hospital, who were more directly engaged in research with patients, during his illustrious career there.[31]

Stadie, in his acceptance of the Kober Medal in 1955, commented on some of those who influenced his career development:

> Warfield Longcope, whom I admired at a distance, was Physician-in-Chief at the Presbyterian Hospital [New York] when I interned there. It was an education to work under him. He taught us the importance of a thorough-going history taking, careful physical examinations, and above all the necessity of delving deeply into contemporary literature in medicine. . . . He represented to me the very epitomization of the consulting physician—experienced, learned, and always polished.
>
> Six years before the advent of insulin, Rawle Geyelin gave me my first insight into diabetes mellitus. He taught me the heroic and inexorable rationale of the contemporary treatment—starvation till the patient was sugar-free. I learned from him how to adjust the diet according to this rationale. . . . This was my first taste of what I considered to be scientific medicine.
>
> In 1917, Bill Palmer came to the Presbyterian. I remember my delight at this event for was not Bill Palmer the very prophet of scientific medicine who had come to us from L. J. Henderson via Van Slyke? Henderson had put the law of mass action into physiology and Van Slyke had crystallized acid-base equilibrium into principles that were appealing to my chemical mindedness. All this Palmer expounded to us, but more than this the solidity of his character, his universal interest in all aspects of medicine, his helpfulness on needed occasions were things which I absorbed with much benefit.[32]

## Isaac Starr

Certainly the most distinguished of Richards's pupils as far as clinical science is concerned was Isaac Starr.[33] After graduation from Pennsylvania, Starr interned at the MGH. Boston medicine was at its best. He learned much from such visiting physicians as Roger Lee, Joseph C. Aub, George R. Minot, and Cecil Drinker.

When the internship was over, Starr joined Richards's laboratory, where he found Wearn, Schmidt, and Joseph Hayman. He did research on the rabbit's kidney with Hayman for several years,[34] but the urge to return to clinical medicine was strong, and Richards was interested in developing clinical pharmacology.

The first medical ward to which he was assigned as visiting physician contained many severe diabetics because insulin, just discovered, was available to the hospital, but not to most practitioners. Since many of these diabetics had advanced peripheral vascular disease, Starr set up Stewart's calorimetric method of measuring blood flow through the feet. Finding that the circulation was reduced in gangrenous and pregangrenous conditions, he studied the effect of therapeutic measures upon it.

Starr's interest in peripheral vascular disease was further stimulated by pharmacological work going on in Richards's laboratory; the actions of new choline derivatives, synthesized by Ralph Major of the Merck Company, were being studied in animal experiments by Simonart. Some of these new drugs proved to be more powerful vasodilators than any known previously, which raised the hope that their action might benefit such cases.

Starr could demonstrate no definite effects of the drugs in patients with peripheral vascular disease. He did demonstrate that the heat cradle, routinely used on such patients, often overheated the limb and could thus be definitely harmful.

In 1928 Starr and Hayman were appointed assistant professors of clinical pharmacology; this was probably the first time that the title was ever used. In Richards's course in pharmacology there was a laboratory exercise in which the students observed the action of a few commonly used drugs on themselves. Starr was put in charge of this section, and it provided him for many years with a source of normal volunteers in whom drug action could be studied, first by existing cardiac output methods and later by the ballistocardiogram.

That an increase in the strength of the cardiac contraction followed exercise and appeared during the action of catecholamines was easily demonstrated by these methods in literally hundreds of normal subjects. Thus, the ability of Starr's methods to detect changes in cardiac contractility qualitatively was established early in his studies.

After the conventional animal experiments had been made by the pharmacologists in Richards's laboratory, Starr studied the clinical pharmacology of all the newer choline derivatives, both in normal volunteers and in patients likely to be benefited by their action. During these studies, the methods used for the detection of drug action in patients were steadily improved. The ballistocardiogram, first studied in the hope that it would provide a noninvasive cardiac output method, soon proved to be closer related to the forces of the circulation, an aspect of cardiac function not studied before.

In his search for better methods of demonstrating drug action in his patients, Starr has scrupulously avoided the invasive procedures that, by frightening or hurting the subjects, might so alter circulation that the demonstration of drug action or of its absence would be difficult.

In 1933, when Starr was named Hartzell Professor of Therapeutic Research, his official relations with the department of pharmacology were severed only in theory. After he had received this chair, Starr's annual budget contained no salaries for collaborators and only $750 for research expenses. He soon found, however, that young doctors were glad to work with him without pay. Some of these collaborators were clinicians, interested by an observation on the wards that could be studied by the methods that Starr had developed. Others were physiologists or pharmacologists interested in applying knowledge gained in animal experiments to patients. Starr himself wondered whether the demonstration that one does not have to have much money to do effective research was not one of his greatest contributions to the medical scene. Starr has always preferred to work by himself; indeed, what he chiefly needed for his research was to be left alone. He had seen too many American scientists who, having asked for and received large financial support, found that the recruitment, training, and administration of a large team took so much of their time that the loss to their research exceeded the gain.

After World War II Starr's financial support grew. The U.S. Public Health Service built him a new laboratory in the university hospital and provided the funds to permit a most fruitful collaboration with H. C. Berger, professor of biophysics at Utrecht, Holland. This collaboration lasted many years and provided mathematical and engineering support of the greatest value. Major technical improvements in the ballistocardiograph (BCG) resulted, and Noordergraaf devised a mathematical theory of the circulation in which the relations of all measurable aspects to one another are defined. Electrical models of the circulation followed, and such studies showed clearly that the BCG has its origin in movements of the body's center of gravity. A physiological explanation for the BCG abnormalities found in cardiac patients was thus provided.

Starr's interest in mathematics has always strongly influenced the direction of his work. He saw clearly that the cardiac studies used routinely in the clinic gave no information about the higher-frequency aspects of the circulation, and those associated with the velocity and acceleration of blood. These aspects seemed to him vital to any proper estimation of cardiac strength, and he lost no opportunity to improve his knowledge of them.

Yandall Henderson had constructed a crude low-frequency ballistocardiograph in 1905 and had published papers on the effects of altitude on the normal circulation. Starr built the first instrument capable of supplying quantitative information and made the first clinical studies; the name *ballistocardiograph* was introduced by him. He reasoned  that, since the heart sets the blood in motion, Newton's laws of motion must apply. In order to describe motion quantitatively, Newton had to invent calculus, and Starr turned to calculus for interpretation of the records obtained by his improved instruments.

Starr was always eager to apply the newer mathematical techniques to his work. Austin first called his attention to Fisher's book on statistical methods; after reading this, Starr always had a calculator on his desk. It is of interest that one of his papers, published in the *Journal of Clinical Investigation* in 1933, was credited by the editors of that journal with being the first clinical paper in which modern statistical methods had been used. The significance of his results has constantly been tested with statistical analyses.[35]

Trained by Richards in the hard school of quantitative methodology, Starr had always been concerned with testing his methods. With such tests in mind, he designed and carried out experiments in which systole was stimulated in fresh cadavers at necropsy. The results revolutionized his thinking about cardiac function; cardiac output was found to be a poor measure of "cardiac" strength; such strength could be much better estimated from the forces generated by cardiac action.

Thus Starr sought a better method of detecting the weak heart in the high-frequency aspects of the heart's performance, those associated with velocity and acceleration of the ejected blood. He planned to assess such aspects in his patients by taking two records simultaneously; one a derivative of the carotid pulse, a pressure record, and the second the force ballistocardiogram, a flow record.[36]

These methods are now used to measure cardiac contractility and the effectiveness of therapeutic means to improve it. For example, the coronary bypass operation is usually followed by improved cardiac performance, though the maximum gain is seldom maintained in its entirety. The operative procedures used before the introduction of the by-pass resulted in no improvement in contractility.

After studies of his patients by the new methods had stimulated Starr's interest in the high-frequency aspects of heart disease, certain common abnormalities began to attract his attention. Abnormal notches and extra waves, never seen in healthy young adults, were found frequently in both the force BCG and the pulse derivative of many cases of heart disease. This finding plainly suggested that the myocardium was not contracting as a unit. The conception was soon supported by results secured in cadaver experiments in which irregularities of "cardiac" ejection, produced experimentally, were accompanied by corresponding irregularities in one or both of these high-frequency records. Additional evidence of the nature of these abnormalities has accompanied the demonstration in many clinics that cines taken after the injection of x-ray opaque material into the cardiac chambers often demonstrated systolic irregularities of the movement of the ventricular silhouette.

It seems evident that this new conception has brought together the anatomical and physiological findings in coronary heart disease in a gratifying way. We can now believe that those parts of the heart poorly supplied with blood contract less strongly than the areas that are well supplied. In contrast to the "smooth" normal contraction, a "rough" abnormal contraction is to be expected in advanced coronary heart disease. Such abnormalities of cardiac function, completely missed by the conventional clinical methods of the past, are extremely common and appear to have great significance.

In recent years, most of Starr's work has been closely correlated with that of the cardiac catheterization laboratory; over four hundred patients have been studied, both by the battery of invasive tests that can be performed only during catheterization, and by his own group of noninvasive tests. By comparing the pulse rate and systolic blood pressure in the two sets of tests, he has been able to eliminate those individuals whose response is affected by the excitement of catheterization. The remainder, those individuals with differences in pulse and blood pressure that do not exceed the deviation of duplicates during the two sets of tests, are accepted as being able to undergo catheterization without excitement and judged suitable for physiological studies. From the large body of data he has secured, Starr has sought correlations of interest by computer techniques. He has found that the heart's work is related inversely to the amount of coronary arteriosclerosis, and that the arterial pulse amplitude provides an excellent noninvasive estimate of left ventricular strength, whereas the amount of venous congestion does not. The search for simple, inexpensive, and more accurate noninvasive methods of estimating cardiac strength and coordination remains a continuing interest of Starr's.

As the best final test of his clinical data, Starr relies on long-term follow-up of his patients, and he has personally followed several series of cases for over forty years. In such long-term studies, both cardiac weakness and cardiac incoordination are accompanied by markedly diminished life expectancy and increased frequency of untoward cardiac events, findings now confirmed in other laboratories.

Starr still works daily in the laboratory, although he passed the normal age of retirement more than a decade and a half ago. He still publishes about two papers per year, as he has done since his first paper appeared in 1919.[37]

## Other Examples of Clinical Investigation at Pennsylvania

### T. Grier Miller and William Osler Abbott

Although the clinical specialty divisions in medicine were on a "geographical" full-time basis, excellent research was accomplished. T. Grier Miller (M.D., Pennsylvania, 1911) served a two-year internship at the

University of Pennsylvania Hospital. He joined Stengel's staff and worked in Pearce's laboratory. Miller organized the gastrointestinal clinic in 1928 and established the Kinsey Thomas Foundation for the Study of Gastrointestinal Disease. Miller's bibliography is impressive in its breadth and depth.[38]

Miller's most outstanding fellow was William Osler Abbott.[39] Beginning in 1934, Miller published a series of papers with Abbott and W. G. Karr, which were made possible by the invention of the double-lumen tube, the well-known Miller-Abbott tube. The story of the development of the tube is interesting. Abbott was frustrated by not being able to keep a distended balloon at a fixed point in the duodenum. Miller suggested that he tie a second open tube to the bag and see if in that way he could readily secure material from the lower small intestine. Thus, almost by accident, a relatively rapid method of intestinal intubation was created.[40] The value of this technique in intestinal obstruction was not, however, at first suspected. Its initial use in this abnormality followed a suggestion by the surgeon Charles G. Johnston, and was accomplished by Abbott.

From 1934 to 1940 Abbott greatly improved the technique of small intestinal intubation, using the fluoroscope to identify the location of the tip of the tube and thus guide its course down the gastrointestinal tract. The hazards of chronic exposure to x-ray were not fully realized at this time; such exposure led to Abbott's tragic death from leukemia in 1943.

## C.N.H. Long and F.D.W. Lukens

In 1932 C.N.H. Long[41] became the first director of the George S. Cox Medical Research Institute of the University of Pennsylvania School of Medicine. He found the institute consisted of a suite of rooms with bare walls, except for a plaque stating that the institute's purpose was to "find a cure for diabetes." He shared the laboratory with a skillful clinician, Francis Lukens.

Long was educated at Manchester University in biochemistry. He received his M.D. degree at McGill University in 1928. A. V. Hill, the professor of physiology at Manchester, who was working on the physical and chemical changes underlying muscular contraction, needed the assistance of a chemist. Long accepted the challenge, and his conversion from chemist to physiologist took place rapidly. After receiving his master's from Manchester in 1923, he joined E. H. Starling's physiology department at University College, London, for two years. Long began to study diabetes and the role of the various endocrine glands on metabolism during its development. During his period at McGill, he was preoccupied with the fate of lactic acid in health and disease and the neuroendocrine control of carbohydrate metabolism.

Francis Lukens (M.D., Pennsylvania, 1925) had three years of medical residency at Pennsylvania and then served as Jacques Loeb Fellow in Medicine at Johns Hopkins (1928–30). After two years in gastroenterology under Miller, Lukens joined Long in 1932. When Long went to Yale in 1936, Lukens assumed the directorship of the Cox Institute, holding this position for thirty years.[42]

Long and Lukens appreciated the importance of Houssay's discovery that removal of the pituitary gland produced amelioration of experimental diabetes. They recalled the clinical observation that diminished function of the adrenal cortex lowers the blood sugar. They knew also that removal of the pituitary is followed by adrenal atrophy, so that they began a study of the possible role of the adrenal cortex in the Houssay preparation. By early 1934 Lukens was able to prepare cats not only pancreatectomized, but having both adrenals removed as well. The first such cat lived twice as long as the usual diabetic cat, and its blood-sugar values were lower than normal without insulin. The significant aspect of this discovery was that the syndrome of diabetes had to be reconsidered in view of the role played by the pituitary and other ductless glands in the events that followed experimental pancreatectomy. In 1936 Long proposed an important concept in endocrine research: "the clinical condition that follows hypo- or hyper-function of an endocrine organ is not merely due to the loss or plethora of that particular internal secretion but is a result of the disturbance of the normal hormonal equilibrium of the body."

Lukens's later work with F. C. Dohan employed a second form of experimental diabetes; namely, that induced by anterior pituitary extracts. This permitted a study of the breakdown and recovery of the Islands of Langerhans under various conditions. For at least one tissue, the beta cells, the value of controlling hyperglycemia was evident under the conditions used. Elementary studies of the relation of growth hormone and insulin to protein metabolism showed that, to enable growth hormone to cause its usual retention of nitrogen, the insulin dosage of depancreatized animals had to be increased three- to five-fold. In Bernardo A. Houssay's animals, growth hormone produced no nitrogen retention, again emphasizing the fundamental place of insulin in anabolism. During these laboratory studies, inpatient and outpatient activities kept alive the constant effort to examine and improve what was done for the patient.

## Eugene M. Landis

Eugene M. Landis (M.D., Pennsylvania, 1926) completed his Ph.D. degree in physiology under Merkel H. Jacobs. From 1927 to 1929, he was a rotating intern at the university hospital. He received a Guggenheim Research Fellowship to work with Sir Thomas Lewis in London (1929–30) and August Krogh in Copenhagen (1930–31).

He returned to Pennsylvania in 1931, as an associate in medicine and pharmacology. In 1939 he became chairman of the department of medicine at the University of Virginia. After four years there, he was appointed Higginson Professor of Physiology at Harvard Medical School (1943–67).

Landis's research dealt chiefly with the physiology and patho-physiology of the capillary blood vessels, particularly pressures, permeability, and fluid movements through capillary walls.[43] In 1926 he began using micromanipulators and micropipettes to measure blood pressures in single capillaries and in immediately connected arterioles and venules. His studies, which focused on both dog and man, provided quantitative support for the Starling hypothesis of fluid movement through the capillary wall. In other studies, the permeability of the capillary wall to isotonic fluid was measured by determining filtration and absorption constants or coefficients first in single capillaries of frogs' mesentery and then in the collective capillary network of the human forearm—the former by micromethods, and the latter by a special pressure plethysmograph. Later he used these techniques to measure how capillary permeability to fluid, certain dyes, and plasma proteins was affected by chemical injury, pH, $CO_2$, severe hypoxia, venous congestion, tissue pressure, muscular contraction, heat, cold, histamine, and transmural differences of osmolality. His studies led him at various stages to the investigation of related aspects of microcirculatory pathophysiology in peripheral vascular disease, congestive heart failure, hypertension, and nephrosis.

## Charles C. Wolferth and the Edward C. Robinette Foundation for Cardiovascular Research

Charles C. Wolferth (M.D., Pennsylvania, 1912) interned two years and spent another year as a resident in clinical pathology. He was the first chief medical resident at the university hospital (1915–16). In 1917 he became interested in patients with cardiovascular disease and, immediately after the war, studied in Lewis's laboratory in England.

By 1919 an electrocardiograph machine had already been obtained at Pennsylvania, and Wolferth was asked to organize a cardiovascular laboratory, which he modeled after the one in London. As director of the Robinette Foundation (founded in 1928), Wolferth had many important associates, including Thomas M. McMillan, Alexander Margolies, Samuel Bellet, Eugene M. Landis, Lewis H. Hitzrot, and Francis Carter Wood. In later years other well-known physician-scientists worked with him, including Hugh Montgomery, William A. Jeffers, Calvin F. Kay, Truman G. Schnabel, Jr., and Harry P. Zinsser.

Wolferth had a variety of interests, including arrhythmias, hypertension, the anginal syndrome, the generation of heart sounds, the diagnosis of myocardial infarction by chest leads, experimental myocardial ischemia, bundle branch block, and subtotal adrenalectomy combined with sympathectomy for relief of hypertension.

Although Frank Wilson had demonstrated that much could be

learned about cardiac electrical phenomena by placing electrodes directly over the heart (precordial leads), eletrocardiographers continued to employ only the three standard leads until the 1930s. At that time, Wood and Wolferth were interested in the electrocardiogram before, during, and after attacks of anginal pain. Wood had performed experimental studies in dogs, taking electrocardiograms before, during, and after brief periods of obstruction of the coronary arteries. With the standard leads, he did not get any changes when the left anterior branch was obstructed. He then put a lead on the anterior chest wall of the dog and saw striking abnormalities. The following day, when a suitable patient appeared, Wood and Wolferth first demonstrated the changes of coronary occlusion by a precordial lead, after no abnormalities had been detected in the standard electrocardiogram.

Francis Carter Wood[44] received his M.D. degree from Pennsylvania in 1926. After a two-year rotating internship at the Hospital of the University of Pennsylvania, he became a fellow of the Robinette Foundation. From 1947 to 1964 he was chairman of the department of medicine. Wood made a number of other important contributions to cardiology, including a description of diastolic heart sound in patients with pericardial disease.[45]

# 11

⚜

# The Cornell University Medical College–
# New York Hospital Medical Center
# and the Lusk School of Metabolism
# and Nutritional Studies

The most significant element in the development of clinical science at Cornell was the Russell Sage Institute of Pathology and its director, Graham Lusk. By relating his early contributions, their significance to the sequence of events at Cornell University Medical College can be put in perspective.

The son of an obstetrician, Lusk followed in his father's footsteps by going to Germany for advanced studies. Because of Lusk's deafness, his father advised him to forgo medical school and study medical chemistry. In Carl Voit of Munich he found a revered master of whose doctrines and techniques he became a devoted disciple (see chapter 1).

Lusk's father, William T. Lusk, was made professor of physiology at the Long Island College Hospital in 1869. In 1870–71, at the request of Oliver Wendell Holmes, he delivered a course of lectures on physiology at the Harvard Medical School and was among the first to use experimental demonstrations. He then accepted the professorship of obstetrics at the Bellevue Hospital Medical College. His textbook, *The Science and Art of Mid-Wifery,* which appeared in 1882, was written with physiology as its background. The elder Lusk was surrounded in New York by physicians of the old school, only a few of whom had any knowledge of the fundamental sciences. It was an era of bitter controversies about medical education. Lusk was a good fighter, and his son received a strong stimulus toward the reform of medical education.

Graham Lusk's first academic position in the United States was in physiology at Yale, where he became an assistant professor in 1895. He was happy there with Chittenden's inspiring group, but was distressed about the state of clinical medicine. The call to the professorship of physiology at New York University and Bellevue Hospital Medical College in 1898 appeared to offer him greater opportunities. He soon found, however, that clinicians there had little interest in advancing medicine along scientific lines.

While New York had distinguished clinicians, their primary interest was medical practice; advancement in a medical college or hospital was conditioned by a system of priority. The steps upward were the tombstones of one's predecessors. To deviate from this pyramidal type of advancement, by entering a laboratory or going to another institution for special work, was equivalent to "professional suicide." A school devoted to scientific endeavor in clinical medicine was unknown in New York. Lusk defined such an institution as "a group consisting of a master surrounded by pupils who in turn become masters."[1] The average physician's ignorance of physiology and biological chemistry made the transition from the atmosphere of the physiology laboratory to that of the clinic a shock for many students. Lusk quickly detected where the fault lay. He accused the old guard, a group who appeared to consider the science and art of medicine as mutually exclusive, of being interested chiefly in maintaining the status quo. In a plea for the development of leaders, he cited the career of his idol Friedrich von Müller and asked why such training was not possible in America. In 1909 he outlined possible sources of the problem: "One is that we are all dollar chasers; the second, that we are intellectually deficient; the third, that our system is rotten."[2] He quickly discarded the first two possibilities, because he had seen his own students, at a financial sacrifice, devote themselves to the science of physiology. Furthermore, he had influenced Theodore Caldwell Janeway to apply the methods of physiology at the bedside, and he had seen him turn aside from unusual opportunities in medical practice to prepare himself for a career as a teacher of clinical medicine. Lusk concluded that the fault in educational methods lay in the system. Although he never neglected physiology, he fought constantly for clinical positions with security. He recommended the migration of directors and assistants from one medical clinic to another as vacancies arose.

Lusk not only trained men who pursued careers in clinical science but also continued his fight for proper research clinics. In 1915 a national committee was considering reorganization of departments of clinical medicine in the United States. The committee consisted largely of practicing physicians, who were not inclined to combine a responsibility for scientific research and the teaching of clinical medicine. Lusk wrote as follows:

> It is impossible in any faculty to approach this subject without hurting the feelings of true and honorable men . . . who are not to blame for the present situation. . . . The truth of the matter is that, as a country, we have produced few men in medical science. This is frankly because the teaching of medicine has not been in accordance with modern science. The staff of

the medical department should consist of men, themselves devoted to medical science, capable of carrying it on, brought up in the air of it and blessed by the enthusiasm of it. Such men should be produced under the leadership of the Professor of Medicine. . . . Other remedies are only temporary palliatives.[3]

Lusk believed that the facilities for medical research in the hospital should be open to all connected with the school. He suggested that the heads of departments of medicine be placed upon a full-time salaried basis, with a prohibition of private practice for five years. At the end of that time, he felt it would be evident whether it was necessary for a master of medical science to have a sharpening of the wits that an outside consulting practice was supposed to produce.

How thoroughly Lusk believed in the necessity of building such a clinic was soon made evident. He helped Dean Pope of Cornell offer such facilities to a few well-chosen men. Lusk's enthusiastic support of this project was a large factor in attracting these men to clinical investigation, and the results were important in the creation of medicine's scientific base in this country.

## The Russell Sage Institute of Pathology

In 1907, through the influence of Theodore Caldwell Janeway, Mrs. Russell Sage endowed the Russell Sage Institute of Pathology, to promote research at City Hospital. The institute was under the supervision of Drs. Theodore Caldwell Janeway, Edward G. Janeway, D. V. Delavan, Simon Flexner, and Graham Lusk; emphasis was placed on clinical pathology and service to the physicians of the hospital.

Because of a series of misunderstandings with City Hospital, the institute was moved to Bellevue Hospital in 1913. In the meantime, Lusk had been offered the professorship of physiology at Cornell University Medical College, which brought opportunities for a research program that had been forming in Lusk's mind while he was revising his book *The Science of Nutrition.*[4] He decided to construct a respiration calorimeter of the Atwater-Rosa-Benedict type, suitable in size for study of the energy metabolism of dogs or small children. His objective was to investigate the specific dynamic action of amino acids.

H. B. Williams was sent to Francis G. Benedict's laboratory in Boston to study the construction of the calorimeter. J. A. Riche, who was trained in Benedict's laboratory, was hired to operate the new device. These two men, together with Lusk, formed a research team of unusual ability, with a firm comprehension of physiological factors, combined with high technical skill. The first work done with this calorimeter was by Howland, who studied the energy metabolism of sleeping children.

## Graham Lusk's Research Contributions

Lusk's scientific contributions are so highly technical that they cannot be detailed in this discussion. They have, however, been well summarized by Murlin.[5] In the 1928 edition of his *Science of Nutrition,* Lusk gave eighty-five references to his own work and quoted Max Rubner twice as often. In a review entitled "Fifty Years of Progress in the Chemistry of Physiology and Nutrition in the United States, 1876–1926," Lusk mentioned briefly his dextrose-to-nitrogen ratio of 3.65 in the fasting and meat-fed dog under the influence of phlorizine. This was the same ratio, Lusk pointed out, that he found in a totally diabetic man. John R. Murlin described Lusk's painstaking search for the cause of specific dynamic action, that rise in metabolism that follows the ingestion of food. Protein, fats, carbohydrates, and the products of their intermediary metabolism were studied in great detail. Lusk's experiments have served as source material for those who make calculations in this field. He used relatively few experiments, basing his conclusions on a small number of reliable tests, rather than on a mass of material treated statistically.

Lusk was interested in fostering among clinicians an appreciation of fundamental scientific work and an understanding that such scientific knowledge was not to be dismissed as purely theoretical. In an address entitled "Scientific Medicine—Yesterday and Tomorrow" (1919),[6] Lusk described the status of clinical medicine at the end of the last century and quoted a letter from his lifelong friend Theodore Caldwell Janeway, then twenty-seven years old. Janeway had hopes that, in coming to teach at Bellevue College, he "could take some part in the advance of true medical knowledge and not merely diffuse what is already known." He concluded his letter: "I trust that it will be possible for me to keep in touch with your work and Dr. Dunham's next winter and especially with your enthusiasm, and that I may be able to persuade the students to regard symptomatology as the physiology of the 'sick life.' It will certainly be a most interesting experiment from my side." Lusk went on to say:

> This letter gives no picture of New York medicine as it was then. One should remember that Meltzer, at the time, was a practicing physician snatching such moments of rapture as were his when he drove down 59th Street, tied his horse to a lamp post near P & S and, with his coachman who acted also as laboratory servant, entered the dingy recesses of that college and ascended to the laboratory of physiology, there to perform some fundamental experiment. Herter had just undergone metamorphosis from a specialist in nervous diseases into a physiologic chemist. Park had established a modern laboratory in the Board of Health. But besides this there was little to encourage the adventurer into clinical science. A few years later the medical faculty to which Janeway was attached refused him a

teaching position in Bellevue Hospital, though the salary had been raised from outside sources. The same faculty held a solemn, special meeting to discipline me because I had publicly (before the students) expressed opinions favorable to the Johns Hopkins Medical School.[7] These were days when there appeared to be no future for clinical science, days in which there was almost no intellectual, social or financial influence making for its welfare, and yet we in this country, since that time, have made great headway in this direction, not on account of the influence of any special men, but because the principle that the primary mission of a medical school, "to take some part in the advance of true medical knowledge and not merely to diffuse what is already known," is everlastingly right.

There are excellent reminiscences of Lusk written by students who later became prominent in clinical science. William S. McCann, the first professor of medicine at the University of Rochester, first entered Lusk's laboratory in 1911:[8]

One soon felt the full force of his admiration for the practice of medicine whenever he mentioned his father, one of the Janeways, Friedrich von Müller or John Howland, all of whom he "admitted to the first rank in the world of heroes with which his mind was peopled...." In his lectures Lavoisier was our daily companion, as were Carl Voit and Max Rubner, while Magendie and Claude Bernard appeared at least once a week. He might for instance pause to quote Lavoisier: "We must trust to nothing but the facts. These are presented to us by nature and cannot deceive. We ought in every instance to submit our reasoning to the test of experiment, and never to search for truth but by the natural road of experiment and observation."

McCann recalled that the humblest task in an experiment was not beneath the professor's dignity. He fed his dogs. In his calorimeter room, he worked as a member of the team, making readings and weighings, checking the observations and calculations of his humbler subordinates, and being checked by them.

Occasionally, according to McCann, he would send for a student: "The proudest day of my life was one in the autumn of 1914, when the professor sent for me to say that Harvey Cushing had asked him to send one of his students to the Peter Bent Brigham Hospital as an intern, and that he had decided to send me. No squire ever knelt to receive the accolade of knighthood with a heart more blithe than mine that day."

Lusk made a vital contribution to American physiology and through the men who trained under him to clinical science.[9]

## Clinical Research at the Institute: Lusk and DuBois

Lusk selected Eugene F. DuBois as medical director of the program of which he (Lusk) was the scientific director. A series of papers were published under the title "Clinical Calorimetry." Lusk wrote the first paper, which described the history of calorimetry, as well as the general principles of the Atwater-Rosa-Benedict calorimeter. The second paper described the construction of the instrument by J. A. Riche and G. F. Soderstrom; and the next two, the metabolism ward and the first experiments on basal metabolism by F. C. Gephart and DuBois.

The fifth paper was by the two DuBoises. Delafield Dubois was an excellent mathematician and engineer who was able to add the techniques of the physical sciences and engineering in the study of clinical problems. The term *biomedical engineering* had not been coined, but the work of the calorimetry unit is an impressive example of the application of physical and engineering principles to the experimental study of human physiology and its alterations in disease. The DuBoises selected the ingenious paper-mould method to measure the body surface and found the normal basal metabolism to be closely correlated with it. Coleman and DuBois contributed two articles on typhoid fever, after which there was an article by Lusk on the diabetic respiratory quotient.

These studies appeared simultaneously, in May 1915, and represented the first three year's work with the calorimeter.[10] Papers on animal calorimetry from the medical school, and clinical calorimetry from the hospital, continued to flow from the laboratory for nearly twenty years. The series constitutes one of the most important scientific contributions ever achieved under unified direction in the related fields of physiology and internal medicine. Here was the application of the German methods for which Lusk had long striven, "and when these methods became actually available for his own direction, jointly with men of clinical training, he was supremely happy."[11]

### Eugene Floyd DuBois

DuBois (M.D., P & S, 1906) served a two-year internship at the Presbyterian Hospital.[12] He planned to study bacteriology at the Pasteur Institute, but a chance meeting with Howland turned his interests to human metabolism. In Kraus's clinic, he and Borden Veeder, under the guidance of Theodor Brugsch, studied the total energy requirements in diabetes. On his return in 1909 to the Presbyterian Hospital, DuBois found that there was little time to do research. In 1913 Lusk appointed DuBois as medical director of the new metabolism ward at Bellevue.

Just after World War I, DuBois was appointed medical director of the second medical service at Bellevue Hospital, with the request that he reorganize the service. He gathered about him several young men just out of the army, including William S. McCann, John P. Peters, David P. Barr, Harry L. Alexander, Russell L. Cecil, and Paul Larson. Peters and Barr were working on the blood gases in relation to the alveolar air and blood flow.[13] Alexander was studying allergies, while Cecil and Larson were working with pneumococcal pneumonias and specific therapy with pneumococcal antiserum.

During this period, when scientific medicine was in the ascendency in various clinics, there was a deep antagonism between the old-style clinicians and the new breed interested in scientific medicine. DuBois had the viewpoint of a medical scientist and emphasized investigation in the teaching of physiology and medicine. This provided the point of friction, as it became obvious that a turning point was being reached. There were many excellent practicing physicians, men for whom everyone had great admiration, who did a wonderful job as bedside teachers, spending a great deal of time at it instructing students and interns. It was good medicine, but it did not take into account the application of scientific knowledge to the daily study of patients, and it did not always effectively build on the background that the students were by then receiving in their first two years of medicine. The emphasis that DuBois and Peters placed on this alarmed those of the "old school." They felt that medicine as they knew it was not being properly emphasized. (This conflict, which was evident in other centers as well, was particularly bitter at Johns Hopkins.)

In 1926 DuBois recognized the first case of hyperparathyroidism in America. The patient had the same pattern of chemical abnormalities that J. B. Collip had reported in animals receiving parathyroid extract (see chapter 12).[14]

In 1932 the Russell Sage Institute's unit at Bellevue was moved in its entirety to new quarters in the recently completed New York Hospital on Sixty-eighth Street. DuBois became physician-in-chief to New York Hospital, and, although his increased academic duties occupied much of his time, the calorimetry work proceeded under his supervision. In 1940, when Detlev W. Bronk resigned as professor of physiology, DuBois accepted the position. Despite DuBois's strong devotion to clinical medicine, he was tied even more to research, and as chief of medicine his opportunity for research was steadily diminishing.

DuBois made a major contribution in popularizing the fundamental principles of metabolism in disease,[15] and the union of theory and practice finds no better example than in his work. As Means pointed out: "In the broad and continuous spectrum which there should be between basic science and clinical medicine, DuBois occupied a central position."[16]

DuBois pointed out, in reviewing fifty years of the contribution of physiology in America,[17] that in the period between 1906 and 1910 there was a growing enthusiasm for research in physiology as applied to medicine. There was a realization that human disease furnished the physiologist with material much more dramatic than that obtained in animal experimentation. After 1910 there was an increasing collaboration between the clinical investigator, the physiologist, the biochemist, and the pharmacologist. DuBois quoted Starling as saying "the physiology of today is the medicine of tomorrow." DuBois added: "Nowadays we may have to admit that the medicine of today is the physiology of tomorrow. Take for example the discovery of insulin or the pioneer studies of Cushing on the pituitary."

The close association between medicine and physiology that was established at the Russell Sage Institute demonstrated the essential unity of science and medicine. It enabled DuBois to occupy a chair of medicine or a chair of physiology with equal appropriateness. The significance of this enterprise was by no means limited to important scientific contributions. To the laboratory came a notable group of young clinical investigators for training, among them Francis W. Peabody, James Howard Means, Joseph C. Aub, William S. McCann, John P. Peters, William H. Olmsted, Edward Mason, Paul Larsen, Soma Weiss, and Samuel Z. Levine; all of whom later assumed positions of importance in the development of medical education, science, and practice. They gained inspiration from DuBois's deep faith in principles and standards of scientific and personal conduct.[18] Aub has described his period with DuBois.[19]

DuBois's view of scientific research was expressed in his acceptance of the Kober Medal Award: "Medical research may be a science but it still has some of the characteristics of the arts and also of geographical exploration. It is hard to believe that the arts of music and painting would thrive with mass projects. The history of geographical exploration shows clearly that the great discoveries were made in small boats. Can we do better by exploring in battleships or fleets of battleships?"[20]

## McCann and the Russell Sage Institute of Pathology

William S. McCann began his work with DuBois on October 1, 1919.

> During these years in DuBois' laboratory I was able to participate in ward rounds and in the teaching of physical diagnosis to the third year clinical clerks. This was valuable preparation for the next step in my career soon to come. He [DuBois] exerted great influence on the development of those who worked with him. He was a man of great modesty who was therefore consistently undervalued in a city like New York where success so often depends on showmanship, on a bold front, and a facile tongue. My first real contact with him had come during my second year in medical school when I took an elective course in pathological physiology, which was without doubt the thing that determined the main direction of my career in medicine. When DuBois became one of the first whole time professors of medicine and chief of a large clinical service he did not shine as the brilliant theatrical bedside diagnostician. This phase of the work of the clinic was carried out brilliantly by others, but the inquiring mind of Eugene DuBois was always seeking to understand the mechanisms by which the symptoms and signs of disease were produced. From the insight which he gained into mechanisms came practical therapeutics. . . .
>
> DuBois had been interested in a statement made once by Friedrich von

Müller, who had noted that patients with exophthalmic goitre lost weight in spite of a good food intake, from which he surmised that their metabolism was increased. But at the time there were no standards by which one could determine what the basal metabolism or "Grund Umsatz" would be. DuBois set himself the task of doing this. The "Grund" or "Basal" condition was established to be that of complete rest and 16 hours after the last intake of food. Measurements were made in the calorimeter over a three hour period, and the results were referred to bodily measurements of the patient or subject, such as weight, height, surface area, sex, and age. Laboriously he had worked out methods for determining the surface area of the body since his results indicated the most consistent correlation of heat production and surface area in normal subjects under basal conditions. Once this basic work was established it furnished clinicians with a diagnostic tool which was soon widely used in the diagnosis and treatment of diseases of the thyroid gland in which it found its widest application.

During World Ward I Dr. DuBois served in the Navy, where he was assigned to the problem of improving submarine ventilation. Here he was able to use the experience gained in the calorimeter to great advantage, so that he was able to maintain a submarine submerged for 96 hours, which was the record for submergence at that time. In one of these tests the submarine collided with a surface vessel and the batteries were damaged. Lieutenant DuBois volunteered to enter the battery compartment, using an improvised gas mask, since gases were being given off which he was able to stop by dumping the batteries into the sea, thereby saving the lives of the entire ship's company. Some years later he received the Navy Cross for this feat.[21]

## Cornell University Medical College and the New York Hospital

The New York Hospital was granted a royal charter on June 13, 1771. Immediately on the opening of the hospital in 1791, the medical staff became a medical faculty and organized for instruction of students. The medical library, established in 1796, became the largest in the country. (As a medical student, William Henry Welch spent all of his spare hours in this library.) In 1877 the hospital occupied a new building, which extended from Fifteenth to Sixteenth Streets, west of Fifth Avenue.

The Cornell University Medical College was founded in 1898, as the result of a disagreement that led part of the faculty of New York University and Bellevue Hospital Medical College to resign and organize a new school. In April 1898, the trustees of Cornell University accepted the offer of this group to form the medical college of the university. The trustees appointed a faculty consisting of William M. Polk, dean and professor of gynecology; Lewis A. Stimson, professor of surgery; W. Gilman Thompson, professor of medicine; Rudolf Witthaus, professor of chemistry and toxicology; Austin Flint, professor of physiology; and H. P. Loomis, professor of materia medica and therapeutics. The professorship of pathology was not filled until the following year, when James Ewing, the famous cancer pathologist, was appointed. In the fall of 1898 the college opened with 245 students, most of whom had transferred from New York University and Bellevue Hospital Medical College. The students occupied a rented building on Bellevue Hospital grounds and used the Loomis laboratory.

O. H. Payne's contribution of $1,500,000 to Cornell University in 1898 and his assurance of further financial support allowed the establishment of its medical college. His original gift was for the erection of a medical school building, and, in the fall of 1900, the college occupied its new quarters on First Avenue between Twenty-seventh and Twenty-eighth Streets, opposite Bellevue Hospital. The New York Hospital and Cornell University Medical College became organically associated on June 14, 1927, when an agreement was signed that formed the New York Hospital–Cornell Medical College Association. The newly constructed buildings were opened in 1932.

## Loomis Laboratory

The Loomis Laboratory, incorporated on May 16, 1887, and connected with New York University and Bellevue Medical College, was divided into four departments, with a director for each as follows: first, materia medica and experimental medicine, W. H. Thomson; second, chemistry and physics, Rudolf Witthaus; third, physiology, W. Gilman Thompson; and fourth, histology, pathology, and bacteriology, Alfred L. Loomis. On May 6, 1899, Payne requested transfer of the laboratory to Cornell. This final transfer came in 1904, and Cornell Medical College, in its beginning, was housed first in this laboratory and in rented buildings. Another laboratory building was subsequently constructed.[22]

## The Department of Medicine

From 1898 until 1916 W. Gilman Thompson was professor of medicine.[23] In 1877 Thompson graduated from the Sheffield Scientific School and then entered P & S, receiving his M.D. degree in 1881. In 1885 he was awarded the Joseph Mather Smith Prize for his essay "Structure of the Heart Valves," and the Harsen Prize of $500 for his essay "Photography of the Living Heart in Motion." After graduation, he served for eighteen months as an intern at the New York Hospital. Thompson was one of the first in the United States to develop an interest in the occupational diseases, publishing a textbook on this subject in 1915. From 1899 to 1905 Charles N. B. Camac[24] served as director of the laboratory of clinical pathology and was Thompson's chief of staff of the outpatient clinic. The clinical-pathology laboratory in the Cornell Medical College was the first laboratory of its type in New York. The outpatient department clinic was the first in which complete histories were taken for each patient, a disease index system was maintained, and an annual scientific report was published. In 1910 Camac was made a professor of clinical medicine. Camac (M.D., Pennsylvania, 1895) did graduate work in physiology at Oxford (under Sir John Burdon-Sanderson) and in medicine at Johns Hopkins. In 1895 he was an intern at the Johns Hopkins Hospital and, the following year, an assistant resident physician.

Another important member of the staff under Thompson was Walter L. Niles (M.D., Cornell, 1902),[25] who had interned at Bellevue Hospital. Niles worked with Carl Wiggers in Lusk's laboratory on the circulation and later studied the use of digitalis in treating pneumonia.[26] In 1918 he was appointed dean of Cornell University Medical College.

Lewis Atterbury Conner[27] graduated from the Sheffield Scientific School of Yale University in 1887 and received his M.D. degree from P & S in 1890. He then served as a house officer at the New York Hospital. In 1898 he was appointed to the original faculty at Cornell. Two years later he became professor of clinical medicine and, in 1916, succeeded W. Gilman Thompson as professor of medicine. Conner was the first editor of the *American Heart Journal* and, from 1925 to 1937, contributed to its growth and expanding influence. Conner never engaged in experimental medicine, but wrote a number of papers on various aspects of circulatory disease.

There were many practicing physicians who contributed significantly to the teaching program at the Cornell Medical College and engaged in some clinical investigation. Frank Sherman Meara[28] received an A.B. degree from Yale University in 1880 and a Ph.D. degree in 1892. From 1890 to 1892 he was an assistant in physiological chemistry under Chittenden. He received his M.D. degree from P & S in 1895. He was made professor of therapeutics at Cornell Medical College in 1909 and, in 1920, became a professor of clinical medicine. Meara excelled as a teacher. He had a faculty for classifying and systematizing what he knew and presenting it in a vivid and interesting form. He had the wit to see that the science and art of medicine are not antagonistic but complementary.[29] It was, however, the art of medicine that interested him, and he was sharply critical of those full-time faculty members at Cornell whom he thought lacking in the art, especially if they regarded themselves as important teachers of internal medicine.

Alexander Lambert,[30] following his graduation from Yale University in 1884, had a year's graduate study with Chittenden, after which he entered P & S, receiving his M.D. degree in 1888. The following year he served as an intern at Bellevue Hospital. Following two years of study in Europe, he worked with T. Mitchell Prudden and William H. Park on tetanus and diphtheria antitoxins. He then joined the faculty of Cornell, where he held the position of clinical professor of medicine. Lambert developed a special interest in alcoholism and narcotic addiction.

Nellis Barnes Foster (M.D., Johns Hopkins, 1902)[31] was an associate physician to the New York Hospital and an instructor in biological chemistry at Columbia University. In 1913 he became an assistant professor of clinical medicine at Cornell. In 1917 he accepted the chair of medicine at the University of Michigan, but soon volunteered his service in World War I. After the war, Foster returned to New York as an associate professor of medicine at Cornell, and he divided his time between private practice and his university and hospital duties. He isolated a highly toxic substance from uremic blood, the identity of which he was never able to determine. He was one of the first to work with insulin in the treatment of diabetes. Graham Lusk considered Foster's monograph on diabetes the best book of its kind in the English language. He was a charter member of the American Society for Clinical Investigation.

During the early 1900s, most of the papers from the department of medicine were case reports. By 1909, however (*Cornell University Medical College Bulletin,* October 1909), the application of laboratory techniques to the study of patients was becoming more evident. Niles had a paper on the cutaneous and conjunctival tuberculin test in the diagnosis of tuberculosis. Theodore B. Barringer, Jr., described a practical hospital polygraph. Thompson reported on his clinical experiments with homologous vaccines in the treatment of septic endocarditis and pyemia.[32] Conner and Joseph C. Roper described the relations existing between bilirubinemia, urobilinuria, and urobilinemia.[33] By 1913 there were even more articles that had a distinct flavor of clinical investigation. E. R. Hoobler published his work on the standardization of blood pressure readings by means of an automatic device for indicating systolic and diastolic pressures in children.[34] Even by this time, however, the published studies were for the most part of a clinical pathological nature, or related to the reporting of unusual cases.

## The Department under Lewis Atterbury Conner

After 1916, when Conner became a professor of medicine, studies from the Russell Sage Institute of Pathology, which was affiliated with the second medical service of Bellevue Hospital (Cornell division), were numerous. In the early 1920s Eugene F. DuBois and Nellis Barnes Foster were associate professors. David P. Barr was an assistant professor, as were Russell L. Cecil, Robert Anderson Cooke, and Cary Eggleston.

Russell L. Cecil (M.D., Medical College of Virginia, 1906)[35] did postgraduate work at Johns Hopkins under Rufus I. Cole (1906–7). Following this, he studied internal medicine and pathology in Vienna. Cecil then became a resident pathologist at the Presbyterian Hospital.[36] From 1910 to 1916 he was an assistant visiting physician and an instructor in clinical medicine. In 1915 Cecil studied experimental arthritis in rabbits, with special reference to the lesions produced by the streptococcus. In 1916 he joined the Cornell faculty and became a visiting physician at the Bellevue Hospital. From 1917 to 1919 he carried out a large field experiment with James Harold Austin on the value of prophylactic vaccination against pneumonia. From 1918 to 1920, with Francis G. Blake, he made an elaborate study of experimental pneumonia in monkeys, establishing the mode of infection and obtaining collaborative evidence of the prophylactic value of vaccines and the curative value of serum in its treatment. From 1920 to 1928 he continued his research on the prevention and treatment of pneumonia for the U.S. Public Health Service.[37] In 1933 he became a professor of clinical medicine. He was one of the first physicians in the United States to select rheumatic diseases as a clinical and research specialty and, in 1922, established one of the earliest American arthritis clinics. In 1931, with E. E. Nicholls and W. J. Stainsby, he noted the capacity of sera of patients with rheumatoid arthritis to agglutinate strains of hemolytic streptococci, now recognized as perhaps the earliest demonstration of rheumatoid factor.

Robert Anderson Cooke (M.D., P & S, 1904)[38] interned at the Presbyterian Hospital under Theodore Caldwell Janeway (1905-7). Cooke, well known for his work in allergy, had asthma in childhood. In 1910 he rode the ambulance manned by the Bellevue Emergency Ward on numerous occasions. Each ride resulted in a sharp attack of asthma—horse asthma. During his internship, a prophylactic injection of diptheria antitoxin had produced a nearly fatal reaction. This personal experience in the fall of 1910, combined with the realities of the protein reaction in sensitized individuals, stimulated his interest in this area of medicine, and, after 1914, all of his energy was devoted to the "sensitized state."

Francis Rackemann, who was working with Longcope on anaphylaxis at Columbia, remembered one night in 1914 when, in spite of the late hour, Cooke agreed to show him some of his work. They went to his dingy laboratory at the New York Hospital on East Sixteenth Street. As early as 1910—the same year that Leonard Noon and, after him, John Freeman published their classic studies on hay fever—Cooke had extracted a "pollen protein" and found that it caused skin reactions in his patients. In 1915 he published his first paper, "The Treatment of Hay Fever," and the next year he and Albert VanderVeer, Jr., presented their important work entitled "Human Sensitization." This paper included the protocols of 623 cases, most of whom had hay fever. It stressed the inheritance of sensitization. After 1916 Cooke wrote about the antibodies in hay fever, constitutional reactions to treatment, drug idiosyncrasy, the familial occurrence of asthma, and the classification of hypersensitiveness. "Infective asthma" and the importance of sinus disease were two of Cooke's favorite topics. When the serum of a patient with ragweed hay fever is mixed with ragweed extract, the antibody is neutralized, and the mixture can no longer transfer the sensitivity to the skin of a normal recipient. After ragweed treatment, however, transfer becomes successful again, because a new antibody blocks the union of ragweed and skin-sensitizing antibody. Cooke's discovery of this "blocking antibody" was a major contribution.

Cary Eggleston (M.D., Cornell, 1907) interned at the New York Hospital. From 1911 to 1921 he worked in pharmacology at Cornell with Robert A. Hatcher. Many of their studies were focused upon digitalis, for which Hatcher had developed a simple method of standardization. Eggleston applied the information obtained in the laboratory to the care of patients in Bellevue Hospital. He used only carefully standardized preparations of digitalis and confined his observations to the effects of oral medication. He was impressed with the unsatisfactory results obtained with small doses of digitalis over long periods and with the desirability of quickly obtaining complete digitalization. He recognized the necessity of adjusting dosage to the weight of the patient and the importance of early recognition of toxic manifestations of the drug. After meticulous study he proposed a formula for rapid, safe, and complete digitalization, which attracted immediate attention, and became known as the *Eggleston method.* His report represented a landmark in the practical management of heart failure and created a model for the clinical study of other important drugs. In 1921 Eggleston joined the department of medicine at Cornell, where he was engaged in teaching and clinical activities until 1953.

Harold E. B. Pardee (M.D., P & S, 1909) took his internship at the New York Hospital. In 1912 he began work in the medical clinic of the New York Hospital, serving there for thirty-four years. At Columbia he worked with Horatio B. Williams, one of the earliest students of electrocardiography in America. Pardee's book *Clinical Aspects of the Electrocardiogram,* published in 1924, remained for many years the standard work in the field. Pardee described the "coronary T wave." Much of his work was done in collaboration with Arthur M. Master. During World War I, Pardee was assigned to the "Soldier's Heart" project of Sir Thomas Lewis.[39]

Among the instructors in medicine in 1924 were William S. McCann,[40] Harry L. Alexander,[41] and Henry Barber Richardson.[42] Alexander published a paper on the precipitin response in the blood of rabbits following subarachnoid injections of horse serum. In collaboration with N. P. Larsen and R. Paddock, he made immunological observations on bronchial asthma.

The effect of fasting in diabetes, as compared with a diet designed to replace the foodstuffs oxidized during a fast, was studied by Richardson and Mason. Henry Barber Richardson (M.D., Harvard, 1914) interned at the Peter Bent Brigham Hospital and was an assistant in medicine at Johns Hopkins from 1916 to 1918. In 1921 he went to the Russell Sage Institute of Pathology. He continued his association with Cornell until his retirement in 1957. He published on the following subjects: infection and the ketogenic balance, ketosis and the respiratory change in diabetes, and the utilization of carbohydrate in a case of renal glycosuria (with William S. Ladd); and exercise and the respiratory quotient in diabetes (with Samuel Z. Levine). In collaboration with Edward Tolstoi, R. O. Loebel, and Levine, he reported on studies concerning the production of lactic acid in diabetes, following the administration of insulin.

The name of Soma Weiss[43] appeared for the first time in a paper, written with R. M. Morris and M. S. Witter, on the sensitizing action of thyroid on the effect of epinephrine in man.[44]

During the 1920s the research productivity of the department was excellent. There were a number of experiments on the physiology of muscular exercise carried out by David P. Barr,[45] Harold E. Himwich, and their collaborators at the Russell Sage Institute. The studies included the following: changes in acid-base equilibrium following short periods of vigorous muscular exercise; comparison of arterial and venous blood following vigorous exercise; development and duration of changes in acid-base equilibrium; blood reaction and breathing; and oxygen relationships in the arterial blood.

In the *Cornell University Medical College Bulletin* for October 1929, there were references to numerous studies by DuBois on problems of naval medicine. The work of Nicholls, Stainsby, and Cecil on the bacteriology of the blood and joints in chronic infectious arthritis began during that year. R. O. Loebel and Ephraim Shorr published a study on the effect of respiratory depressants on the respiratory quotient of excised tissues.

Ephraim Shorr received many honors at Yale University and Yale School of Medicine. After his internship at Mount Sinai Hospital, he associated himself with Lusk and DuBois. His numerous contributions included studies of parathyroid diseases; examination of creatine metabolism in maladies of the thyroid; influence of the pituitary on the pathogenesis of diabetes; calcium and phosphorus disturbances in diseases of bone; urinary stone formation; the action of sex hormones on citric acid excretion; the effect of menstruation and varying clinical states on epithelium of the vaginal tract; and the action of adrenal hormones in shock and hypertension. During the last decade of his life, he studied substances formed in the liver and the kidney during anaerobiosis and their action on the circulation. This work led, among other things, to definition of the functions of ferritin. Some of this important work was presented in 1954 in his Harvey Lecture.[46]

It was in 1929 that Arthur M. Master and E. T. Oppenheimer published a simple exercise-tolerance test for circulatory efficiency, with standard tables for normal individuals.[47]

## DuBois as Chairman of the Department of Medicine

With the opening of the new buildings of the New York Hospital–Cornell Medical Center, Eugene F. DuBois became the chairman of the department of medicine. In his report as physician-in-chief, dated June 6, 1935, DuBois described the total operation of the department:

> The metabolism unit contained six beds and was used for study and treatment of patients requiring careful dietary supervision. This ward was a direct continuation of the metabolism ward which was operated on the second (Cornell) medical division of Bellevue Hospital from 1913 until the move into the new center building. The Bellevue unit had attracted much attention throughout the country and its methods have been copied in a large number of hospitals. This small group of six patients provides research material for four or five doctors and three technicians. The work is coordinated in such a manner that several research problems can be carried out on the same patient. These studies are invaluable in the estimation of the effects of treatment. They entail no hardships on the patient; in fact it is difficult to induce the patients to leave the metabolism ward and go to another part of the hospital.

Studies were made to establish the fundamental laws of heat loss through radiation, conduction, and vaporization. These studies have an important bearing not only on questions of clothing and ventilation but also on the phenomenon of fever. In the course of these studies, James Hardy of the Russell Sage staff developed two physical instruments of great accuracy—a radiometer for the measurement of heat loss from the human skin, and an infra-red spectrograph that made possible the detailed study of radiation of the wave lengths emanating from the human body.

Richardson and Shorr, in collaboration with George N. Papanicolaou of the department of anatomy, made great practical advances in the study of female sex hormones, developing a test that made it possible to study the effects of hormones by means of vaginal smears.

In the field of cardiovascular disease, Harold J. Stewart and two assistant residents, Norman Crane and John E. Deitrick, were studying the volume output of the heart and the efficiency of the circulation in a wide variety of conditions, as well as making quantitative observations of the effects of various drugs.

Harold J. Stewart (M.D., Johns Hopkins, 1919)[48] received an M.A. degree from Johns Hopkins in 1923 and held a Bingham Fellowship in Medicine (1921–22). He then spent ten productive years at the HRI. Together with Alfred E. Cohn, A. Baird Hastings, and others, he carried out fundamental studies on the blood gases, the pathologic physiology of various cardiac arrhythmias, the treatment of congestive heart failure, the pharmacology of digitalis, and the effect of heart failure on renal function.

When Stewart moved to DuBois's service at the New York Hospital–Cornell Medical Center in 1932, a clinical division of cardiology was developed, but Stewart continued to spend time in the laboratory. Studies of the circulation in pericardial disease, in various arrhythmias and in valvular heart diseases were pursued. Important contributions on the surgical treatment of heart disease were published. George Heuer wrote on pericardial constriction; Frank Glenn, on mitral stenosis.

Richardson and Shorr were studying the metabolism in Graves's disease and continuing their work on the respiration and metabolism of small portions of surviving tissue. Paul Reznikoff, of hematology, was interested in polycythemia.

Of particular interest was the work of Harold George Wolff, of the neurology clinic, who had gathered a staff, which included Ade T. Milhorat, to study the metabolism in diseases of the nervous and muscular systems. Wolff and his collaborators also carried on research work in the department of physiology.

Harold George Wolff (M.D., Harvard, 1923)[49] interned at Roosevelt Hospital and trained in neurology under Foster Kennedy and Stanley Cobb. Later he studied psychiatry under Adolph Meyer at Johns Hopkins; neuropharmacology with Otto Loewi in Austria; and neurophysiology with Ivan Pavlov in Russia. After this extensive preparation, he returned to New York in 1932 as head of the department of neurology at the New York Hospital–Cornell Medical Center, a position he held for the remainder of his career.

He made careful studies of the cerebral circulation, of neuromuscular transmission, and of the metabolism of muscle; later devoting himself increasingly to those aspects of nervous function for which the only possible experimental subject is man. In his classical studies on pain and on the mechanisms of headache, the experimental subject was often himself; through rigorous observation he was able to endow subjective experiences with a clarity and reliability ordinarily found only in objective data. Probably his most significant contributions were his conception of the mind-body relationship; his conception of disease related to "defensive reaction patterns" against environmental threats; and his extensive documentation of the relevance of these concepts to common diseases such as peptic ulcer, essential hypertension, bronchial asthma, and migraine.

Wolff was interested in migraine because he suffered from it. His first important contribution was to establish what had been proposed by others: that cranial arterial dilatation was fundamental to the mechanism of pain in migraine. He perceived in migraine patients a striking personality pattern, and he learned that talking with patients about their way of life could often mitigate their symptoms and sometimes abolish their headaches altogether. This stimulated his interest in psychosomatic medicine.

One of Harold George Wolff's outstanding students was Stewart Wolf, who provided the following description of his training and his work under Wolff:

> The practice in Eugene DuBois' Department of Medicine was for the assistant residents to be assigned to ward service only half the year and for

the other half to work directly in research with OPD experience in one of the sub-specialties which then were cardiology (Harold Stewart), neurology (Harold Wolff), endocrinology and metabolism (Ephraim Shorr, Harry Richardson and Ade Milhorat), pulmonary (Claude Forkner), hematology (Paul Reznikoff) or syphilis and infectious diseases (Bruce Webster).

I started with Harold Wolff and J. D. Hardy in 1939. They, with Helen Goodell, were studying pain perception and reaction in humans. I began participating in the "blackened forehead" pain threshold work and did a year long project on cold pain with Hardy. Then I began studying gastrointestinal pain on my own, mainly with healthy volunteers who were swallowing balloons for me. It was in 1940 that I learned through Charles Kunkle, another resident assigned to Harold Wolff, of the existence of Tom. A letter had come to Miss Helen Lincoln, director of the record library, requesting information on a patient operated on in the Old New York Hospital in 1895. The patient was Tom at 9 years of age and the operation was one of the first gastrostomies done in the country. The story of the encounter with Tom is described on pages 29 to 35 of the book *The Stomach.*[50]

The "Tom" work made it clear that bodily changes associated with psychological and social stresses could be measured and to some extent, quantified. It led to the work that I did on the measurable effects of placebos and, after the war, to the formation of Medicine A, a fellowship training program supported by the Commonwealth Fund. I was put in charge and although David Barr, then Chairman of Medicine, wanted me to make an independent section of it, I preferred to operate under the general supervision and guidance of Harold Wolff. I recruited Herbert S. Ripley, Jr., a talented psychiatrist. (Among the outstanding fellows in this program were Theodore Treuting, David Graham, Lawrence Hinkle, Thomas Holmes, Robert Schneider, Ian Stevenson, Charles H. Duncan, Adrian Ostfeld, Albert Stunkard, Harry Stalker, and Morton Bogdonoff.)

We studied a great many psychophysiological responses and diseases. Everyone worked in a special clinic in the morning and in the afternoon worked in the laboratory. We collaborated with specialists in a number of surgical and medical fields and wrote papers on gastric and colonic function, nasal function, hemodynamic responses, skin, ocular, bladder, and genital responses and metabolic alterations as well.

Harold was a superb chief but he wasn't for everybody. Many considered him cold and demanding. He required the unrestrained best efforts of his colleagues and students. Only a few were willing to give that much. On many occasions when I thought I had turned out an excellent experiment or test of a hypothesis, he would shake his head and say: "Why don't you dive down and try to come up with something better?" Every ten minute presentation at a meeting was rehearsed for hours with Harold Wolff sitting on the front row, often commenting at the end: "I haven't the slightest idea what you are saying." I worked with him for 14 years, minus the 3 years of the war. I learned from him respect for evidence, courage to sail on uncharted seas and precision in using the language in writing or speaking. Over his desk was the motto: "Fixity of purpose requires flexibility of method."[51]

In 1935 the department of medicine had nine doctors on a full-time basis, paid from a joint budget contributed to equally by the hospital and the medical school; and, in addition, six research workers, paid by other funds. The great depression of the 1930s had a profound influence on medical colleges, and practically no new appointments were made. This interfered greatly with the flow of personnel, which was such an important part of the system before 1929. When there was active competition between the different medical schools and hospitals for the services of the best men, promotion came much more rapidly. During the thirties, there was great stagnation throughout the United States. Many of the older men were gradually forced into private practice, abandoning their research careers. Many promising young men could not find proper opportunity for advanced training.

DuBois spoke about the full-time system:

> The old controversy about the advantages of the part-time system and the full-time system in the department of medicine has quieted down although it is still active when it concerns some of the other branches of the medical sciences. The physician-in-chief [DuBois] has served Cornell for two periods on a part-time basis and for two periods on a full-time basis. As far as he can tell his work has been of the same quality throughout. Under the part-time system a doctor has somewhat more freedom. On the full-time system he is supposed to be in the hospital all day and devote much time to executive work. He becomes the target for all sorts of committee meetings, conferences, interviews, and so forth. The executive officers of his own institution and of innumerable medical and charitable groups throughout the country have the impression that since he is on full-time basis he is available for any and every worthy project. Somewhat the same attitude prevails with physicians in that community who come to him for advice. Unless measures are taken to counteract this tendency the full-time professor who has made his name as a clinician-teacher and investigator will become nothing more than an executive, a sort of hospital superintendent, living on his past reputation. This is far from the ideal of a chief who can act as the leader of a highly trained group of younger men.[52]

# 12

# Clinical Science in Boston[1]

On September 26, 1906, new buildings of the Harvard Medical School were dedicated. President Charles W. Eliot,[2] who gave the principal address, spoke of the importance of medical research:

> When we consider what has already been learnt about the production, transmission and prevention of smallpox, cholera, yellow fever, the black death, typhoid fever, diphtheria, anthrax, rabies and tetanus we cannot resist a conclusion that in the future medical science must include the study of causes and consequences. . . .
>
> Students of disease must, therefore, be competent to utilize in their great task every aid which natural science can furnish. How vastly is the range of medical science and medical education broadened by this plain necessity.[3]

## The McLean Hospital

The organization of the Harvard laboratory of physiology by Henry Pickering Bowditch has already been described (see chapter 3).

In 1879 Dr. Edward Cowles[4] became medical superintendent of the McLean Hospital. The hospital's laboratory work, which began in 1889,[5] combined neurological studies in the departments of psychiatry and physiological psychology and explored their relations with anatomical and chemical pathology. There were eight rooms devoted to psychological, chemical, and pathological work. A study by William Noyes on certain peculiarities of the knee-jerk in sleep in a case of terminal dementia was published in the *American Journal of Psychology* (4: 343, 1892). Early on, there was a report on urinary excretion in insanity, with special reference to urea and uric acid. Observations of the blood cells in certain mental diseases were carried out by Joseph A. Capps. Capps was an intern at the McLean Hospital when he first used the red cell volume index to classify anemias.[6]

Cowles made the following remarks in characterizing the work and aims of the laboratory:

> The purpose of establishing and developing the laboratory has been carried on under much difficulty, naturally due to the newness of the attempt to combine with psychiatry the other departments of scientific medical research.... Also, in the dependence in these changes upon general physiological processes, and in order to take into account all the elements of vital activity involved, it is supremely necessary to study both physiological and pathological chemistry in their direct and indirect relation to mental changes.[7]

Cowles himself had taken an extended course in psychology at the Johns Hopkins University. August Hoch was sent abroad to study with Emil Kraepelin in order to prepare to assume directorship of the laboratory (1894). Angelo Mosso, in whose laboratory Hoch also studied, was one of the most productive of Ludwig's pupils. Hoch, a native of Switzerland, was a resident in William Osler's medical service in Baltimore.

The chemical laboratory was established in 1900. Otto Folin was its director until 1908, when he became a professor of biological chemistry at Harvard (see chapter 3). The psychological laboratory was opened in 1904, with Sheppard Ivory Franz as its head. In 1921, John C. Whitehorn, a pupil of Folin's, came to the McLean Hospital to continue biochemical researches in the field of mental disease.[8]

## The Carnegie Nutrition Laboratory

The Carnegie Institution of Washington, D.C., was founded by Andrew Carnegie in 1902. In its early stages, the Institution supported a wide range of specific studies. Later, the support went to major projects, the solution of which required longer periods.

The Carnegie Nutrition Laboratory, organized in Boston in 1907, was directed by Francis G. Benedict.[9] Benedict became the foremost investigator of gaseous metabolism of his time. After studying at Harvard, he received his Ph.D. degree at Heidelberg under Victor Meyer in 1895. Then he became a research assistant to Wilbur O. Atwater in the chemistry department at Wesleyan University (1895).

Benedict made what he regarded as his most important contribution to science in 1907:

> The development of the closed circuit respiration apparatus and calorimeter at Wesleyan University is, in my judgment, the most important mechanical contribution I have been privileged to make. This was developed from the ground up based on the idea that if the actual amount of oxygen absorbed by the human body could be directly measured, such a measure would have great significance in comparison with the simultaneous heat production.[10]

The importance of Benedict's researches with the calorimeter was recognized by Welch and Billings. It was largely through their initiative that the Carnegie Institution established the Nutrition Laboratory in Boston. Built next door to Harvard's medical school, it became one of the leading research laboratories in America.

Benedict built two small calorimeters of the Atwater-Rosa type and devised several smaller instruments for measuring oxygen consumption as a means of estimating energy production. One such device was the *Benedict apparatus,* used for many years to measure the basal metabolism of patients.

Benedict and his collaborators added much to our understanding of heat production and heat regulation, particularly the conditions requisite for measuring the "basal" metabolism in man. In an intensive study of the respiratory metabolism in diabetes, Benedict and Elliott Proctor Joslin showed that during severe diabetes there is a distinct increase in the basal metabolism. The abnormal breakdown of food materials results in an excessive production of beta-oxybutyric acid, which directly stimulates the cell to greater activity. With treatment, "particularly with the new remarkable Allen treatment, this increased metabolism entirely disappears."[11]

Elliott Proctor Joslin (M.D., Harvard, 1895)[12] studied under Russell H. Chittenden at Yale, and his first paper on diabetes was presented before the Boylston Medical Society in 1893, while he was a medical student. After a year in Germany and Austria (1896–97), he interned at the MGH and reviewed the records of 172 diabetic patients admitted from 1824 to 1898. In 1898 he again visited Europe, where he met Naunyn, Minkowski, Magnus-Levy, and Gerhardt. Joslin was an assistant in physiological chemistry at Harvard from 1898 to 1900. He advanced through various academic grades to clinical professor of medicine in 1925. Joslin recognized the value of Frederick M. Allen's concept of undernutrition in the treatment of diabetes (1914–22) and with this starvation diet kept many patients alive and in reasonable condition. In 1922 Joslin was invited to Toronto to study the clinical use of insulin. He was the first to treat diabetics with insulin in Boston (among them George R. Minot). In 1932 he was awarded the Kober Medal of the Association of American Physicians.[13]

Benedict also studied, with Fritz Talbot,[14] the metabolism of infants in the first hours of postnatal life, showing the importance of knowing the energy requirements and the character of the combustion in newborn infants.

## The Massachusetts General Hospital

Laboratory work began at the MGH when James Homer Wright[15] joined the faculty as a pathologist in 1896. In addition to the bench space for the pathologists, there were sixteen benches in Wright's laboratory for research by members of the clinical staff. Each staff member paid $25 a year for the privilege of working there.

Wright,[16] who studied with Welch and Councilman, was an active leader in pathology from 1896 to 1925. He devoted much of his time to methods and techniques in pathology and bacteriology. He was the first to recognize the plasmacyte as the cell typical of multiple myeloma. Some credit him as the first to describe the bone marrow origin of blood platelets; for this description, he received a fine accolade from William Henry Welch. Thus, Wright was the man who formed the rallying point for the scientific work at the MGH before the arrival of Edsall.

One of the medical practitioners who began research in bacteriology under Wright was Frederick Taylor Lord, whose special area of interest was pulmonary disease.[17]

In 1904, to further encourage investigation at the hospital, the trustees made the following announcement:

> Believing that in promoting scientific medical research they will encourage the broadest of charities, your trustees have attempted by creating this department not only to stimulate the interest and cooperation of scientific men, but also to attract the attention thereto of possible benefactors of the hospital who will recognize that by giving to this cause they are promoting knowledge—the basis of both prevention and cure of human suffering.
>
> Although there has been established during the past few years by benefactors special funds and institutions for medical research, we believe that a large part of such research must be carried on in close proximity to patients, and that this hospital, with all its marked advantages for such studies, should be generously provided with the means of carrying them all on successfully.[18]

Thus, a department of scientific research was established, and a gift of $5,000 was accepted as the nucleus of a fund for its support. Unfortunately, this development was not followed up at the time. After David Linn Edsall's arrival at the hospital in 1912, clinical research laboratories were organized apart from the pathology laboratory.

Specific opportunities for clinical research at the MGH became available with the appointment of the Dalton scholars and, later, the Walcott fellows.[19] The first Dalton scholar (1894–95) was Richard Clarke Cabot, whose thesis was entitled "Minute Examination of the Blood." The first Walcott fellow (1910–11) was Charles H. Lawrence, who worked on hypertension and had four beds placed at his disposal for this study.[20]

Clinical hematology was introduced at the MGH by Cabot as early as the middle 1890s.[21] Interest increased with the arrival of Wright.[22] Others who contributed in this area were Roger I. Lee, Beth Vincent (a collaborating surgeon), and, finally, George R. Minot, who returned to the MGH in 1915, after two years with Thayer and Howell in Baltimore. Problems of blood coagulation first engaged his attention, then pernicious anemia and other anemias. Oswald H. Robertson[23] also had a hematological orientation (1915), studying urobilin and urobilinogen excretion in blood diseases. Another was Andrew Watson Sellards,[24] who worked with Minot.

## The Birth of Modern Clinical Science in Boston: David Linn Edsall

An important event for clinical science in Boston was the appointment, in 1912, of David Linn Edsall as Jackson Professor of Medicine at the MGH (for a description of Edsall's early career, see chapter 10). Edsall's first relations with Harvard were between the years 1905 and 1909, when he developed a friendship with Edwin Allen Locke[25] and other Boston members of the Interurban Clinical Club. In 1908 Locke concluded that Edsall might succeed Frederick C. Shattuck, then Jackson Professor and head of a medical service at the MGH. Cabot was the logical successor to Shattuck, but Locke perceived that a new era for medicine was coming and felt that the MGH and Harvard needed a different type of medical chief; a man whose purpose was learning the mechanisms involved in disease.

Locke wrote his own account of these developments some thirty years later: "I had known Edsall rather intimately for a few years prior to 1912 and had come to consider him as one of the very few brilliant young medical men in the United States. He was one of the original young teachers of medicine chosen by Osler in 1905 to form the Interurban Clinical Club."[26]

Locke arranged to have Edsall meet informally with representatives from the trustees of the MGH and the administration of Harvard College. After several conversations with Locke, Shattuck became convinced of the importance of trying to bring Edsall to Boston. Locke told Cabot of these developments. His reply was that he had always expected to succeed Shattuck and that his whole life had been planned with that in view. He went on, however, to say that this was of no importance if Edsall was a better man for the position than he and that he would be happy to serve under him.

Edsall's arrival in 1912 was labelled as "a minor medical revolution." Cabot wrote for the *Boston Transcript* of the new developments in Boston medicine.[27] Of Edsall he spoke as follows: "His special technical equipment represents something rather new in clinical medicine. He does not represent a clearly defined new order of things, with a division so sharp as that which Lister brought into the practice of surgery; yet in a very real way he does stand for that new combination of chemical and pharmacological research which is the most striking and most promising movement in the medical world today."

Cabot then outlined the changes necessary at the MGH in order to bring Edsall to Boston:

> Hitherto ... it was impossible to call from the outside the man whom the faculty of the school might most desire, because the school had no way of

providing him with the hospital material necessary for purposes of instruction. In Dr. Edsall's case the generous cooperation of the staff and the trustees of the MGH has made it possible for the school to call a strong man from outside, and assure him of adequate hospital material. A similar situation is already assured in the Peter Bent Brigham Hospital, where the school nominates the men for the positions of surgeon and physician to the hospital.

Edsall's important goal was to study the mechanisms of disease—the physiological approach to medicine. He had a great talent for selecting promising young physicians to work at the MGH, who then went on to obtain research training in the best possible places. These young men, upon completion of their studies, returned as members of the staff of the MGH, and most became distinguished clinicians and investigators. James Howard Means and Cecil Kent Drinker[28] were sent to Denmark to study respiratory physiology with August Krogh. Edsall urged George R. Minot to go to Baltimore, where he became interested in hematology; an experience that lay the groundwork for his later studies in pernicious anemia. Paul Dudley White[29] went to England to work with James M. MacKenzie and Sir Thomas Lewis on cardiac problems. W. W. Palmer remained in Boston to work with Lawrence J. Henderson. Francis Rackemann[30] journeyed to New York to study allergy under Longcope, and Joseph C. Aub went to the Russell Sage Institute to work under Lusk and DuBois.

The areas of interest selected were varied. Oswald H. Robertson[31] was sent to New York to work with Rufus I. Cole at the Rockefeller Institute on the bacteriological aspects of pneumonia. Carl A. L. Binger went to study pharmacology with Abel at Hopkins and then to the Rockefeller Hospital to investigate therapy in pneumonia. Stanley Cobb took his internship with Harvey Williams Cushing, although he never planned to be a surgeon.[32] It was Edsall's idea of good preparation for Cobb's eventual career in neurology and psychiatry, which he then trained for at Johns Hopkins, under Adolf Meyer and William Henry Howell.

## Edsall Pioneers in the Study of Industrial Disease

In 1917 Edsall spoke as follows: "If in a brief time I can give a superficial suggestion of the general relations of medicine to industry and can combat what I think I may fairly call the common academic aloofness of medicine toward these things ... I shall have accomplished my main purpose."[33] The medical profession in general had scarcely recognized the complexities and importance of industrial disease. Edsall changed this situation by establishing an industrial disease clinic at the MGH.

The clinic was directed first by Harry Linenthal and then by Wade Wright. Within six months, they studied 276 cases related to industrial exposure out of 1507 male medical admissions to the outpatient department. Cases of poisoning with benzine, brass, naphtha, turpentine, and benzol were uncovered, which had been incorrectly diagnosed (with labels ranging from apprehension to appendicitis). So many cases of lead poisoning were found that the hospital issued their famous "lead slips"—"Advice to Persons Working with Lead" and "Precautions for Printers." Shattuck provided money for a medical fellow in industrial disease and a social worker, who checked every patient admitted for possible industrial exposure.[34]

## Facilities for Research

When the administrative offices moved to the Mosley Building, Edsall arranged to keep space in the Bulfinch Building for research. Means wrote about this period: "The organization of a laboratory for clinical investigation was made possible in the spring of 1918 when the old offices on the ground floor of the Bulfinch Building were vacated; the collection of equipment having been started as early as the spring of 1916. Reconstruction was begun immediately. Six rooms became available which now constitute a fairly satisfactory laboratory for about 12 workers. Before the organization of this laboratory, clinical research had to be conducted in any corner that the investigator could find."[35]

Among the more important studies during this period were those on blood gases, by Arlie Bock and Henderson;[36] pathology of the blood, by George R. Minot and his colleagues; metabolism of bile pigments, by Chester M. Jones;[37] thyroid disease by the Thyroid Committee (involving the medical and surgical services); measurements of respiratory metabolism, under Means and Aub;[38] clinical calorimetry of infants, by Fritz Talbot; bacteriology of pneumonia, by Frederick Taylor Lord; blood and urinary chemistry in diabetes and nephritis, by Reginald Fitz; and the work in Rackemann's anaphylaxis clinic.

In 1918 Edsall became dean of the Harvard Medical School; before he left the hospital, he found the money to add an ell to the Bulfinch Building, in order to house the famous Ward 4 and other needed research facilities.

## James Howard Means as the Second Jackson Professor

One of the earliest influences on the career of James Howard Means was the intellectual impact derived from William T. Sedgwick, professor of biology at the Massachusetts Institute of Technology (MIT), who was a pupil of Henry Newell Martin in Baltimore. During Means's undergraduate period at Harvard, the most influential of his teachers was Lawrence J. Henderson.

The new Johns Hopkins medical school was only fifteen years old, and, to meet the challenge of its dramatic innovations, Eliot had appointed a new dean—Henry A. Christian, who had graduated from Johns Hopkins in 1900. Means's first meeting with him was at the autopsy table of the Carney Hospital in South Boston. Christian, known as "the boy dean," was ardently in love with teaching; a love that he firmly planted in Means.[39]

Another important influence on Means was Walter B. Cannon, who at that time was recording the movements of the alimentary canal, in order to study the effect of the involuntary nervous system and the emotions upon them. Means sensed that the work of Henderson and Cannon had great meaning for clinical medicine. Otto Folin, a professor of biochemistry, was another teacher who made a great impression on Means.

Means has vividly described the way he and other medical students at Harvard spent their time (1907–11). In the third year, for five afternoons a week, Means had to attend three, sometimes four, hour-long lectures, one after another. The fourth year student could walk the wards of hospitals, but not in any such responsible role as that enjoyed by the clinical clerks of later years at Harvard. Means could recall nothing being said to students about research or research careers during his clinical years there.[40]

Edsall's approach to the development of clinical investigation is best exemplified by the peregrinations of Means, who was one of his early protégés.[41] Means was first sent to the Carnegie Nutrition Laboratory to learn the use of the apparatus designed to measure the exchange of pulmonary gases. Later, Means went to work under August Krogh, in circulatory physiology. Means recognized that he was preparing for clinical research by acquiring methodology, rather than by really coming to grips with basic principles—perhaps not the best approach, but the one that he was led into by Edsall. After leaving Krogh, Means visited the physiological laboratory at Cambridge, where he saw Sir Joseph Barcroft's work on the blood gases. When Means returned to the MGH, in December 1913, Edsall provided him with a research fellowship and a small laboratory. Means had equipment of the type used by Krogh and Barcroft as well as a Benedict universal respiration apparatus. After getting them in working order, Means felt like a small boy with a new tool kit, looking for problems that could be attacked by the methods at hand. Obviously, imagination was needed, and, in the beginning, Means said that his "was not outstandingly well developed." Starting with problems his clinical experience brought to mind, he probed in a variety of fields. He struck up a friendship with Louis H. Newburgh, later a professor of medicine at Michigan, who had finished his internship at the MGH in 1908. Newburgh's first love was research. In the physiological laboratory of Professor William T. Porter, Means and Newburgh made observations on respiratory function in experimental pneumonia and worked on blood flow in patients with respiratory and cardiac abnormalities. Newburgh taught Means what research in medicine was about, and his devotion to it was contagious.

Means ultimately developed a major interest in diseases of the thyroid. He had already been making determinations of the metabolic rate with the Benedict apparatus when he heard a paper by DuBois on basal metabolism at a meeting of the American Society for Clinical Investigation in 1914. In 1916 Means spent three weeks with DuBois working in the Russell Sage Institute, learning the techniques of the respiration calorimeter. When Aub returned from his training under DuBois, he and Means worked on metabolic problems until 1917, when the war brought an end to their collaboration.[42]

In 1921 Means was promoted to an assistant professor. The activity at the MGH for "full-time clinicians" (geographic full-time) entailed three essential functions—practice, teaching, and research. It was felt that one could be neither a sound clinical teacher nor a well-oriented clinical investigator unless one was exposed to the important influence of direct responsibility in patient care. Means made rounds with the house staff and ward clerks and also had some private patients. In 1923 Means succeeded Edsall as Jackson Professor of Clinical Medicine and became chief of medical services at the MGH.

## The Clinical Research Ward: Ward 4

As already indicated, Edsall had obtained a grant from the Rockefeller Foundation that was sufficient to reconstruct half of the basement of the Bulfinch Building (the original MGH) and to add an ample ell in the rear. Means had the opportunity to work out the plans for the new construction. While the building was being completed, Means had a semisabbatical year, which he spent in London with Sir Francis Fraser, Arthur Hurst, Arthur W. H. Ellis, and Hugh MacLean.[43]

In 1925 the new clinical research facility of five two-bed rooms, designed by Means, began operation. Because of his repeated benefactions toward the support of the ward, it was named in honor of Edward Mallinckrodt, Jr., of St. Louis. Adjoining this ward, which was initially called Ward 4, two chemical laboratories were installed, and other laboratories for physiological and bacteriological work were placed in every nook and cranny that could be found from attic to cellar. A penthouse for animals was erected. It was not until 1951, when the present five-story research building was opened, that the investigators at the MGH were given the use of a modern animal farm. Thus, although Edsall initiated the clinical research ward at the MGH, it was Means who supervised its growth and development.

Edsall had added a new position entitled "Medical Resident" in 1913. W. W. Palmer was the first resident and Paul Dudley White the second. Their time was largely free for research, although they were available to advise the interns upon request. Means increased the teaching functions of the residents, but they still had a portion of their time for research. In 1930 he added, somewhat in the Johns Hopkins tradition, a "chief resident," who became the head of the medical house staff. This resident tied the whole service together, at the student and house officer level, into a smoothly running enterprise. In addition, a new category of workers—research fellows—made their appearance, increasing rapidly in number.

## The Thyroid Clinic

Means's research involved the measurement of metabolism in patients with thyroid disease. Thus he was able to follow the effect of treatment using the basal metabolic rate (BMR) as a measuring stick of thyroid function. Clinicians from other departments joined Means's medical group, including Edward P. Richardson, the first full-time chief of the surgical service at the MGH, and George W. Holmes, chief roentgenologist. Means's first research fellow was Harold N. Segall of Montreal; the second was M. Paul Starr, then of Chicago.

Early studies centered on iodine and the thyroid parenchyma's special need for this element. Thus, the biochemical study of thyroid hormone and its precursors became a major interest. In 1928–29 Means sent one of his gifted residents, William Thomas Salter, to work at the University College of London under Charles R. Harington, who had earlier synthesized thyroxine. Salter learned the techniques of producing various fractions of thyroglobulin, and, together with Jacob B. Lerman, he assayed these on patients with myxedema.[44] They soon found that any substance possessing thyroid hormonelike activity must contain iodine and that its calorigenic activity is related to the amount of iodine it contains.[45]

Under Means, the development of special clinics associated with research laboratories became a recurring pattern at the MGH. This furnished the substrate for long-term clinical investigation, in which physicians, surgeons, clinical specialists, and basic scientists often joined hands in solving problems of common interest. This type of research activity attracted an increasing number of professional visitors, including fellows both from the United States and abroad, and thus had a valuable role in training investigators, as well as accomplishing important investigative work. During Means's tenure at the MGH as Jackson Professor, the major investigators were Joseph C. Aub, Chester M. Jones, Walter Bauer, and Fuller Albright.[46]

## Research Projects on Ward 4

The prototype of Ward 4 was the metabolism ward at Bellevue Hospital, organized by Lusk and DuBois. Both Means and Aub[47] had worked in this metabolism unit before World War I.

Edsall had already interested Aub in the study of lead poisoning.[48] Aub's animal studies disclosed that in the body lead is carried in the blood stream as a colloidal lead phosphate. When it reaches bone it is removed from the blood and deposited in the bone as insoluble lead phosphate. Aub showed that lead thus tucked away in bones is essentially harmless.

In 1924 Aub returned full-time to the MGH to extend his lead studies to man. When Ward 4 was opened he was the major user of its facilities. He demonstrated that giving acids or acid-producing salts caused a marked increase in the output of both lead and calcium. With a high calcium intake, the elimination of both lead and calcium rapidly declined. A high serum calcium led to a redeposit of both lead and calcium in the skeleton. These results were of great importance for the treatment for both acute and chronic lead poisoning.[49]

While Means was abroad, Aub recruited as resident physician Walter Bauer, who had graduated from Michigan in 1922 and had interned at the Long Island College of Medicine. Bauer attempted to isolate the active principle of the adrenal cortex and soon was studying patients on Ward 4. While abroad, Means met Donald Hunter and recruited him for work at the MGH, where he became part of Aub's program. In 1925 Collip isolated parathormone and demonstrated its role in the regula-. tion of calcium metabolism. Hunter found that parathyroid hormone causes the withdrawal of lead from the bones.

### Studies on Calcium in Health and Disease

Aub and Bauer were joined by Fuller Albright in their further studies of calcium metabolism. They discovered that bone trabeculae mechanically strengthen the bone and chemically respond to the body's need for calcium. Parathyroid hormone pulls calcium out of the trabeculae first and, if lead is deposited there, pulls that out too. These basic facts were of great value in understanding the various bone diseases in man.[50]

### Hyperparathyroidism

One of the dramatic stories of research on Ward 4 is that of Captain Charles Martell. Martell developed the classical manifestations of hyperparathyroidism and entered Bellevue Hospital, on January 15, 1926, under the care of Eugene F. DuBois. DuBois recognized that Martell was suffering from a bone disease described by Friedrich von Recklinghausen in 1891. DuBois's studies disclosed a high calcium level in the blood, a high output of calcium in the urine, and a low level of phosphorus in the blood. Knowing of Aub's work with Collip's parathyroid extract (parathormone), DuBois decided to transfer Martell to Boston.[51] Studies on Ward 4 confirmed the diagnosis of hyperparathyroidism, and on May 16, 1926, Edward P. Richardson carefully explored Martell's neck, but could find no tumor. Unknown to this group was Mandl's successful removal of a parathyroid tumor from a patient with this type of bone disease. This operation, which was performed on July 30, 1925, resulted in remarkable improvement. In 1932 after this patient's neck had been explored on six occasions, Edward Churchill performed a sternum-splitting operation, and a tumor was found in the mediastinum.

Other basic studies were done by Aub, including the effect of acid-producing substances on the metabolism of calcium and phosphorus.[52] Two young men who worked on this project with him later became important members of the research community: William Thomas Salter graduated from Harvard in 1925 and became a professor of biochemistry at Yale, and Ray Fletcher Farquharson became a professor of medicine at the University of Toronto.

### Fuller Albright and Clinical Endocrinology

Fuller Albright was an outstanding endocrinologist.[53] In 1934 Albright, Aub, and Bauer reported on the first seventeen patients at the MGH who were discovered to have hyperparathyroidism.[54] These and other studies done mainly on Ward 4 clarified the disease entity. Albright studied hypoparathyroidism and its treatment, including the use of vitamin D.[55] Soon a better agent was found—a synthetic substance known as dihydrotachysterol, or AT 10. This work on the parathyroid gland formed a foundation upon which Albright subsequently developed a conceptual system applicable to all bone disease. He emphasized that bone is constantly being formed in some places and destroyed in others. An important distinction stressed by Albright was between osteoporosis (excessive porousness of bone) and osteomalacia (softening of bone). Osteoporosis is the condition that develops when osteoblasts lay down too little bone matrix or osteoid.[56] What matrix is formed is normally calcified, because there is no abnormality in calcium or phosphorus metabolism. Osteomalacia is the condition in which, although osteoblasts form plenty of matrix, there is an impediment to its calcification resulting in softening of the bone.

The extension of Albright's studies to the pituitary-gonad axis in 1929 was stimulated by Professor Bernhard Zondek of Berlin. In 1927 Selmar Aschheim and Zondek showed that, within the first two weeks and through the fourth month of pregnancy, large amounts of gonadotropic material are found in blood and urine. Albright set up a laboratory in which he performed the Aschheim-Zondek and other endocrinological tests for the routine purposes of the hospital. Albright was, however, no routinist. The results that came out of these examinations were not only used diagnostically by practicing physicians but also served as important research information.

Albright organized two ambulatory clinics: an Ovarian Dysfunction Clinic and a Stone Clinic. In the former, diagnostic and treatment services based on principles derived from his research were provided for women with menstrual disorders or other abnormalities due to faulty ovarian function. Many of these patients were selected for study in Ward 4. In this way, new patterns of disease were recognized, from which basic endocrinological knowledge was acquired. In the Stone Clinic, new cases of hyperparathyroidism were found, and Albright extended his interest to the study of all types of stone formation in the urinary tract.

The pituitary-gonad axis became a major advance in the endocrinological structure erected by Albright. This was later reinforced by the pituitary-adrenocortical axis, as biochemical knowledge of adrenal cortical function increased in the middle 1930s. Albright separated primary myxedema from hypothyroidism of pituitary origin, and he recognized an analogous relationship with respect to the pituitary and adrenal cortex in Cushing's syndrome.[57]

Albright was a master at unravelling the endocrine enigmas that he encountered in the clinic. He had an extraordinary capacity to fit various pieces of information together and construct a complete clinical picture. He exemplified better than any other clinical investigator the complete blending of research and practice in all that he did. His characterization of clinical pictures was in terms of excessive, insufficient, or normal action of hormones. Thus, his diagnoses would come out as hyper-this, or hypo-that and iso–the other.

Albright had a great capacity to use any technique at hand that would illuminate the subject he was investigating. First came careful history-taking and bedside observation of patients. In the laboratory, hormone assays of various sorts were made on blood and urine; blood chemistry and balance studies, and the use of x-ray and removal of bits of tissue for microscopic examination were all utilized effectively.

He observed directly the effects of hormones on their target organs or tissues—skin, bones, hair, nails, breasts, sex organs, and so forth. His careful observations often changed the view of the pathogenesis of a clinical syndrome. For example, ovarian agenesis, characterized by short stature and the absence of the ovaries, had been considered to be caused by a lack of the growth hormone of the pituitary, resulting in retardation of bodily growth; a lack of pituitary gonadotropic hormone, with consequent failure of ovarian stimulation. Albright found that there was instead a great excess of gonadotropin. The pituitary had not failed but was doing its best to make ovaries that actually were not there function.

Albright had a succession of able disciples, many of whom became distinguished in their own right, including Frederic C. Bartter, Charles H. Burnett, Reed Ellsworth, Anne Forbes, Russell Fraser (of London), William Parson, Edward Reifenstein, and H. Sulkowitch.

## The Third Jackson Professor: Walter Bauer

An important participant in clinical investigation at the MGH was Walter Bauer, who later became the third full-time Jackson Professor of Medicine.[58] When Ward 4 opened, Bauer and Hunter were Aub's associates in the study of lead poisoning. In 1927 Bauer received a fellowship for study with Henry Hallett Dale at the National Institute for Medical Research in London. With Dickinson W. Richards, he investigated the control of the circulation through the liver. The following year Bauer accepted Cecil Kent Drinker's invitation to head the Robert W. Lovett Memorial Unit for the Study of Crippling Diseases. He soon organized (at the MGH) a vigorous program of research on diseases of the bones and joints, which remained his major interest.

After a productive contribution to the war effort, Bauer returned as an associate professor of medicine at Harvard and succeeded Means in 1951 as Jackson Professor. In his arthritis research unit much significant work was done, and he trained many talented workers in this field, including Charles Short, Marion Ropes, Evan Calkins, Stephen Krane, and others.

## The Birth of Cancer Research in Boston[59]

The months John Collins Warren spent in Vienna with Alfred Biesiadecki and in Berlin with Virchow and Cohnheim, studying pathological histology, awakened his scholarly interest in cancer, which he maintained throughout his life. In 1899, when Mrs. Caroline Brewer Croft made a bequest to Harvard University for the study of cancer, Warren was named chairman of a committee of investigators organized to make use of the fund. Support was given for studies carried on in the pathological laboratory of the medical school on Boylston Street and, to some extent, at the new clinico-pathological laboratory of the MGH. The first annual report of the Croft Fund Cancer Commission to the surgical department of the Harvard Medical School was issued on October 23, 1900. In his introductory remarks, Warren noted that the surgical department was not able "to undertake a systematic investigation into the origin of cancer" and also indicated that the report represented tangible evidence of "the policy of this department in devoting its energies, not only to the teaching of surgery but to original research in some of the many inviting fields which are offered to well trained and well organized bands of scientific investigators."[60] This report appeared during a period when the parasitic origin of cancer was being debated and histological and bacteriological techniques were being applied to cancer tissue in an attempt to identify some specific infecting organism.

In 1909 the Croft Fund Cancer Commission was renamed the Cancer Commission of Harvard University. In the following year, the commission decided to undertake the study of living cancer in human beings. At a meeting of the commission, on April 13, 1910, Warren emphasized the importance of turning more actively to the clinical side of the cancer problem, indicating that "we had been training scientific men in our laboratories who have become experts in the work to which we have referred. We wish now to place these experts in intimate contact with living cancer in human beings.... It might be asked if among all the hospitals that are going up it would not be perfectly easy to obtain permission from the Trustees for accommodations for the patients in some of their wards. The answer is that we want to have this little hospital entirely under our own control independent of any other organization so that we can study the cases to the greatest possible example."[61] President Eliot fully endorsed the plan to have a special cancer hospital. Through the efforts of Warren and his colleagues, $292,885 was raised for this purpose. Because of Mrs. Huntington's generous gift for cancer research, the new institution, which opened in March 1912, was named the Collis B. Huntington Memorial Hospital for Cancer. In the words of Frederick C. Shattuck, credit for the organization of this hospital belonged to Warren alone: "He was the father and mother." The hospital was operated under the control of the Cancer Commission and the directorship of E. E. Tyzzer, who had general supervision of the research work of the commission.

In the first annual report of the hospital (for the year ending June 30, 1913), Warren stated: "It is much to be desired that a laboratory building should be constructed in close physical relation to the hospital where investigations along different lines of science can be pursued. . . . A certain amount of chemical research on cancer problems has already been carried on in the laboratories of the Huntington Hospital and the department of biochemistry in the medical school. Much more could be done if better facilities were provided in the chemical laboratory in close relation to the hospital."[62] The laboratory building became a reality in 1922, largely through Warren's fund-raising efforts; by action of the Harvard Corporation it was named the John Collins Warren Laboratory.

Among the early directors of research at the Huntington Hospital was Francis W. Peabody. In 1923, when Peabody was invited to become director of the new Thorndike Memorial Laboratory, George R. Minot succeeded him, and, in 1928, Aub succeeded Minot. Aub proposed to attack the problem in a fundamental way, by regarding cancer as an aberration in growth control. This was a bold course on which to set an entire laboratory effort, since it involved a search for normal control mechanisms as well, and the short-term relevancy of such studies to the cancer problem was not immediately apparent. Almost a generation passed before this forward-looking point of view met general acceptance among the cancer research laboratories of the world.[63] The Huntington Hospital was finally closed in 1941, and Aub moved his laboratory back to the MGH. Even after his retirement as a professor of research medicine at Harvard in 1956, Aub undertook a fresh study of the surface of the tumor cell. He was honored by the presentation of the George M. Kober Medal of the Association of American Physicians in 1966.

## The Peter Bent Brigham Hospital

The Peter Bent Brigham Hospital was envisaged as early as 1900; it became the key factor in the overall design of the Harvard Medical School complex on Longwood Avenue.[64] The site finally chosen was the

Ebenezer Francis estate in Roxbury. Over 1,100,000 sq. ft. of land were purchased, of which Harvard reserved about 500,000 sq. ft. for the new medical school; somewhat more than 400,000 sq. ft. for the Brigham executors; and about 200,000 sq. ft. for the Children's Hospital. The new Brigham Hospital, which was designed by John Shaw Billings (designer of the Johns Hopkins Hospital), won an architectural prize. Ground was broken on August 7, 1911, and in 1913 the hospital was opened. Because of this long period of gestation, the hospital was born with stature and staffed from the beginning with well-qualified teaching and research physicians and surgeons.

Henry A. Christian[65] became the first physician-in-chief. Harvey Williams Cushing,[66] a graduate of the Harvard Medical School who received the major portion of his surgical training and did his early research in Baltimore, was named surgeon-in-chief.

A graduate of Randolph Macon College, Christian took his M.D. degree at Johns Hopkins in 1900. He had served as physician-in-chief at the Carney Hospital in South Boston since 1907, before accepting his appointment at the Brigham in 1913. On May 26, President Emeritus Eliot wrote to him:

> Now that you and Cushing have been put at the head respectively of the two departments of the Brigham Hospital I feel as if the medical school were entering on a happier future. Ever since I have been a member of the medical faculty I have seen clearly what a handicap on the school it was that the university had no hold on hospital appointments. Hereafter the school will be able to search all over the country for the very best men to fill vacancies.[67]

Christian's specialty was diseases of the heart and kidneys, but his writings also cover the general field of internal medicine.[68] Samuel A. Levine wrote of him:

> He is one of the few remaining illustrious medical figures in this country who stemmed from the early Osler days of the Hopkins Hospital. He was primarily a clinician of the descriptive type, with a thorough background of pathology. His era antedated the great period of physiological and chemical emphasis that prevails today. Although in his early years he conducted animal experimentation, studying nephritis and myocarditis in rabbits, thereafter his attention was entirely directed to bedside medicine. Many of the young residents and fellows working under Christian made notable research contributions.[69]

Christian, who was made dean of the Harvard Medical School at the age of thirty-two, "was among the early leaders to stimulate a spirit of research in the medical faculty." According to Levine, it was because of Christian's wisdom in the development of the medical clinics that the Peter Bent Brigham Hospital assumed a predominant position throughout the world. He incorporated a scientific spirit with one of care for the patient that was a model for academic institutions. He was among the first to institute the system of residency training in the United States. He was meticulous about recording observations, both clinical and laboratory, so that they might be available for research purposes.[70]

## Francis Weld Peabody

Peabody[71] was the first resident physician at the Peter Bent Brigham Hospital. At the end of his third year in Harvard Medical School (1906), he was urged by Reginald Heber Fitz to pursue a career in "academic medicine." When Joseph Hersey Pratt[72] returned to Boston, after training at Johns Hopkins with Osler, and in Germany with Ludolf Krehl, he offered an elective course in clinical investigation for fourth year students, in which Peabody enrolled.

Pratt described that year (1906–7): "We took a bare room in the newly opened building and fitted up a bacteriological laboratory. The problem assigned to Peabody was to isolate typhoid bacilli from the dejections of typhoid patients. He had to go from his home in Cambridge each morning to the MGH to collect the feces of typhoid patients and bring them to the school . . . he had to make the culture media, and do all the other work aided only by an untrained laboratory boy."[73] During his internship at the MGH, Peabody developed a method of growing typhoid bacilli from the blood. He reported these studies before the AMA in June 1908.[74] Pratt could "recall no other intern who has reported original work in clinical medicine at a meeting of our national society."[75]

His research with Pratt gave Peabody his first real enthusiasm for medicine—it showed him that medicine was a "growing thing." Immediately after his internship, he set out on a training program, which in the next six years made him one of the best-educated internists in America. Two years at Johns Hopkins, in the newly established full-time physiological division in the department of medicine under Arthur D. Hirschfelder, were followed by a year in Germany, where Peabody studied organic chemistry with Emil Fischer and Georg Fresenius. Then he spent time with Krogh in Copenhagen. In 1911 he worked as a resident at the HRI.

Thus, Peabody became one of the first to undertake what he called "making clinical applications of the methods of physiology" to diseases of the heart and lungs. In the years 1913 to 1920, while a member of Christian's full-time staff, Peabody and his associates established the importance of the vital capacity as a measure of pulmonary reserve and also showed the mechanism by which vital capacity is decreased in heart failure, emphysema, and other diseases.[76]

## Other Members of the Brigham Staff

One of the early members of the Brigham hospital staff was Isaac Chandler Walker[77] (M.D., Johns Hopkins, 1909), who interned at the

Carney Hospital. In 1913 he worked with Homer Fordyce Swift at the Hospital of the Rockefeller Institute. In 1915 he began the study of asthma and in 1917 published his first summary paper, followed by a clinical study of four hundred patients with bronchial asthma.[78] He was a pioneer in the field of allergy.

Channing Frothingham[79] (M.D., Harvard, 1906) became second in command under Christian. He interned at the Boston City Hospital and then spent four years (1908–12) as an assistant visiting physician at the Carney Hospital. After World War I, he returned to the teaching staff of Harvard Medical School, was chairman of the executive committee of the departments of medicine[80] for many years, and served as an associate clinical professor of medicine from 1928 to 1933. Early in his career, he published papers on trichinella infestation both in man and in the experimental animal. He also studied the behavior of proteolytic enzymes in tissue and attempted to produce arterial lesions experimentally.[81] In later years he was concerned with the social and economic aspects of medical practice.

Clifford Lambie Derick[82] (M.D., McGill, 1918) began his clinical training at the Montreal General Hospital in 1919, under H. A. Lafleur, Osler's first chief resident physician. In 1922 he was awarded a National Research Fellowship, which he spent in the departments of medicine and biochemistry at the Harvard Medical School. His first publication, in collaboration with Otto Folin, dealt with gout. In 1924 Derick went to the HRI to work with Swift on rheumatic fever and bacterial allergy.[83] In 1928 he returned to the Brigham, as an assistant and then an associate professor.

James P. O'Hare[84] (M.D., Harvard, 1911) worked with Christian as a student and developed a life-long interest in diseases of the kidney. His knowledge of renal physiology, bacteriology, and pathology provided a resource for his young colleagues, who later improved the original artificial kidney machines and made renal dialysis practical. He established the renal division at the Brigham, which he had on a firm basis by the time that John Merrill succeeded him as its head. Throughout his career, he maintained an interest in hypertension and renal disease.[85]

Samuel A. Levine (M.D., Harvard, 1914) had his postgraduate training at the Brigham and continued to serve there throughout his career. He became a clinical professor of medicine at Harvard University in 1948. After James B. Herrick (1912), Levine was the next to recognize coronary thrombosis, and, in 1919, he and C. L. Tranter published an important paper on the differential diagnosis of acute cholecystitis and acute myocardial infarction. Most of his research contributions were concerned with heart disease, including the relation of hypertension to mitral stenosis, Lead IV with special reference to the findings in angina pectoris, temporary relief of anginal pain by carotid sinus stimulation, and the "chair" treatment of acute coronary thrombosis.[86]

Philip Grabfield[87] (M.D., Harvard, 1915) was a medical house officer at the Brigham in 1916–17. He went from an instructor to an associate professor of pharmacology and medicine at Harvard from 1921 to 1946. He was a member of the American Society for Clinical Investigation. His fields of research included the effects of endocrine products; the effect of iodide on nitrogen metabolism; nitrogen and sulfur metabolism in Bright's disease; gout; and uricosuric drugs.[88]

Reginald Fitz (M.D., Harvard, 1909),[89] the son of Reginald Heber Fitz, served on the resident staff of the MGH, the Johns Hopkins Hospital, and the Peter Bent Brigham Hospital. In 1915 he went to the HRI as an assistant resident, where he devised a new method for the determination of beta-hydroxybutyric acid. Studies in diabetics were designed to investigate the relationships between the amounts of fat, carbohydrate, and protein burned, and their effect on the formation of oxybutyric and diacetic acid. In 1920 he became a staff physician at the Mayo Clinic, but in 1922 returned to the Peter Bent Brigham, where he maintained his laboratory until 1936. From 1936 to 1939 he was a professor of medicine at Boston University.

William P. Murphy[90] (M.D., Harvard, 1920) was an assistant resident physician at the Brigham in 1922. He remained as a part-time member of the staff and was associated with George R. Minot. It was Murphy who carefully followed the patients with pernicious anemia during Minot and Murphy's demonstration of the effectiveness of liver therapy. He received the Nobel Prize with Minot and George Whipple in 1934.

## Soma Weiss

When Christian retired in 1939, Soma Weiss[91] became Hersey Professor and physician-in-chief at the Brigham Hospital. Weiss attended the Royal Hungarian University at Budapest, where he was a research fellow in the institute of biochemistry. He came to the United States in 1920. While studying for his B.A. degree (Columbia University, 1921) and for his M.D. degree (Cornell, 1923), he held the position of an assistant in pharmacology at Cornell, working with Robert A. Hatcher.[92] After graduation, Weiss interned at the Bellevue Hospital. In 1925 he went to the Thorndike Memorial Laboratory, where he collaborated with Herrman Blumgart in studies of the velocity of blood flow in man. During the next seven years, his research interests were in cardiovascular disease and problems in clinical pharmacology and therapeutics. He and his colleagues contributed to our knowledge of left-sided heart failure, carotid sinus disorders, syncope, hypertension, beriberi heart disease, chronic pyelonephritis, and toxemias of pregnancy. The list of his disciples includes Robert W. Wilkins, Richard Capps, E. B. Ferris, Jr., and G. P. Robb.

Weiss often generated the concept of a disease mechanism by shrewd observation at the bedside and later documented it by the application of an appropriate laboratory technique, in the selection of which he possessed the "sense of the craftsman for the right tool." He gathered about him at the Brigham a group of young associates, including Eugene Stead, Paul Beeson, Charles Janeway, and John Romano, who created an ever-expanding school of clinical investigators in various areas of medicine. If one considers these four men as the first generation, the second, most of whom trained with Weiss at the Brigham as house officers, includes J. D. Myers, J. B. Hickam, Robert Grant, Louis Heppleman, Clement Finch, Philip Bondy, and J. V. Warren. Almost all of these men have served as chairmen of a department of medicine and each have protégés, including Ivan Bennett, James Leonard, Arnold Weissler, Samuel Martin, William Hollingsworth, Norton Greenberger, Wallace Jenson, Leighton Cluff, Robert Petersdorf, and Joseph Ross.[93] Weiss was also instrumental in bringing E. B. Astwood to Harvard. At Harvard, Astwood discovered the antithyroid activity of thiouracil, just before he took a post at Tufts School of Medicine. Soma Weiss died on January 31, 1942, at the age of forty-three, thus cutting short the career of one of the most stimulating clinical investigators on the American scene.

### The Boston City Hospital and Clinical Research

When the Boston City Hospital (BCH) opened on June 1, 1864, Harvard supplied five house officers: two medical, two surgical, and one ophthalmological.[94] In 1867, when he became Professor Emeritus at Harvard, Henry I. Bowditch, Jackson Professor of Clinical Medicine, joined the staff. Many other distinguished members of the Harvard faculty served at the BCH, including George B. Shattuck, Henry Jackson, and Thomas M. Rotch.

In 1899 the following statement appeared in the annual report of the trustees: "A large metropolitan hospital not only serves as a hospital for the care of the sick, but also is an institution for education in medicine and the pursuit of medical science . . . the trustees feel that it is their duty to assist this most laudable work."

In 1914 a committee was appointed to study professional support for the BCH, leading to an agreement with the three Boston medical schools that their chiefs of service would be appointed after joint conference between the BCH and the institutions concerned. The new Fourth Medical Service began a Harvard affiliation; G. G. Sears, a clinical professor of medicine at Harvard, was placed in charge.[95] After World War I, William Richard Ohler, who was aided by private funds for research, began studies on patients with nephritis and diabetes. Late in 1918, following the influenza epidemic, a ward service was organized to care for cases of influenza-pneumonia. Under the direction of Edwin Allen Locke, a resident physician, Henry M. Thomas, Jr.,[96] of Baltimore, was placed in immediate charge, followed a year later by F. Dennette Adams. The research laboratory attached to this "special service" was supported by the department of hygiene at Harvard and later provided a base for Maxwell Finland's studies of the specific serum treatment of pneumonia.

In July 1919 the medical staff assigned all hematologic cases to the First Medical Service and established a laboratory for research, supervision of blood donors, and transfusions, which was headed by Ralph B. Larrabee (M.D., Harvard, 1897), a visiting physician since 1912. The research was done by Thomas E. Buckman and four technicians.

## The Thorndike Memorial Laboratory under Francis Weld Peabody[97]

In 1912 David Linn Edsall developed an interest in the organization of an "academic clinic" at the BCH. Peabody pointed out that without full-time leadership such a clinic could not rank with those at the Brigham or the MGH. In 1919 the bequest of George L. Thorndike, in memory of his brother Dr. William H. Thorndike, visiting surgeon of the BCH from 1866 to 1884, was turned over to the City of Boston. The trustees added to this a loan appropriation of $150,000. On July 1, 1921, the trustees, acting on Dean Edsall's nomination, voted "to appoint Francis Weld Peabody as director of the Thorndike Laboratory." Harvard also appointed him as a professor of medicine. Peabody, who was then on temporary assignment as a visiting professor of medicine at Peking Union Medical College in China, returned to assist in the planning of the new research laboratories. The basement and first floor were occupied by the x-ray department; the patients were on the second floor; and the third and fourth floors housed laboratories and offices. An animal house was added. In August 1923, Peabody and his staff occupied the new quarters. There were three assistants: Henry Jackson, Jr.,[98] Robert N. Nye, and Gulli Lindh Muller, the first woman to graduate from the College of Physicians and Surgeons. Goronwy O. Broun, Carl F. Pelkan, and Herrman Blumgart were resident physicians.

On November 15, 1923, the Thorndike Laboratory was formally dedicated and thus became the first clinical research facility in a municipal hospital in this country. In 1924 Charles A. Doan and Perrin Hamilton Long, and in 1925 William B. Castle, Joseph T. Wearn, and Soma Weiss, received appointments. The group was very productive in research.[99]

From biopsies of the tibial bone marrow made before and after liver feeding, Peabody correctly concluded that in pernicious anemia "the bone marrow shows a cellular hyperplasia but is functionally inefficient."[100] Doan, fresh from Florence Sabin's laboratory at the Rockefeller Institute and from Johns Hopkins, studied the phagocytic activity of leukocytes in supravitally stained preparations. Blumgart and Weiss employed radioactive materials in their pioneer studies defining the velocity of blood flow in normal subjects.[101]

Joseph T. Wearn[102] trained under Henry A. Christian and later worked with A. N. Richards at Pennsylvania, where he was the first to obtain glomerular filtrate from the frog kidney by micropuncture. At the

Thorndike Laboratory, he was interested in the Thebesian vessels of the cardiac septum and the problem of collateral circulation. Jackson was working on nephritis in rats and in patients, as well as on the nucleotides of human blood. Millard Smith was concerned with metabolic studies in diabetes and with the factors permitting minimal nitrogenous metabolism.

In 1924 Peabody became physician-in-chief of the Fourth Medical Service, where he emphasized the coexistence of medical science and the healing art in the training of physicians for careers in medical practice or in academic medicine. Peabody believed that the general ward was the backbone of the medical unit and should be the meeting place of teachers, practitioners, and researchers.

On October 13, 1927, Peabody died of cancer at the age of forty-seven. Harvard created the Francis Weld Peabody Fellowship and, in 1963, established the medical school's first faculty professorship in his honor.

### Peabody's View of the Chief of the Clinic

Peabody recorded his thoughts regarding the ideal qualifications for the chief of the clinic in a letter to Warfield Theobald Longcope:

> One hears a great deal about research ability as a qualification for the professor of medicine. . . . Ability to do good, conscientious, independent work, interest in stimulating and assisting others to carry on research, and an appreciation of the role that research plays in the medical clinic are more important than great personal research genius. The professor must keep in close touch with the work of his staff, guiding where he can, suggesting and encouraging, and he should always try to keep up some independent work if only for his own intellectual satisfaction so that he may set an example to the staff and may have some little field in which he excels his assistants.
>
> One may reasonably question whether the large proportion of the budget of the department of medicine that is devoted to research and the great stress that has been laid on research ability in the selection of teachers is entirely justified when one considers that much of the research output is of a routine nature. . . . My feeling is that it is justified, although I think the pendulum has swung too far in the matter of choice of professors . . . there is a . . . tendency to pay too little attention to broad clinical experience, something that is acquired only by many years of hard work, and too much attention to research ability. . . .
>
> There is a common tendency to attempt to select assistants in a department of medicine whose training represents the different preclinical sciences, physiology, organic chemistry, physical chemistry, physics, bacteriology, and so forth;—so that one may have a well-rounded clinic. . . . These men, thoroughly trained in one direction, quite naturally look for their research problems in the fields in which they are trained. . . . The approach of the internist to the study of disease in man should be quite different. He is, first of all, absorbed by an interest in the problem and then

seeks the type of tools necessary to solve it. This is the intellectual rather than the technical, method of approach. Once given an absorbing passion for the solution of a clinical problem, the man who has had a good general scientific training can usually acquire in a few months or in a year or so, enough of any of the fundamental sciences to enable him to tackle it. The clinical investigator, with his knowledge of disease in man, thus finds the problem first and determines the practical way to study it, turning to his colleagues in the fundamental sciences especially for technical experience. . . . The medical clinic should encourage its staff to use methods of any sort, no matter how difficult or specialized, that are needed for the solution of their immediate problems, but their first interest should center about the general subject of disease in man. The first interest of the "scientist," on the other hand, is and should be in the development of his own particular field. Each has his proper and legitimate role, but in the medical clinic it is better to have an inspired internist than a skilled chemist.[103]

In later years, William B. Castle expressed similar views in his presidential address before the Association of American Physicians (see chapter 7).[104]

Alfred E. Cohn of the HRI saw Peabody's letter and made the following comment:

The difference between Peabody and me is that to him the center of interest in medicine is practice and the care of the sick; to me it is the enlargement of the confines of knowledge. His is not an unworthy object. But its center of gravity is not one which places the medical clinic in the heart of a university. His might be a preparatory or an apprentice school. It makes of the professor the father of his children and knowledge a decoration. But in a university knowledge is not a decoration but a passion and indeed life itself. The university does not neglect the care of the sick nor ignore teaching how this end may be accomplished—it has a function here just as it has assumed one in respect to engineering; at the same time though it cares for mathematics and physics. . . .

The wards are not "the backbone of the clinic"—at least of a university clinic. They represent merely one of the vertebrae. Whatever part of the argument depends on this assumption must go the way of all syllogisms based on incorrect premises. The description of "the head of the clinic" is trivial. This conception of the professor is more like that of a YMCA secretary than of a person with vital purposes in life.[105]

## The Second Director of the Thorndike Laboratory: George Richards Minot

Minot, who had just found a "cure" for pernicious anemia, succeeded Peabody as director of the Thorndike Laboratory.[106] Minot was physician-in-chief at Huntington Hospital. On April 1, 1928, he became a professor of medicine at Harvard. Joseph T. Wearn was appointed associate director of the Thorndike, but served only one year before going to Western Reserve (1929). Within a few months after Peabody's death, Blumgart also left the Thorndike, to become director of medical research at the Beth Israel Hospital at Harvard. In 1930 Soma Weiss became associate director of the Thorndike.[107] Weiss was instrumental in guiding the initial work of a biochemically trained associate, F. H. L. Taylor.

Under Minot's directorship, productive research continued to flow. Jackson began work on the lymphomas and in 1947, with Frederick Parker, Jr., published a classic monograph, *Hodgkin's Disease and Allied Disorders.*[108]

In 1929 William B. Castle[109] (M.D., Harvard, 1921), who had interned at the MGH, published the first of his studies on the etiologic relationship of achylia gastrica to pernicious anemia. This work, begun in 1927, demonstrated erythropoietic effects in pernicious anemia patients, using mixtures of normal human gastric juice (intrinsic factor) and beef muscle (extrinsic factor). The supervision and dietary control of these patients would not have been possible without the use of the Thorndike ward, where clinical trials of the potency of liver "fractions" prepared by Edwin Cohn, professor of physical chemistry at Harvard, or by G. H. A. Clowes, of Eli Lilly and Company, were also conducted. In 1931 the first practical liver extracts for intravenous and intramuscular use in pernicious anemia were developed and used by Taylor and Maurice B. Strauss. A few months later, Castle demonstrated their therapeutic value in tropical sprue in Puerto Rico.

W. D. Sutliss (M.D., Cornell, 1924) joined Finland, in 1929, in a series of studies on antibody development in untreated and in serum treated cases of pneumococcal pneumonia. Maxwell Finland[110] (M.D., Harvard, 1926) was an intern and then a "pneumonia resident" under W. H. Robey, physician-in-chief of the Second Medical Service. Chester S. Keefer (M.D., Johns Hopkins, 1922) joined the unit in 1930, as an assistant professor of medicine at Harvard.[111] Keefer turned his attention to the degenerative and infectious types of arthritis, both streptococcal and gonococcal.[112] In 1933 H. F. Dowling (M.D., George Washington, 1931), subsequently a professor of medicine at the University of Illinois, joined Keefer's group for two years.

The research fellows were assigned, in accordance with their interests, to work under various staff members of the Thorndike, of which Castle had become associate director in 1932. James M. Faulkner, a part-time staff member, supervised the electrocardiography, emphasizing the importance of precordial leads in the diagnosis of myocardial infarction. Weiss was studying pulmonary, peripheral, and venous blood flow with G. P. Robb; carotid sinus syncope with Richard Capps and E. B. Ferris, Jr.;[113] oxygen requirements of exercise in cardiac patients with L. B. Ellis; arterial hypertension with Capps;[114] and beri-beri heart disease with Robert W. Wilkins. With Parker, a pathologist, Weiss investigated the nature of the pulmonary vascular changes in chronic mitral stenosis. In 1933, in a pioneer effort at angiocardiography, Robb persuaded an intern in the x-ray department to inject 20 cc of uroselectan into his (Robb's) antecubital vein while the pulmonary vessels and heart were observed under the fluoroscope. In 1931 Minot began studies of the iron deficiency anemias. With S. R. Mettier, he showed that iron was better absorbed by achlorhydric patients when presented in an acid medium strongly buffered with beef muscle. With C. W. Heath, he performed studies of the effects of iron therapy upon both reticulocytes and blood regeneration in hypochromic anemia. In 1932 Heath and Strauss[115] demonstrated that parenterally administered iron caused a corresponding increase in circulating hemoglobin in hypochromic anemia, thus showing that the principal ingredient of food substances responsible for hemoglobin regeneration in Whipple's chronically bled dogs was iron. In 1935 Strauss established a nutritional basis for the macrocytic and hypochromic anemias of pregnancy, and he demonstrated that alcoholic polyneuritis could be cured by dietary supplementation despite continued use of spirits. In 1936 Paul Kimmelstiel, of the pathology laboratory, and Clifford Wilson, a Rockefeller Traveling Fellow from London, demonstrated the well-known syndrome in diabetes with which their names are associated.[116] In 1934 T. Hale Ham (M.D., Cornell, 1931) came from a residency at the New York Hospital to work in hematology.[117] In 1937 he published the first of a series of papers on the mechanisms involved in hemolytic anemias, describing for the first time the sensitivity to acid hemolysis of the red cells of patients with paroxysmal nocturnal hemoglobinuria. Later studies were done in this area in collaboration with John H. Dingle. In 1936 Arthur J. Patek, Jr., and R. P. Stetson showed that the coagulation defect in hemophilia could be corrected by a platelet-free plasma globulin factor. This initiated a series of studies of defective blood coagulation involving hypoprothrombinemia, platelet deficiencies or fibrinolysis carried out over the next ten years by F. J. Pohle, E. L. Lozner, R. Kark, A. W. Souter, Henry J. Tagnon, Charles S. Davidson, Jessica Lewis (Mrs. Jack Myers), and others in collaboration with F. H. L. Taylor.

By 1938 Minot was the head of a well-balanced research unit with Castle, Keefer, and Weiss as senior and Finland and Ham as junior members. In 1939 Weiss went to the Peter Bent Brigham Hospital. Keefer replaced him as director of medical services for one year before becoming Wade Professor of Medicine at Boston University, where he was soon joined by Faulkner, who later became dean. In later years, Robert W. Wilkins, P. B. Emerson, and F. J. Ingelfinger, as well as other former members of the Harvard Medical Unit, were attracted to Keefer's department. Keefer was ultimately succeeded as Wade Professor by Wilkins.

Castle, who had become a professor of medicine at Harvard in 1937, became director of the Harvard Medical Services. New young men were recruited, including Robert H. Williams (M.D., Johns Hopkins, 1934), who founded an endocrine clinic in 1942 and published studies on Simmond's disease and the treatment of thyrotoxicosis with thiouracil. He also studied alterations in the biological oxidations of the thyroid, hirsutism in females, obesity, and other metabolic problems.

In 1941 Charles S. Davidson was appointed a research fellow. Davidson (M.D., McGill, 1939) served as a house officer for two years at the San Francisco General Hospital. His first research activities at the Thorndike were in collaboration with Tagnon and Taylor on the activation of plasmin by chloroform, and the fibrinolytic effects of intravenous injections of trypsin and thrombin in animals. In 1942, while caring for survivors of the Coconut Grove, Florida, fire, Davidson became involved in problems of sepsis, protein depletion, and anemia in patients with burns. One of these studies on abnormal nitrogen metabolism stimulated his later interests in malnutrition and in the parenteral use of protein hydrolysates, homogenized fat, and other nutrient mixtures. Davidson's research was for a number of years concerned with various problems of liver disease.

In 1947 Minot developed a hemiparesis, and Castle took over his adminstrative responsibilities. Minot died in February 25, 1950, and, in 1957, the George Richards Minot Professorship of Medicine at Harvard University was established.

## The Third Director: William Bosworth Castle

William B. Castle contributed outstanding work on the pathogenesis of pernicious anemia.[118] Castle's description of this work is exciting:[119]

When I attended the Harvard Medical School (1918–21) and read *Osler's Textbook,* it seemed clear that effective therapy was limited. Indeed, Richard Cabot a decade earlier had said that there were only 12 efficacious drugs; and the rest seemed to be used as palliatives of uncertain value. Most diseases other than blood disorders and bacterial and parasitic infections were recognized by symptoms, signs and course rather than by a specific laboratory test. By way of contrast anemia, leukemia, thrombopenic purpura, and hemophilia could be relatively reliably diagnosed by study of the peripheral blood. Nonetheless, of these only one—chlorosis—was curable. For the treatment of infections there were only three specifics: quinine, diphtheria antitoxin, and salvarsan.

During our second year E. V. McCollum from Baltimore talked about "water soluble B" and "fat soluble A," miniscule non-identities that nonetheless completely prevented or cured experimental conditions in animals due to their lack. Also I had heard that rice polishings cured Oriental beri-beri, orange juice scurvy, and meat and milk pellagra. There was for me great attraction in the completeness of such restorations and so a possible area of effective application to other human diseases of what Casimir Funk in 1913 had called, a "vitamine." You will understand that this was by no means clearly defined in my cortex, but was nevertheless a sort of "gut feeling."

Later on in a clinical lecture somebody described pernicious anemia . . . and said that invariably there was no acid in the stomach. I thought that just *had* to mean something about its cause. Then as an intern at the MGH while working in the neurological outpatient department somebody said that all patients with combined system disease who usually were anemic also had no acid in the stomach. The bell rang again, but I slid down no brass pole to go to the fire. The current British explanation (by Arthur Hurst) was streptococcal infection of the bowel.

After the internship Osler's evaluation of clinical medicine did not urge me to try to join somebody in a Back Bay practice. I went for two years into Cecil K. Drinker's department of physiology and learned from Harold Himwich that research requires dedication and hard work; also that our research on the R.Q. of dog muscle was not my idea of how to study human disease.

By great good fortune Francis Peabody at the Thorndike, prompted by Joseph Wearn, offered me a job there in 1925. I helped Peabody by persuading patients with pernicious anemia to submit to tibial bone marrow trephines. . . . What really interested me was the regularity of this response [liver in pernicious anemia] to an unknown dietary component. This sounded like the behavior of another dietary deficiency disease much more than the cure of an intestinal infection. I tried feeding dried yeast; no luck, yet liver worked every time.

The "idea" of a functional relationship between effective gastric digestion and pernicious anemia happened to formulate itself in terms of an experimental approach at a particular moment in 1927. Of course, all the necessary data had been known to me for some months or even for years, such as the nearly universal incidence of achylia gastrica.

Nevertheless, I recall very clearly that sometime early in 1927, I was leaving the Thorndike to go across town to a meeting of the American Academy of Arts and Sciences, at which Dr. Minot was to speak about the present state of his work with liver extracts. My lease of life at the Thorndike, having been generously extended during that year by Francis Peabody and Joseph Wearn on the basis of no tangible accomplishment on my part, caused me to feel some urge to make a favorable impression on Dr. Minot, some of whose liver fractions we were testing at the Thorndike. At any rate, I left the laboratory on the fourth floor of the Thorndike . . . without any specific plan in mind. However, while descending in the "back elevator" the idea of digesting beef steak in the human stomach and administering it subsequent to a control period of beef muscle alone did occur to me. The reticulocyte response that we were using in the evaluation of liver extracts meant that a "yes or no" answer could be obtained in 20 days, only the last 10 of which would involve any personal inconvenience. Our observations began in February, 1927. They were first reported in May, 1928 to the Young Turks. I sat up all night in Boston preparing my ten minute talk and saw the dawn. While shaving, I noticed that my hair had turned gray at the temples.

It is important to emphasize that without the "useless" observations of reticulocytes by Paul Ehrlich and the finding by Minot[120] that their increase heralded remission in pernicious anemia, the length of time required for a single study on the effect of beef muscle, plain and then predigested, would probably have been two months—a length of time too fraught with danger for the patient to have embarked on the study.

Castle did not know until later that in 1860 Austin Flint, Sr., was aware that Handfield Jones had recently published an account of the microscopic findings in one hundred human stomachs examined postmortem, of which fourteen showed considerable atrophy of the secretory glands. In a lecture on anemia to medical students, Flint referred to the "idiopathic anaemia" described by Thomas Addison of Guy's Hospital only five years before as follows: "I suspect that in these cases there exists degenerative disease of the glandular tubuli of the stomach . . . fatal anemia must follow on account of degenerative disease reducing the amount of gastric juice so far that assimilation of food is rendered wholly inadequate for the wants of the body."[121]

Castle stated the following:

> Viewed in the historical perspective of Flint and Fenwick's conclusions, my own hypothesis concerning the cause of the disease scarcely seems original. The inability of 200 grams of beef muscle given daily to cause erythropoietic effects in pernicious anemia (such as were readily obtained with beef muscle recovered from the normal human stomach or with 200 grams of liver alone) seemed consistent with the idea that digestion of beef muscle normally produced a different substance present also in liver.
>
> In the subsequent article of this series observations were reported that clearly showed that contact between a normal dietary (extrinsic) factor and a normal gastric (intrinsic) factor were necessary for the erythropoietic effects observed. The necessity for this contact between beef muscle and gastric juice together with the demonstrated requirement that it take place at or near neutrality in the alimentary tract seemed then to characterize some type of hitherto unrecognized gastric enzyme activity. This mistaken idea I cherished until many years later, when it became clear that the active principle of beef muscle and liver (vitamin $B_{12}$) differed only in quantity. William Dock had pressed upon me in correspondence the correct interpretation: namely, that gastric juice merely increased the uptake of a preformed active erythropoietic principle present in beef muscle as in liver. . . .
>
> In conclusion, a general comment. Knowledge of pernicious anemia began with descriptive study of disease, led to active clinical investigation of patients, and only subsequently continued on to derivative animal and test tube experiments. Let us never forget that nature is the most original of all experimenters and that it is the patient's physician who is privileged to learn most directly from her sometimes cruel, but never meaningless, clinical presentation.[122]

In 1957 Castle was made the first George Richards Minot Professor of Medicine at Harvard. Space does not allow recitation of the many other researches of William B. Castle, which were principally made in collaboration with Maurice B. Strauss, T. Hale Ham, and James H. Jandl.

## The Influence of the Thorndike Laboratory

The influence of the Thorndike Laboratory on clinical science has been enormous. Maxwell Finland, in his update of figures forty years after the opening of the laboratory, found that of 872 alumni of the Harvard Medical Services and/or of the Thorndike during that period, 402 had held the academic rank of assistant professor or higher. Of the 791 alumni then living, 141 had achieved the rank of full professor. Their departmental affiliations in clinically oriented subjects other than medicine included preventive medicine, 28; pediatrics, 18; bacteriology, 16; psychiatry, 14; pathology, 10; surgery, 7; radiology, 6; obstetrics and gynecology, 4; dermatology, 2; and ophthalmology, 1. The full professors of preclinical subjects totalled 27.[123]

There were also many distinguished academic leaders in medicine in foreign countries who had worked at the Harvard medical unit, including John Brock of Capetown, Pierre Dustin of Brussels, Henry Egana of Santiago, Harold Fullerton of Aberdeen, Scotland, J. Groen of Jerusalem, Kenneth Hetzel of Adelaide, Australia, Alberto Hurtado of Lima, Henry J. Tagnon of Brussels, Dame Janet Vaughan of Oxford, Clifford Wilson of London, and Mohsen Ziai of Shiraz, Iran. Other graduates were or had been chairmen of the departments of medicine at the medical schools of Alabama, Albany, Arkansas, Boston University, the University of California at Los Angeles, Duke, Illinois, Iowa, Louisville, New Mexico, New York University, State University of New York (Brooklyn and Buffalo), North Carolina, Pittsburgh, St. Louis, South Carolina, Medical College of Virginia, University of Washington, Western Reserve, and Wisconsin. Other alumni were chosen to head the departments of medicine at Harvard-affiliated Boston hospitals, including Herrman Blumgart at Beth Israel and Soma Weiss at Brigham. In 1964 Robert Ebert became head of the department of medicine at the MGH and, shortly thereafter, dean of the Harvard School of Medicine.

## Pioneer in Clinical Investigation in Neuropsychiatry: Stanley Cobb

Stanley Cobb[124] was by temperament a "nature lover." His earliest papers describe the behavior of birds, and, in later life, he returned to this interest. Cobb's fondness for the natural environment was reflected in his way of life.

His internship at the Peter Bent Brigham Hospital under Harvey Williams Cushing gave him experience with patients, colored his later formulations, and tempered his interpretation of mental events. With Adolph Meyer he learned about disorders of behavior. It was probably Meyer who inspired Cobb's later attempts to develop a unified concept of body and mind. Training completed, he joined the Harvard medical faculty and was rapidly promoted to Bullard Professor of Neuropathology. For the next thirty years, he studied and taught the related disciplines of neuroanatomy, neuropathology, clinical neurology, and psychiatry, making contributions in many fields. He first did much to define the neurophysiology of the human nervous system by applying electrophysiological techniques. Thus, he was able to explore the nature of clonus, spasticity, fatigue, convulsions, and many other neurological manifestations.[125] He next demonstrated variations in the blood supply of the brain, depending on local needs and reflex effects. One of the principles that evolved was that increased brain function is linked with increased blood flow.

Another significant contribution related to epilepsy. Cobb and W. G. Lennox[126] demonstrated that photic driving or a given type of retinal stimulation can so disturb excitation as to induce epileptic seizures. Cobb later showed that much that was attributed to the effects of alcohol followed insidious starvation and deprivation of vitamin B.

Backed by a life of bedside experience and the realization that much of psychiatry is the understanding of human motivation, Cobb turned his energies to studies of man in this context and the pertinence of this relationship to disease. He was challenged by the opportunity of making psychiatry both scientific and dynamic, and this he did in a significant way.

In his acceptance of the Kober Medal of the Association of American Physicians for 1956,[127] Cobb recalled the intellectual stimulation that he received in those centers of excellence where he worked. First, of the Johns Hopkins Hospital in the period just before World War I, Cobb spoke as follows:

> Many physicians speak of an earlier time as the "golden age of medicine" when Osler, Welch and Halsted developed a great center of American medicine. In 1915, we still had Halsted, Howell and Abel with Barker, Howland, Thayer, Janeway, Meyer, and McCollum. They were the teachers who drew us to Baltimore and inspired us. But it was the young men who made that time so exciting. Blackfan, Park, Gamble, Marriott, and Powers at the Harriet Lane; Bloomfield, Austrian, Levy, Thomas, Pincoffs, and King in medicine; Heuer, Reid, and Dandy in surgery; Moore, Watson, Richter, Lewis, and Greenacre at the Phipps; and across the street in the medical school laboratories: Drinker, Lamson, Binger, Bayne-Jones, Rivers, Richardson, Wilson, Weed, and Clark. After the war, of course, these men were dispersed as investigators and teachers over many centers.

Of Harvard he said:

> At Harvard in the years around 1930 there was grouped together one of those rare combinations of men deeply interested and active in the advancing field of neurology. Monthly meetings describing each other's current researches were held. From physiology came Cannon, Alexander Forbes, Bard, Fulton, Rosenbluth, and Davis; from surgery Cushing, Putnam, Bailey, and Mixter; from clinical neurology Ayer, Viets, Crothers, and Soloman; and from neuropathology Lennox, Wolfe, Harry Forbes, Morrison, Gibbs, Fremont-Smith, and Gildea.

## Herrman Blumgart and the Beth Israel Hospital[128]

The Beth Israel Hospital, a nonsectarian hospital supported by the Jewish community of Boston, was opened in 1916. It rapidly outgrew its facilities, and, by the middle 1920s, its trustees decided to build a new hospital near Harvard Medical School. After consultation with Dean David Linn Edsall, an agreement was reached to establish a Harvard affiliation at the Beth Israel.

In 1928 the new hospital opened, and Herrman Blumgart (M.D., Harvard, 1921) was appointed an associate professor of medicine, head of the Harvard teaching service in medicine, and director of medical research.[129] Blumgart had trained at the Peter Bent Brigham Hospital, under Henry A. Christian; and at the Boston City Hospital, under Francis W. Peabody. He spent a year in England with Sir Thomas Lewis. Blumgart brought A. Carlton Ernstene, who later became chief of medicine at the Cleveland Clinic, with him. Samuel L. Gargill, later head of endocrinology, and Dorothy Rourke Gilligan, who became chief chemist of the medical research department, were also recruited.

Blumgart described the early days of the hospital:

> In 1928 I accepted the position ... but the buildings were completely finished. No space for research laboratories ... had been planned. The Out-patient building had been built before the main hospital, and a boiler room was necessary to provide heat for it before the main buildings were completed; but now that the main building was finished, the boiler room was removed from the basement of the Out-patient Department, linoleum placed on the floor, several dogs were bought, and research was inaugurated. Our total budget, including salaries totalled $20,000 per year. ... But those were the days! A room of one's own ... and only the world to conquer.[130]

Blumgart started a new course, entitled "The Application of Physiological Principles to Medicine," for first year students. This course included lectures, and demonstrations of patients with atrial fibrillation, angina pectoris, congestive heart failure, and heart block. The series was subsequently enlarged to include the study of other organ systems and the biochemical principles of disease.

Research began slowly. At the Thorndike Laboratory, Blumgart had studied the velocity of blood flow in man. He and Gargill extended these studies and developed the concept that induction of hypothyroidism might be useful in the treatment of intractable angina pectoris, congestive heart failure, and supraventricular arrhythmias. Anatomic and pathologic studies of the thyroid gland were completed, and a surgeon, David D. Berlin, specially trained in thyroid surgery, joined the team. On December 15, 1932, the first total thyroidectomy was done on a patient with intractable congestive heart failure, resulting in improvement. A variety of studies were completed on the effects of total thyroidectomy on the heart and lung, on diabetes mellitus and carbohydrate metabolism, on parathyroid and pituitary gland function, and on chronic lymphatic leukemia. Several hundred patients were thyroidectomized at the Beth Israel Hospital, and larger numbers throughout the world.[131]

Harvard students who selected the department for work on a variety of problems included Hebbel Hoff, Louis H. Nahum, and Mark Altschule. Altschule subsequently joined the laboratory full-time and was responsible for cardiac physiology. Benjamin Alexander,[132] Paul M. Zoll, A. Stone Freedberg, and others later came to work there.

In 1936 Blumgart, with Hebbel Hoff and Monroe Schlesinger, the chief pathologist, began a series of studies of experimental coronary occlusion. Later experiments with Freedberg and Zoll demonstrated the development of intercoronary collateral circulation following chronic coronary artery narrowing. These experiments led to an extended study of factors (nitrites, anemia) favorably influencing the rate of development of coronary artery collateral circulation.

In 1946 Blumgart became a professor of medicine and physician-in-chief. He encouraged practicing physicians to undertake clinical investigations. Several did outstanding work, including Joseph E. F. Riseman, who developed a standardized exercise tolerance test to study the effect of drugs on angina pectoris. David Davis, who had been studying hypertension, joined Blumgart and Schlesinger in a clinical-pathological study of angina pectoris; a classic paper resulted.[133] Louis Wolff (of the Wolff–Parkinson–White syndrome) became head of the electrocardiography laboratory. The number of full-time physicians in the medical research department increased from under ten to thirty or more.

The availability of radioisotopes, particularly $^{131}$I, led to the restudy of $^{131}$I-induced hypothyroidism in intractable heart disease. Confirmation of the therapeutic benefit observed after total thyroidectomy was obtained. M. W. Hamolsky and Freedberg soon developed a diagnostic test of thyroid function: namely, red cell uptake of $^{131}$I triiodothyronine, which had wide use as the resin $^{131}$I $T_3$ uptake test.

Stanford Wessler developed a technique for study of plasma factors involved in accelerated intravenous clotting and began the study of experimental pulmonary embolism. Zoll worked on the transmission of external electrical currents into the heart and developed the first clinically effective method of initiating cardiac impulses in patients with repeated syncopal seizures due to Stokes-Adams disease using external electrodes. He later developed an internal pacemaker; the surgical technique was worked out by Howard A. Frank.

The department expanded significantly during the early 1940s. Freedberg, Altschule, and others began a series of studies of the cardiovascular effects of fever and of infectious shock. Alexander, who had joined the department as head of hematology, was at first involved in studies of amino acid metabolism in shock, but later established a coagulation laboratory, which served as a training center for investigators from all over the world.

Blumgart retired in 1962. Over fifty physicians and basic scientists obtained part of their training in the medical research department; professorial status was obtained by a majority of these individuals. Many were elected to the American Society for Clinical Investigation, the Association of American Physicians, and other scientific groups. In addition, many of the medical house officers who were trained at the Beth Israel Hospital went on to academic careers in medicine.

## Lawrence J. Henderson and the Harvard Fatigue Laboratory[134]

Lawrence J. Henderson, who had been at Strasbourg, returned to Harvard as a lecturer in the medical school department of biochemistry in 1904. Two years earlier, Carl Alsberg had returned from a similar period of study in Europe to become an assistant in the department of physiological and pathological chemistry at Harvard. In 1905, after the death of Edward S. Woods, department chairman in chemistry, Henderson and Alsberg for the succeeding three years undertook, with some success, to bring new concepts into the teaching of biochemistry. It was they who introduced the term *biological chemistry* and wrote a manual,  *Laboratory Practices in Biological Chemistry,* for the use of the first year course in the Harvard Medical School. For help in the laboratory, they invited Folin, who had recently published his papers on urine analysis, to give instruction in analytical procedures. In 1907 Folin was appointed an associate professor of biological chemistry and, in the next year, was advanced to the Hamilton Kuhn Chair of Biochemistry.

Henderson moved to Cambridge and developed an interest in physical chemistry. By 1925, however, he had almost divorced himself from the laboratory of physical chemistry, turning it over to his protégé Edwin Cohn. Henderson initiated studies on the physical-chemical properties of blood, research that was carried on in a laboratory at the MGH under the direction of Arlie Bock. Bock had been a Moseley Traveling Fellow with Barcroft in Cambridge. There he learned how to derive oxygen and carbon dioxide dissociation curves of blood. Henderson provided support for Bock to join Barcroft's high-altitude study. When Bock returned to Boston from Peru in 1922 he was assigned two rooms in the Bulfinch Building of the MGH. By 1924 Bock had published papers on carbon dioxide dissociation curves and gas equilibrium in the lungs and, in addition, had provided data for Henderson's *Blood as a Physical Chemical System: II,* of which Bock was a joint author.

In 1925, when Bruce Dill joined the group, a series of studies on muscular exercise was done, using as the subject the famous Boston marathon runner Clarence DeMar. Bock also had capable residents working with him during that period, including Lewis M. Hurxthal, John S. Lawrence, Thomas Coolidge, and John H. Talbott.[135]

The concept of the Fatigue Laboratory took form in Henderson's mind in 1925. He consulted Wallace Donham, dean of the Harvard Business School, and the professor of industrial research, Elton Mayo. Henderson saw the possibility of a bond resulting from the interest of Mayo and his associates in the sociological aspects of business management, and his own interest in what he later described as the study of man in his everyday life. Donham agreed to set aside rooms in Morgan Hall for offices, and space in the semibasement for a laboratory. Henderson received funds from the Rockefeller Foundation to equip the laboratory and $500,000 for ten years to support its work. The work of the Fatigue Laboratory was an attempt, by means of research and collaboration with others, to make contributions toward the establishment of "human biology." It was believed that the study of man's activities in their condition of interrelatedness would be eventually recognized as bearing upon human welfare in the normal business of life, as similar studies bear upon the treatment of the sick.

John Talbott, after his residency at the Presbyterian Hospital in New York, played a major role in the laboratory and its field studies until 1935, when he was given responsibility for Bock's laboratory at the MGH. Talbott worked on the first high-altitude study in 1929 and on the first desert study in 1932, was responsible for the study of heat-related illnesses in the steel industry at Youngstown, Ohio, in 1934, and was a clinical investigator in another high-altitude study in 1935.

Henderson attracted many foreign fellows. Another category of participants included physiologists from the United States, postdoctoral fellows, and degree candidates. Among these were W. H. Forbes, R. E. Johnson, Ancel Keys, Ben Jones, and J. W. Thompson. There were also opportunities for students in the Harvard Medical School to work in the Fatigue Laboratory, and to many this experience was an important factor in their careers. Among them were Richard Riley, W. B. Wood, Eliot V. Newman, Bernard D. Davis, Clifford A. Barger, Norman Zamcheck, and John Maier. Another group joined in collaborative efforts. Notable in this category were Walter B. Cannon, Ashton Graybiel, Earle Chapman, A. N. Pappenheimer, Jr., Bryan Matthews, and E. F. Adolph. Members of the Fatigue Laboratory made distinguished contributions to applied research during World War II. The laboratory finally closed its doors in 1946, four years after the death of Henderson. Many of those who worked there created new centers of research in one or another field of applied physiology; one example was the Laboratory of Physiological Hygiene, established at the University of Minnesota by Ancel Keys.

# 13

✦

# The Washington University School of Medicine

Following Abraham Flexner's inspection of the Washington University medical department in 1909, the school underwent a complete reorganization. Convinced that Flexner's criticisms were justified, Robert S. Brookings quickly accepted his advice to abolish the school and to form a new faculty, reorganize clinical facilities "from top to bottom," and raise an endowment that would enable him to "repeat in St. Louis what president Gilman [had] accomplished in Baltimore."[1] Brookings envisioned that the new medical school, which would serve the Southwest, would "have the finest standards of excellence." After consulting with Henry S. Pritchett, of the Carnegie Foundation, Flexner, and William Henry Welch, Brookings accepted the Johns Hopkins University School of Medicine as his model.

A committee formed in December 1909 presented a plan of reorganization that in a general way determined the future policies of the university. What evolved was the creation of a large medical center dominated by the Washington University School of Medicine. The committee recommended that the first step in this creation was to secure a professor of internal medicine whose training was thoroughly scientific, who had recently been in touch with well-organized medical schools and teaching hospitals, whose eminence as a physician was recognized, and who would assume immediate responsibility under the board and chancellor for the execution of the board's plans. In December David Linn Edsall visited the school but ultimately, after presenting an important and detailed memorandum[2] of what should be done, turned the position down. Harvey Williams Cushing likewise declined the professorship of surgery.

After Brookings returned from Europe in 1910, having visited hospitals and medical schools abroad, progress was rapid. Funds were obtained from a number of St. Louis sources, including Adolphus Busch, Edward Mallinckrodt, Jr., William K. Bixby, and Brookings himself. The provision for hospital teaching facilities was worked out with the trustees of the Barnes Hospital and with the directors of the St. Louis Children's Hospital. In 1905 Barnes Hospital purchased a site on Kingshighway and, in 1908, commissioned architects to plan the hospital. Brookings convinced the trustees that if the hospital was used for teaching, its service should be greatly broadened and that a staff controlled by the professors of the medical school was essential. The hospital became affiliated with the medical school in 1910; the hospital agreeing to provide the facilities for university clinics, including teaching and research, and the university agreeing to furnish facilities for an outpatient department and a school of nursing and to assume the costs of facilities required for teaching and research.[3]

## George Dock's Tenure as Professor of Medicine[4]

George Dock became a professor of medicine and dean. Eugene L. Opie was appointed a professor of pathology; John F. Howland, of pediatrics; Joseph Erlanger, of physiology; Philip A. Shaffer, of biological chemistry; and Robert J. Terry, of anatomy. These six, who constituted the executive faculty of the medical school, had their first meeting on June 10, 1910, approximately one year after reorganization began.

George Dock[5] received his M.D. degree at Pennsylvania Medical School in 1884, when William Osler and William Pepper II were on the faculty in medicine. He came under the influence of the cardiologist K. F. Wenckebach when he studied at Leipzig, Berlin, Vienna, and Frankfurt-am-Main. He perfected himself in the then new methods of clinical laboratory diagnosis; Osler remarked that "he knew more about clinical laboratory procedures at that time than any man in the United States." In 1887 Dock was an assistant in clinical pathology at Pennsylvania. From 1888 to 1891 he was a professor of pathology at the University of Texas. He was then called to Michigan, where he served as chief of medicine (which at that time included psychiatry, pediatrics, and pathology) until 1908 (see chapter 18).

Victor Vaughan, the dean of medicine at Michigan, wrote in his book *A Doctor's Memories* that "from 1891 to 1908 Dock served as Professor of the Theory and Practice of Medicine [at Michigan]. As a teacher he initiated his students in scientific investigations and demonstrated the value of research work in the treatment of disease."[6] It was at Washington University, however, that Dock reached the peak of his career. In order to make generally available Dock's method of running the medical service of Barnes Hospital, George R. Herrmann wrote *Methods in Medicine: The Manual of the Medical Service of Dr. George Dock*, first published in 1924.

Dock was the school's stimulant for twelve years. He helped assemble a full-time faculty and was himself one of the first full-time professors of medicine in the United States, giving up all practice. While at St. Louis, Dock trained men who were to hold chairs as professors of medicine at seven U.S. medical schools.

Roger Sylvester Morris[7] became an associate professor at Washington University in 1911. Morris had been a pupil of Osler. After graduation from Johns Hopkins, he spent two summers with Friedrich von Müller in Munich. He then worked under Thomas R. Boggs in the clinical laboratory at Johns Hopkins. In 1912 he became director of medicine at the Clifton Springs Sanatorium in New York. In 1913 he was appointed the Frederich Forschheimer Professor of Medicine at Cincinnati.

George Canby Robinson[8] arrived in St. Louis as an associate professor in September 1913 and took over the course in clinical chemistry and microscopy taught by Morris. Robinson also conducted the course in physical diagnosis and offered an elective course in electrocardiography. The medical department had purchased an Edelmann string galvanometer two years before. It had been set up by J. S. Brotherhood (a Johns Hopkins graduate who was Dock's resident physician during 1910–11), but was stored after he left. The electrocardiograph was carefully reassembled, and various members of the resident staff worked with Robinson on special cardiac problems: Hugh McCullough, who later had an outstanding career in pediatrics in St. Louis and Chicago; Drew Luten, for many years one of the leading teachers of the school; Joseph F. Bredeck,[9] who became commissioner of health in St. Louis; Fred J. Hodges, later a professor of radiology at the University of Michigan and then at Chicago; and George R. Herrmann, who became a professor of medicine at the University of Texas. Robinson's outstanding associate was Frank Wilson, who was an instructor in medicine in 1916. Later, as a professor at the University of Michigan, he was recognized as a national leader in fundamental studies of electrocardiography, being the one who first developed the precordial lead.

Dock gave Robinson responsibility for the outpatient department and delegated to him many of the details of organizing the medical service. Robinson also took a special interest in the laboratories of the medical department. Here were facilities for chemical, bacteriological, and physiological research closely related both to the patients and to the teaching laboratory of clinical chemistry and microscopy.

Frederic M. Hanes (M.D., Johns Hopkins, 1908)[10] was a house officer at the Johns Hopkins Hospital and then an associate in pathology at the College of Physicians and Surgeons [P & S] from 1909 to 1912. The following year, he was an associate at the Rockefeller Institute and, in 1913, became an associate professor of medicine at Washington University. After studying neurology at Queens Square Hospital in London for one year, he returned to the United States as a professor of therapeutics at the Medical College of Virginia. At the end of World War I, he resumed practice in Winston-Salem, where he set up a clinical laboratory. When Duke University School of Medicine was organized in 1930,

Hanes accepted the professorship of neurology and became a professor of medicine in 1933.

Ralph A. Kinsella (M.D., St. Louis University, 1911)[11] received his house training at the St. Louis City Hospital (1911–14). His interest in infections, particularly the streptococcus, continued throughout his career. From 1914 to 1917 he published papers on hypersensitivity to streptococci, on rheumatic fever, and on endocarditis while working with Homer Fordyce Swift at the P & S. During World War I, he was involved with Evarts A. Graham in a study of empyema and, in 1919, became a professor of experimental medicine at St. Louis University. In 1921 he moved to Washington University as an associate professor of medicine and became acting director in 1922, after Dock's resignation. He held the latter position for two years before returning to St. Louis University as a professor of medicine (1924–53). He received the first federal grant ever awarded to the St. Louis University School of Medicine and developed the school's first full-time faculty. He produced an experimental model of infective endocarditis in dogs, which was used to study the routes of bacteria entering the blood stream and their deposition on injured heart valves.[12] In 1930 (with Omar Hagebush), he demonstrated the blocking effect of sodium salicylate on hypersensitivity to hemolytic streptococci. The Center for Experimental Medicine at St. Louis University is dedicated to him.

## The Full-time Plan

With the help of a grant from the General Education Board, the full-time plan was put into effect on July 1, 1916. Dock was professor of medicine. The venture received a temporary setback with the advent of World War I, because it was difficult in 1916–17 to find men suitably trained for academic positions. Some excellent appointments were made, however; that of Frank Wilson has already been mentioned. Alan M. Chesney[13] was called from the Hospital of the Rockefeller Institute to the full-time staff in medicine. Chesney later became dean of the Johns Hopkins University School of Medicine. There were excellent appointments in other departments.

Fred T. Murphy, the first professor of surgery, who had directed the organization of the base hospital that Barnes organized for overseas service in World War I, was not fully in sympathy with the full-time plan. An account of the appointment of Murphy's successor was given by Philip A. Shaffer:

> At that time, members of the staff of Base Hospital #21 from Washington University were also returning from France . . . Dr. Fred Murphy, chief surgeon of Base Hospital #21, was also professor of surgery in Washington University and head of that department. During his absence

the full-time system had been adopted for heads of the clinical departments. This plan displeased Murphy and led to his retirement.

In 1916, I had been drafted as dean . . . and, in that capacity, went to Chicago in search of a candidate for our department of medicine. My friend Dr. Rollin T. Woodyatt, whom I consulted, told me that if I had wanted a surgeon he could have named an excellent candidate. He cited the talents and accomplishments of Evarts A. Graham, who, however, had just accepted appointment to a clinic in Mason City, Iowa.

In 1917 . . . I received the resignation of Murphy as professor of surgery . . . I recalled the praise of Woodyatt and others of a young surgeon whose name I had forgotten. My files, however, disclosed it. Dr. Graham was located at Fort Sheridan and a committee was sent to confer with him as to his qualifications and interest in the position in St. Louis. He was invited to visit the school which he did on June 6 and 7, 1919. The corporation approved his appointment as professor of surgery effective July 1, 1919.[14]

## Evarts A. Graham as Professor of Surgery

After completing his studies at Princeton, Graham[15] pursued medicine at Rush Medical College, the first two years of the medical course being given at the University of Chicago. At Chicago, he was exposed to the inspiring teaching of A. J. Carlson, H. Gideon Wells, and R. R. Bensley. He received his M.D. degree in 1907 and interned at the Presbyterian Hospital in Chicago, where he came under the influence of Rollin T. Woodyatt. Woodyatt had just returned from a year of post-graduate study with Friedrich von Müller, an able chemist and a leading internist. Woodyatt developed in Chicago a scientific clinic patterned on that of von Müller's. He advised Graham to secure more training in chemistry.[16]

In 1918 Graham joined the army and became a member of the empyema commission. Methods were devised for closed drainage of these cavities without permitting air to enter and to collapse the lungs.

Graham's early research in St. Louis was concerned with the gall bladder. Peyton Rous and Phillip McMaster had demonstrated that the thin bile from the liver was stored in the gall bladder between meals and concentrated there by the absorption of water by the gall bladder mucosa. Abel and Rowntree had discovered that phenoltetrachlorphthalein was selectively removed from the blood by the liver and excreted in the bile. A similar compound, phenoltetrabromphthalein, was being used to test liver function. Graham speculated that if iodine, which was opaque to x-rays, could be substituted for the chlorine, the gall bladder could be visualized. He began work on animals, in collaboration with Warren Cole and Glover Copher. Although they were able to visualize the gall bladder in dogs, when they first administered the drug to patients with gallstones or suspected gallstones, no visualization occurred. Fortunately, they later gave the drug to patients without symptoms of gall-bladder disease and found that the gall bladder visualized perfectly. If the gall-bladder mucosa was normal, it concentrated the bile; the concentrated bile containing the drug was visualized by x-ray. When the gall-bladder wall was diseased and did not concentrate the bile, there was no visualization of the gall bladder.

Graham's department became one of the leading centers for thoracic surgery. At that time, removal of a lobe of the lung was occasionally done in patients with localized cancer. Graham was operating upon a fellow physician when exploration revealed that the cancer involved more than one lobe. He proceeded to remove the entire lung. The patient recovered and was cured of his disease. This operative triumph in 1933 electrified the surgical world.

## The Disciples of Evarts A. Graham

Barney Brooks (M.D., Johns Hopkins, 1911) interned under William Stewart Halsted. In 1912 he went to Washington University as a member of the surgical house staff. While there, he organized a surgical pathology laboratory and a course in surgical pathology, which served as a model for other institutions.

Brooks's best work in investigative surgery was concerned with regeneration of bone; intestinal obstruction; Volkmann's contracture; and arteriography. His studies in the growth, regeneration, and repair of bone established beyond question the fate of transplanted bone, and the value of the use of bone grafts in surgery was more fully realized.

Brooks pointed out that the presence or absence of strangulation, as well as the portion and length of intestine involved, influence the rate and degree of mucosal damage, which in turn determines the rapidity and amount of toxin absorbed.

In 1882 Richard von Volkmann described the paralysis and contracture of muscles that follows application of a constricting bandage to an extremity. In 1922 Brooks concluded that the cause was the increased tissue pressure that resulted from an open artery and an occluded vein.

In 1924 Brooks was the first to perform arteriography on patients, when he injected sodium iodide into the femoral artery. Until that time there had been no accurate means of determining the location and extent of arterial occlusion in the extremities of a living patient.

Robert Elman (M.D., Johns Hopkins, 1922)[17] remained at Johns Hopkins for one year and then spent two years at the Hospital of the Rockefeller Institute. He joined the faculty at Washington University in 1928 and became an associate professor in 1936. In that year, Elman was the first to demonstrate the serious deficit in serum protein resulting from extensive burns, providing the foundation for treatment by plasma administration. In 1937 he published his first article describing attempts to increase the blood proteins by the intravenous injection of amino acids. In 1945 he received the Samuel D. Gross Award for this work.

Elman was the first to show that a depletion of protein from the liver caused the structural changes that were formerly thought due only to loss of carbohydrate. Elman was also the first to test pancreatic function by estimating the amount of diastase in the blood. He made other important contributions to the development of our knowledge of water and electrolyte metabolism.

Men trained in Graham's department were called to head surgical departments elsewhere. Among these were Barney Brooks, to Vanderbilt; Edwin R. Schmidt, to Wisconsin; Alton J. Ochsner, to Tulane; and Edwin P. Leaman, to Virginia.

## David P. Barr as Professor of Medicine

During Kinsella's term as the acting head of the department of medicine, efforts to secure a permanent successor were difficult. The position was first offered to Eugene F. DuBois, who, on Lusk's advice, declined. The position was then offered to Woodyatt and Russell Wilder, both of whom also declined. Barr,[18] the next candidate, accepted the appointment in 1925. He had had only six years of preparation for this important academic post.

Barr (M.D., Cornell, 1914) interned for one year at Bellevue and then took a fellowship with DuBois. Using the calorimeter, Barr studied the chills produced by malaria (1917).

After World War I, when the new Second Medical Division team was organized at Bellevue under DuBois, John P. Peters and Barr worked together in the Loomis Laboratory.[19] It was altogether a successful year in Barr's development. He learned a great deal from Peters, including how to write papers. The difficulties of being in the field of academic medicine—with its demands in research, teaching, and patient care—are well brought out by Barr's experience:

> When I worked with Peters, the same situation occurred [referring to research stimulus when he worked with DuBois]. If you were going to do this work with Peters, do it well, get the most out of it, [the research] was really a full-time job so when I did get into the ward, or when I was studying for my class, it was an interruption of the other [the research]. That double pressure pursued me forever afterward and I've never gotten over it. I have always felt that if I spent as much time as I wanted to in the development of an idea [in research], I was neglecting something that was very dear to me and that was the care of people, and also, not only the care of people but learning about . . . disease so that I had that [double pressure] all the time, as early as from the time I went with DuBois. Before that I was a man who had a good deal of peace of mind. They are just two things that are quite different, very difficult to choose between.[20]

In 1920 Barr and Peters published three papers on the respiratory mechanism in cardiac dyspnea, and three the following year on the carbon-dioxide absorption curve and carbon-dioxide tension of the blood in normal resting individuals, in cardiac dyspnea, and in severe anemia.[21]

After Peters's departure, Barr worked with Harold E. Himwich, who later became a professor of physiology at the Albany Medical College. Their studies on the physiology of muscular exercise covered the following: the changes in acid-base equilibrium following short periods of vigorous muscular exercise; the comparison of arterial and venous blood following vigorous exercise; the development and duration of changes in acid-base equilibrium; blood reaction and breathing; and the oxygen relationships in the arterial blood. There were additional observations on the effect of exercise on diabetes, including changes in acid-base equilibrium and their relation to the accumulation of lactic acid and acetone, and another on lactic-acid formation in phlorhizin diabetes.[22]

From 1922 to 1924, Barr was deeply engrossed in his research. He wrote a short paper on the fallacy of considering the hydrogen-ion concentration as the only factor affecting the breathing rate. He submitted the paper to Van Slyke, the editor of the *Journal of Biological Chemistry,* who did not want to publish it, because it was heresy at that time. Everyone believed that pH made the respiratory center work. The paper was finally published in that journal, in its original form, and the theory turned out to be correct.[23] In 1924 the offer came to go to St. Louis.

## The Department of Medicine under Barr

Barr found the department very disorganized, but the school of medicine essentially healthy. Barr asked for four assistants to help him run the clinic. The provision for the department was inadequate, so that he was allowed one assistant, who would receive $8,000 annually. He eventually had two more assistants, one whose salary was $6,000, another whose salary was $5,000. That was the full-time department, and Barr had to depend heavily on part-time help.

Because he needed a man interested in bacteriology and immunology, Barr tried to recruit Harold L. Amoss from the HRI, but he was unsuccessful. Barr made an excellent move when he chose Harry L. Alexander, who was especially interested in clinical immunology and allergy and also had a good knowledge of clinical bacteriology.

Harry L. Alexander (M.D., Columbia, 1914)[24] spent two years on the medical service of the Presbyterian Hospital in New York City, where Warfield Theobald Longcope stimulated his interest in allergy.[25] Alexander then worked with Chandler Walker, another pioneer in the study of allergic disorders, at the Peter Bent Brigham Hospital. He returned to the Presbyterian Hospital as resident physician and later continued his research there. After World War I, he joined the department of medicine at Cornell, where he first met Barr.

Alexander's career at Washington University spanned forty-five years. He became a professor of medicine in 1934 and was acting chairman of the department during the year after Barr's departure for Cornell. He organized and directed the private medical service at Barnes Hospital and directed the activities of the allergy laboratory. He played a significant role in the emergence of allergy as a major branch of internal medicine and remained in the forefront of the discipline for over half a century. He contributed to the characterization of blocking antibody, to the definition of anaphylactic purpura as a clinical entity, to the understanding of bronchial asthma, and to the study of emphysema.[26]

Barr next tried to recruit Joseph T. Wearn, who declined. Barr then recruited Francis Smith, who later became head of the metabolism division of the Scripps Metabolic Clinic in California. Lawrence D. Thompson, one of Barr's students, accepted one of the full-time positions, and Barr took advantage of his tremendous capacity for work. Paul S. Barker took charge of cardiology, but later left to join Frank Wilson at Michigan.

A great difficulty for Barr was that the department of medicine had to run the hospital's routine clinical laboratories, for which activity it received no income. This had a very damaging effect on the development of the clinical departments, as recorded in a letter written on June 2, 1936, by Barr, Graham, and Shaffer to M. B. Clopton, President of the Corporation of Washington University.[27]

## Barr's Research in St. Louis

Barr's published papers during his tenure at Washington University deal for the most part with clinical subjects. There were a series of research papers in 1928 and 1929 on which Barr's name appeared. These included a paper on inhibition of lactic acid formation in muscle by extracts of desiccated pancreas; one on the inhibitory action of an extract of pancreas upon glycolysis of malignant tumors,[28] and another on the effect of pancreatic inhibitors on the glycolysis of muscle tissue and muscle extract.[29]

On November 23, 1928, Barr read a paper on hyperparathyroidism before the Central Society for Clinical Research; this paper was published in the *Journal of the American Medical Association* on March 23, 1929, with Harold Aten Bulger and Henry H. Dixon as coauthors. They stated that "in the literature on osteomalacia, on multiple cystic tumors of.bone and on parathyroid tumors, there is a clinical picture, found occasionally under all of these titles, which seems to deserve description as a separate clinical entity. The study of the case reported here first called our attention to this disease." A parathyroid adenoma was found and removed. This patient and two others were described by Bulger, Dixon, and Barr in a classical study that did much to make the disorder familiar to American physicians.[30]

At the end of Barr's paper in the *J.A.M.A.*, the following paragraph appeared: "The finding of the parathyroid tumor and the effects that followed its removal seemed to complete the chain of reasoning necessary to implicate the parathyroids in the causation of the symptoms. . . . With the assembling of all the evidence, *it seems justifiable to introduce the name of hyperparathyroidism* [my italics] and to consider under this heading the various cases as constituting a clinical entity as definite and distinct as parathyroid tetany or exophthalmic goiter." Thus the term *hyperparathyroidism* was first introduced by Barr.

Harold Aten Bulger (M.D., Harvard, 1920) served on the resident staff at the Peter Bent Brigham Hospital. From 1922 to 1925, he worked with John P. Peters. In 1926 Bulger moved to Washington University as an associate in medicine. His interest was in carbohydrates and electrolytes in health and disease.[31]

Barr's other contributions included clinical papers on multiple myeloma, thyrotoxicosis, myxedema, hemochromatosis, obesity, and disorders of the pituitary. When Barr returned to New York as a professor of medicine at Cornell, he published, in collaboration with Howard Eder and Ella Russ, a series of papers concerning the protein-lipid relationships in the plasma of normal individuals and those with atherosclerosis and diabetes mellitus. The abnormalities predictably associated with atherosclerotic disease were described, and the influence of estrogens, other hormones, and diet on the distribution of cholesterol between the heavy and light lipoproteins was noted. The importance of these findings was indicated by George V. Mann in 1977: "Measurement of the cholesterol in these dense 'alpha-lipoproteins' is several times more predictive for coronary artery disease than measurement of low-density lipoprotein. The irony is that in 1951 Barr, Russ and Eder made just such a proposal. They were ignored in the rush to the fashionable thinking about lipoproteins. We kept the bath water—threw out the baby."[32]

## The Department of Pediatrics

The department of pediatrics was organized in 1912 under John F. Howland; however, Howland left during that same year for Johns Hopkins. From 1912 until 1917, Borden Veeder was acting head of the department. In 1915 the St. Louis Children's Hospital moved to its new quarters on Kingshighway, and, for the first time, facilities for research became available.

In 1918 W. McKim Marriott became the director of the department.[33] At age fifteen, Marriott entered the University of North Carolina, where he majored in chemistry under Charles Baskerville. In 1904 he went with Baskerville to teach chemistry at the City College of New York. Soon afterward he became an assistant to C. G. L. Wolf in physiological chemistry at the Cornell University Medical School, where he spent six years assisting in laboratory instruction and attending enough classes to obtain his M.D. degree in 1910. He took no further clinical training.

In 1910 Marriott went to Washington University as an instructor in biochemistry. After Marriott taught for four years there, however, he wished to apply his biochemical knowledge to the direct study of clinical problems and therefore accepted an offer to become Howland's assistant in pediatrics at Johns Hopkins. He applied his biochemical knowledge to Howland's clinical problems and devised the technical methods that led to their joint work on acidosis in infancy (see chapter 8).

In a memorandum of April 21, 1917, a tentative plan for the organization of the department of pediatrics on a full-time basis had been outlined.[34] A professor was to receive a salary of $5,000; Borden Veeder, an associate professor who was not on full-time, but who was to continue his role of directing the department in Marriott's absence, a salary of $2,500; Philip Jeans, an associate professor, a salary of $2,500 to $3,000; and McCulloch, an instructor, a salary of $1,800. This totaled $17,620, leaving approximately $13,000, from which the following positions were to be filled by Marriott as soon as feasible: $2,500 for an associate in bacteriology; $2,000 for an instructor in chemistry; $3,000 for two assistants.

Scientific investigation became an important activity in pediatrics under Marriott. He attracted excellent men, many of whom later became professors of pediatrics.

Although Marriott made significant contributions while in St. Louis, his most important scientific work centered on the toxic condition in infancy known as *alimentary intoxication*. Marriott showed that it was not a result of food poisoning or of infection, but a syndrome brought about by a reduction in blood volume due to water loss.

Another contribution concerned infant feeding. For years, in line with the teaching of Thomas Morgan Rotch of Boston and L. Emmett Holt of New York, infant feeding in the United States had been dominated by the so-called "percentage method." This system, which was a complicated one involving mathematical formulas, was scientifically unsound. Marriott, with his uninhibited biochemical approach, introduced simplified procedures based on inexpensive evaporated milk and corn syrup. The *Marriott method* was a major factor in placing the artificial feeding of infants on a sound basis.[35]

In 1923 Marriott became dean and found administrative duties to his liking. As a result, his research interests waned. In 1936 he left St. Louis to become dean and professor of research medicine at the University of California Medical School in San Francisco. Soon after his arrival, he died at the age of fifty-one of a fatal streptococcal infection.

Marriott served as a stimulus to his successor at Washington University, Alexis Frank Hartmann.[36] Hartmann received his B.S. degree from Washington University in 1919. During his period in medical school, Hartmann was attracted by Marriott's work and entered pediatrics. This, combined with a still earlier stimulus from Shaffer, the professor of biochemistry, led to his winning the Gill Prize in Pediatrics in 1921. He received his pediatric training under Marriott while serving as an intern, an assistant resident, and a resident at the St. Louis Children's Hospital from 1921 to 1924. He rose to the rank of an associate professor in 1927 and succeeded Marriott in 1936.

Hartmann, along with James L. Gamble, Daniel C. Darrow, and Allan M. Butler, were the "extracellular fluid" pioneers. Hartmann's early publications revealed his primary interest in biochemistry and metabolism. He published four papers on chemical changes occurring in the body as the result of certain diseases, three of which were written in collaboration with Darrow. The three publications that brought Hartmann international fame appeared in 1932; their general theme was the metabolism of sodium racemic lactate.[37] Hartmann was among the first to stress the importance of alkali therapy in severe acidosis. He was also one of the first to show the difference in the effect of vomiting and diarrhea on the serum electrolyte pattern. The therapeutic approach he outlined, which stressed the concomitant need for restoration of body fluid volume and replenishment of other extracellular ions in addition to sodium, was widely adopted. The basic thrust of Hartmann's lactate-Ringer's solution was the need for more sodium than chloride in parenteral fluid solutions. So-called Hartmann's solution (lactate-Ringer's solution) became universally used. Hartmann's paper with Jaudon on neonatal hypoglycemia remains a classic. Hartmann was also well aware of the needless deaths of infants due to salicylate intoxication and stressed the value of alkali in treatment. It was Hartmann's enthusiastic search for an answer that led Carl and Gerty Cori into their classical studies of glucose-6-phosphate in glycogen storage disease.

In 1962 the section on pediatrics of the AMA conferred upon Hartmann the first Abraham Jacobi Award "in recognition of outstanding achievements in pediatrics." Among Hartmann's students were H. L. Barnett, M. R. Behrer, R. J. Blattner, M. J. Carson, Gilbert B. Forbes, and David Goldring.

# 14

## The Medical Institution of Yale College

After Ezra Stiles became president of Yale University in 1777, he outlined a program of medical education. The first step in this program was taken in 1806 when the Yale Corporation appointed a medical professor: Benjamin Silliman, trained in chemistry, anatomy, and midwifery by the medical professors of the University of Pennsylvania and the University of Edinburgh.[1]

In 1810 the Assembly of Connecticut incorporated the Medical Institution of Yale College under the joint auspices of the College and the State Medical Society. Silliman was named a professor of chemistry and pharmacology. Nathan Smith became a professor of the theory and practice of medicine, surgery, and obstetrics. The medical institution opened in 1813 and the New Haven Hospital in 1833.

A new charter, obtained from the legislature in 1879, allowed the faculty to determine the length of the term and the methods of instruction. The course of study was lengthened to three years, each year consisting of two terms of eighteen weeks each. Admission examinations were required. Physiology was separated from anatomy. In 1885 a plan of reorganization was instituted, and the faculty responded with a request for $400,000 to endow instruction in the rapidly expanding medical sciences.

In an address at Yale in 1888, William Henry Welch declared that medicine should always be regarded as a department of a university: "There must be a union in spirit as well as in name. . . . In no other direction could this university expand with greater promise of usefulness and of renown than in the line of liberal support of the highest and most scientific medical education. The decision of the corporation to accept the medical school as an integral part of the university is assurance that the future of the medical institution in the 20th century will be secure."[2]

In 1910 George Blumer was appointed a professor of medicine and dean.[3] At that time the school was at a low ebb; the faculty was made up largely of local physicians who volunteered their services. Although the period from 1910 to 1920 was one of unrest, and struggle for improvement in the face of inadequate resources, Blumer and a small group of colleagues held the school together. Notable among Blumer's achievements was the appointment of several individuals who would assume prominence in the years to come, including Samuel C. Harvey, Milton C. Winternitz, and Charles E. A. Winslow. Winternitz was made dean of the school in 1920.[4] With the strong support of James Roland Angell, who assumed the presidency of Yale in 1922, the school moved forward rapidly.

William Henry Welch is reputed to have stated that he knew of nothing in modern medical education so remarkable as "the recent transformation of the Yale School of Medicine from the old type into a modern medical school." Important were the Brady gift, which built the Brady Memorial Laboratory in 1917, and the Sterling gift, which led to the construction of the Sterling Hall of Medicine in 1923. Little could be accomplished in medical research until these facilities became available. A gift from the General Education Board of the Rockefeller Foundation made possible the inauguration of full-time appointments in clinical departments.

## The Leadership of Milton C. Winternitz

Hebbel E. Hoff has characterized the influence of Winternitz in Yale's development as follows:

> In the catbird seat, a vast office of almost Napoleonic splendor . . . , flanked by a series of devoted secretaries . . . was that pluperfect, prestissimo, grand master of all Deans, Milton Winternitz. Coming to Yale as Professor of Pathology, with an almost apocalyptic vision of what a great medical school ought to be and the energy and drive to accomplish its purposes, he had, virtually single-handed, devised a program for the new school's activities, planned its building, sought and obtained the support of the Rockefeller Foundation and enlisted the faculty . . . Winternitz had the concept of a . . . medical center that would offer exemplary medical care in an atmosphere of scholarship and investigation, with a full and free flow of ideas in an unbroken self sustaining loop of laboratory, bedside studies, practice and teaching.[5]

Winternitz retired as dean in 1935 and was succeeded by Stanhope Bayne-Jones,[6] a 1910 graduate of Yale College, who had joined the faculty as a professor of bacteriology in 1932. Both of these men were graduates of the Johns Hopkins University School of Medicine and received their early postgraduate training there. Bayne-Jones was succeeded as dean by C. N. H. Long, then a professor of physiological chemistry, who was responsible for reassembling a strong faculty and restoring operations to an even keel during the postwar years.

## The Department of Medicine

### Francis Gilman Blake

An important step taken by Winternitz was the recruitment of Blake[7] as professor of medicine. Blake spent seven years at the Harvard Medical School and the Peter Bent Brigham Hospital, where he became a resident in medicine. He joined the staff of the HRI in 1919, after wartime service at the Army Medical School. While at the Rockefeller Hospital, he and James D. Trask placed the nasopharyngeal secretions of a patient with measles directly into the trachea of monkeys. The animals developed typical measles; by first passing the secretions through a bacteria-retaining filter, Blake and Trask proved that measles was a viral infection.

When Blake went to New Haven, a number of medical schools were establishing full-time clinical faculties. At Yale the experiment worked from the start. Blake recruited men of unusual talent, including William C. Stadie and John P. Peters, to develop the metabolic field; H. M. Marvin, to head cardiology;[8] and his own associate Trask. He was effective in raising money for their researches and leaving them alone to pursue their own interests.

Blake turned his attention to several special research projects: first, the application to clinical medicine of Dochez's discovery that certain strains of hemolytic streptococci produce an exotoxin and at times a demonstrable toxemia that could be treated successfully by scarlatinal antitoxin; second, the possible use of pneumothorax in the treatment of acute pneumonia; and third, the use of chemotherapeutic agents and antibiotics. During World War II, as president of the Army Epidemiological Board, Blake accompanied a team of investigators to New Guinea to study scrub typhus. He was a primary mover in the organization and director of the Army Epidemiological Board, which was established in 1941.

### John Punnett Peters

It was at the HRI that Peters[9] met Blake, Trask, and Stadie. It was a return home for Peters when, in 1922, he became an associate professor of medicine at Yale. He had entered Yale College at the age of sixteen, graduating in 1908 with a B.A. degree. He received his M.D. degree at the College of Physicians and Surgeons in 1913. After two years of internship, he was a Coolidge Fellow in Clinical Medicine under Longcope and Rawle Geyelin. From 1919 to 1920, Peters was a fellow at the Russell Sage Institute of Pathology. The following year, while at the

Hospital of the Rockefeller Institute, he accepted an appointment at Vanderbilt University School of Medicine as an associate professor of medicine. While Peters was waiting for the reorganization of the school in Nashville, the offer came from Blake.

At Yale, Peters made important contributions to various diseases of metabolism; electrolyte and acid-base equilibrium; nephritis and water exchange; the interrelation of proteins, carbohydrates, and lipids in metabolism; and the role of the thyroid in health and disease. Although Peters emphasized clinical studies, his investigative work was based on a profound knowledge of physical chemistry and biochemistry. He represented the modern approach of medicine in the study of disease, an approach in which signs and symptoms are regarded as aberrations of normal biochemical processes. This concept of medicine, so universally accepted today, had its beginnings at the end of the World War I, when an enlightened group of young clinicians saw and applied the work of such men as Van Slyke, Folin, and Benedict to the problems of the clinic. Peters and the young men that he trained made a major contribution to this development. They devised new methods, such as those for the determination of the bases in body fluid and for the microdetermination of iodine, that became standard for such analyses.[10]

Peters had conservative views on the use of these new tools in practice. He insisted that they be employed only by those who clearly understood the physics and chemistry involved. His views on this were well summarized in an address he gave to the New York Academy of Medicine in 1934.[11]

The list of Peters's trainees is impressive: H. A. Bulger, A. J. Eisenman, Evelyn B. Man, David M. Kydd, Paul Lavietes, Alexander Winkler, Theodore S. Danowski, Joseph R. Elkinton, Belton A. Burrows, Philip Bondy, Louis G. Welt, Donald Seldin, and Maurice B. Strauss, among others. Winkler, whose premature death deprived medicine of one of its best minds, and clinical chemistry of one of its most productive exponents, remained at Yale, as did Gerald Klatskin and Lavietes.[12]

Medicine was almost two departments at Yale, held together by the pride and permissiveness of its chairman, Blake; and by the fundamental loyalty of its most distinguished member, Peters. Together they made the department one of the truly great centers for medicine in the United States.

## John R. Paul

John R. Paul[13] headed "clinical epidemiology" as a division of the department of medicine. He related how he entered this area of medicine:

> This fervent interest started when as a second year medical student, I was privileged to attend a session of the Federation of Biological Sciences [1916]. . . .

I ... was certainly engrossed in ... hearing ... these great men, who were engaged in recounting their efforts to attempt to solve the problem of epidemic poliomyelitis, applying the very weapons which we had been taught to use in our first years at medical school.

As a rapt listener, the idea first dawned on me that the religion of the true physician was incomplete without having the concept of prevention thoroughly engrained in him. My immature reasoning, which I never lost, was that, together with attempts to cure this pestilence, there should be attempts to control it, and this should be done by clinicians who knew the disease best.[14]

In 1938 Paul spoke as follows:

The term, clinical investigation in preventive medicine is cumbersome and so I will not use it. ... It presupposes the existence of a so-called sister science in curative medicine. ... Clinical investigation in epidemiology is better for the purposes at hand; clinical epidemiology is best, and really what I mean ... it is a science concerned with circumstances, whether they are "functional" or "organic" under which human disease is prone to develop. It is a science concerned with the ecology of human disease. It must face the question of "why" as well as "how." The clinical epidemiologist starts with a sick individual and cautiously branches out into the setting where that individual became sick ... to analyze the intimate details under which this patient became ill ... to search for other members of the patient's family, or community group who are actually or potentially ill ... to thus place his patient in the pattern in which he belongs, rather than to regard him as a lone sick man who has suddenly popped out of a healthy setting. ... It is also his aim to bring his judgment to bear upon the situation, as well as on the patient.[15]

Paul accepted the title "professor of preventive medicine" in 1940, under the condition preventive medicine would be a section in the department of medicine, rather than an independent department. Its activities were directed toward the epidemiology of disease in the family, in the local community, and in factories; attention was also paid to clinical and environmental virology, including the role of insects and animals as vectors of human disease. Thus, throughout his career, Paul held a conviction that "clinical medicine means more than the practice of the techniques of diagnosis and therapeutics."

From the work of Blake and Trask on scarlet fever, various lines of research developed in which Paul was involved; one on the epidemiology of rheumatic fever was begun before the role of the hemolytic streptococcus was appreciated. On the basis of the way in which rheumatic fever spread through families, it was concluded that respiratory infection of some kind precipitated the acute attack.[16]

In 1929 it was reported that agglutinins to sheep cells were present in  cases of serum sickness. These results were quickly confirmed at Yale. Control sera from individuals suffering from a variety of other clinical conditions were examined. It was discovered that antibodies capable of agglutinating sheep cells were present in the serum of patients with infectious mononucleosis. Thus, discovery of the Paul-Bunnell test for infectious mononucleosis is an example of serendipity, which Greene paraphrased as "the finding of the farmer's daughter while searching for a needle in the haystack."[17]

## Part-time Clinical Scientist: Louis H. Nahum

In the early 1930s, Hebbel E. Hoff returned to Yale to work in Fulton's new laboratory of physiology. While at Oxford, Hoff studied the pacemaker of the heart. At Fulton's weekly seminars in physiology, Hoff was struck with Louis H. Nahum's[18] acquaintance with the work of Sidney Ringer. He soon learned that Ringer and Nahum had much in common; each earned his living in private practice and, despite its demands, worked regularly in the laboratory. Nahum was familiar with Hope's work on heart sounds. Sir Thomas Lewis was one of the stars in his scientific firmament. He recognized that Lewis had missed a major value of the electrocardiogram by not paying more attention to the S-T segment and the T waves. Hoff and Nahum soon began restoring to function an archaic Hindle electrocardiograph. Static electricity was much in evidence, and, at more than one crucial point, the string was attracted to the lens and stuck there. Nahum was adept, however, at plucking a hair from his head, attaching it to a splint in a toothpick, and gently encouraging the string (a quartz thread some 6 $\mu$ in diameter) to "leave the lens and return to duty." Nahum and Hoff used acetyl beta-methyl choline in a number of studies on ventricular fibrillation after electric shock. They soon became aware of its action in atrial fibrillation, converting flutter to fibrillation, and arresting atrial tachycardia. They correlated Lord Adrian's supranormal period in the frog's heart with the U-wave in the mammalian heart. They also produced S-T segment displacements by superficial application of potassium chloride, and they adapted this technique to mapping out the representation of the cardiac surface in the limb leads.

Nahum's experience as a cardiologist brought new ways of viewing old problems. Nahum was, in essence, modeled after Samuel James Meltzer. He had a wide circle of friends in medicine, law, business, and politics, and moved freely between town and gown, playing an important part in reducing tensions. He was effective in interpreting the importance of experimental medicine to the practitioners of the art.

## The Department of Pediatrics

### Edwards A. Park

Winternitz again chose well when he selected Edwards A. Park as the first chairman of the newly created full-time department of pediatrics in 1921.[19] Funds were allocated for a small full-time staff, a modest new laboratory and office building, and the conversion of an attic into a ward for general pediatric patients. With funds given by the General Education Board, a research laboratory building was erected. Laboratories for biological and chemical research occupied the entire ground floor.

The 12 o'clock rounds were a high point in the development of the spirit of this department. One of the interns of those early days, Daniel C. Darrow, described them:

> To an intern, Park presented the picture of the scholar rather than the practitioner as a professor of pediatrics. He always wanted to know first what students of the disease under discussion had written. Second, he wanted to know how observation of the patient could advance the knowledge of disease.... I believe we all got the feeling that each patient presented an opportunity to learn from the literature and, if we were smart enough, from planned observations of the patient or in laboratory experiments. The highlight of Park's service to pediatrics while at Yale lay in the fine quality not only of the scientific study of disease but in the emphasis on the broad implications, social relationships and public health correlations of child care.[20]

The department of pediatrics at Yale under Park was research-oriented at all times. The written evidence, revealed in the bibliography covering the six years Park spent at Yale, is of pathological studies of experimental and human rickets; chemical studies of electrolyte disturbances in rickets and other diseases; clinical studies; and projects relevant to the social and public health aspects of pediatrics. Park's special interest was on the effects of radiant energy, cod liver oil, and bile on rickets in infants and in experimental animals. The major studies in electrolyte metabolism, led by Alfred T. Shohl, dealt with hydrogen ion concentration of gastric and intestinal secretions in various clinical conditions and electrolyte disturbances in infantile and experimental rickets and tetany.

An outstanding contribution to public health was a three-year project undertaken in cooperation with the New Haven Health Department and the Visiting Nurse Association, with the support and sponsorship of the Children's Bureau of the U.S. Department of Labor. The purpose was to demonstrate whether or not infantile rickets was an eradicable disease. The study provided a positive answer at a time when rickets was rampant in babies living in northern latitudes.

Park was a vigorous proponent of women in medicine, and his first resident was Martha Eliot. During his tenure at Yale, some thirty to forty women physicians worked full-time in one capacity or another in his department. Most of them achieved positions of leadership in some aspect of the broad domain of child health.

## Grover Powers

In 1927 Edwards A. Park became a professor of pediatrics at Johns Hopkins. He was succeeded by another of Howland's pupils, Grover

Powers, who came from Baltimore with Park in 1921.[21] Powers had graduated from Johns Hopkins in 1913 and received his residency training there. Although Powers made substantial contributions to scientific problems in pediatrics, these appear as almost incidental by-products of the care of sick children and were often not published. Under Park and Powers, a department was organized that emphasized care of the patient, training of students and house staff, and research in the laboratory and on the wards, in an effective combination.

Powers's great contribution was his ability to solve clinical problems and to suggest suitable fields of research to his associates, who had skills he did not possess. He published a simple, straight-forward analysis of the principles of infant feeding, and, from clinical observations, he established a successful regimen for the care of premature infants. At the suggestion of Lafayette B. Mendel, he administered liver extract as a source of possible unidentified vitamins in celiac disease; but these observations, presented before the New England Pediatric Society, were never published. In 1926 Powers did publish a description of his comprehensive plan for the treatment of infantile diarrhea.

Powers persuaded Trask[22] to leave adult medicine and take charge of infectious diseases in the department of pediatrics. He and Powers gave the description of age and previous infections as the explanation of the different manifestations of streptococcal infections.

Powers also had an influence on chemical research. A series of papers on the physiological disturbances in diphtheria by Herman Yannet and Darrow arose from Powers's statement that glucose was sometimes beneficial in toxic cases.[23] The studies that the group did on deficit of extracellular electrolytes grew out of his asking Darrow why hypodermoclyses of 5 percent solutions of glucose were irritating and often made children sick. Yannet and Darrow were surprised at the magnitude of the physiological disturbances produced by intraperitoneal injections of isotonic solutions of glucose.[24] Harrison's paper on the nitrogen and calcium balances of infants fed condensed milk was undertaken because Powers felt that, contrary to current reasoning, the protein intake of this food was inadequate. A paper on acidosis produced by protein milk followed his statement that he did not understand why protein milk was not tolerated by young infants. Thus, Powers carried on in the Park tradition and presided over a pediatric department that made many excellent contributions to the development of clinical science.

## Research in Metabolic Disease

Research in metabolic diseases was led by Daniel C. Darrow.[25] Among his important coworkers were Herman Yannet, Edward Pratt, Harold E. Harrison, and Robert E. Cooke. In 1916 Darrow graduated from Cornell University and in 1920 from the Johns Hopkins University Medical School. It was at Johns Hopkins that Darrow received his initiation into the experimental field of which he was later to become a master—that of electrolytes and acid base physiology. In 1922 he became a pediatric intern under Park and Powers. During the following two years (1923–25), he was an assistant resident and a resident on the pediatric service of Thomas Buckman at the Boston City Hospital. The next three years were spent as an instructor in pediatrics, under Marriott and Hartmann, at Washington University Medical School, where he developed a keen interest in the problems of dehydration and acute streptococcal infections in children.

In 1928 Darrow returned to Yale, where he spent the next twenty-five years. It was Darrow who put intracellular fluid and its principal cation, potassium, on the medical map. What Marriott and Hartmann had done in emphasizing the importance in disease of plasma volume and extracellular acidosis and what Gamble and Butler had done for extracellular fluid, Darrow and his associates did for water and electrolytes inside the body cells. Darrow used two main investigative techniques, balance studies and the direct analysis of tissue—especially skeletal muscle—for its electrolyte and water content. In 1935 Darrow and Yannet demonstrated, by injections of solutions of dextrose and water into the peritoneal cavity of dogs, and subsequent withdrawal after electrolyte equilibration, that water shifted into cells when the extracellular electrolyte concentration was lowered. In 1942, with Miller, he showed the potassium depletion of muscle resulting experimentally from low potassium diets and desoxycorticosterone administration and clinically in patients from adrenocortical insufficiency. In 1945 he published his classic review in the *New England Journal of Medicine* on body fluid physiology.[26]

In 1945 Darrow studied a case that was most important for his subsequent research. A very young child had congenital alkalosis due to chloride-wasting diarrhea. By balance measurements, he demonstrated that the extracellular chloride deficit and bicarbonate excess were associated with a loss of potasssium and a gain of sodium in the intracellular phase of the body fluid.[27] From this study stemmed the investigations that led to two of his greatest scientific achievements: the life-saving use of potassium-containing infusions in patients suffering from potassium depletion, especially infants with diarrhea; and elucidation of the intimate relationship between extracellular acid-base equilibrium and ionic composition of body fluid. In the summer of 1945 Darrow, treating infants with diarrhea at Johns Hopkins, showed that the administration of potassium chloride produced a dramatic fall in mortality rate. Potassium therapy was here to stay, and Darrow's solution became known the world over.[28]

## Poliomyelitis

In 1931 there was a severe epidemic of poliomyelitis in Connecticut. Since Yale had the only research unit in the state with experience in the clinical investigation of virus diseases, the problem fell to Blake and Trask. At that time, however, they were poorly prepared to handle virus research. When it appeared that the epidemic would last for some time, the Yale Poliomyelitis Commission was created, under the direction of Trask, with the first objective of isolating the virus from acutely ill patients. When a deluge of minor illnesses struck Connecticut at the height of the 1931 epidemic, most physicians would not believe they were examples of "abortive" poliomyelitis. The studies of the Yale unit during the summer of 1931 revealed that out of twelve oropharyngeal washings obtained from children who were in the early and midstages of suspected "abortive" poliomyelitis, two yielded polio virus. These experiments reestablished the fact that a poliomyelitis epidemic is not restricted to the diagnosed and officially reported cases, but that actual infections far exceed this number.[29]

## Influence of the Department

One can see the breadth of Park and Powers's influence by examining a survey of the subsequent activities of the members of the department of pediatrics at Yale from 1921 to 1951. As of 1952, seventeen had become full professors of pediatrics, and one each professors of bacteriology, psychiatry, and physiology. Of these twenty, sixteen took all or part of their resident training at Yale and four were fellows. Twenty became senior members of medical faculties—associate professors devoted to full- or part-time teaching and research—and two became deans of medical schools. A former resident became head of the Children's Bureau, and at least five former residents were directors of important institutions that were engaged in research or specialized pediatric service, but not associated with universities.

# 15

# The Vanderbilt University School of Medicine

The Flexner Report of 1910[1] led to the closing of more than half of the existing medical schools and the reorganization of the remaining schools to an acceptable standard. Generally, the factor that determined whether to close or reorganize a school was its underlying strength; its background, tradition, existing support, ideals and concepts, and, above all, the foresight, vision, determination, and dedication of one or more of its leaders. Vanderbilt was fortunate in that Chancellor James H. Kirkland had an interest in medical education.[2] Vanderbilt had already undergone two reorganizations, each of which was a step in the direction of excellence. This background attracted the Rockefeller, Carnegie, and other foundations to Vanderbilt as the site for the development of a modern medical school in the mid-South. Important was a plan of medical education that included a core of full-time faculty in the clinical subjects. By 1920 sufficient funds were at hand, and George Canby Robinson, then at Washington University Medical School in St. Louis, was selected as the new dean and professor of medicine.[3]

## Reorganization under Robinson

George Canby Robinson (M.D., Johns Hopkins, 1903) spent two years in pathology at the Pennsylvania Hospital. He served as a resident physician there for a similar period, after which he studied physiology in Europe and attended Friedrich von Müller's teaching exercises in Munich.[4]

Robinson was Rufus I. Cole's resident physician when the HRI opened in 1910. He remained there for three years and then accepted a position as an associate professor in medicine at Washington University, where he played a major role in organizing the department of medicine (see chapter 13).

From 1922 to 1928, Robinson's efforts were focused on the Vanderbilt University School of Medicine. A hospital had to be built, a staff assembled, and the curriculum revitalized. In order to carry out the modernization, the General Education Board contributed $4 million to Vanderbilt University in 1919. All members of the faculty resigned in order to make possible a complete reorganization of the teaching staff. It was soon evident that the medical school should be on the campus of the university, and, to provide the necessary funds, the Carnegie Foundation and the General Education Board each contributed $1.5 million. In 1921, the sum of $8 million was available for the new school.

Robinson proposed a bolder, more far-reaching, and more expensive plan than anticipated. It involved the transfer of the school to the west campus and the abandonment of buildings on the south campus, including an uncompleted new hospital, and the provision for a new university hospital that would be an integral part of the medical building. The distinctive features were the unitary construction of medical school and hospital with departments, wards, outpatient facilities, a library, and administration space, all designed from a functional point of view. The library was placed as centrally as possible. The preclinical departments of biochemistry, physiology, and pharmacology connected directly with the medical wards on two floors; the offices for the full-time staff in medicine were located in between. Those of anatomy and pathology had the same relation to the surgical wards. Bacteriology, now considered microbiology, was a division of pathology, and pediatrics was a division of medicine. With its clinical laboratories under the charge of the related department heads; the latest equipment; many innovations in the various service areas; an adequate operating room suite; and animal quarters on the top floor, the hospital provided a facility commensurate with the aims and plans of the new school.[5] Plans similar to those of the new Vanderbilt medical school were drawn up independently for the new medical school of the University of Rochester.

A new feature was the provision of facilities for research in the clinical departments, so that investigation related to patients could be closely correlated with the preclinical departments. In order to foster research that would not be confined to a single department, thought was given to correlating the teaching and research of the laboratory and clinical departments. Thus, in the department of medicine, a laboratory of clinical bacteriology adjoined the department of bacteriology; laboratories of medical chemistry and physiology led into the departments of biochemistry, pharmacology, and physiology; and the surgery laboratory was next to the departments of anatomy and pathology. These special arrangements were intended to break down barriers between departments, so that the influence of the medical sciences would be felt constantly by the clinical staff and students and that the knowledge and training gained in the laboratories would be carried into medical practice. This arrangement also served to keep laboratory teachers aware that the ultimate aim of medical education was the application of their sciences to the practice of medicine.

## The New Faculty

By the fall of 1924 the following new professors had been apointed: anatomy, R. Sydney Cunningham; biochemistry, Glenn Cullen; pathology, Ernest Goodpasture;[6] preventive medicine, Waller S. Leathers; and, as associate professors: C. Sidney Burwell and Hugh J. Morgan in medicine; James M. Neill in bacteriology; and Horton R. Casparis in pediatrics. Cunningham had been an associate professor at Johns Hopkins, where he had worked with Florence Sabin. Cullen, who had been associated for some years with Donald D. Van Slyke in the HRI—where he had developed a special interest in the biochemical problems related to disease—had recently been appointed an associate professor of research medicine at the University of Pennsylvania. Goodpasture had been on the faculties of Johns Hopkins and Harvard and had served as a professor of pathology in Manila and then as director of the Singer Memorial Laboratory in Pittsburgh.

C. Sidney Burwell[7] graduated from the Harvard Medical School and interned at the MGH. As a research fellow with Paul Dudley White, he developed a continuing interest in diseases of the heart and circulation. In 1921 he was chief resident in medicine at Johns Hopkins while Robinson was professor of medicine pro-tempore. He remained at Johns Hopkins, where he continued his research with Francis Dieuaide and Robinson, and in 1923 became interested in new methods of determining cardiac output.[8] He was recruited by the Vanderbilt medical school and spent 1924 in Europe observing teaching and research programs.

In 1925 he began his ten-year association with the Vanderbilt medical school; from 1928 to 1935 he served as professor of medicine and head of the department. Here he introduced medical students to the concept of physiological response of the host to disease, in contrast to the old-time nosological teaching methods. He also pursued avidly the study of diseases from the point of view of physiological alterations; his researches being primarily directed toward the circulatory diseases and the adjustments of the circulation during pregnancy.[9]

In 1935 Burwell returned to Harvard as dean and professor of research medicine. He was visiting physician at the Boston Lying-In Hospital, where his interest in heart disease and pregnancy culminated in a book cowritten with James Metcalfe. In 1955 he became the first Samuel A. Levine Professor of Medicine.

Hugh J. Morgan, a Johns Hopkins graduate (1918), had his residency training at the Johns Hopkins Hospital. He then joined the staff of the

HRI (1919–21), where he worked in infectious disease with Avery.[10] Neill had also served at the Rockefeller in bacteriology under Avery. Casparis was a member of Howland's pediatric department at Johns Hopkins. Again one can see the benefits of these centers in supplying excellent scientists and clinicians to new or reorganizing medical schools.

During 1924, Barney Brooks, a Johns Hopkins graduate, was brought from Evarts A. Graham's department in Washington University (see chapter 13) as a professor of surgery. Paul D. Lampson, who had been an associate professor of pharmacology at Johns Hopkins under John J. Abel, was called to fill that chair. Walter E. Garrey, who had worked with Joseph Erlanger, was made a professor of physiology.

Barney Brooks soon recruited Isaac Bigger from Virginia, and Beverly Douglas (a native of Nashville) from Yale. Two years after the school opened, John B. Youmans,[11] who did outstanding research in the field of nutrition, became the director of the outpatient service. Youmans recruited Rudolph Kampmeier, then at Louisiana State, who had been a colleague at Michigan.

The research laboratories of the medical department consisted of the physiological division, under Burwell; the infectious disease division, under Morgan; and the chemical division, under Harrison. Each assistant resident physician worked half-time in one of these laboratories.

## The Early Residents in Medicine and Surgery

In 1925 two important additions were made to the faculty, which illustrate how clinical science was evolving. Tinsley R. Harrison[12] was appointed as resident physician and Alfred Blalock as resident surgeon. Blalock and Harrison worked closely together, and Blalock's contributions to the pathogenesis of shock were outstanding, as were those of Harrison relating to cardiac function and heart failure.

### Tinsley R. Harrison

At an early age, Harrison graduated from the University of Michigan with an A.B. degree and a year's advanced study in medicine. He joined the class of 1922 at Johns Hopkins. After graduation he spent two years at the Peter Bent Brigham Hospital, where he had close contact with Samuel A. Levine, William Dock, Samuel Grant, Henry A. Christian, and others.

One of the men who stimulated Harrison to do research was Samuel Grant, a young physician who had developed his investigative interest while a medical student,[13] and who as a house officer at the Brigham showed that insulin restored to the body tissues the power to burn glucose.[14] When Grant left Boston, Harrison moved into the laboratory that the former had developed for the study of blood flow by the Fick method. Harrison, in collaboration with William Dock, measured blood flow in rabbits with arteriovenous fistulae and artificial pneumothorax.[15]

After two years in Boston, Harrison returned to Baltimore as an assistant resident physician. Here he worked with Alfred Blalock, William Resnick, George Canby Robinson, and C. Sidney Burwell. The research started in Boston continued, and the cardiac output in dogs with pneumonia and other conditions such as anemia, hemorrhage, and thyroidectomy was studied. The following year, Harrison moved to Nashville. Here he achieved his full potential and advanced to the forefront as a leader in clinical investigation. The results of his research were published in many scientific papers and in his book, *Failure of the Circulation,* which is a classic in its field.[16]

After sixteen productive years at Vanderbilt, Harrison became the first professor of medicine at the new four-year medical school at Bowman-Gray. Harrison by this time had developed his own ideas about establishing a medical school along university patterns rather than in the traditional way. He recognized the need for breaking down sterile departmentalization and emphasized the interdependence of thought, ideas, and institutions.[17] Although his experience at Winston-Salem was short, he had a tremendous impact on the development of the school. As a professor of medicine, his ideas attracted considerable attention, and soon he was invited to become the first dean of the newly established Southwestern Medical School. He succeeded in establishing sound ideals in this school, which has become one of the outstanding institutions in the United States. After two years as dean, he devoted his full attention to the department of medicine.

Harrison—cosmopolitan teacher, investigator, author, and physician— returned home to Alabama after thirty-five years at these various institutions. During the ensuing years he had a great influence on the evolution of the medical school of the University of Alabama as a major U.S. institution.

## Harrison and Blalock[18]

In the annals of clinical investigation there is no more outstanding example of effective mutual stimulation toward success than that between Alfred Blalock, surgeon, and Tinsley R. Harrison, internist. In 1918 Blalock entered the freshman class of the Johns Hopkins University School of Medicine. The following year, Harrison transferred to Johns Hopkins. Tennis was his hobby, and he had played on the University of Michigan tennis team. One or two days before classes started in Baltimore in September 1919, on the tennis courts he encountered another southern country boy whose "Georgia accent could be cut with a knife." There is no record of who won their match, but it was close. The two men became close friends and roomed together their remaining three years in Baltimore. After graduation Harrison joined the house staff at the Peter Bent Brigham Hospital, while Blalock, disappointed at not receiving an internship on Halsted's surgical service, accepted one in urology at Hopkins.

When Harrison returned to Baltimore after two years in Boston he and Blalock renewed their friendship and their tennis rivalry, and decided to do research together. They measured cardiac output in dogs, studying the effects of drugs and various other factors.[19] The following summer, they left for Vanderbilt on the same day to join the resident staff there and, sixteen years later, left Nashville on the same day. When the Nashville City Tennis Championships were played in September 1926, Blalock and Harrison won the doubles and played the singles finals against each other.

Blalock developed tuberculosis in 1927 and Harrison accompanied him to Saranac Lake. On the day they left for the sanatorium together, Blalock realized that there would be no more tennis for him, and Harrison hung up his racket and did not play again. Blalock remained in Trudeau's Sanatorium for a year and then spent a few months in the department of physiology in Cambridge, England, working under the direction of G. V. Anrep and Sir Joseph Barcroft.

In the *Review of Surgery* for July 1964, Blalock recalled his work on shock as follows:[20]

> On my return to Vanderbilt [after his year with tuberculosis] in the latter part of 1928 some studies were performed with the aid of Hubert Bradburn in which the oxygen content of blood withdrawn from veins in various parts of the body was determined in shock produced by several different methods including the injection of histamine and trauma to an extremity. The difference in the oxygen content from the various areas sampled led to the following statement: "These observations suggest a local accumulation of blood at the site of trauma to a large area such as the intestinal tract or an extremity, and are evidence against the action of a histamine-like substance that produces a general bodily effect." The prevailing theory at the time was that traumatic shock was due to a toxin, possibly histamine. The strongest evidence that had been put forward in favor of the toxic theory was derived from the experiments of Cannon and Bayliss, in which they concluded that shock resulting from trauma to the extremity of the cat could not be accounted for on the basis of the local loss of whole blood and plasma. In brief they traumatized one posterior extremity and, when shock resulted, they amputated the two posterior extremities and determined the difference in weights. After completing the studies on blood gases, I repeated the experiments of Cannon and Bayliss using anesthetized dogs. Shock was produced by trauma in the experiments of the same duration as those of Cannon and Bayliss. It was noted that the swelling extended to a higher level than the upper most limit of the trauma and suggested that they had not performed their amputations at a sufficiently high level. In my experiments the posterior part of the animal was bisected and the difference in the weights of the traumatized and non-traumatized parts was determined. A comparison of this dif-

ference with the results of other experiments in which shock was produced by the slow withdrawal of blood showed that the trauma produced a sufficient loss of whole blood and plasma to explain the development of shock. In my paper published in 1930 entitled "Experimental Shock: The Cause of the Low Blood Pressure Produced by Muscle Injury"[21] it was stated: "The experiments which are presented in this paper offer no evidence that trauma to an extremity produced a toxin that caused a general dilatation of the capillaries with an increase in capillary permeability and a general loss of fluid from the bloodstream. These and many other experiments . . . removed most of the support from the toxic theory and played a significant role in the more copious use of whole blood and plasma in the treatment of various forms of trauma and burns."

Harrison recalled Blalock's hospitalization at Saranac as follows:

In the meantime he had completed his work on hemorrhagic shock and it was in process of publication. He had already finished his initial studies on traumatic shock but had not written the paper. When he bemoaned that it would be at least two years before the doctors would let him write it I asked him where the data were. He told me and I volunteered to write the paper. He told me where the data (all completed) were and he handed me the keys to his desk. He insisted that my name go on it too. I refused. We argued for an hour or more about it, but I was adamant. During a friendship of almost half a century this was the only strong quarrel we ever had. The featherweight (Harrison) won that. Al always gave me more credit than I deserved. He never spoke of the other side of the picture. After about three years of joint work, first as undergraduates and later as assistant residents, we had decided to split up and work independently but still to advise each other and to continue to visit each other's laboratories frequently. He decided to work on peripheral circulatory failure or surgical shock and I on heart failure which is only occasionally—the cardiogenic type—a major problem in shock. I had previously found indirect evidence that heart failure of the usual type is mainly due to elevated pressure, within the cardiac chambers, the veins and the capillaries rather than to altered blood flow. I call this "elevated intracardiac pressure" rather than using the more eloquent term, since then introduced by Harold Dodge, "diminished ejection fraction."

It was Blalock's observations on dogs with peripheral circulatory failure that confirmed my own, as yet incomplete, evidence that severe dyspnea was absent in dogs with very reduced cardiac output. Such dogs exhibited impaired alertness, tachycardia, postural hypotension, decline in urine volume, etc.—but they were not severely dyspneic.

In 1940 Dean Lewis retired as a professor of surgery at Johns Hopkins, and Blalock was selected as his successor. Blalock was then interested in the surgical treatment of hypertension, vascular surgery, pulmonary physiology, and shock. He did pioneer work in the field of congenital heart disease, an effort in which Edwards A. Park and Helen Taussig played a major role. In 1944 Blalock and Park described the surgical treatment of experimental coarctation (atresia) of the aorta.

Later, Blalock anastomosed the subclavian artery to bypass an atresia of the pulmonary artery.[22] This and his operation on closure of the patent ductus arteriosus, which had already been described by Gross, were classical contributions to the field of heart surgery, which has had a logarithmic growth since that time.

Among Harrison's collaborators in Nashville who also worked with Blalock was Morton Mason, who worked on the biochemical aspects of the problems under study. Mason later moved to Southwestern Medical School in Dallas when Harrison became a professor of medicine there.

During Harrison's last eight years in Nashville, John Williams joined him in studies on hypertension and various aspects of renal pathophysiology. Williams accompanied Harrison to the Bowman-Gray School of Medicine.

After Harrison's departure, George Meneely came to Vanderbilt from Rochester, New York. He became involved with John B. Youmans in studies on the relationship of sodium chloride to hypertension.

The second resident physician was John S. Lawrence, a University of Virginia graduate with extensive hospital training in Boston. He was appointed an associate professor of medicine at the University of Rochester and, in 1947, became a professor of medicine at the University of California in Los Angeles. Lawrence had a continuing influence on the department of medicine at Vanderbilt. Edgar Jones (M.D., Vanderbilt, 1929), after interning at Western Reserve and serving as an assistant resident at Vanderbilt,[23] obtained a Josiah Macy fellowship in 1931 to work with Lawrence at Rochester. After his return to Nashville, Jones, working closely with William J. Darby, made several important contributions: he helped to discern the cellular changes in blood in chronic infections; the physiologic variations of leucocytes; the greater effectiveness of ferrous over ferric salts in iron deficiency; the lasting stores of hematopoietic substances in patients previously treated for pernicious anemia; and the effectiveness of vitamin $B_{12}$ in pernicious anemia.

## John B. Youmans and Nutrition

In 1930 Youmans published several papers on his experimental and clinical observations on ergotamine. He extended his studies to the physiological factors influencing the exchange of fluid between the blood and the tissues and their relation to the occurrence of edema in patients; a publication in 1935 on some clinical aspects of dietary deficiencies gave evidence of the future direction of his research interests.[24]

The studies on nutrition by Youmans and his associates, including dietary and nutritional surveys in a rural county in Tennessee, are classics and are being applied in the Third World nations today. The first application in the field was in "unoccupied France" in 1941–42, under the Rockefeller Commission. Youmans next applied his methods in the American zone in Germany in 1945. Working with him in these studies were Charles S. Davidson, Julian Ruffin, Frederick Stare, William Robinson, and Rudolph Kampmeier. After the war, studies were carried out, as part of the work of the International Council on Nutrition, in some fifteen countries in the Near East, the Orient, and South America. Among his collaborators in this work were William Dodd Robinson, William J. Darby, E. White Patton, and Marvin Corlette.

Youmans's classic contribution in the field of nutrition was his recognition of the importance of protein malnutrition occurring in hospitalized patients, which led him to carry out his series of nutrition surveys in middle Tennessee; the influence of which was so far-reaching in determining the methodologic pattern that characterized later national and international nutritional surveys. Youmans was head of the Armed Forces Nutrition Services for the Office of the Surgeon General during World War II. He established with C. S. Robinson, of the department of biochemistry, a required nutrition course for medical students, laying the foundation for the strong division of nutrition at Vanderbilt, which was developed by Darby.

## Other Research in the Department of Medicine

The various investigations in this new stimulating atmosphere created by George Canby Robinson can be seen in the Report of Publications (October 1925–December 1938) of the Vanderbilt University School of Medicine. In 1926 there were seven publications from the department of medicine. All of the problems that were taken to the laboratory were generated from experience with patients. The following year there were fifteen publications. Nine concerned the regulation of the circulation, for the most part representing cooperative studies between medicine and surgery and involving Harrison and Blalock. C. Sidney Burwell published a report on the effect of digitalis upon the output of the heart in normal man. One of John S. Lawrence's many studies concerned the elliptical and sickle-shaped erythrocytes in the circulating blood of white persons. Most of these papers were published in excellent journals; four in the *American Journal of Physiology* and three in the *Journal of Clinical Investigation*.

In the next few years the research output continued at a high level, both in quality and in quantity. Striking were the evidences of cooperative effort between various departments of the school—a reflection of the functional arrangement that George Canby Robinson created in the construction of the hospital and the medical school.

## Robinson's Departure

George Canby Robinson accepted the directorship of the New York Hospital–Cornell Medical College Association in July 1927, with the understanding that although he would remain at Vanderbilt for another year, he would participate in the architectural and other planning in New York as needed. Waller S. Leathers was appointed associate dean, and Youmans was brought from Michigan as an addition to the medical department. Burwell later succeeded Robinson as a professor of medicine. Morgan was appointed a professor of clinical medicine and succeeded Burwell as head of the department in 1935.[25]

In 1925 Morgan joined the faculty of the Vanderbilt University School of Medicine as an associate professor of medicine and played an important role in the reorganization of the school. From that time until his death in 1962, Morgan was a major influence in the department of medicine at Vanderbilt.[26] He retired as head of the department in 1958.

# 16

❧

# The University of Rochester School
# of Medicine[1]

In 1921 George Whipple[2] was invited to be the dean of the new medical school to be organized at the University of Rochester.[3] The original proposal for the school came from the General Education Board of the Rockefeller Foundation through Abraham Flexner. Five million dollars was given by the Rockefeller Foundation, $4 million by George Eastman, and $1 million for the University Hospital by the daughters of Mr. and Mrs. Henry Strong. Whipple accepted on the condition that he be given enough assistance to enable him to continue with his teaching and research. Freida Robscheit-Robbins joined him one year later, and their work on experimental anemia and hemoglobin production as influenced by diet—for which Whipple received the Nobel Prize for Medicine or Physiology in 1934—was continued without serious interruption.

One important decision was that the school and its teaching hospital would be under one roof. The Vanderbilt Medical School was also making plans for a new building, and both schools incorporated the same general architectural plan. The building consisted of two major axes, about one hundred feet apart, extending north and south, and two other axes of similar type pointing east and west. Related clinical departments and hospital wards were placed on floors adjacent to the various preclinical departments.

## William S. McCann: The First Professor of Medicine

William S. McCann[4] was appointed as chairman of the department of medicine in 1924. He studied medicine at Cornell Medical College and served as a Cabot fellow in Harvey Williams Cushing's laboratory of surgical research at Harvard. After World War I, he returned to New York as a research fellow in the Russell Sage Institute of Pathology. This training with Graham Lusk and Eugene F. DuBois provided an important base for his future career.

In 1922 he went to Johns Hopkins, where he headed the metabolism division and did outstanding work on diabetes mellitus with R. R. Hannon.[5] His background in chemistry enabled him to study disease in precise terms. At Rochester he established the metabolism unit that subsequently became the clinical research center of the medical center.

McCann recalled the Rochester appointment and the formation of the first faculty in his unpublished memoirs:

> Early in the fall we were visited [at Johns Hopkins] by three representatives of the University of Rochester. . . . The visitors were President Rush Rhees, Dean George H. Whipple, and Professor of Biochemistry Walter Bloor. I observed our visitors calling on one after another of the numerous associate professors in the department of medicine. . . . Being the junior to them all it never occurred to me that they might consider me. However, President Rhees spent some time conversing with me in my office, about general subjects of interest, and Walter Bloor came into the laboratory making measurements and sketches of the layout. . . . To my surprise, I received a letter from Dean Whipple asking me to come to Rochester in consultation, as there were some problems concerning the department of medicine on which they needed my advice.
>
> Two days were spent going over plans and blue prints, and discussing general problems of teaching and hospital organization. As the second day wore on George Whipple asked me if I would like a look at the city of Rochester, so we took a tour of the town in Whipple's car, finally pulling up to the curb on a side street looking straight ahead to a view of two tall smoke stacks emitting yellow smoke, which I learned was the main Eastman Kodak plant. There we remained in silence, which was broken after what seemed a long time by Whipple's question, "How would you like to be the professor of medicine in the new medical school?" I replied that I would, and he said "that is settled. . . ." All of the initial group (professorial team) were graduates of Johns Hopkins, except Faxon, Bloor, Fenn, Wilson, and me. Both Wilson and I had a substantial part of our teaching experience in Johns Hopkins, so it is fair to say that the new school in Rochester was formed by simple fission from the famous institution in Baltimore.[6]

## Full-time Professors in the Clinical Departments

Like their preclinical colleagues, the heads of the clinical departments, including medicine, surgery, pediatrics, and obstetrics-gynecology, were to be university professors devoting all of their time to their university work, without private practice. While Whipple was a staff member at Johns Hopkins, the influence of Mall, Barker, and Welch served to imbue the idea of full-time clinical professors in his mind. The adoption of the full-time system by the University of Rochester was implicit in the university's acceptance of half of its endowment from the General Education Board.[7]

## Organization of the Department of Medicine

In organizing the department of medicine, McCann recognized that the ideal internist is a general consultant. He had seen the tendency of medical clinics to be subdivided into specialties, such as tuberculosis, syphilis, cardiology, metabolic disorders, dermatology, and neurology, without the basic provision that all men in training as internists have a broad experience with some knowledge of all of these fields.[8] The personnel of the department of medicine for the year 1926–27 consisted of one professor, one associate professor, one instructor, two assistants, and five interns giving their whole time to the department. Nine other physicians in active practice in the city served as part-time instructors. Of these men, two were concerned chiefly with pulmonary tuberculosis, one with cardiac disease, one with gastrointestinal problems, one with dermatology, and two others were general practitioners.

The members of the whole-time staff were engaged in various fields of investigation (see Appendix C).[9] One of the assistants studied the general problem of the secretion of urine and its applications to renal disease. Another worked in electrocardiography. The resident physician, Lawrence A. Kohn, who had the rank of instructor, studied pneumonia. Stafford Warren, the assistant professor in charge of the department of roentgenology, worked on the effects of radiation, with a view to its use in therapy. The associate professor, Richard Lyman,[10] devoted special attention to neurology and to various physiological investigations. He was attempting to perfect methods for the graphic registration of sound and, with the assistance of one of the students (P. F. Metildi, a member of the first class), carried on studies of the acoustics of the chest. He collaborated with McCann in making preparations for the study of the reactions of patients with various diseases to muscular activity. In this connection he was instrumental in developing a new ergometer and a new apparatus for the rapid, complete analysis of air by the measurement of thermal conductivity.

There were two good-sized laboratories. The respiration laboratory was equipped with spirometers, an ergometer (dynamometer), and a portable metabolism apparatus. In the adjacent room, the gas analyses were carried out. In the same wing was a four-bed metabolism unit, which consisted of two bedrooms on either side of a special diet kitchen. In this unit it was possible to carry on accurate metabolic studies involving the careful measurement of food intake and of excreta. There was a heart station equipped with a string galvanometer for electrocardiography and a polygraph. There was also a room for routine diagnostic work in bacteriology, which was under the charge of the resident physician. On another floor, a laboratory was equipped for the physiological investigations of the associate professor in charge of neurology. This equipment consisted of an oscillograph, an electric stethoscope, and apparatus for psychogalvanic reactions, for Barany tests, and so forth.

In 1927 R. R. Hannon came from Baltimore as an associate professor of medicine, but resigned at the end of one year to accept a post at the Rockefeller Institute. He was succeeded by Paul Garvey. During his short stay, Hannon left a lasting imprint on the service by his careful revision of many therapeutic procedures. In 1929 John S. Lawrence was made an associate professor of medicine. Lawrence came from the Thorndike Memorial Laboratory in Boston, having previously served on the faculty at Vanderbilt Medical School.[11] He devoted himself to the organization of a hematologic laboratory, which became an active center of investigation. Lawrence's particular interest was in leukocytes, and he discovered and studied intensively a spontaneous form of agranulocytosis in cats.

In 1930 the first grant was made for a comprehensive study of the effects of diathermy and fever. Drs. Charles M. Carpenter and Ruth A. Boak were appointed as research assistants. These studies, in cooperation with the subdepartment of radiology, included observations on the effect of temperatures between 29° and 42° C on bacteria, especially the gonococcus and *Treponema pallidum*.

The department was fortunate in having a number of excellent fellows supported by the Rockefeller Foundation. The first was Yauso Ikeda from Tokyo, who spent a year doing metabolic studies. Alberto Hurtado of Lima, Peru, conducted important studies of the functional disturbances in chronic pulmonary disease from 1931 to 1934.[12] W. D. W. Brooks from Oxford spent a year in the study of cardiac output in chronic pulmonary diseases, and Kintaro Yanagi of Tokyo completed two years of work on the colloid osmotic pressure of the blood plasma.[13] Konrad Dobriner engaged in a study of the urinary porphyrins in disease.[14]

A Rockefeller Foundation grant was available in 1934 for work on respiratory adaptations to anoxemia and a study of the physiological mechanisms involved in treating lobar pneumonia by artificial pneumothorax. The cardiorespiratory laboratory (1931–35) was supported by a number of industrial organizations interested in the study of the pneumokonioses.

## Research of William S. McCann[15]

McCann set out to develop a program of research in mineral metabolism in disease, which received support from the Fluid Research Fund provided by the Rockefeller Foundation. Under his direction, studies were made of the nature of the mineral exchanges during periods of blood regeneration in pernicious anemia and during rapid blood destruction produced by phenylhydrazine in erythremia; in the dropsical state and during diuresis produced by potassium salts. An important collaborator was Samuel H. Bassett, who was in charge of the chemical laboratories of the medical clinic. There were also students who participated in the research, including C. A. Elden, who was a well-trained chemist.

Alberto Hurtado, who was interested in the physiological adaptations to high altitude exhibited by the Andean natives, came to the department in 1931, when Doran J. Stephens and McCann were investigating some cases presenting the Ayerza syndrome and clinical conditions associated with sclerosis of the pulmonary arteries. Hurtado, as already mentioned, with the assistance of Charles Boller, accumulated much data regarding the lung volume, blood volume, and circulatory reactions of these patients. The following year, Hurtado was joined by W. D. W. Brooks, a fellow of the Medical Research Council of England and assistant director of the medical unit of the St. Mary's Hospital, London. Brooks combined a study of the blood flow through the lung with the lung volume studies in progress. An important collaborator in this work was Nolan Kaltreider, one of the assistant residents (1932–33).

Thus McCann, by continuing participation in research, even if to a very limited degree, provided an important stimulus to the development of clinical investigation in this newly emerging department of medicine. His philosophy was expressed in a lecture, "The Present Status of Clinical Investigation," in 1937: "Science proceeds both by observation and experiment, yet we are sometimes prone to slight the disciplines which develop observation, without which experiment frequently remains sterile."[16]

## Research Divisions in the Department

McCann organized the laboratory of clinical chemistry and the metabolism ward, but their direction was subsequently transferred to Samuel H. Bassett, the second resident physician. Later Bassett was joined by Henry Keutmann,[17] who became a full professor in 1958. Bassett and Keutmann did important research on the dietary factors governing the regeneration of serum proteins in nephrotic states. They also conducted metabolic investigations of idiopathic steatorrhea and electrolyte exchanges in pneumonia and other fevers.[18]

Among the earliest associates in hematology were Doran J. Stevens,[19] a graduate of the first class at Rochester, and Edgar Jones,[20] who later became the hematologist at Vanderbilt. Others who had training in this division were Clement Finch, who later organized the department of hematology at the new school in Seattle, and William Valentine and

William Adams, who accompanied John S. Lawrence when he assumed the chair of medicine at the University of California in Los Angeles in 1947.[21]

Conrad E. Birkhaug was appointed an associate in bacteriology in 1924. He had received his M.D. degree at Johns Hopkins, interned at the Sydenham Hospital in Baltimore, and, while a fellow in medicine there in 1924–25, developed an interest in infectious diseases. He received the Rochester Award (for an act or service contributing to the public interest) during 1925 for his development of a serum treatment for erysipelas.

While an assistant resident in medicine (1936–37), Gerald Klatskin, later to become a professor of medicine at Yale and an international authority on diseases of the liver, published an experimental study of the action of crystalline vitamin $D_2$ (calcified) in chronic parathyroid tetany.[22] Other important products of the program in the department of medicine were Marsh Tenney, who made major contributions in respiratory physiology and later went to Dartmouth as a professor of physiology and dean; and Arthur Kornberg, who did a study on jaundice in medical students with McCann.

## Industrial Medicine

For a number of years the department of medicine engaged in physiological studies of silicosis. Liaison was arranged with the Saranac Laboratory, under Leroy Gardner, and with the Trudeau Sanatorium. Gardner, Fred H. Heise, Arthur J. Vorwald, and George W. Wright of the Trudeau staff held appointments on the medical school faculty. There were extensive studies of occupational disease due to dust and its relation to tuberculosis. George W. Wright, an associate in medicine, established a laboratory of clinical investigation at the Trudeau Sanatorium at Saranac Lake.

The cardiorespiratory laboratory also took up problems related to aviation medicine. A study was made of the effect on the heart and lungs of low oxygen tensions at normal and at low barometric pressure. It was hoped from these beginnings that an institute of industrial medicine would ultimately be formed in which the clinical, experimental, and engineering aspects of industrial hygiene could be studied. Meneely, who collaborated with Kaltreider on studies of blood volume and extracellular fluid using radioactive sodium,[23] was one of the first to use this radioisotope in medical investigation.

From 1941 to 1942, several members of the department engaged in research on military problems. McCann and Romansky collaborated with Brian O'Brien of the Institute of Optics in the study of scotopic vision. There were collateral problems in connection with this work in which E. B. Millard, Jr., H. A. Friedman, Arthur Kornberg, and Nolan Kaltreider participated. Wright and Kaltreider set up a cardiorespiratory laboratory at Mineville, New York, in the Hospital of the Republic Steel Corporation. These arrangements were made under the general direction of Leroy Gardner.

## The Buswell Fellows

During 1943 and 1944, McCann served in the navy, and the department was ably directed by John S. Lawrence. After the war there were many returning veterans who were eager for help in gaining research experience. A special fund for research fellowships was provided by a generous donor, Ralph Hochstetter, in memory of Henry Clarke Buswell and Bertha Hockstetter Buswell.

The first of these Buswell fellows to reach faculty status was Lawrence E. Young, who was made assistant professor in charge of hematology when Lawrence became the professor of medicine at the University of California in Los Angeles. Young had a vigorous program of research dealing with immunological aspects of hematology related to transfusion of blood and the hemolytic anemias. William Valentine, William Adams, and Charles Craddock investigated the radiological effects of atomic energy on the blood and blood-forming organs and the hemorrhagic disorders, including hemophilia. This program was integrated with, and supported by, the department of radiation biology.

Ralph Jacox, a Buswell fellow, studied certain plasma protein fractions that were related to nonspecific immune reactions and that also entered into the complex mechanisms governing blood coagulation.

Herbert R. Brown, Jr., also a Buswell fellow, was engaged in a navy-sponsored study of the effects of cold on the circulation. He used the ballistocardiograph and carried out ingenious experiments aimed at a better understanding of the ballistic movements of the body induced by the heartbeat. He made simultaneous records of the ballistocardiogram, the electrocardiogram, and the intraventricular pressure changes occurring in the right ventricle of the heart.

In 1946-47 a splendidly equipped laboratory with a large treadmill ergometer was set up in the municipal hospital. In cooperation with W. O. Fenn's laboratory, studies were made on the composition of the respired gases by a continuous physical method of gas analysis.

The program of the metabolism ward continued up to January 1948, under Samuel H. Bassett, who was engaged in work in the field of atomic energy. In January, studies of beryllium poisoning were initiated; Howland, Keutmann, and Christine Waterhouse were engaged in this interdepartmental project. Waterhouse was a Buswell fellow who had been studying the physiology of the kidney and assisting Keutmann in his studies of Addison disease and Bassett in a study of the body's utilization of purified plasma albumin. Keutmann, who had been a member of the department since 1929, was promoted to professor in 1958. Assisting him in endocrinological problems was Robert Burton, a Buswell fellow who devised new analytical methods for the determination of keto-steroids.[24]

# 17

⤔

# Western Reserve University School of Medicine and the Cleveland Clinic[1]

An early step in medical science in Cleveland was the formation of a section of experimental medicine within the County Medical Society in 1903.[2] Torald Sollmann, a professor of pharmacology at Western Reserve, viewed this section as a platform "for the informal exchange of views on research subjects . . . having a bearing on medicine." As late as 1910, J. J. R. Macleod, a professor of physiology at the university, said: "At present we are just on the border of this mysterious field of research. But the general physician, if he is intelligently to apply rational therapeutics . . . must know something of the general principles of chemistry upon which it is all based."[3] The first significant move to develop research at Western Reserve came in 1906, with the endowment of a department of experimental medicine.

## The Henry Kirke Cushing Laboratory of Experimental Medicine

In 1906 H. M. Hanna and Colonel Oliver H. Payne, in letters addressed to Dr. Edward F. Cushing, offered to contribute the sum of $100,000 each for a laboratory of experimental medicine.[4]

George N. Stewart was appointed head of the new laboratory. Stewart received his M.A. degree from Edinburgh in 1881 and his M.D. degree in 1890. He became a professor of physiology at Western Reserve in 1894. He was on the staff at the University of Chicago from 1903 until his return to Cleveland.

His chief innovation at Western Reserve as a professor of physiology was the laboratory course. At that time laboratory exercises in physiology were given in but two schools and consisted almost entirely of some nerve-muscle work and a few test-tube experiments on digestion, saliva, and urine. Stewart was one of the first to make mammalian experiments a part of the regular course. As a result of this experience, Stewart wrote his *Manual of Physiology, with Practical Exercises,* one of the best available physiology manuals at that time.[5]

The need for research in clinical departments had not yet been widely appreciated. There were no clinical chairs in America that carried more than a nominal salary. One alternative was to establish a department of experimental medicine, which would have the task of building bridges between the research laboratories of the basic sciences and the clinic. Unfortunately, because of the way things were arranged, Stewart lost contact almost entirely with students; his greatest asset was his ability to teach. Of interest is Stewart's note to the trustees of the Cushing Laboratory on December 8, 1906:

> The experimental medical sciences were originally developed and taught by clinicians. In the evolution of medical research and instruction the necessity for greater and greater specialization has gradually led to the establishment of separate chairs of anatomy, physiology, pharmacology, pathology, and so forth, filled by men who have no time to take any direct share in clinical work; and of separate chairs of medicine, surgery, obstetrics and so forth, filled by men who in general have no time to devote to the systematic investigation in the laboratory. While this specialization is bound to become even more marked in the future, it has created the necessity for some synthesizing agency to bridge the gulf between the laboratory and the clinical branches. I conclude that the chair of Experimental Medicine should fulfill this function not usurping the province of physiology or pathology on the one hand or of clinical medicine or surgery on the other. *It should find its field of research and instruction in the systematic application of the experimental results of the sciences to clinical problems, and the systematic investigation of clinical problems by laboratory methods* (italics mine). To do this effectively the chair should have an official *locum standi* both in the laboratory and in the hospital.[6]

Stewart was a pioneer in the field of electrophysiology. Among his contributions were papers on the electrophysiology of cardiac nerves; hemolysis; circulation time; action of hemolytic agents; agglutination of blood cells; permeability of animal cells; measurements of skin temperature; cerebral anemia; shock; and resuscitation. For a number of years his chief work, in collaboration with J. M. Rogoff,[7] was on the adrenals. They produced an extract that contained the active principle of the adrenal cortex, publishing their report simultaneously with that of F. A. Hartman and his group at the University of Buffalo.

Stewart summarized his studies on the circulation in a Harvey Society Lecture in 1912.[8] He pointed out that it is more important to know the rate at which the blood is flowing in an organ—the so-called mass movement of blood—than to know the pressure in the artery supplying the organ or part. He worked out a method permitting the quantity of blood passing through a part of the body such as the hand to be easily determined with approximate accuracy. His method depended upon the fact that the amount of heat produced by a part of the body such as the hand during rest is negligible in comparison with the heat conveyed to it by the arterial blood (see Hewlett's plethysmographic studies, chapter 18). He described extensive observations in normal individuals and in a wide variety of disease states, including situations in which there were obvious differences between the hands or feet caused by local interference with the circulation; in various anemias; in patients with fever due to various causes; in diseases of the heart; in peripheral vascular diseases; in diseases of the nervous or respiratory systems; and in miscellaneous cases.

## David Marine

Perhaps the most distinguished scientist in the Cushing Laboratory of Experimental Medicine in terms of the relevance of his work to clinical medicine was David Marine (M.D., Johns Hopkins, 1905).[9] After graduation, Marine accepted a post under W. T. Howard, Jr., at Western Reserve. On his arrival in Cleveland, he walked to the hospital from the railroad station and noticed that many of the dogs roaming the streets had swollen necks. When Howard raised the question of a suitable research problem, Marine, remembering the stimulus provided him by Halsted's work on the thyroid and having just seen the canine goitres so prominently displayed, chose to study goitre. He found a direct relationship between epithelial hyperplasia and iodine content of a given gland.[10] The lower the iodine concentration, the greater the hyperplasia. He found also that the morphological appearance of a goitrous canine gland could be altered by partial removal, just as Halsted had shown in the normal animal. If enough of a colloid goitre was excised, hyperplastic areas would appear in the remainder. Furthermore, he found that the structure of the hyperplastic gland could be modified by the administration of iodine in vivo. He advanced the following hypothesis concerning the pathogenesis of colloid goitre:

> That lack of iodine leads first to increase in size of the thyroid epithelial cells or hypertrophy; as the process continues the cells increase in number, that is, hyperplasia occurs. Associated with these changes are a decrease in the amount of colloid in the follicles and an increase in vascularity of the tissue. Whenever iodine is returned to the gland it reverts to normal. However, it cannot return to its original size. The closest state to normal is colloid goitre. The complex histological character of glands from endemic regions is explained by a series of cycles of hyperplasia and involution to the colloid state.

Marine recognized that many goitres were due to iodine deficiency and, in 1909, labeled goitre as a nutritional disease. He also made the prophetic statement, however, that some goitres were associated with "one or more chemical substances which are antagonistic to or inhibit the normal absorption or assimilation of iodine."[11] Thus, he anticipated the chemical agents that are recognized today as goitrogens and are used in the treatment of Graves's disease.

Marine conceived of the potential value of the prophylactic administration of iodine in endemic goitre areas. He showed that iodine preparations were effective in treating the family members of his professional associates. In 1910 the Commissioner of Health arranged for him to visit a school board, before which he stated the case. Afterward the chairman, a doctor, told the other board members that Maine wanted "to poison our children." Here the matter rested until 1916, when Marine was lecturing to a class in pathology. He stated that any doctor who did not prescribe iodine for children with thyroid enlargement was guilty of negligence. After the class. a student asked why he had not done more to institute a program of iodine prophylaxis. After Marine told of his difficulties, the young man said that he had taught school in Akron, Ohio, knew all of the local politicans, and felt that he could arrange a clinical trial in the public school system. The dramatic results from the trial in Akron, carried out by Marine and O. P. Kimball, a second-year medical student, proved that the prophylactic administration of iodine could reduce the prevalence of goitre. These findings eventually led to the introduction of iodized salt.[12]

## The Department of Medicine

### Charles F. Hoover

The man who had the opportunity to advance scientific medicine at Western Reserve was Charles F. Hoover (M.D., Harvard, 1892),[13] a member of the department of medicine from 1894 and its chairman from 1909 until his death in 1927. From 1890 to 1894 he worked with E. von Neusser in Vienna and studied under Friedrich Kraus in Strasbourg. Hoover began the practice of medicine in 1894 in Cleveland. From 1894 to 1907 he was a teacher of physical diagnosis and a visiting physician to the Cleveland City Hospital. He contributed a number of papers on alveolar air, functions of the diaphragm, and the significance of "acro-ataxia" and "proximo-ataxia." Hoover was especially interested in cardiorespiratory, neurological, and hepatic diseases.

Hoover's contacts in the European schools that harbored the influence of Skoda and Laennec explain his interest in bedside examination. Two physical signs are named for him: first, observations on movements of the costal margins and consequent conclusions about underlying pulmonary structure and function; and second, a method for differentiating true hemiparesis of the leg from malingering by notice of pressure of the opposing heel of the supine person as the patient attempts to raise the affected leg.

Hoover's studies also introduced him to German physiological chemistry and experimental research. Although he was not associated with the department of experimental medicine, he did conduct experiments in his own laboratory. He failed, however, to stimulate actively clinical investigation within his department and among his associates—this failure reflected his obsession with clinical medicine.

Upon Hoover's death in 1927, Marion A. Blankenhorn was acting chairman for two years. Blankenhorn (M.D., Western Reserve, 1914)[14] left in 1935 to become chairman of the department of medicine at the University of Cincinnati. Tom Douglas Spies,[15] who was doing research on pellagra and the efficacy of niacin therapy, joined Blankenhorn at the University of Cincinnati.

## The Department under Joseph T. Wearn

In 1928 Joseph T. Wearn was appointed professor of medicine and director of medicine at Lakeside Hospital. He suggested that the new hospital, then in process of being built, be redesigned to include research laboratories close to the medical patients. Wearn brought with him Joseph M. Hayman, Jr., and Gerald Shibley as associate directors of the department.[16]

Joseph M. Hayman, Jr. (M.D., Pennsylvania, 1921) interned at the Pennsylvania Hospital, was an assistant resident at the Boston City Hospital in 1926, and then became an assistant professor of pharmacology and an associate in medicine at Pennsylvania. He was a contemporary of Isaac Starr, another pioneer in the field of clinical pharmacology. He participated in the classical studies of A. N. Richards on the physiology of the kidney.

At Western Reserve, Hayman continued his research in renal disease and took an active role in teaching.[17] After a distinguished war record, for which he received the Legion of Merit, he returned to Western Reserve and became a professor of medicine in 1948. In 1953 he went to Tufts University School of Medicine as dean and professor of medicine.

Gerald Shibley, who had his research space in the Cushing Laboratory of Experimental Medicine,[18] received his M.D. degree from the College of Physicians and Surgeons in 1916, and from 1919 to 1922 he was an associate professor of medicine at Siang-Ya Medical School (the Yale of China). He was an instructor from 1923 to 1925 and an assistant professor of medicine from 1928 to 1930 at Columbia. Shibley's work on infectious disease, particularly pneumococcal pneumonia, was underwritten by the Rockefeller Fund.[19]

Wearn's first resident physician was Reece Berryhill, who later became dean of the school of medicine at Chapel Hill. Two other key individuals were Austen Weisberger and the outstanding scientist Paul Zamecnik, who were both interns. The internship, patterned after that at the Peter Bent Brigham Hospital in Boston, was essentially the first months of a residency in internal medicine. There was no rotation through other services. Although research was not obligatory, everyone in medicine was expected to engage in it, and house officers understood that advancement in the department depended considerably on interest in clinical investigation.

Wearn was well prepared to advance the cause of clinical investigation in American medicine (see chapter 12). He continued his work on blood vessels of the heart, showing that the valves, even of normal adults and especially of children, are frequently vascularized. In studies of the capillary bed of animal and human hearts, he made the fundamental observation that as the organ hypertrophies under stress, the muscle fibers enlarge, but the capillaries do not multiply. Consequently, oxygen or other nutrients have farther to go in attempting to supply the greater metabolic needs of the hypertrophied muscle fibers.

During World War II, Wearn became a staff member of the Committee on Medical Research of the Office of Scientific Research and Development. He also served as chairman of the Subcommittee on Blood Substitutes of the National Research Council, and the battles involving shock, blood substitutes, and blood preservation were not all in the front lines. Wearn's wide knowledge of men and affairs in academic medicine enabled him to allocate urgent research problems to those best equipped to study them. In his talks with young medical officers he found that much of what they had learned in medical school had been of little value in guiding their performances as doctors in the armed forces, and would not be especially useful on their return to civilian practice. This confirmation of his own previous impressions convinced him more than ever that a long, hard look at the medical curriculum was needed.[20] He had this opportunity when he returned to Cleveland and assumed the deanship, as well as continuing as head of the department of medicine. His return coincided with the almost simultaneous retirement of eleven senior department heads. Wearn appointed outstanding new chairmen; among them were Douglas Bond, John Dingle, Hymen Friedell, Arnold Welch, and Harland Wood. He also recruited a strong group at the Metropolitan Hospital, including Charles Rammelkamp,[21] Frederick Robbins, and Frank Simeone. He soon launched an impressive effort to construct an entirely new type of curriculum and recruited T. Hale Ham as the program director. This venture was very successful and Wearn was the first to receive, after John M. Russell, the Russell Award of the Markle Scholars (1963). At Western Reserve there stands the Joseph Treloar Wearn Laboratory of Clinical Research—a magnificent tribute dedicated to him in 1961 and jointly sponsored by the university hospitals and the school of medicine for the use of all clinical departments.

In 1950 Wearn became John H. Hord Professor of Medicine. In 1956 he relinquished the responsibility of this title, as well as that of director of medicine, to Robert Ebert, while continuing as dean until 1959 and, for a year thereafter, as vice-president of medical affairs. In 1965 he was awarded the Kober Medal of the Association of American Physicians.[22]

In the period between 1935 and the beginning of World War II, some new faces appeared among the full-time members of the department of medicine. Men such as Robert Parker, in microbiology and infectious diseases; Robert Heinle, in hematology; Paul Glenn, in gastroenterology; Max Miller, in diabetes and metabolism; Reginald Shipley, in endocrinology; and Walter Pritchard, in cardiology, carried on active research programs and conducted clinical teaching.

Elliott C. Cutler had arrived in Cleveland as a professor of surgery, bringing with him Claude S. Beck, a graduate of the Johns Hopkins University School of Medicine. This was just at the time of their experimental and clinical studies on the surgical treatment of mitral stenosis. Beck established the first surgical research laboratory devoted to cardiovascular disease. His major problems for study were constrictive pericarditis, conduction of the cardiac impulse, and coronary heart disease. An important contribution was his demonstration that the heart was susceptible to surgical attack and that the mortality was reasonably low.

One of the great strengths of the department of medicine at Lakeside Hospital in its relationship to the university was the involvement of clinical practitioners in teaching and clinical research. Harold Feil, who did research in cardiology with Carl Wiggers at Western Reserve and with Sir Thomas Lewis in London, contributed importantly to the activities of the department. Horace Korns introduced the first electrocardiograph service in the hospital. When Korns moved to Iowa, Feil assumed the responsibility for this laboratory.

## The Department of Medicine at Cleveland Metropolitan General Hospital

Edward Perkins Carter (M.D., Pennsylvania, 1894) served as a resident under Osler and as a fellow in pathology at Johns Hopkins. In 1898 he became the first resident physician at the Lakeside Hospital. He studied in Vienna in 1899 and then returned to practice in Cleveland. In 1912 he withdrew from practice and spent the next two years in London with Lewis and at the laboratory at Saranac Lake. When Western Reserve assumed responsibility for the Cleveland City Hospital in 1914, Carter became full-time chief of medicine. In 1918 he accepted a faculty position at Johns Hopkins.[23]

From 1919 to 1929, Samuel Webster, a practicing physician, served as department chairman. In 1929 Roy W. Scott succeeded Webster and soon gained recognition as an investigator and teacher of cardiovascular disease.[24] A division of pulmonary disease was developed by Raymond McKay, and Robert M. Stecher established a division of rheumatology.

## Harry Goldblatt

An important discovery in terms of its influence on clinical science was Harry Goldblatt's method of producing experimental hypertension.[25] Carrie Derrick, McGill's first woman professor, stimulated Goldblatt's interest in biology. He was appointed a demonstrator of biology, where he came into contact with premedical students. It was this association that led to his entering McGill University Medical School, from which he graduated in 1916. While resident pathologist under Howard Karsner at Western Reserve University, he became interested in experimental pathology. He worked at the Lister Institute of Preventive Medicine in London, where research on rickets won him a Beit Fellowship.

As a pathologist, Goldblatt noted that some individuals with normal blood pressure had extensive atherosclerosis without kidney involvement, whereas others had hypertension and atherosclerosis almost limited to the kidneys. These observations led to his experiments with a silver clamp used to constrict the renal artery. He found that if only one kidney had its blood supply impaired, the subject still became hypertensive. Early release of the clamp or removal of the ischemic kidney resulted in resolution of the hypertension.[26]

Irvine H. Page evaluated the impact of Goldblatt's work:

> Up to 1934, clinical and experimental hypertension were the poor stepchildren of cardiology. Many believed that elevated blood pressure was "benign" and some even thought it was a good thing, the rise in pressure compensating for thickened blood vessels that required higher pressure to force blood through them. To lower pressure could be disastrous—a very convenient theory indeed, since no one knew how to lower arterial pressure permanently in patients.
>
> Goldblatt's discovery came at the right time. He established beyond doubt a method which was to prove infinitely useful in unraveling the complexity of hypertension.[27]

From Goldblatt stemmed a family of investigators, the best known of whom are Leonard Skeggs, Joseph Kahn, and Erwin Haas. Skeggs and his long-time associate Kahn made unique contributions to the knowledge of the chemistry of the humoral agent, angiotensin. They not only described the amino acid sequence of the angiotensin molecule, but showed the conversion of angiotensin I, a weakly active pressor substance, to angiotensin II, the most powerful pressor substance known. Further, they partially clarified the nature of the angiotensin-converting enzyme that performs this hydrolysis.

Their synthesis of one renin substrate, the tetradecapeptide, provided a firm base from which to study the kinetics of angiotensin formation. Skeggs's later work was concerned with a penetrating analysis of renin, the kidney enzyme that cleaves angiotensin I from renin-substrate. Skeggs, who also developed the automatic multiple analyzer, received his Ph.D. degree in biochemistry from Western Reserve University in 1948. Haas's primary interest was in the complex task of purifying renin.

## Irvine H. Page and the Cleveland Clinic

Page's research began at the Rockefeller Institute with Donald D. Van Slyke in 1931. Arthur C. Corcoran, a graduate of McGill, joined him in 1936. The use of clearance methods for study of renal blood flow during changes in blood pressure, the effects of anterior nerve root section (in 1931), and beginning work on extracts of kidney—called *renin*—constituted the first phase of their studies.

Corcoran was both a clinician and an experimental scientist. The first to apply the clearance methods to the more intimate analysis of renal function in hypertension, he was quick to see the major 'problem—whether the kidney is the culprit or the victim of hypertension. His interest later spread to the adrenal cortex, at a time when its relationship to hypertension was not appreciated. Corcoran worked with Page until 1959; he then became head of the department of clinical investigation at St. Vincent Charity Hospital and, in 1964, a professor of medicine at Michigan.

Page moved to Indianapolis in 1931 and discovered angiotensin in 1938, concurrently with Eduardo Braun-Menéndez and his group in Argentina.[28] The clinical delineation and experimental treatment of patients constituted the remainder of his work.

In 1944, when Page left Indianapolis, it was clear that hypertension was a treatable and reversible disease. Corcoran and Page—at the invitation of William E. Lower and Russell Haden—organized the Research Division of the Cleveland Clinic in 1945. They were joined by James McCubbin, Harriet Dustan, Merlin Bumpus, Hans Schwarz, Georges Masson, and Maurice Rapport. Studies on serotonin and the synthesis of angiotensin II followed.

The chief contribution of Bumpus was the purification and synthesis of angiotensin. In this he had the assistance of Schwarz. Subsequently, he entered the rapidly developing field of antiangiotensin blocking agents. The experience of Bumpus and Schwarz illustrates the value of eliciting the interest of first-rate young persons trained in pure chemistry. As a result of Bumpus's interest in the renin-angiotensin system, important advances in our understanding of humoral mechanisms were made.

## Other Research at the Cleveland Clinic

After World War I, Frank E. Bunts, George Crile, and William E. Lower completed their plans for the organization of the Cleveland Clinic Foundation. They were convinced that there should be broad coverage of medical services and, therefore, invited John Phillips, an associate professor of medicine at Western Reserve, to join them as chief of medicine. The plan was to organize a clinic, hospital, research institution, and teaching unit.

Phillips was chairman of the division of medicine for eight years (1921–29); a period of transition in the practice of medicine. The trend away from house calls and a practice based in the office and in the institution had begun.

In September 1930, Russell L. Haden,[29] a professor of experimental medicine at the University of Kansas School of Medicine, was appointed chairman of medicine. The contrast between Haden and his predecessor is striking. Phillips was interested primarily in the clinical aspects of disease, whereas Haden was the clinic's first laboratory-oriented medical scientist.

Haden's primary interests were the purpuras, deficiency anemias, and hemolytic anemias. He was the first to demonstrate that the spherocytic shape of the erythrocytes in congenital hemolytic anemia is responsible for their increased osmotic fragility. Although the clinic was still heavily oriented toward surgery at the time of Haden's appointment, the number of medical patients was increasing rapidly, and he quickly foresaw that therapeutic and technologic advances would necessitate progressive departmentalization and specialization in the division.

The first appointment made by Haden was A. Carlton Ernstene, who in 1932 organized the department of cardiorespiratory disease.[30] Ernstene, a graduate of the Iowa State Medical School, was a resident and a research assistant at the Boston City Hospital. He then spent four years at the Beth Israel Hospital, where he and Dorothy M. Rourke developed a method for determination of the sedimentation rate. Ernstene was one of the first researchers to point out the shoulder-hand syndrome following acute myocardial infarction, and he and his associate William L. Proudfit described the electrocardiographic changes of hypokalemia.

# 18

*cᵗᵖ*

# The University of Michigan
# School of Medicine

The University of Michigan School of Medicine, founded in 1850, was from the start a scientific, in contrast to a practical, institution.[1] For twenty-five years it had no hospital.[2] Ambulatory patients brought to Ann Arbor were given free consultation, provided that they submitted to demonstration before the students.

James D. Angell, a contemporary of Daniel Coit Gilman and Charles W. Eliot, became president of the medical school in 1871. He appreciated the importance of science in university education. During his tenure there were many important advances: stiffer requirements for admission; increase in time required to obtain an M.D. degree; and graded as well as postgraduate courses. A hospital was built, laboratories of hygiene and bacteriology were founded, and new facilities for histology, physiology, and surgery were developed.

By 1900 Henry Sewall,[3] a professor of physiology and a former student of Henry Newell Martin in Baltimore, had demonstrated for the first time immunity to a chemical agent. George Dock had made a number of important investigations in the clinical laboratory. Arthur R. Cushny had published a monograph on the action of drugs of the digitalis class; Frederick G. Novy had made important observations on hog-cholera and plague; Aldred S. Warthin had completed his studies on the hemolymph glands; and G. Carl Huber had published his observations on degeneration and regeneration of nerve fibers. Thus, the school at Ann Arbor was one of the first to recognize the value of research. No other state university equaled its accomplishments at this period, and it was considered to be in the same class as Johns Hopkins, Harvard, and Columbia.[4]

An important appraisal of the University of Michigan School of Medicine was given by J. G. Adami in 1901:

Your university has been well to the fore in this matter of laboratory training. Since 1856 . . . there has been a chemical laboratory, for 25 years histological and physiological laboratories have been established; your laboratory of medical chemistry was the first of its kind in America, as was that in electrotherapeutics, as was, again, your laboratory of clinical medicine. . . .

Let me tell you that there is no state university that has the same reputation as you have; nay more, that among those interested in medical science you take a stand equal to that of far older and far wealthier institutions. . . .

The veritable medical renaissance in this country . . . dates from Newell Martin's appointment as professor of physiology at Johns Hopkins, and from his pregnant enthusiasm in physiological experimentation. His work, ably seconded later by Welch, has had the greatest influence in stirring up the love for medical research throughout this continent.[5]

## George Dock

From 1891 to 1908 George Dock[6] served as a professor of medicine. Osler's pupil in Philadelphia, Dock studied in Germany from 1885 to 1887. Dock has given a fascinating description of the medical school at Michigan during his tenure as professor:[7]

In the earlier era, teaching on medical cases was limited to people from a distance who . . . were examined by the professor . . . were lectured upon by the professor, prescribed for, and returned home. . . .

The house staff consisted of a steward. matron, house-surgeon and physician in one person, a most efficient orderly . . . and an equally efficient pharmacist. . . . There were . . . no trained nurses until 1891, when we organized a school. . . .

There was no one available as an assistant, no salary to bring one from another school, but I was fortunate to find in the graduating class one who was willing to undertake the job. It was Aldred S. Warthin, who . . . got his degree in medicine and continued to work for a degree of Doctor of Philosophy. . . . In Ann Arbor we had women in every class . . . and some became eminent . . . as investigators, including Alice Hamilton and Lydia Dewitt. . . .

Instrumental examinations (such as aspiration, use of stomach tubes) were often done in the clinical hour. Also chemical tests, as for bile, albumin, diacetic acid and acetone, Ehrlich's diazo reaction, etc., were made there, sometimes by the student. . . . If percussion were needed, I did it with hammer and pleximeter, marking lines with wax pencil, and having the student in charge, or another, describe the results.

From the beginning we eschewed the almost universal polypharmaceutic treatment for heart disease, but after a brief observation period gave digitalis as tincture or leaf. Our heart patients were always seen with Arthur Cushny, a pioneer in the scientific treatment of such cases. . . .[8] We insisted the future of heart patients could only be based on careful and thorough efforts at treatment.

The clinical laboratory was well equipped from the beginning of my tenure, and space and apparatus increased with the service. We had one of the first centrifuges for medical work, a German model worked by hand power and friction wheels. Before buildings were furnished with suction, we used Chapman pumps. We were credited with introducing leucocyte counts in suspected appendicitis. As soon as James Mackenzie announced his polygraph we had an attachment made and used it with satisfaction. . . . We got one of the earliest machines for getting blood pressure estimations through Joseph L. Miller.

Many medical students, stimulated by Dock's teaching, later came to occupy positions of prominence in the United States. Aldred S. Warthin became a professor of pathology at Michigan, and David Murray Cowie served as a professor of pediatrics and infectious diseases there. James Rae Arneill became a professor of medicine at Colorado; Rogert Sylvester Morris, a professor of medicine at Cincinnati; and James Gerrit Van Zwaluwenburg, a professor of roentgenology at Michigan.

In 1908 Dock accepted the professorship of medicine at Tulane University, and later the chair of medicine at Washington University.

## Albion Walter Hewlett, Professor of Medicine, 1908–1916[9]

The modern practice of medicine is, to a large extent, applied physiology. Since 1900, physicians have remolded the major concepts upon which the care of the sick is based. At times the science of medicine pushed the art of medicine into a secondary position. One of those who successfully combined the two was Albion Walter Hewlett, a trained physiologist who developed into a skillful practitioner.

Hewlett attended the Cooper Medical College in San Francisco for one year and then transferred to Johns Hopkins in 1897. His interest in research began early, and, according to Ray Lyman Wilbur, he did volunteer work in the physiology laboratory at the Cooper Medical College. His first scientific study was, however, conducted in collaboration with Joseph Erlanger during his second year at Johns Hopkins. This resulted in a paper published in the *American Journal of Physiology* in 1901.[10]

They found that dogs from which 70 to 83 percent of the combined jejunum and ileum had been removed lived indefinitely after operation. On a diet poor in fat, the dog with a shortened small intestine absorbed the fat as well as a normal dog. With a high-fat diet, 25 percent of the ingested fat appeared in the feces, whereas in normal dogs only about 4.5 percent appeared.[11]

After graduation in 1900, Hewlett interned at the New York Hospital. From there he went to Tübingen (1902–3), where he studied under Ludolf Krehl, who was among the first to emphasize abnormal function (pathological physiology) as opposed to pathological anatomy. In 1905 Hewlett translated Krehl's book on clinical pathology. William Osler, in his introduction to this work, said: "In this book, disease is studied as a perversion of physiological function. The title, 'Clinical Physiology,' expresses well the attempt which is made in it to fill the gap between empirical and scientific medicine." The translation of Krehl's book was only the beginning of his important publications; the first edition of Hewlett's own *Pathological Physiology of Internal Diseases: Functional Pathology* appeared in 1916.

While at Johns Hopkins, Hewlett learned of Flexner's work on the occurrence of a fat-splitting ferment in peritoneal fat necroses.[12] It seemed reasonable to assume that this ferment was the pancreas' fat-splitting enzyme, which escaped as a result of the pancreatic disease. Hewlett demonstrated lipase in the urine of dogs in whom pancreatic disease had been experimentally produced.[13]

In Hewlett's next study he examined the effect of bile upon the ester-splitting action of pure pancreatic juice obtained from dogs by injections of secretin and pilocarpine, and he concluded that the bile acted as an accelerator upon the fat-splitting ferment.[14]

One of Hewlett's most impressive studies was that on the effect of amyl nitrite inhalations on the blood pressure in man.[15] He found that besides being a vasodilator, amyl nitrite was an active cardiac stimulant.

In 1907 C. I. Young and Hewlett studied the normal pulsations within the esophagus.[16] They introduced a stomach tube over the end of which a small rubber balloon had been fastened, and they studied abnormal heart action by this method. In the same year, Hewlett studied heart block in patients receiving digitalis. All these studies were done before any electrocardiograms had been taken in the United States.

In 1907 Hewlett also published his study on the *positive venous pulse,*[17] a term used to indicate a regurgitant venous pulsation due to a stream of blood being forced back into the veins from the heart. He found that three conditions gave rise to a positive venous wave in early ventricular systole: first, the simultaneous contraction of auricles and ventricles; second, tricuspid insufficiency; and third, paralysis of the auricles.

In 1908 Hewlett published his clinical observations on absolutely irregular hearts.[18] The characteristics of the absolutely irregular heart were: first, absence of normal auricular contractions; second, the total irregularity itself; and third, its permanency. To the existing criteria, Hewlett added the presence of an auricular wave on the cardiogram obtained from within the esophagus. Atrial paralysis was first observed experimentally by von Frey and Krehl in 1890, and in man by Sir James Mackenzie (1894), using venous tracings. The final proof came when Hewlett demonstrated it by means of esophageal tracings.

At Michigan, Hewlett developed an interest in the peripheral circulation. With Van Zwaluwenburg, he devised a method for estimating blood flow in the arm.[19] They noted that the most important factor is the rate of blood flow. T. G. Brodie had estimated the blood flow in an organ in the dog by suddenly occluding its efferent vein and measuring the change of volume with an oncometer.[20] The arterial blood entered the organ with undiminished speed at first, but soon the flow was re-tarded by the rise of pressure in the veins and capillaries. The organ therefore swelled rapidly at first and progressively more slowly. The earliest portion of this curve represented the rate at which the blood entered under normal conditions. Hewlett used Brodie's principle to determine the rate of flow in the arm of man with a plethysmograph. The rate of flow was found to vary in different individuals and, to a less extent, in the same individual under different circumstances.[21]

Hewlett and Van Zwaluwenburg found that application of heat to the body as a whole increased the rate of flow through the arm.[22] Among those with slow rates were severe diabetics and patients with nodular sclerosis of the radial arteries, or with valvular heart disease with abso-lutely irregular rhythm and partial heart block. The fastest rate was in exophthalmic goitre.

In 1912 Hewlett, Van Zwaluwenburg, and J. H. Agnew developed a new method for studying the brachial pulse of man.[23] When the venous outflow from the arm is obstructed by suddenly inflating a circular cuff to a pressure somewhat below that which prevails in the arteries, the arm swells, owing to the entrance of arterial blood. Volume tracings of the arm taken at that time show the arterial pulsations; and just as the average rate of inflow is recorded by the average rate at which the arm swells, so the inflow during each portion of the pulse cycle is recorded by the momentary variations in arm volume. Since the chief inflow to the arm is through the brachial artery, Hewlett, Van Zwaluwenburg, and Agnew obtained an approximate record of the volume flow in the brach-ial artery during each portion of the pulse cycle. The average blood flow in the arm depended in part upon the average blood pressure, but chiefly upon the degree of constriction of the finer arterioles controlling the escape of blood from the arterial reservoirs to the capillaries and veins. Nitroglycerin produced characteristic changes in the pulse form due to a relaxation of the larger arteries of the arm without a corre-sponding effect upon the arterioles.[24]

Hewlett later studied the effect of pituitary substance upon the pulse form of febrile patients.[25] The pulse changes were precisely opposite to those that he had described following a therapeutic dose of nitroglyce-rin.

When Hewlett held the chair of medicine, there was widespread interest in the irregularities of the heartbeat. Electrocardiograms were first taken at the university hospital in 1914. Frank Wilson (M.D., Michi-gan, 1913) installed and operated the instrument, which was placed in Hewlett's private office. A tiny darkroom was available for the develop-ment of the records. In spite of these meager facilities, many interesting observations were made.

Before Hewlett left Michigan he summarized the course of develop-ments during his eight years there.[26] He emphasized that a university clinic should devote itself to teaching, to patient care, to testing new methods of diagnosis and treatment, and to the scientific study of disease. "The clinic which is not adding to the sum total of medical knowledge is already falling in the rear. . . . Members of the clinical staff must devote a portion of their time to research; and facilities for such research must be furnished by the hospital or by the university . . . if the members of the clinical staff are to do research in addition to their hospital and teaching duties, there will be relatively little time for private practice."

During those eight years, no private offices were opened in the business district of the city. The plan proved effective in centering the major interest of the staff upon hospital and university duties. Two disadvantages of the plan, however, became apparent. It was not possible to pay the assistants sufficiently large salaries to retain them for an indefinite period with the university; and with no private wards in the hospital, the assistants were deprived of the experience that comes from contact with private patients. These objections did not in his mind outweigh the advantages. Hewlett felt that "from the standpoint of the students there is a disadvantage in bringing them in contact solely with men who devote themselves to the scientific side of medicine." He thought that this difficulty could be easily overcome by having on the staff certain men who were engaged in private practice.

> The problems confronting internal medicine at the present day involve not alone the usual clinical observations of patients but the study of these patients by the various methods that have been developed in biochemistry, physiology, bacteriology, and immunology. These methods are often costly both in time and money and they require laboratory space, special apparatus, and the services of technical assistants. . . . Herein it seems to me has been the most serious defect in my department. Our facilities for the study of cardiovascular disease have been excellent but only beginnings have been made along other lines. . . . In the leading clinics, new ideas are being originated . . . and so far as internal medicine is concerned this means work in a clinical laboratory equipped for chemical, bacteriologic, and physiologic work. The University Hospital has reached a size that is adequate . . . for its university purposes and . . . the time is at hand when more effort should be made toward its development as a center for clinical research.

Hewlett was at the forefront of those who helped to create medicine's scientific base through the development of clinical investigation. He was a charter member of the American Society for Clinical Research and in 1925 served as its president.

## Nellis Barnes Foster[27]

Hewlett was succeeded in 1916 by Nellis Barnes Foster (M.D., Johns Hopkins, 1902), who had pursued postgraduate studies at various European institutions before joining the Cornell Medical College.

Foster found the department of medicine established in the old medical ward. A small room provided the only available space for experimental work. In order to provide much needed space, the dean permitted Louis H. Newburgh, who had recently joined the department, to work in the Hygienic Laboratory in the basement of the West Medical Building.

Foster was later assigned additional room in an old building that had formerly housed the hospital laundry, and the regents appropriated $2,000 for the purchase of laboratory equipment. The room was situated over the hospital furnace, and it was so dark that it was necessary to have the lights turned on in the middle of the day. The L-shaped room was partitioned off and divided into four small laboratories. Small experimental animals, such as guinea pigs and rabbits, were kept at one end.

Foster had served for only six months when the United States entered World War I. Shortly afterward he suddenly left the university, because of a misunderstanding with Dean Vaughan, and joined the Medical Corps of the United States Army.

## Louis H. Newburgh[28]

When Foster left, Newburgh was made acting head of the department, but was not given control of the budget or the privilege of recommending new appointments.

Newburgh (M.D., Harvard, 1908) came to Michigan in 1916 as an assistant professor of medicine. Following a medical internship at the MGH and a period of study under Hans Eppinger in Vienna, he entered practice in Cincinnati (1910), but soon returned to Boston, where he began his lifelong career in clinical investigation. He received encouragement from David Linn Edsall, but opportunities were limited for a clinical investigator in those days. Support for young men wishing to spend their full time in research was almost nonexistent, and Newburgh had to do some private practice. He served for four years as an assistant at the Harvard Medical School. His major studies concerned respiration, circulation, and the effect of strychnine on the blood pressure of patients with pneumonia.[29]

At Michigan, Newburgh developed an experimental nutrition laboratory that functioned as a unit of the department of medicine. He studied such chronic problems as diabetes mellitus, nephritis, and obesity.[30] The university hospital afforded him excellent facilities for calorimetry, and many studies on the exchange of energy and the metabolism of foodstuffs were carried out. With John M. Sheldon,[31] he perfected methods for determining total heat balance, both by indirect calorimetry and from the insensible heat loss. Newburgh was assisted in his studies of nephritis produced by diets rich in protein by Theodore L. Squier, Phil L. Marsh, Arthur C. Curtis,[32] Sarah Clarkson, and Margaret W.

Johnston (see footnote 30 for specific studies). Richard H. Freyberg[33] was concerned with recoverability from the injury produced by the diet.

Newburgh had become interested in the kidney as early as 1919.[34] In 1930 he and F. H. Lashmet[35] published an important paper on the specific gravity of urine as a test of kidney function.[36] Newburgh's work on kidney function led to further studies on water metabolism. In 1935 he constructed a remarkable balance scale in a closed chamber, in which the subject lived for indefinite periods of time, allowing accurate body water and caloric exchange measurements.

To study obesity, methods for measuring the exchange of energy and of water were devised with the help of Frank H. Wiley. Newburgh and Johnston demonstrated that obesity is always caused by an inflow of energy greater than the outflow and can be overcome by appropriate dietary methods.

In 1920 Newburgh and Marsh presented evidence supporting the use of the high-fat, low-carbohydrate, low-protein diet, for the dietary regulation of diabetes.[37] Newburgh, Johnston, Jerome Conn,[38] Florence White, and Elizabeth B. Stern made elaborate studies of the normal and abnormal metabolism of carbohydrate.

Newburgh was appointed a professor of clinical investigation in medicine in 1922. In June 1956, he was awarded the Banting Medal of the American Diabetes Association.

Cecil Striker described his period with Newburgh, which dated from 1924:

> There was very little insulin available and almost all diabetic patients were living on an undernutritional diet. Dr. Newburgh was convincingly demonstrating that nitrogen equilibrium could be maintained and ketosis controlled by putting patients on diets very low in carbohydrates and low in protein but high in fat. For example, the Newburgh Four, as it was called in those days, was a diet of 35 gm. of carbohydrate, 55 gm. of protein and 220 gm. of fat. . . .
>
> I shall never forget the daily rounds at the old University Hospital where along with the human interest in the patient, Dr. Newburgh led a very objective discussion of the chemical phenomena that were going on in each patient. As every investigator exemplifies an unsatisfied individual, so Dr. Newburgh always propounded the eternal question of why, why, why.[39]

Alexander Leaf, who worked as a fellow under Newburgh, has given a penetrating analysis of the man and his scientific accomplishments:

> Dr. Newburgh . . . had his internship and residency here at the MGH. Shattuck was Chief of Medicine and when he arrived in frockcoat each morning to make rounds in the Bulfinch Building, his residents were lined up to greet him with the intern tagging at the tail of the entourage.
>
> At that time typhoid fever was prevalent in Boston and patients were treated with the Shattuck regimen; they were starved during the febrile phase of the illness. Many died. Covering the ward one evening young Dr.

Newburgh noted the clear evidence of wasting and starvation in one of the typhoid patients and provided her with a beef steak. The next morning on rounds Dr. Shattuck noted the patient's improvement and asked Newburgh how the patient had been treated. When told, he had a near tantrum and almost fired Newburgh on the spot. Newburgh's subsequent career was characterized by high suspicion of accepted dogma and always a willingness to try fresh solutions to a problem.

He insisted on precise numbers to describe physiological and clinical phenomena. He was always fussing about how some clinical parameter could be measured. He was outspoken in his intolerance of the anecdotal response and the "clinical impression." Things had to be measured and he was always measuring everything.

In those early days, renal function, fluid, and electrolytes as well as metabolic parameters could be most readily quantitated. Thus ... he engaged in laborious, precise balance studies and demonstrated the relationship of the insensible loss of fluid to metabolic energy production. He built a whole body calorimeter and respirator in which his subjects would reside for days while oxygen consumption, carbon dioxide production and body weight were carefully followed while eating a diet which Dr. Newburgh had measured for calories in a bomb calorimeter and for chemical composition by means of direct quantitative analyses. By a series of such meticulous measurements he was able to refute a then popular theory for obesity, the Luxoskonsumption hypothesis of Rubner....

At a time when authorities denied that the First Law of Thermodynamics, the conservation of energy, could be applied to human metabolism, Dr. Newburgh proved irrefutably by meticulous determination of calories in and calories out that this natural law applied to man as well as to inanimate matter.

He was one of the first to realize that the volume of extracellular fluid was determined by the quantity of sodium salts in the body and was virtually independent of water intake. He was treating edema by a low sodium diet long before clinical colleagues recognized the relationship of sodium retention to extracellular fluid volume. In quantitating the sodium balance he included measurement of the insensible loss of sodium from the skin of non-perspiring subjects. This required careful extraction of sodium from prewashed sheets upon which his naked subjects reclined and a daily wash down of each subject with distilled water from a wash bottle. This was done in the days before flame photometer when each sodium determination made by uranyl nitrate precipitation was practically a research procedure.

He described the entity of adult onset diabetes and noted the differences in the clinical course from that of juvenile diabetes. This led to a longstanding friendly controversy with F. N. Allen who insisted they were both the same condition.

Following my military service he arranged for me to join him as a Research Fellow. When I arrived he showed me our laboratory and admonished me, "Come talk to me any time about your work. Only one topic is prohibited—never ask me what you should be doing. If I knew, I wouldn't have invited you here, I'd have done it myself!"[40]

## Louis Marshall Warfield

Dean Hugh Cabot recommended Warfield[41] (M.D., Johns Hopkins, 1901) to succeed Foster as professor medicine.

Warfield interned under Osler and, after spending a year in Germany, entered practice. In 1911, only ten years after his graduation, he became a professor of medicine at the reorganized Marquette Medical School. His major interest was in circulatory and pulmonary diseases. Warfield served as head of the department of medicine at Michigan from 1922 to 1925.[42]

Preston Manasseh Hickey, a professor of roentgenology, was then temporarily in charge, and James Deacon Bruce directed the department from 1926 to 1928. During the latter's regime, a tuberculosis unit was started, an allergy service was developed, and the Simpson Memorial Institute was built.

## Cyrus C. Sturgis

From 1928 to 1958 Cyrus C. Sturgis[43] served as a professor of medicine and director of the Simpson Memorial Institute. Sturgis (M.D., Johns Hopkins, 1917) interned at the Peter Bent Brigham Hospital. He was a member of the group under Francis W. Peabody, who studied "the irritable heart" in soldiers (see chapter 12).

After the war, he returned to the Brigham as an assistant resident physician for two years and then became chief medical resident. He was appointed a physician to the hospital and, in 1925, was made an assistant professor of medicine at Harvard. It was during this time that he carried on his studies of hyperthyroidism and myxedema.[44]

The department of medicine had previously been divided into several divisions: a service in metabolism, headed by Newburgh; a cardiology service, under Wilson; a private medical service, supervised by Bruce; and a tuberculosis service, chaired by George A. Sherman.[45] Sturgis combined these services with general medicine. This allowed Newburgh, Wilson, and their staffs increased time for experimental work.

Sturgis vigorously supported the work of Frank Wilson[46] and his group.[47] As mentioned, in 1914 Wilson assembled the first electrocardiograph at Michigan. In 1917 a group of cardiologists from the United States was chosen to work with Sir Thomas Lewis in England; Wilson was the youngest member of the group. Lewis recognized his genius and was later instrumental, along with Willem Einthoven, in encouraging Wilson to continue his career in cardiology. Following World War I, Wilson worked at Washington University and collaborated with George R. Herrmann, a Michigan graduate, on a study of bundle branch block.[48] Included were some fundamental observations concerning the electrical field as it is produced by the heart, which acts as a volume conductor. In 1920 Wilson returned to Ann Arbor, but adequate facilities were not available for his research until 1922, when Herrmann joined the staff. When the new laboratory was completed in 1922, Lewis visited the university; this visit stimulated interest in electrocardiography. In 1924 Einthoven visited Ann Arbor and agreed to construct a galvanometer designed to record two electrocardiographic leads simultaneously. The heart station was moved to the new hospital in the autumn of 1924. Herrmann was succeeded by Paul S. Barker.[49]

During these years, Wilson studied the repolarization process in the heart. He discovered that the form of the T wave of the electrocardiogram of normal persons was influenced by the drinking of iced water. This was only the first of other important observations on the T wave, which had a profound influence on interpretation of electrocardiograms.[50]

In 1927 Sturgis relieved Wilson of all academic responsibilities in order to give him more time for his research. Meanwhile, a prolonged illness presented a second hiatus in Wilson's career. This in the end proved beneficial in that during his convalescence Wilson mastered mathematics, knowledge of which enabled him to make his later important contributions. A further aid to Wilson's later work was based on one of Barker's cases. A patient of Barker's was admitted with purulent pericardial disease requiring surgery, and the exposure of the heart permitted electrocardiographic studies never before performed in the human. When the surface of the exposed heart was stimulated electrically by Barker and Macleod, complexes were produced of a type not in keeping with the then generally accepted concept of bundle branch block. Developed by Lewis, this concept had been based on experimentally produced lesions in dogs. What we now know to be *left* bundle branch block was then called *right,* and some of the instances of what we now know to be *right* were then labeled *left* bundle branch block. Lewis's concept had been challenged by Oppenheimer and Pardee in 1920, as a result of pathological findings in human cases, and Fahr had objected also, on theoretical grounds. Until that time, however, Wilson had gone along with the accepted teaching, and there had been many a friendly argument with Oppenheimer concerning it. During one of these arguments Wilson had stated that he would accept Oppenheimer's view if stimulation of the exposed right ventricle produced diphasic complexes of the kind Oppenheimer attributed to left bundle branch block. Barker's case provided the conditions for which Wilson had asked.[51]

The years from 1930 to 1940 were the most productive in Wilson's career. Fortified with his knowledge of mathematics and intrigued by the new concept of bundle branch block, he set out to study anew the process of ventricular excitation. Needed for these studies was a direct lead for animal use and a semidirect, precordial lead, as nearly unipolar as possible, for use in man. To meet this need Newburgh developed the central terminal; this device utilized an indifferent electrode connected to each of the three extremity leads through resistances of 5000 ohms. Using unipolar electrocardiography, Wilson and his associates soon established that the Lewis concept of what was right and what left bundle branch block was reversed. He also did important studies relating to myocardial infarction, which led to further systematic elucidation of the phenomena of normal ventricular excitation. Much of what we now know concerning endocardial potentials, the intrinsic deflection, and Q waves has been derived from this research.

In 1932 Franklin D. Johnston joined the staff. He not only took an active part in many of the studies mentioned but also did a great deal of work on the registration of heart sounds and on the adaptation of the cathode-ray oscillograph to the study of the electrocardiogram.[52]

## The Thomas Henry Simpson Memorial Institute for Medical Research[53]

When the Simpson Memorial Institute was established in 1927,[54] its first director was Cyrus C. Sturgis. Although the original goal of the institute was for research on pernicious anemia, it was later expanded to include the whole of hematology. Sturgis's research interests were leukemia and pernicious anemia. He demonstrated that material from the wall of the hog's stomach, *ventriculin,* was effective in producing remissions in pernicious anemia.[55]

### Raphael Isaacs[56]

Sturgis appointed Raphael Isaacs as an assistant director of the institute. Isaacs (M.D., Cincinnati, 1918) joined George R. Minot's research team at the Huntington Memorial Laboratory in 1923. Weekly conferences between the groups in Boston conducting research on pernicious anemia brought him into contact with William P. Murphy, Cyrus C. Sturgis, Francis W. Peabody, Joseph T. Wearn, and William B. Castle.

In 1924 Issacs studied the effects of exercise on the distribution of corpuscles in the blood stream, the properties of young erythrocytes in relation to agglutination, and their behavior in hemorrhage and transfusion. He made a quantitative analysis of hemagglutination and hemolysis. In 1924 Minot and Isaacs published the first definitive article on the effect of x-ray on malignant lymphoma. They found no prolongation of life.[57]

From 1927 to 1940 there was a continuing flow of hematologic studies from the institute; largely the result of the close collaboration between Sturgis and Isaacs.[58] Isaacs described the *Isaac granule*—the last vestige of reticulum in the maturing red cell before it attains its full hemoglobin complement.[59]

## The Second Director of the Institute: Frank H. Bethel

Frank H. Bethel (M.D., Johns Hopkins, 1929) was appointed an instructor in medicine and a research assistant at the institute in 1931. He was named assistant director in 1942, associate director in 1954, and succeeded Sturgis as director in 1956. His promotion to a professor of medicine came in 1948. In addition to investigations of pernicious anemia, his early work centered on nutritional anemias and the anemias of pregnancy.[60] He received the Henry Russell Award, a university-wide prize for outstanding investigation, in 1939. Beginning in 1943, much of his effort was devoted to an Atomic Energy Commission project on the biological effects of irradiation on bone marrow and the reticuloendothelial system. He was also a pioneer in the investigation of the hematologic effects of adrenocortical steroids.

## Other Clinical Investigators in the Department of Medicine

Henry L. Field, Jr.,[61] came to Michigan from the MGH in 1927. He remained at Ann Arbor until 1944, when he joined the clinical faculty at Buffalo. He was a member of the American Society for Clinical Investigation.

Millard Smith[62] came to Ann Arbor in 1927 as a research associate at the institute and an instructor in medicine. Smith (M.D., Harvard, 1923) worked for two years at the Thorndike Memorial Laboratory, developing an interest in rheumatic diseases. He returned to Boston in 1930 to enter private practice.

Herman Harlan Riecker[63] came to Michigan from Cornell in 1927 and left to enter private practice in 1943. His research interests were in rheumatic fever and various aspects of gastrointestinal disease. He was a member of the American Society for Clinical Investigation.

John Blair Barnwell[64] became director of the tuberculosis unit in November 1928. He had been a research instructor in pediatrics at Pennsylvania and a fellow and an acting first assistant of the Trudeau Foundation. He left Ann Arbor in 1946 to become director of the tuberculosis section in the Veterans Administration.

Charles L. Brown[65] graduated from the University of Oklahoma School of Medicine and received further training at the Peter Bent Brigham Hospital. He came to Michigan in 1928 and left in 1935 to become chairman of the department at Temple University. William Dodd Robinson[66] received his M.D. degree from Michigan in 1934. During his residency he became interested in shifts in water between the intracellular and extracellular compartments and joined Newburgh's group. Although not much progress could be made on his problem using the existing techniques, Robinson learned a great deal from Newburgh at a time when the quantitative thinking of physical chemistry was beginning to be applied to clinical problems. Robinson joined Field's laboratory group, which was studying nutrition. Thiamine was investigated in normal subjects and in a variety of clinical situations. In 1940 Robinson worked in nutrition with Youmans at Vanderbilt. In 1944 Robinson returned to Michigan as an assistant professor of medicine, was made a professor in 1952, and served as chairman of the department from 1958 to 1975. His research interest was arthritis.

Michigan's outstanding contribution to clinical science was aptly summarized by William Henry Howell, a Michigan graduate and the first professor of physiology at Johns Hopkins:

> When the methods of the experimental sciences began to penetrate into the field of medicine, some of the older and more influential schools failed to adjust themselves to the new conditions and thereby lost gradually their prestige. The Medical Department of this University, on the contrary, was among the first to adopt the newer methods of instruction, and early enrolled itself among the progressive schools in this country. It adds much, I think, to the credit of the University that all of its good work in this direction was done quietly and modestly without undue flourish of trumpets. Its behavior in this respect contrasts favorably with that of some of our eastern schools, which, when forced by the pressure of competition to modernize their methods, have been quick to make a virtue of their necessity and have attempted to claim among their own clientèle the advantages of leadership, when as a matter of fact all they have been entitled to has been a high privacy in the rear rank.[67]

# 19

⚜

# The Emergence of Chicago as a Force
# in Twentieth-Century Medicine

By 1900 Chicago was a center of attention in the medical world. Its rapidly progressive growth from a frontier outpost to a busy city led to a revolution in medical as well as in cultural and scientific life in general.[1]

Surgery was the first specialty to advance, and among many outstanding surgeons was Christian Fenger. Fenger studied at the University of Copenhagen under Peter Ludwig Panum, a pupil of Claude Bernard. Fenger arrived at Chicago in 1877, and his lectures at the Cook County Hospital soon became famous. At the West Chicago Medical Society meeting in 1879, he demonstrated the bacterial nature of endocarditis—the first demonstration of pathogenic bacteria in Chicago. Fenger attracted many important students, including such celebrated surgeons as J. B. Murphy and William J. Mayo. Three of his trainees later became eminent pathologists: Ludwig Hektoen, E. R. LeCount, and H. Gideon Wells. Hektoen was one of the most influential pathologists in the development of medical science in Chicago.[2] James B. Herrick interned at the County Hospital under Fenger, as did Frank Billings, who later played a vital role in developing Chicago as a medical center. When Rush Medical School became affiliated with the University of Chicago in 1898, Billings was made a professor of medicine. He soon became dean of the school, where for the next twenty years he developed the clinical work at Rush and at the adjoining Presbyterian Hospital. It was largely through Billings's influence that in 1902 the John McCormick Memorial Institute for Infectious Diseases was established.[3]

Another outstanding figure in early Chicago medicine was the surgeon Nicholas Senn, who graduated from the Chicago Medical College in 1868. Senn recognized early the importance of clinical microscopy, animal experimentation, and antisepsis. He organized his own experi-

343

mental laboratory. Senn was among the first to report the x-ray treatment of leukemia.[4] In 1878 Senn was appointed a professor of surgery at Rush.

## Early Facilities for Clinical Research in Chicago

### The John McCormick Memorial Institute for Infectious Diseases

The McCormick Institute was organized in 1902 by Billings, Herrick, and Hektoen, who was its director. The record of the institute and the associated Anna Durand Hospital for Contagious Diseases, whose medical service was headed by George Weaver, was excellent. The *Journal of Infectious Diseases* was started and, under Hektoen's editorship, immediately took high rank as a scientific publication. The institute, which was affiliated with the University of Chicago, was transferred to its campus in 1941.

Ludwig Hektoen was a professor of pathology at Rush Medical College from 1898 to 1933 and head of the department of pathology at the University of Chicago from 1901 to 1930. Between 1903 and 1937 his research was concerned with the typing of blood, antibodies, allergy, and experimental measles.[5] Hektoen was among the first to suggest that by properly selecting blood donors the danger of blood transfusion could be averted. His first laboratory, located in the basement of the old Rush Laboratory Building, was a haven for scientific work of quality. The new institute laboratory on Wood Street and the Anna Durand Hospital later provided opportunity for fundamental studies on blood transfusion, scarlet fever, measles,[6] pneumonia, and streptococcal infection.

#### Scarlet Fever

The studies of George and Gladys Dick on scarlet fever were done under Hektoen's supervision. The discovery of the etiology of scarlet fever can be traced from the 1919 study of Dochez, Avery, and Lancefield on the antigenic relationships between strains of *Streptococcus hemolyticus*.[7] Hemolytic streptococci from human sources were shown, by agglutination reactions with immune sera prepared in animals and by protection tests, to fall into at least four biological types.

Walter Bliss found that about 80 percent of strains of hemolytic streptococcus from patients in the first week of scarlet fever were agglutinated by four different antistreptococcic sera made from similar organisms. He concluded that the streptococci from scarlet fever comprised a specific type.[8] Future work showed his view to be incorrect, but it was a stimulus to further studies, including the definitive human inoculation experiments of the Dicks.

The Dicks swabbed the tonsils of two volunteers with a forty-eight-hour culture of hemolytic streptococcus isolated from the throat of a scarlet fever patient. One volunteer developed typical scarlet fever, with sore throat, fever, leukocytosis, rash, desquamation, etc. The authors concluded that "since the streptococci used in these experiments have fulfilled the requirements of Koch's laws, it may be concluded that they cause scarlet fever."[9]

Although the Dicks deserve credit for the final proof that streptococcus is the cause of scarlet fever, the logical approach to the problem by Dochez and his associates was equally important.

The observations of the Dicks on soluble toxins in scarlet fever were of fundamental importance in leading to the final understanding of the disease. Simultaneously with their work, Dochez expressed the view that the "principal localization of the infection is in the throat in most instances and ... there the streptococcus in question elaborates a toxin which is absorbed and produces the rash and general symptoms."[10] It was, however, the Dicks who first prepared a usable "toxin" from filtrates of cultures of streptococci obtained from scarlet fever patients; they showed that an intracutaneous injection of this filtrate practically never produced a skin reaction in people convalescent from scarlet fever or with a history of a previous attack, whereas persons who had no previous history of scarlet fever had a positive test. This was the basis of the Dick test.[11]

The Dicks's next communications dealt with the production of an antitoxic serum by immunizing a horse with the toxic filtrate of cultures.[12] It was ultimately shown that the antitoxin acted mainly on the rash and perhaps certain toxic symptoms, but did not have the antibacterial action necessary to eliminate the streptococcal infection.

George Dick served as chairman of the department of medicine at Chicago from 1933 to 1946.[13] He graduated from the Rush Medical School, interned at Cook County Hospital, and did postgraduate work at the universities of Vienna and Munich. After World War I, he became head of the department of medicine at Rush and remained there until 1933, when he moved to Chicago.

Another of Hektoen's associates was Howard Taylor Ricketts, who made brilliant contributions to the study of the pathogenesis of this disease and of Rocky Mountain Spotted Fever[14] before his premature death from typhus fever.

## The Otho A. Sprague Memorial Institute[15]

Although the Sprague Institute had no laboratories and no paid staff, it aided greatly in the development of clinical investigation in the Midwest.[16]

Otho A. Sprague, who died of tuberculosis in 1910, had bequeathed securities to his brother Albert, to be used in the relief of human suffering. Albert Sprague obtained a charter, on June 30, 1910, for the Otho A. Sprague Memorial Institute. The board decided to concentrate support in the Chicago area and selected H. Gideon Wells,[17] a professor of pathology at the University of Chicago, as the "Director of Research." The trustees of the institute held their first organizational meeting on January 6, 1911. At that time, only eighteen foundations of all types existed in the United States, and probably none was devoted exclusively to medicine. (The Rockefeller Foundation was not established until 1913.) The Sprague trustees decided to provide support for investigators already working in hospitals and medical schools. Assisting Wells on the advisory council were Frank Billings, E. R. LeCount, Ludwig Hektoen, Joseph Miller (an internist), E. O. Jordan (a bacteriologist at the University of Chicago), and Julius Steiglitz (chairman of chemistry at Chicago).

A distinguished group of investigators was selected: Rollin T. Woodyatt, Henry F. Helmholz, Evarts A. Graham, and Henry Corper. Helmholz later became head of pediatrics at the Mayo Clinic. Graham, who became chairman of surgery at Washington University, devised the Graham-Cole test for visualization of the gall bladder and was the first surgeon to remove a human lung for cancer. Corper was research director at the Municipal Tuberculosis Sanitorium in Chicago.

### Rollin T. Woodyatt

Rollin T. Woodyatt,[18] after research training under Nef and Steiglitz at Chicago and then under Friedrich von Müller of Munich, was chosen as the principal investigator at the Presbyterian Hospital. Woodyatt organized his laboratory adjacent to eight research beds, all fully subsidized by Sprague funds. This was one of the first clinical research facilities in the United States.[19] The center operated effectively for about twenty-five years and was chiefly concerned with various problems of carbohydrate metabolism. Many important fellows received their training there, including Wilder, Sansum, Colwell, and Keeton. In 1912 Woodyatt was appointed an associate professor of medicine at Rush.

One of Woodyatt's research interests was the study of diabetes. He found the Allen method of treating diabetes by fasting not altogether satisfactory. In severe cases, the patient was reduced to a skeleton. Woodyatt dealt a serious blow to the Allen treatment by pointing out that the important thing was not what one fed the patient in terms of protein, carbohydrate, and fat, but what the patient burned, that is, the composition of the metabolic mixture.

After 1923 Woodyatt devoted his attention to the use of insulin. In studying the diabetic defect he sought to identify the products of dissociation of glucose within the body by using as a model the in vitro studies of Nef on the dissociation of glucose in alkaline solutions.[20]

Arthur Ralph Colwell, Sr., a long-time associate of Woodyatt's in the practice of medicine, wrote of him as follows: "According to my standards, his was the finest medical mind this city has produced in this century, and many of his colleagues and students have been profoundly influenced by it. . . . Rollin Woodyatt was completely satisfied with the results which he knew and saw. . . . He was amply rewarded, I know, by the certainty that he exerted constructive forces at fundamental levels."[21]

Another of Woodyatt's pupils, Robert Wood Keeton[22] (M.D., Northwestern, 1916), served as an assistant in pharmacology for two years. His interest then turned to physiology. He completed a study of the secretion of gastric juice after parathyroidectomy under the direction of A. J. Carlson. Thereafter he worked on such varied problems as diabetes, obesity, metabolism, toxic hepatitis, hyperthyroidism, and the physiological adjustment to changes of environment. Appointed an assistant professor of pharmacology at Illinois, Keeton transferred in 1925 to the department of medicine as an associate professor and in 1933 became head of the department.

In 1915 the combined staff of the Sprague Institute consisted of twenty members who were engaged in significant research relating to clinical problems. Graham[23] studied the toxic effects of anesthetics;[24] Helmholz was concerned with the pathways of sugar metabolism in the infant; and Corper and Wells searched for a chemical substance that would destroy or inhibit the tubercle bacillus.

Maude Slye, another recipient of Sprague support, pointed out the possible relationship of cancer and heredity. By her thousands of selective breeding experiments in mice, she was able to produce some sixty-five mice with liver tumors, showing the feasibility of breeding for a tumor of a single organ.

After World War I, a number of clinically oriented projects were supported. Robert Clark worked on kidney disease at the Presbyterian–St. Luke's Hospital. Theodore B. Schwartz studied hormonal influences on cell activity; and Samuel G. Taylor searched for agents for the treatment of breast cancer. The fund also established fellowships and traineeships at the Presbyterian–St. Luke's Hospital.

The institute in 1938 changed its policy of giving grants to private medical schools and hospitals in Chicago for the support of special research projects. With the advent of more federal funding for specific research, the institute devoted most of its income to term grants and supplementary single payment grants to a limited number of Chicago institutions.

## James Bryan Herrick

Herrick[25] graduated from Rush Medical College in 1888. His internship at Cook County Hospital, and ten years of general practice in the horse-and-buggy days, provided his clinical background.

Herrick realized early that chemistry was destined to play an important role in medicine and, in 1904, although forty-three years of age, matriculated at Chicago for courses in this subject. He took a laboratory course in physical chemistry under Julius Steiglitz, then one in organic chemistry under J. U. Nef. He also attended a class in physical chemistry conducted by Alexander Smith, who advised him to pursue the subject further with Emil Fischer in Berlin, which he did for three busy months. At that time, Fischer was studying polypeptides, splitting proteins into their constituent parts, and trying to construct synthetically a compound that approached the complex albumin molecule. Two colleagues from Chicago, Wells and LeCount, also worked in this laboratory. Herrick gives a delightful account of Fischer as a person and the work in the laboratory in his *Memories of Eighty Years.*[26]

Thus, this general practitioner, turned consultant in internal medicine, recognized the importance of clinical science and the application of the techniques of the basic sciences to its study. As a result, in 1908, when the Presbyterian Hospital admitted a patient whose blood examination showed a peculiar crescentlike shape of the red cells—a condition now known as sickle cell anemia—Herrick was ready for the challenge. He appropriately delayed his report until a battery of tests to exclude artifacts had been done and repeated.[27]

Recognition of the symptoms and the signs that characterize coronary occlusion was Herrick's most important accomplishment. Scientific curiosity as to the meaning of what he saw, his expertise in physical diagnosis, and his clinical acumen guided him to the correct conclusion. Sudden obstruction by a thrombus of the coronary artery supplying the muscle of the heart was known as a cause of sudden death. It had been shown that ligation of a coronary artery in animals likewise caused sudden death, although some survived for a few hours or days. After reviewing these facts in his classic paper of 1912, Herrick continued: "But there are reasons for believing that even large branches of the coronary artery may be occluded—at times acutely occluded—without resulting death, at least death in the immediate future. Even the main trunk may at times be obstructed and the patient live. It is the object of this paper . . . to describe some of the clinical manifestations of sudden yet not immediately fatal cases of coronary obstruction."[28]

Herrick's first published paper on the subject in 1912 aroused virtually no interest. In 1918 he read his second paper on coronary thrombosis before the Association of American Physicians, included two more cases with autopsies, and told of the studies of Fred M. Smith on coronary artery occlusion in dogs.[29] Herrick wistfully asked, "Why is it that work done in the laboratory on a dog attracts more attention than that done in the ward on a human being?" From that point on, physicians woke up, and coronary thrombosis soon became a household word.[30]

Before 1917 Herrick had no help from the electrocardiograph. A Cambridge instrument was installed in the Presbyterian Hospital through the generosity of Mrs. Cyrus H. McCormick, and Herrick installed one in his office. Fred M. Smith began his pioneer experiments in ligating the coronaries in dogs, with electrocardiographic studies. Herrick at first outlined the experiments for Smith, with suggestions as to technique. Smith rapidly became independent, however, and published his first important paper on the subject in 1918.[31]

As soon as Smith's studies were underway, he and Herrick searched for a suitable patient to study. Such a patient appeared on May 3, 1917. James R. Greer, Herrick's office assistant, took the electrocardiogram and, after studying it, ventured a diagnosis of acute coronary obstruction—in which diagnosis Smith concurred. This case furnished proof that patients might live for many days after coronary occlusion and that the clinical picture was typical enough to permit a diagnosis during life.

In 1930 Herrick became the sixth recipient of the Kober Medal of the Association of American Physicians;[32] he joined the distinguished company of the previous recipients—Hideyo Noguchi, Theobald Smith, William Henry Welch, Victor Vaughan, and George R. Minot. Fred M. Smith[33] had a fine record as head of the department of internal medicine at the University of Iowa.

## Joseph Almarin Capps

Another who contributed to clinical investigation as a by-product of his medical practice was Capps[34] (M.D., Harvard, 1895). While a student, he demonstrated that leukocytosis occurred during convulsions, and, as a resident at the McLean Hospital, he used a volume index to classify the anemias. Capps obtained an appointment at Rush Medical College, where he rose from an instructor to a professor of medicine.

Over a period of twenty years, Capps carried out studies on the sensory pathways for pain from the pleura, pericardium, and peritoneum. In patients who needed removal of fluid from these body cavities, Capps would insert a wire through the needle and map out the sensitive areas on the serous membrane surfaces.[35]

Capps was a founding member of the Central Society for Clinical Research, a founding member and president of the American Society for Clinical Investigation, and president of the Association of American Physicians. The annual Joseph A. Capps Award for the best original investigation by a young graduate of a Chicago medical school was established in his honor by LeCount in the Institute of Medicine.

## The Development of Medicine in the University of Chicago[36]

One of President Rainey Harper's keenest desires when the University of Chicago was founded was to develop a great medical school. As a beginning, an affiliation was effected in 1898 between the University of

Chicago and Rush Medical College. In 1901 the trustees of Rush Medical College requested that the University of Chicago receive students in the first two years of medicine to do their work in the university laboratories. To this the university agreed, and, after that time, Rush Medical College made no provision for work in the preclinical branches of medicine.

President Harper recruited a bevy of outstanding scientists, including Michelson, Whitman, Mall, Donaldson, and Nef, to Chicago in time for the school's opening in 1892. They were soon joined by Jacques Loeb, Lewellys Franklin Barker, and others; thus, a great faculty in both the physical and biological sciences was created essentially overnight.

It was during his tenure at Chicago that Mall (see chapter 4) crystallized his ideas on medical education as an integral part of the university. On February 28, 1902, Barker,[37] then a professor of anatomy at Chicago, gave an address, undoubtedly stimulated by the influence of Mall, in which he emphasized that the university hospital clinic should be staffed by men possessed of the same talents as other university professors and that these men should give their whole time and energy to teaching and to investigating the nature of disease, that is, they should not engage in private practice. This was certainly among the first explicit American references to research as a function of the departments in the clinical branches of medicine and to the principle of "whole-time" appointments in university hospitals.

Also in 1902, John M. Dobson,[38] dean of medical students in Rush Medical College and the University of Chicago, published an important paper in which he stated that "the medical school must be made an intimate, integral part of the university" and that "this means, in the first place, the provision of a corps of teachers in each of the clinical branches who, divorced entirely from the labors and distractions of active practice, may devote themselves unreservedly to teaching and investigation in their several departments." In 1903 Frank Billings, then a professor of medicine and dean of Rush as well as a lecturer in medicine at Chicago, made a plea for research in the clinical branches in his presidential address before the American Medical Association. Billings proposed that "the hospital should be constructed with a definite idea of teaching students and of making researches into the nature, cause, and treatment of disease."[39] In 1905 President Harper appointed Billings as a professor of medicine in the University of Chicago, a position he held without portfolio until he reached emeritus status in 1924.[40]

From 1900 until his death in 1906, Harper made a determined effort to get the support of John D. Rockefeller for the medical school and hospital. The plans temporarily attracted the attention of F. T. Gates, but there was keen competition from a group in New York supporting the interests of the newly created Rockefeller Institute for Medical Research. The balance turned toward the New York enterprise.

In 1916 President Harry Pratt Judson invited Abraham Flexner to make recommendations concerning the program in medicine. Flexner suggested that new departments with appropriate clinical facilities should be created in close physical and administrative relationship with the preclinical departments. This plan was accepted by the board of trustees, and $5.3 million had been raised by 1917; however, there was a long delay due to World War I.

In 1923 a committee was appointed from the university senate to advise President Ernest DeWitt Burton on medical developments. Their report stated that "the aim of the University of Chicago Medical School should not be primarily to increase the number of practitioners . . . further progress in medicine depends upon the advancement of medical knowledge and it is believed that the University of Chicago is in a peculiarly favorable position for promoting research and training investigators in the medical sciences."[41] Thus the principles were clear: first, that clinical departments should be established at the university; second, that these departments should be university departments, in every sense of the word; and third, that the departments should have for their "chief aim the advancement of the medical sciences," as to both teaching and research. The person who should receive major credit for making these plans a reality was Billings. The success of the fund-raising campaign was largely due to his personal efforts. He secured a contribution of $1 million from the Billings family for the establishment of the Albert Merritt Billings Hospital.

President Burton devoted much of his energy to the development of medical education at the university. Appointments to the new clinical departments were made, and plans for the medical building were gotten underway. The objective was to provide close relationships between the clinical departments and the Ogden Graduate School of Science. The medical faculty was later incorporated into the new division of biological sciences.

Franklin C. McLean (M.D., Rush, 1908) was chosen as professor of medicine and later as director of the university's clinic.[42] He interned at Cook County Hospital and, in 1911, became a professor of pharmacology at the University of Oregon, a post he held for three years, during which time he published the first quantitative method of determining blood sugar in health and disease.[43] In 1913 he worked with Otto Loewi in Graz, Austria. McLean then accepted an appointment as an assistant resident at the HRI. There he remained for two years, working with Van Slyke on the application of chemical methods to the study of human disease and with Alfred E. Cohn on clinical problems. He studied chloride excretion in pneumonia and urea clearance in nephritis.[44] To his tutors at the Rockefeller Institute, he represented a model of the new medical scientist who would solve problems of disease with the instruments of physics and chemistry.

In 1916 McLean was appointed professor of medicine and director of the Peking Union Medical College, which had been established by the Rockefeller Foundation. His interest in the study of blood as a physicochemical system was initiated when he spent several months in 1919–20 with Lawrence J. Henderson. When the Peking Union Medical College was ready for its first class in 1920, he took up his responsibilities there. In 1922 Van Slyke joined him as a visiting professor, and they, together with Hsien Wu, completed their classic studies of gas and electrolyte equilibria in blood.[45]

McLean returned to Chicago in 1923 and, while the new buildings were under construction, spent his time on the organization and selection of a professional staff. Among those recruited were Emmet B. Bay, Lester R. Dragstedt, Paul C. Hodges, Charles B. Huggins, C. Phillip Miller, Louis Leiter, Richard Richter, Walter L. Palmer, and Chester A. Keefer (the first chief medical resident). Patients were admitted and instruction in the clinical departments was begun on October 3, 1927.

The University's statement in 1923 made it clear that it was entering the field of medical education and research with goals well in advance of those of most other schools. This led some to believe that the university would not concern itself sufficiently with the instruction of medical students or with the quality of medical service to patients, so that the following statement was issued: "It does not imply a neglect of teaching, with which all departments are concerned, or of the care of patients, which responsibility the clinical departments must assume in addition to their teaching and research activities, but does imply that, by limitation in numbers of students and of patients, both time and means may be conserved for research activity."[46]

The first clinical departments—medicine and surgery—and subsequent ones were unique. The university had established departments in the basic sciences some twenty-five years before it undertook to make direct provision for the clinical branches of medicine. The preclinical departments were incorporated within the Ogden Graduate School of Science, together with other departments in the biological sciences, as well as those in the physical sciences. Thus these departments were firmly entrenched as university rather than medical school departments. The science faculty of the university was convinced that the same ground rules that had kept the preclinical departments within the framework of the scientific activities of the university should also apply to the new clinical departments. When the university was reorganized into divisions in 1930, all of the departments concerned with medicine, together with zoology and botany, were incorporated into the new division of biological sciences. This organization afforded the clinical branches of medicine the same opportunity of developing into productive scientific departments that was provided earlier for the preclinical branches.

## Full-time Clinical Professorships

The faculty was organized on the full-time principle. William Henry Welch said, in a convocation address at the University of Chicago on

December 17, 1907, that "the heads of the principal clinical departments, particularly the medical and the surgical, should devote their main energies and time to their hospital work and to teaching and investigating without the necessity of seeking their livelihoods in a busy outside practice and without allowing such practice to become their chief professional occupation."[47]

Even before acceptance of a grant from the General Education Board in 1917, the program was based upon the original Johns Hopkins plans; a stipulation written into the contract with the board. The Johns Hopkins plan depended, however, on the availability of a hospital with large "charity" services and was not suited to the conditions in Chicago. Before the clinic opened in 1927, it became necessary to develop a new plan, which was without precedent. Basically this plan rested on an adaptation of the group practice of medicine to medical education. It provided that every member of the clinical faculty be paid a salary by the university, in return for which he gave his entire professional time to his university duties. In the beginning, the hospital offered medical services to all economic classes. The concept was successful at first, but, by the mid-thirties, the United States was in the midst of the Great Depression, and it became obvious that patient income alone would not be sufficient. At that time the charity patient, or the patient supported by public funds who had been cared for because his condition was important for the purposes of teaching and research, virtually disappeared from the clinic, except where special funds were available for the study of a particular disease. Soon the clientele was almost entirely derived from that middle-income group who either paid their own way or whose charges were met by a third party, such as Blue Cross.

Throughout this period, the fundamental concepts of the medical center continued to be those described in 1931 by Franklin C. McLean. The concepts may be summed up as follows:

1) Scientific, clinical and experimental investigation, a superior quality of medical education and the best possible practice of medicine constitute the three functions of the clinical departments. These three activities—research, teaching and the practice of medicine—are mutually dependent upon one another, for teaching and the practice of medicine are best carried out in an atmosphere of research . . . 2) . . . The primary functions of a university are teaching and research. It engages in clinical medicine for two purposes only: to acquire patients as teaching and research material and to help those patients whose particular ailment put them beyond the skill and facilities of individual medical practice. The full-time plan, in relieving the faculty member of many worries and responsibilities relevant to private practice, provides him with more time for research and better facilities for investigation . . . 3) The clinical departments do not constitute a unit by themselves but form part of the larger division of the biological sciences. Such an organization has the effect of integrating the studies and interests of the clinicians with those of the preclinical faculty . . ."[48]

The faculty's performance was outstanding, as shown by the many awards that they received. At that time, the National Academy of Sciences generally reserved its honors for those engaged in abstract research, but a number of the University of Chicago faculty were made members, including Paul Cannon, professor and chairman of the department of pathology; Lowell T. Coggeshall, dean of the division of the biological sciences and Frank H. Rawson Distinguished Service Professor of Medicine; Charles B. Huggins, professor of urology; O. H. Robertson, professor of medicine; Lester R. Dragstedt, Thomas D. Jones Distinguished Service Professor and chairman of the department of surgery; C. Phillip Miller, professor of medicine; and others in later years.

## The Department of Medicine

Russell Wilder described the organization of the department of medicine in 1931: "For the purpose of carrying on its clinical and teaching duties and research the Department is subdivided into sections ... the advantages of the specialization which this subdivision involves outweigh the disadvantages; the patient benefits from it materially ... and the advancement of knowledge should be promoted more effectively."[49] The men in charge of these divisions were mature clinical investigators and leaders in their fields: renal and vascular disease, Louis Leiter;[50] gastroenterology, W. L. Palmer; pulmonary disease, Robert Bloch; metabolism, Russell Wilder; infectious disease, Oswald H. Robertson and C. Philip Miller; and cardiology, Emmet B. Bay. The department also was responsible for such major specialties of medicine as neurology, dermatology, radiology, preventive medicine, and public health; and it encompassed such diverse fields of investigation as enzyme chemistry, histochemistry, and the history of medicine.

The research areas included:

1. in the biological division (Robertson and Miller), intensive studies of the patient from the immunological, physiological, and chemical points of view, with correlated observations on the disease produced experimentally in animals. An attempt was made to gain information about the metabolic activities of the etiological agent and certain physiological alterations occurring in the diseased individual. Miller studied the growth requirements of the gonococcus as well as the cell constituents and immunological reactions of this microorganism[51]

2. in the metabolism division, Wilder studied the action of the parathyroid hormone in chronic experiments stimulated by observations on clinical hyperparathyroidism. A study of the effect of environment on the histology of the thyroid was made by Allan T. Kenyon

3. in the renal-vascular section, studies concerned such fundamental problems as the relation of low plasma proteins to experimental

edema; the physiology of purine-induced diuresis with reference to the modern theories of urine formation; and the question of the role of allergy to bacterial products in the experimental production of diffuse nephritis

4. in gastroenterology, Palmer and his group were chiefly concerned with the problem of peptic ulcer, the mechanism of gastric pain, and the effect of alkalis on the acid-base balance of the blood. T. E. Henry studied the effect of insulin on gastric motility and hunger. The division studied the disturbed physiology of the colon in disease states. An effort was made to produce chronic ulcer in dogs—work done in collaboration with W. J. Gallagher of the department of physiology

5. in the pulmonary disease section, clinical studies were made with tuberculin prepared on synthetic media by Esmond Long and Florence Seebert; on the behavior of the heart and mediastinum in lung collapse; and on the effects of lung collapse in rabbits kept continually under artificial pneumothorax

The successive chairmen of the department of medicine were Franklin C. McLean, Russell Wilder, Oswald H. Robertson (pro tempore), George Dick, Lowell T. Coggeshall, Wright Adams, and Leon Jacobsen.

In 1933 Franklin McLean,[52] aged forty-five, left medical administration completely and, for the ensuing thirty-five years, studied calcium, its metabolism, and the physiology of bone as a tissue.[53] He determined for the first time calcium-ion concentration in body fluids and demonstrated that calcium and plasma proteins combine according to the law of mass action. He also developed the feed-back hypothesis for the mode of action of parathyroid hormone, a theory that, though incomplete, led indirectly to the later discovery of calcitonin.[54]

In the early period, Robertson and his group made extensive studies of pneumonia. In 1906 Oswald H. Robertson[55] entered the premedical course at the University of California, where as a first-year student he studied the complement fixation test for rabies in the laboratory of Frederick P. Gay. He entered Harvard Medical School and later won a Dalton Scholarship Award to study pernicious anemia at the MGH, where he interned in 1913–14. He then became an assistant in pathology at the Rockefeller Institute for Medical Research, where he continued his studies on the physiology of blood in the laboratories of Peyton Rous. He interrupted his work to join the Harvard team led by Harvey Williams Cushing in France in World War I and was assigned the task of finding ways to reduce the risks of transfusion. Robertson created the "first blood bank" by using a fluid devised by Rous in the laboratory to preserve human blood cells in vitro. He showed that such cells were, indeed, an acceptable substitute for fresh blood. On his return to the Rockefeller, his studies were in the field of infectious diseases, first with

Noguchi and then with Avery. In the latter's laboratory, he became interested in the pneumococcus and pneumonia, the study of which held his attention for more than twenty years. He accepted an offer from Peking Union Medical College to become an associate professor of medicine; he became a professor of medicine and remained in China for eight years.

Robertson's classic work at Chicago was on the pathogenesis of pneumococcal pneumonia.[56] In collaboration with Coggeshall and Terrell, Robertson demonstrated in the dog that the pneumococcus was carried in infected edema fluid, from alveolus to alveolus, from lobule to lobule and from lobe to lobe. When the discovery of the sulfonamides indicated that simple effective therapy of pneumonia was possible, Robertson turned his attention to prevention. Beginning in 1939, his group elucidated the factors of air-borne infections and especially the techniques for aerosol disinfection. In this period many outstanding young men and women were trained, including Edward Bigg, Morton Hamburger, Henry Lemon, Clayton Loosli, Benjamin and Zelma Miller, and Theodore Puck.

Russell Wilder became chairman of the department in 1929.[57] During his tenure, he worked on osteitis fibrosa cystica, obesity, Addison's disease, and epilepsy. In 1931 he returned to the Mayo Clinic.

When George Dick became chairman of the department in 1933, the subspecialty system was already well established. Dick was regarded as a superb clinician. He endorsed and nurtured the subspecialty concept, but identified himself as a general internist and established the "Professor's service," which was in essence his own general medical service. During his long tenure as chairman, tension developed between the subspecialty services and the new general internal medicine service. In 1938 the general medical service occupied 20 of the 120 beds,[58] but by 1945 this service utilized about one-third of the beds assigned to the department. The departmental attitude toward this service is reflected in the action taken at the first faculty meeting following Dick's retirement in 1945. The faculty voted to disband the general medical service, and the beds were reallocated to the subspecialty groups.[59]

New talent continued to be added over the years to the department. These new additions illustrate once again the interrelationship between the important institutions working toward the development of clinical science in this country. For example, Alf Sven Alving[60] (M.D., Michigan, 1927) worked from 1929 to 1934 with Van Slyke at the Rockefeller Institute. He then received an appointment at Chicago, achieving the rank of professor of medicine in 1944. From 1934 to 1962 he was head of the section on renal-vascular disease. Areas in renal physiology to which he contributed include renal blood flow, and the effects of anoxia, acidosis, hypertension, and diet.

The importance of medical science to other national activities is illustrated by a virtually new career into which Alving was launched during

World War II—the chemotherapy of malaria. The famous Malaria Project was established at Statesville Penitentiary. Alving headed this project from 1944 until his death in 1966. The project represented a union of the highest order between so-called theoretical and applied research. What started out to be practical research turned up many new scientific facts of basic importance. Study of the chemotherapy of malaria ranged from investigations of the compounds under field conditions to fundamental investigations into the mechanism of drug toxicity—leading to the discovery of glucose-6-phosphate dehydrogenase deficiency. One of the high points in this twenty-year program came in 1947, when primaquine was reclaimed from the chemical archives and used for the first time in primate malaria.

## Surgery

One of the important foci of clinical investigation in surgery has been in Chicago. Dallas B. Phemister became the head of surgery at Chicago in 1925, when Dean Lewis was called to Johns Hopkins. Among the important members of the department was Lester R. Dragstedt, whose clinically oriented investigations made him famous in the field of physiological surgery of the gastrointestinal tract.

There are two other "greats" in surgery whose roots began in Chicago—Evarts A. Graham and Charles B. Huggins. Graham graduated in 1907 from Rush Medical School. Graham's primary interest at that time was the effect of anesthesia upon tissues and physiological processes. Graham's early background in Chicago made him one of the few surgeons of the decade 1910 to 1920 with the type of training that research committees were looking for to head full-time departments of surgery.

Huggins was a professor of urology. His outstanding contributions, particularly to the physiology of reproduction and the study of the hormonal influences on carcinoma of the prostate, need no elaboration. These were recognized by the award of the Nobel Prize, which he received along with Rous, of the Rockefeller Institute. A penetrating analysis of the research process was given by Huggins when he received the annual award of the American Urological Association in 1948 for his research on the male reproductive tract.[61]

# 20

❦

# The University of Minnesota School
# of Medicine[1]

On April 7, 1887, it was recommended to the board of regents of the University of Minnesota that a school of medicine of good quality be established. On June 8, 1888, the faculty held its first meeting.

Abraham Flexner, after his visit to the medical school in 1909, concluded that its affairs had been handled effectively under the first two presidents of the university: "Minnesota is perhaps the first state to have solved the most perplexing problems connected with medical education and practice. . . . It is, indeed, still too early to realize its plans for an adequate clinical establishment of modern character; but . . . this is only a question of time."[2]

Shortly after Flexner's report, three individuals joined the university who were to shape the successful course of the school: President George E. Vincent; Guy Stanton Ford, dean of the graduate school; and Elias P. Lyon, professor of physiology and dean of the medical school.

Three outstanding achievements resulted: the teaching of the basic medical sciences was greatly improved; the graduate school activities in medicine were advanced with the cooperation of William J. Mayo, who became a member of the university's board of regents; and the clinical departments were strengthened.

## Evolution of the Basic Sciences

For many years, the department of anatomy, which was led by Clarence M. Jackson from 1912 to 1941, was the most distinguished. Jackson's work concerned inanition and growth. Other outstanding members were Hal Downey, in hematology; Andrew Rasmussen, in neuroanatomy; and E. A. Boyden, who studied gallbladder physiology and segmental anatomy of the lung.

In 1936 Elias P. Lyon was succeeded in physiology by Maurice Visscher, who not only did significant work in intestinal and cardiovascular physiology but also selected surgical residents to work in his laboratory, thus laying the foundation for important advances in gastrointestinal and cardiovascular surgery.

E. T. Bell headed the department of pathology. Pharmacology was directed by Arthur D. Hirschfelder, who had trained under Abel at Johns Hopkins and was interested in cardiology. The department of microbiology, headed by Dr. Winifred Larson, was strengthened by Arthur Henrici, whose book *Molds, Yeasts and Actinomyces* remains a classic.

There was a close relationship both intellectually and geographically between the basic and clinical sciences. Thus, the brilliant cluster of basic scientists at the university contributed greatly to the success of clinical science at Minnesota.

## The Graduate School

On December 19, 1905, the board of regents formally established a graduate school. In the *University Bulletin* (1909–10), it was stated that "the degree of master of arts or master of sciences is open to graduates of the College of Medicine and Surgery who are also bachelors of arts or sciences. Candidates must pursue approved courses in the College of Medicine and Surgery for at least one year after taking the degree of doctor of medicine." Along with the research activities in the department of anatomy, under Jackson, which began in 1913, the graduate fellowship program stimulated research in the clinical departments. On December 4, 1913, the administrative board appointed Drs. Hirschfelder, J. B. Johnston, and Frank Corbett to a Committee on Research and, on January 9, 1914, recommended a classification of students: (1) graduate students who are not doing research; (2) physicians and others who are doing research but are not candidates for degrees; and (3) candidates for advanced degrees granted by the graduate school who are finishing their research in the College of Medicine.

In July 1914, the Committee on Research made the following recommendations regarding the graduate school of medicine: (1) that requirements for admission to graduate work include the possession of an M.D. degree from a recognized medical college or university as well as one year's internship in an approved general hospital or an approved equivalent of service; (2) that the graduate course cover a period of three years, leading to the degree of doctor of science (that is, doctor of science in surgery); and (3) that a candidate for the degree should be required to do at least the last year's work in the University of Minnesota. The committee also recommended a graduate medical student program of three nine-month academic years. Students in this program would not be assigned any teaching or other service and would be allowed a free range of graduate medical study. Tuition fees would be $150 a year.

Another important step was affiliation with the Mayo Clinic. When this was first proposed by President Vincent in 1913, it created a storm of protest from many private practitioners; but their opposition was successfully dealt with, and an antiaffiliation bill died in the legislature. The Mayo Foundation was incorporated in 1915, and, in 1917, the Mayo Foundation for Medical Education and Research became affiliated with the graduate school of the University of Minnesota.[3]

When Guy Stanton Ford became dean of the graduate school in 1912, only two persons had previously been granted the Ph.D. degree in the field of medicine. It was the original plan to have medical graduate work directed by the medical school; however, Dean Ford encouraged and welcomed the plan of having this work conducted in the graduate school, as was done by other departments and schools of the university.

Each student, with the assistance of his advisor and the approval of the dean, mapped out a program best fitted to his individual needs, both laboratory and clinical. The graduate student worked largely under the direct personal guidance of his supervisor, thus preserving the advantages of the preceptor or apprentice system. A thesis was required, in connection with which the student was trained for scientific work in his special field. The extent of the thesis research varied according to the degree sought. For the degree of doctor of philosophy, an extensive original study, representing a substantial contribution to knowledge, was necessary. From 1914–15 through 1930–31, a total of 429 graduate degrees in the medical specialties, including both medical and laboratory subjects, were conferred. Of this number, 177 were at the university, including 123 master's and 54 doctor's of philosophy degrees; 252 were at the Mayo Foundation, including 238 master's and 14 doctor's of philosophy. The graduate school granted 41 of these degrees during 1930–31; 12 were master's and 5 doctor's of philosophy at Minneapolis, and 24 were master's at the Mayo Foundation. Of the graduates who took degrees in laboratory science, some went into clinical work, but many continued their careers in laboratory teaching and research at Minnesota and other universities. Examples of the latter are Cecil J. Watson, who became chairman of the department of medicine at Minnesota, and Owen H. Wangensteen, who headed the department of surgery there.

## Evolution of the Clinical Sciences

Following the Flexner Report of 1910, teaching and research in the basic sciences continued at a high level, but the clinical teachers carried on part-time practice as their dominant activity, and clinical science was lacking.

Charles L. Greene graduated from the University of Minnesota College of Medicine and Surgery in 1890, after which he took some postgraduate courses in Europe. He became a professor of the theory and practice of medicine at Minnesota in 1903 and head of the department of medicine when it was established in 1909. Cardiovascular diseases were his particular interest, and he developed a plan for rehabilitation of cardiac patients. He resigned when the affiliation with the Mayo Clinic was established.[4]

## Medicine under Leonard G. Rowntree

After Greene's resignation as chief of the department of internal medicine, the administrative board decided, on September 13, 1915, that the new chief should be placed on a full-time basis with only restricted consultation practice allowed, and no private off-campus practice. On November 1, Leonard G. Rowntree[5] of Johns Hopkins became the first full-time clinical department chief.

In 1906 Rowntree, after finishing his internship, entered general practice in Camden, New Jersey. In the autumn of 1907 he became a voluntary student in the department of pharmacology at Johns Hopkins. By 1913 he was an associate professor. Rowntree studied the cathartic action of certain phthalein compounds in a joint investigation with Abel.[6] They discovered that some of these compounds were excreted by the kidney and others by the liver. Out of this observation came the phenolsulfonephthalein test for renal function[7] and, later, the tetrachlorphthalein test for hepatic function. When the first full-time staff in internal medicine was organized at Johns Hopkins in 1914, Rowntree joined as associate professor.

Rowntree spent sixteen years in Minnesota; the early years on the campus in Minneapolis and, from 1919 to 1932, in the Mayo Foundation and Clinic at Rochester.

When Rowntree became a professor, Millard Hall (the medical school building) was a spacious three-story, red brick building, with large rooms and unusually high ceilings. On the next square, mounted on the bluff overlooking the Mississippi, stood the University Hospital (the Elliott Hospital), which contained approximately 170 beds. There were additional clinical facilities in the Minneapolis General Hospital and in the Ancher Hospital in St. Paul. Hirschfelder was continuing his pharmacological studies on digitalis, with the aid of the electrocardiograph. Kingsbury was interested in hippuric acid as a test of liver function. S. Marx White[8] had been the acting professor of medicine. The medical department had fifty-eight staff members, but, beside Rowntree, only one other full-time individual. This was Francis G. Blake, who later became a professor of medicine at Yale. Archie Beard came from the Peter Bent Brigham Hospital as Rowntree's first resident physician.

In Baltimore, Rowntree had become interested in the standardization of digitalis. In Minneapolis, the School of Pharmacy was cultivating digitalis plants, and Rowntree learned that digitalis grew wild in some of the western states. A project was developed in which Boy Scouts shipped digitalis to the School of Pharmacy. Standardized tinctures were made, which opened up a source for the drug in the United States. Rowntree developed a technique for the graphic recording of tendon reflexes. His major interest was, however, blood pH and the role of buffers in acidosis and alkalosis. He and Leo Hart, of the Mayo Clinic, found that alkalosis not infrequently develops in patients under treatment for peptic ulcer. Rowntree made pioneer studies of basal metabolism with Albert M. Snell and Francis Ford.

In 1919 Rowntree joined the staff at the Mayo Clinic in Rochester (see chapter 21). He was succeeded by White.

## The Department of Medicine from 1919 to 1945

S. Marx White, who was chairman (on a part-time basis) from 1919 to 1925, received his M.D. degree from Northwestern in 1897 and came to Minnesota in 1898 to teach bacteriology and pathology. He studied in Vienna in 1904. In 1908 he transferred to the department of medicine, under Greene. He brought the first electrocardiograph to the University of Minnesota in 1914, after studying under Sir Thomas Lewis. In 1921 he participated in the formation of the Nicollet Clinic in Minneapolis. He concluded that a full-time chief was required and resigned in 1925, although he continued as a part-time clinical professor.

In 1921 George Fahr joined the faculty at Minnesota and, by 1923, was the only full-time member of senior rank in the department. He was, for a short time, on the staff of the University of Wisconsin, following a long sojourn in Europe, where he had worked under von Müller in Munich and Einthoven in Leyden. He fully shared von Müller's philosophy that a professor of medicine should not be highly specialized, except in his own personal research. In 1927 Fahr was made chief of the medical service at the Minneapolis General Hospital and established an excellent unit for teaching and research. Zondek was probably the first to draw attention to "myxedema heart," but Fahr extended his observations. Fahr found that digitalis produced no definite change in the cardiac status, whereas thyroid extract caused remarkable reversal toward normal function.[9]

After White's resignation, Hilding Berglund, a Swedish medical scientist, was brought from the Peter Bent Brigham Hospital as chairman of the department. His thesis for his M.D. degree in 1920 was titled "The Secretion of Urinary Tissues"—a study inspired by the work of Volhard and Fahr. From 1921 to 1923 he served as a fellow and an assistant in biochemistry, under Otto Folin. His main interest was in the plasma proteins, cystinuria, and gout.[10] At Minnesota he studied uric acid metabolism, secretion of gastric juice, pernicious anemia, and renal function. In 1928 he went to the Peking Union Medical College as a visiting professor for nine months.[11] On his return in 1929, he recruited Hobart A. Reimann, whom he had known in China, and who had had extensive training and experience in infectious disease and had worked at the HRI.

Berglund organized a superb international symposium on renal disease, the first of its kind, which was held in Minneapolis in 1930. The papers were published in a classic monograph that was coedited by Berglund, Grace Medes, Carl Huber, Warfield Theobald Longcope, and A. N. Richards.[12] Personal difficulties led to Berglund's resignation, after which he returned to Sweden in 1933.

In the 1930s, stability entered into the full-time appointments of the clinical staff, which resulted in first-rate clinical science. In 1933 the department was composed of three divisions: internal medicine, neuropsychiatry, and dermatology. John Charnley McKinley, director of the division of neuropsychiatry, became the department's acting head in 1933 and the permanent head a year later. He served in that capacity until the formation of the department of neurology and psychiatry, of which he became chief in 1943.

Hobart A. Reimann served as director of the division of internal medicine from 1933 to 1936, when he became professor of medicine at the Jefferson Medical College.

Moses Barron made important contributions to the clinical teaching of the department over many years. His early training as a pathologist greatly enhanced his ability at clinical-pathological correlations. His work in pathology brought him fame for providing the initial stimulus to Frederick Banting to isolate insulin successfully.[13]

Cecil J. Watson[14] joined the department in 1932. Watson was awarded the M.D. degree from Minnesota in 1924. He then studied under E. T. Bell, professor of pathology, and wrote his thesis on periarteritis nodosa. Watson reported the first case of histoplasmosis recognized in the United States. In 1928 he received his Ph.D. degree; his thesis was on splenic disorders. In 1930 he took advanced courses in organic chemistry before leaving for Munich to work in the laboratory of Hans Fischer. In that laboratory, he accomplished the isolation of crystalline stercobilin. While in Munich, he attended the medical clinics of Friedrich von Müller. In 1932 Watson returned to Minneapolis as an assistant resident at the Minneapolis General Hospital and at the University Hospital, continuing his studies in the field of bile pigment-porphyrin chemistry. In 1936, while an associate professor of medicine, he was named director of the division of internal medicine. Watson was promoted to full professorship and became head of the department in 1942. He was also president of the American Society for Clinical Investigation and the Central Society for Clinical Research. In 1958 he was elected to the National Academy of Sciences. In 1966 Richard Ebert, head of the department of medicine at the University of Arkansas, succeeded Watson.

Wesley Spink became an assistant professor in 1937. Spink was a graduate of Harvard Medical School (1932) and, as a medical student, had done research in the department of comparative pathology on the clinical and immunological features of trichinosis.[15] Spink was an intern and resident on the Fourth Medical Service, which was associated with the Thorndike Memorial Laboratory. Spink, whose major interest was in infectious diseases, worked principally with Chester A. Keefer. Spink's scientific contributions included studies on the pathogenesis of strep-tococcal[16] and gonococcal diseases.[17] These studies were carried out just before the sulfonamide-antibiotic era. At Minnesota, his chief investigations were on sulfonamides,[18] antibiotics, and brucellosis.[19] Spink served as president of the American Society for Clinical Investigation, the Central Society for Clinical Research, and the American College of Physicians. He was made a professor of medicine in 1946. A number of Spink's trainees have had outstanding careers in the field of infectious diseases.[20]

For a number of years after 1937, expansion of the department of medicine was relatively slow, both in terms of facilities and full-time staff members. Additions were made largely by selecting outstanding young men who had served as interns and residents, one of whom, Frederick W. Hoffbauer, became a professor of medicine. His outstanding contributions to research were terminated by his premature death in 1965. Another was Edmund Flink, who subsequently became head of the department of medicine at the University of West Virginia.

## Owen H. Wangensteen and the Department of Surgery

The builder of the department of surgery was James E. Moore, who succeeded James A. Dunn as professor of surgery in 1904. He was a strong proponent of the Mayo affiliation and was the leader in formulating and instituting proposals for graduate study and degrees in the clinical fields. Moore was responsible for pointing out that suppurative arthritis of the hip joint usually had its origin in osteomyelitis of the neck of the femur. Most young surgical house officers using the Moore gall-bladder spoon are unaware that its origin traces back to Moore.

Moore wrote the following letter to Dean Lyon on February 8, 1915, in relation to full-time medicine:

> After 32 years of professional life in Minneapolis I've concluded to retire from private practice on March 1, 1915. I would not feel justified in retiring yet were it not for the salary paid me by the university. I have now been in the university for 25 years, the first 16 without salary. Each year my interest in the university has increased; until now, it is my first interest and the joy of my life. . . . Therefore I wish to tender through you, to the Administrative Board, the whole of my time after March 1. . . .
>
> I am influenced . . . by the fact that the trend in medical education seems to be toward a few full-time clinical teachers and this move will afford the University an opportunity to try out this principle without expense.[21]

Arthur C. Strachauer, who succeeded Moore in 1918, continued support of the graduate training program. In the early 1920s there were already extensive research laboratories in the department of surgery, used for the most part by J. F. Corbett, Conrad Jacobson, Augus Cameron, and Arthur Zierold.[22]

Owen H. Wangensteen succeeded Strachauer as chairman in 1930. Wangensteen received his M.D. degree (1922) and his Ph.D. degree (1925) from Minnesota. His doctoral thesis was entitled "The Undescended Testicle: An Experimental and Clinical Study."

The story of Wangensteen's outstanding contributions to the University of Minnesota and to surgery are best told in his own words.

My identity with the Department of Surgery dates back to the completion of my internship at the University Hospital in 1922. My primary investigative efforts have related to the alimentary tract. One might well say that I have spent most of my life essentially as a plumber of that long tube, having worked at both ends, but primarily with the problem of intestinal obstruction, for which I received the Samuel D. Gross Award in 1935. ... Similarly, we have demonstrated that appendicitis with perforation is primarily a phenomenon relating to lumenal obstruction of the appendix. This was first shown in rabbits, and subsequently in the chimpanzee, and finally, in man. Internal secretory pressures within the appendix of these creatures regularly exceeds that of diastolic blood pressure, perhaps the highest internal secretory pressure of any organ in the body.

The most important contribution of my Department to surgery's advance during my tenure (1930 to 1967) related primarily to the close relationship cultivated ... with Maurice B. Visscher ... probably Ernest Starling's last pupil ... I had a hand in persuading Maurice Visscher to come here in ... 1936.... I discussed with Maurice the matter of a weekly surgical-physiologic conference to which he readily assented. The first significant windfall from those weekly discussions was acquisition of a monitoring device to reveal the concentration of inhaled anesthetic gases during surgical operations. Our anesthetists in that period [the late 1930s] were administering simultaneously a large number of anesthetic gases, without knowing the concentration of any of them.... Maurice knew of the work of Alfred Nier [of Minnesota] who subsequently discovered 235 Uranium and had developed a mass spectrograph ... he consented to give us one of his original models, which we installed in the operating rooms. Within a week, it became evident that our surmise that anesthesiologists were responsible for occasional deaths on the operating table was correct. Nier has since developed a small portable apparatus to assess concentration of inhaled anesthetic gases. ...

The second great windfall ... was the development of a well-organized team of intracardiac surgeons. Paracardiac surgery came essentially through Robert Gross of Boston and Alfred Blalock of the Hopkins. Progress with intracardiac surgery, however, was slow. John H. Gibbon, Jr. of Jefferson Medical College, Philadelphia, was the first to come forward in the late 1930s with the thesis that inflow stasis of the superior and inferior vena cava, could be tolerated for brief periods of time with employment of a cardio-pulmonary oxygenator pump.

The first success in man with a formal intracardiac operation was closure by F. John Lewis here, September 2, 1952, of an inter-atrial septal defect under systemic hypothermia, an operation which he concluded within seven minutes.

Personally, I have had no experience with intracardiac surgery. . . . In the development of intracardiac surgery, I was essentially the regimental water carrier . . . I recognized early that the problem needed the attention of the physiologist. Visscher consented to our sending men interested in this segment of surgery . . . for a period of training from one to three or four years in the knowledge of the circulation. . . . Persons like Clarence Dennis, Richard Varco, the two Lillehei's [C. Walton and Richard], Merendino, Gott now at the Hopkins, Castenada, successor to Robert Gross as the cardiac surgeon at the Children's Hospital in Boston, McLean of the University of Montreal, Norman Shumway of Stanford University, Chris Barnard of Groote Schurr Hospital at the University of Cape Town—all these and several others were products of that combined training in surgery and in the physiology of the circulation . . . many of the early corrective procedures for congenital cardiac defects, as well as for acquired cardiac lesions, evolved as contributions from this great group of surgeons. . . .

In essence . . . this summarizes . . . the significant contributions to surgery's advance during my years of tenure as Chairman of the Department of Surgery at the University of Minnesota. . . .

I should . . . add [that] one of the great developments during my tenure here at the Medical School was . . . one of the strongest departments of Pediatrics that has existed anywhere in the 20th century. [This department was] under the direction of Irvine McQuarrie. He probably trained more pediatricians for the academic arena than anyone else in this century. Similarly, Leo Rigler, now at U.C.L.A., developed a strong department of Radiology here, and his many trainees occupy perhaps as many chairs in the radiologic academic arena as any American medical school has provided.[23]

## Irvine McQuarrie and the Department of Pediatrics[24]

Irvine McQuarrie attended the University of California at Berkeley, where he spent two years with Whipple at the Hooper Foundation, after completing the first two years of medical school.

After receiving a Ph.D. degree in experimental pathology and biochemistry, McQuarrie moved to Johns Hopkins, receiving his M.D. degree in 1921. After weekly ward rounds with Edwards A. Park and Grover F. Powers, and exposure to the lectures of James L. Gamble on infant metabolism and nutrition, McQuarrie chose pediatrics as his field. He interned at the Henry Ford Hospital and, two years later, was made director of endocrinology and metabolism there. The hospital decided to develop a special division of pediatrics and offered McQuarrie a year's leave in order to prepare himself for the position. Park, who had just accepted (in 1921) the professorship of pediatrics at Yale, offered him an instructorship. While in New Haven, McQuarrie accepted Whipple's offer to join the new school of medicine in Rochester. After four productive years there, McQuarrie accepted the professorship of pediatrics at Minnesota, an assignment that occupied him for the next twenty-five years.

When McQuarrie arrived there were six full-time staff members. Building the Variety Club Heart Hospital was one McQuarrie's outstanding efforts in the development of the department. This hospital was devoted to the investigation and treatment of children and adults with cardiovascular disease. At the end of World War II, the American Legion Division of Minnesota established an endowed Heart Research Professorship in pediatrics, which was first occupied by Lewis Thomas and then, beginning in 1954, by Robert A. Good, a student of McQuarrie's. Another important addition was the McClure Metabolic Ward for Teaching and Research on pediatric problems; the first director of this ward was Robert A. Ulstrom, another of McQuarrie's students.

McQuarrie's record shows a stream of productive research. He directed energies to the study of metabolic diseases and the metabolic aspects of disease in general. His investigations covered a broad spectrum, however, including protein, fat, and carbohydrate metabolism; mineral and water metabolism; and the endocrine control of metabolism. His most important contributions were to the understanding of the relation between water balance and seizures, as well as to the relation between sodium, potassium, and carbohydrate metabolism, which represented new thinking of a high order. Certainly his studies on idiopathic hypoglycemia warranted naming that condition *McQuarrie's disease.*[25] Much of his work was carried out with the aid of young associates; perhaps this group of young pediatric academicians that he trained represents his greatest contribution.

# 21

⚜

# Clinical Science at the Mayo Clinic: The Concept of Team Research[1]

William Worrall Mayo, the father of the founders of the Mayo Clinic, learned chemistry from John Dalton in Manchester, England. The elder Mayo mortgaged his home to buy a microscope, and he found time in his busy practice not only for clinical microscopy but also for histopathologic study of his own surgical specimens. This determination to utilize all of the techniques available for the solution of clinical problems explains the fact that when the clinic was gaining international fame, medical research was supported on a greater scale than at most universities.

Early in the development of the clinic, it was obvious that assistance would be needed in setting up laboratories to aid in the diagnostic work.[2] A diversified genius, Henry Stanley Plummer, was instrumental in organizing such laboratories. After graduation, Plummer (M.D., Northwestern, 1898) returned to Racine, Minnesota, to practice with his father. In 1900 William J. (Will) Mayo was called by Dr. Albert Plummer, Henry's father, to see a patient in consultation. When Dr. Mayo arrived, Albert Plummer was ill, and Henry accompanied Mayo to see the patient. Henry made smears of the patient's blood, which the two doctors examined. These smears were compared with those made from the hired man, and a diagnosis of leukemia was established. Mayo was so impressed by Henry Plummer's scientific approach to medical problems that he placed him in charge of the clinic laboratories, then largely devoted to examinations of urine and blood. Plummer soon became a pioneer in the development of x-ray diagnosis, an activity that led to burns of his hands. Lye strictures of the esophagus, relatively frequent in those days, interested Plummer, as did other esophageal lesions. He made improvements in their treatment by using a previously swallowed silk thread as a guide for bougies of increasing size, which were passed through the strictures. Plummer also became adept at bronchoscopy and developed instruments for the removal of foreign bodies from the bronchi.

## Pioneer Work on the Thyroid Gland

Plummer detected differences as early as 1913 that led to the characterization of one group of patients with hyperthyroidism as having Graves's disease or exophthalmic goitre, and another group with adenomas in their thyroids, but without the eye changes and the characteristic tremor of Graves's disease. In 1921 Plummer concluded that the excessive thyroid hormone in patients with goitre and hyperthyroidism was deficient in iodine. He administered iodine (Lugol's solution) to patients with exophthalmic goitre, and the beneficial effects were immediately obvious. Surgical mortality figures fell to less than 10 percent.[3]

There were others who helped to make the clinic an outstanding center for thyroid disease. Louis B. Wilson[4] came to Rochester in 1904 as a pathologist and bacteriologist. From 1908 to 1922, he published a number of studies relating the size and abnormal histology of the thyroid gland to the clinical condition of the patient.[5]

In 1914 Wilson received an inquiry from Edward C. Kendall of New York City, a young research chemist looking for a new position. While working for a pharmaceutical manufacturing concern, and later in a minor post at a New York hospital, Kendall was trying to isolate the active hormone of the thyroid gland. Nellis Barnes Foster suggested that the Mayo Clinic might be the place for him. The possibility of isolating the active product of the thyroid was of great interest to Plummer and Charles Mayo, so that Kendall was invited to come in February 1914. He arrived carrying in his pocket a test tube full of a whitish substance that he had obtained by treating thyroid glands with sodium hydroxide. On Christmas morning of 1914, Kendall dissolved some material of high iodine content from the thyroid gland in ethanol, which contained a small amount of sodium hydroxide. Addition of a few drops of acetic acid precipitated a pure material in fine crystalline form. This was the hormone of the thyroid gland, later named *thyroxin*.[6]

Walter M. Boothby[7] came to the clinic in 1916 to establish a metabolism laboratory. For four years he had been in charge of the metabolism and respiration laboratories of the Peter Bent Brigham Hospital. With Boothby came Dr. Irene Sandiford and later her sister, Kathleen Sandiford, who became a fellow in biochemistry. Boothby introduced a procedure for determining the basal metabolic rate and carried out early studies of respiratory metabolism, particularly in reference to diseases of the thyroid gland. Boothby and Irene Sandiford did extensive studies that were the basis for the Mayo Foundation standards for basal metabolic rates.[8]

Other of Boothby's experiments showed that insulin does not increase the rate of heat production and, therefore, that it is not a true calorigenic agent, such as thyroxin or epinephrine; however, Boothby also showed, with Wilder, that when the sugar of the blood is depressed by insulin to a level that provokes the symptoms of hypoglycemia, the rate of heat production increases abruptly, as if epinephrine had been injected.

Boothby was interested in pulmonary physiology, particularly in problems relating to altitude, before World War II. As a result of this early work and its application to aviation, Boothby, W. Randolph Lovelace, Captain Harry G. Armstrong, and the airlines of the United States, were given the Collier Trophy for 1938. In 1942, while continuing as head of the metabolic laboratories of the Mayo Clinic, Boothby assumed the duties of director of the Mayo Clinic Aeromedical Unit. In 1950 and 1951, Boothby was advisor for research and consultant in physiology in the Air Force Medical School at Brooke Field, Texas.

In 1921, Samuel F. Haines, after receiving his M.D. degree from Harvard and completing an internship at the MGH, started a fellowship in medicine at the clinic. His interest in the thyroid was established early and continued during his long association with Plummer. Perhaps his most important role was in the general development of clinical endocrinology at the clinic; first as head of one endocrine section and then as chairman of the division.

## Development of the Clinical Laboratories

Under Plummer's supervision, suitably trained men were recruited for the various sections.[9] Russell E. Carmen, a St. Louis physician, was engaged to take charge of the x-ray division. Frank Smithies, demonstrator of clinical medicine at the University of Michigan, was employed to manage the gastric analysis laboratory of St. Mary's Hospital. A clinical pathologist was needed, and, in 1911, Arthur A. Sanford opened a second clinical laboratory for work in bacteriology, as well as in serology and parasitology.

Although these various laboratories were for the purpose of aiding in clinical diagnosis, research was an inevitable by-product. Findings from thousands of blood counts and other specimens demanded analysis and to research of this sort the Mayos gave wholehearted encouragement. Development of independent research based on experimentation came slower. Will Mayo recognized the validity of Plummer's contention that a research program was necessary to the vitality of the group and would keep the practice from becoming static at the present level of knowledge.

## The Institute of Experimental Medicine

Shortly after his arrival at the clinic, Louis B. Wilson[10] began work in experimental pathology, keeping his animals in the basement of St.

Mary's Hospital. Wilson built a new barn at his farm home in 1908 and, with financial assistance from the Mayos, a laboratory facility for experimental animals was included. Frank C. Mann[11] was put in charge of it, and experimental medicine at Rochester was underway.

The Institute of Experimental Medicine grew steadily to a staff of nine scientists and more than twenty expert technicians. It provided excellent facilities for experimental surgery, pathology, biochemistry, biophysics, bacteriology, and physiology. Any clinician could use its facilities for his research. Institute teams made outstanding contributions to the physiology and pathology of the liver, as well as to the mechanism of production of peptic ulcers. The use of plasma for surgical shock was described in 1918, and experimental transplantation of the heart in 1933.

The team concept of the research laboratory made possible participation by physicians primarily engaged in clinical medicine and surgery. Many of the investigations involved extensive surgical procedures on animals. These researches, carried out under the demanding conditions of preantibiotic surgery, were part of the training of some of the outstanding surgeons of the clinic. One of the many significant innovations of the laboratory was the addition of a veterinarian (William H. Feldman) to provide care for the animals and to conduct research in animal diseases.

## The Division of Biophysical Research

It was the x-ray and radium that first introduced the physicist into medical practice, and it was the need for a radium plant to permit this type of therapy that led to the establishment of a physics laboratory at the clinic. In 1923 Charles Sheard, professor of physics at Ohio State University, became the head of a division of biophysical research. Sheard and his associates contributed to the group's research problems by devising the necessary apparatus and techniques for accurate physical measurement of bodily functions.[12] They helped in solving some of the practical problems of the chemical laboratories, including the development of the Sanford-Sheard Photolometer, which performed some fifty chemical tests mechanically.

## The Rowntree Group for Teaching and Clinical Investigation

It was decided in 1919 to extend the facilities for bedside teaching and clinical investigation. A major step was the recruitment of Leonard G. Rowntree[13] and Henry F. Helmholz. Rowntree supervised the training of fellows in medicine and directed clinical research; the same responsibility in pediatrics was assigned to Helmholz.

Rowntree brought Norman M. Keith from Johns Hopkins, Reginald

Fitz from Harvard, and, a short time later, George E. Brown from Miles City, Montana, and C. S. McVicar from Toronto. Carl H. Greene joined the group in 1921, and Bayard T. Horton arrived in 1925.[14] Beds on the second and third floors of the Stanley Hospital were provided for their patients until the spring of 1921, when the Rowntree group moved into the remodeled Olmsted Hotel. They remained there until July 1922, when the surgeons who had occupied the older wings of St. Mary's Hospital took over a newly constructed surgical pavilion. The research group was given their former space after it had been remodeled. The old operating rooms were converted into laboratories.

This new staff in medicine was responsible for the development of the work associated with the graduate school of the University of Minnesota. Rowntree, who also took charge of one of the Clinic's sections, had Louis A. Buie and Eric Larson as his assistants. The section, which occupied a floor of the clinic, included six hospital services—Rowntree's own; the diabetic service, under Russell Wilder;[15] the kidney service, under Keith; the vascular disease service, under Brown;[16] gastroenterology, under McVicar; and intestinal diseases, under Jay Bargen. The laboratories were devoted mostly to clinical investigation and were headed by Greene. Grace Roth, who took her Ph.D. degree at Minnesota, became a valuable member of the staff. Rowntree developed a new type of seminar that was handled in rotation by the section chiefs. A patient, preferably one with diagnostic or therapeutic problems, was presented. The section chief brought the participants up to date on current knowledge, then the problem was thrown open for discussion and suggestions as to how, by critical analysis and by experimentation, one might advance the current knowledge about that particular problem.

In 1923 Rowntree, by means of roentgenography, outlined the pelvis of the kidney, the ureters, and the bladder, following the injection of sodium iodide solutions. In the same year, he observed that a large intake of water caused serious intoxication—an early stimulus to other investigations at the clinic on water and electrolyte problems.[17] Rowntree also developed an interest in blood and plasma volume, and in Addison's disease. Rowntree was ultimately made chief of the medical department of the Mayo Foundation, director of clinical investigation, and professor of medicine in the graduate school of the University of Minnesota.

## Rowntree's Associates

Norman M. Keith[18] pioneered the use of dilution technique for measuring blood volume, initially using Evans blue dye and later sucrose. He also appreciated at an early stage the role of potassium in biologic processes. A third endeavor was to bring some order into the classification of vascular disease. With Henry Wagener and others, he developed the Keith-Wagener grouping of hypertension.[19]

George E. Brown[20] (M.D., Michigan, 1909) interned in the Northern

Pacific Hospital in Brainerd, Minnesota, and then practiced medicine in Miles City, Montana. His ten years in Miles City were broken by brief study periods at Harvard in 1914, and at Johns Hopkins in 1916. In 1921 he joined the Mayo Clinic and in 1930 was appointed chief of a section of the medical division. He became a member of the American Society for Clinical Investigation and gained national standing for his research in peripheral vascular diseases.

Edgar V. Allen[21] was a fellow under Brown. In 1929 he received a National Research Council fellowship to work with Irvine H. Page. Returning to the clinic, he became head of a section of medicine in 1936 and a professor in 1947. His bedside appraisal of diseases of the peripheral circulation was outstanding. He introduced the coumarin anticoagulants into clinical medicine and vigorously explored various drugs for the control of hypertension. He received the Distinguished Service Medal of the American Heart Association (1957) and the Albert Lasker Award for Scientific Achievement (1960). He was president of the Central Society for Clinical Research in 1948.

Reginald Fitz[22] (M.D., Harvard, 1909) served on the resident staff at the Massachusetts General, Johns Hopkins, and Peter Bent Brigham hospitals, and then worked on metabolic problems at the HRI. He devised a method for the determination of betahydroxybutyric acid and investigated in diabetics the amounts of fat, carbohydrate, and protein burned by the body, and their relation to the formation of oxybutyric and diacetic acid. After World War I, he returned to the MGH as resident physician. In 1920 he joined Rowntree's group; after only two years, however, he returned to Boston as associate professor of medicine at Harvard.

Bayard T. Horton came to the Mayo Clinic in 1925 and, while still a fellow, received an award from the A.M.A. for his exhibit on pyloric block. After obtaining his M.D. degree from the University of Virginia, he interned and then was professor of biology and physician at Emory and Henry College. As early as 1927, he gained recognition for his research on hypersensitivity to cold. In 1932 he was the first to demonstrate arteriovenous fistulae by means of arteriography. He described two new diseases: histaminic cephalalgia (Horton's headache) and temporal arteritis.

## Progress in Clinical Investigation

Clinical investigation at the clinic continued to grow in the 1920s. Efficient organization of the diagnostic services brought clinical advantages to each of the sections in terms of broadening the clinical experience of the staff and their opportunity to make clinical research contributions. Hospitalization was available for continued observation and for controlled studies.

Will and Charles Mayo traveled frequently and brought back some medical innovation from every trip. Will Mayo's journey to Australia in 1924 was fruitful. He met John Hunter, an anatomist at the University of Sidney, who was studying the effects of the sympathetic nervous system on muscle tone. On the basis of Hunter's findings, M. D. Royle, the orthopedic surgeon, had achieved good results in treating spastic paralysis by sympathectomy. Will described Royle's operation to A. W. Adson, the clinic neurosurgeon, who promptly used it in his next case of spastic paralysis. Adson observed that the temperature of the skin of the feet was higher after than before operation. Adson surmised that sympathectomy might prove an effective treatment for diseases of the peripheral vascular system.

George E. Brown studied the patients on whom Adson performed sympathectomy, leading to a successful trial of this procedure in peripheral vascular disease.[23] Brown carefully analyzed his patient observations until he was able to differentiate the various diseases with confidence. He and his associates studied the effect of every proposed treatment from drugs to postural exercises in order to learn more about the response of the vascular system and to find some therapy less radical than surgery. For the severe types, the neurosurgeon had to provide the treatment; sometimes, however, the operation did not work, so that some means was needed to predict the result from surgery. Brown used typhoid vaccine to induce fever and found that if the rise in the skin temperature of the foot was greater than the rise in oral temperature, the patient would benefit from the operation. Fundamental in all this work was the measurement of variations in skin temperature. The devices available were not adequate, so Brown sought assistance from Sheard, the biophysicist, who constructed an electrothermometer. Thereafter, Sheard participated actively with the group, contributing techniques and apparatus for many of the mechanical treatment methods that were tried.[24] When it became evident that more rigidly controlled room conditions were needed for these studies, Sheard devised equipment for keeping the room temperature and humidity constant. These studies led to the first sympathectomies for hypertension.[25] Sympathectomies were also done for Buerger disease and Raynaud syndrome.

With the assistance of Brown and of Grace Roth, Rowntree studied blood and plasma volume and introduced the terms *normovolemia, hypervolemia,* and *hypovolemia.*[26]

In 1929 the Rowntree program encountered difficulties. Will Mayo became disillusioned with what had come to be known as the *Rowntree Empire,* with the result that much of the unit's support was withdrawn.[27] The research laboratories were reduced, all chemistry was centralized in a section of biochemistry in the main area, and all investigation that involved the use of larger animals was restricted to the Institute of Experimental Medicine. S. Franklin Adams and William P. Finney, associates on the diabetic service, were assigned elsewhere, and Frank N.

Allen was placed in charge of diabetes. Other members of the Rowntree group were scattered among other sections of the clinic.

Rowntree resigned in 1931 and later became director of research at the Philadelphia Institute for Medical Research. In 1937 Rowntree received the Gold Medal of the American Medical Association for demonstrating that malignant tumors were produced in rats fed with wheat germ oil. During World War I, he was executive officer for research medicine on the Medical Research Board of the Air Force and was engaged in the study of the medical problems of aviation and aviators. In 1940, when the National Selective Service was organized, Rowntree was appointed chief of the medical division. He was also president of the American Society for Clinical Investigation and had an important role in organizing the Central Society for Clinical Research.

### Russell Wilder[28] and the Development of Clinical Endocrinology at the Mayo Clinic

Although the clinic soon became an outstanding center of thyroidology, the emergence of clinical endocrinology as an identifiable specialty in Rochester and elsewhere came later. For many years, clinical endocrinology was not a respectable specialty because much of its diagnostic and therapeutic content was lacking in scientific validity. At the Mayo Clinic, wise leadership, a basic conservatism, and skeptical colleagues encouraged a sound practice in this field and did much to improve the national status of the specialty. One of those chiefly responsible for this development was Russell Wilder.

During his student days at Chicago, Wilder worked with Howard Taylor Ricketts and played a part in the discovery of the microorganisms causing typhus fever, later named *Rickettsia.*[29]

Wilder came to the clinic, in 1919, to develop more bedside teaching and clinical investigation. He carried out metabolic studies in diabetic patients and stimulated Henry Wagener's interest in the complications of the eye caused by the disease. Early in 1921, the Olmsted Hospital provided larger, but still temporary, quarters for the diabetic service and the dietetic department. A laboratory was organized, and it was there that the chemical determinations in Wilder and Boothby's famous study of the diabetic patient "Bessie B." were performed.

Wilder also had an interest in the thyroid's effect on the metabolism of carbohydrates in diabetes. Woodyatt, Wilder's mentor in Chicago, devised a precision instrument with which fluids could be injected continuously at timed rates, and Wilder determined the amounts of dextrose excreted by dogs when the inflow of sugar was maintained at a steady rate. Thus the rate of utilization could be measured with accuracy. They tried the effect of Kendall's crystalline thyroxin and unexpectedly found that the rate of utilization of glucose was lowered, as was the tolerance.

This was also demonstrated in patients. Wilder's later studies with Boothby revealed that although tolerance to dextrose was lowered by thyroxin, the respiratory quotient after dextrose rose even more abruptly than normal. They concluded that the lower tolerance to dextrose of hyperthyroid patients was not indicative of true diabetes mellitus. The two diseases may, however, accompany each other.[30]

## Hyperinsulinism

Frank C. Mann and P. B. Magath described the symptoms of hypoglycemia induced by total removal of the liver. Frederick Banting and Charles Best, on the basis of this description, recognized the nature of the convulsive disturbances that their first pancreatic extracts induced in dogs. Seale Harris of Birmingham, being shown this phenomenon on a visit to Toronto in 1923, deduced that similar symptoms occasionally observed in nondiabetic patients might be related to spontaneous overproduction of insulin. He found lower blood sugar levels in such patients and came to the conclusion—without any proof—that he was dealing with "hyperinsulinism." Wilder and his group provided positive proof that hyperinsulinism could occur. On October 29, 1926, a man who appeared to be in "shock" from an overdose of insulin was brought to St. Mary's Hospital. The man had never taken insulin and had previously had several similar episodes. When Will Mayo exposed the pancreas, it contained a carcinoma with nodules in the liver. The microscopic sections showed pancreatic islet tissue. M. H. Power demonstrated the presence of insulinlike activity in the pancreatic tumor and in the hepatic metastases.[31]

## Hyperparathyroidism

The group at the clinic also diagnosed one of the early cases of parathyroid tumor. In 1928 David P. Barr of St. Louis reported at a meeting, which Rowntree and Allan were attending, what was probably the third case recognized. They asked Wilder to consider this possibility in a case then under study with Power. The diagnosis was confirmed at operation; Frederick W. Rankin removed a parathyroid tumor. Wilder's interest in the subject continued.[32] A human subject was treated experimentally, first with parathormone and then with parathormone and viosterol. The characteristic disturbance of calcium and phosphorus metabolism was produced, as well as bone pain and muscle weakness. "The result of these... experiments confirms the view that the pathogenesis of osteitis fibrosa osteoplastica, as this disease is observed spontaneously in man, is an oversupply of parathyroid hormone and that this disease bears no relation, etiologically, either to osteomalacia or rickets."[33]

In 1929 Wilder received an invitation to become the chairman of the department of medicine at Chicago. He accepted, only to return to Rochester in the fall of 1931. During the mid-thirties, Wilder and his group, including R. G. Sprague, Benjamin B. Blum, A. E. Osterberg, and Edwin J. Kepler, made extensive studies of slow-release insulins such as Hagedorn's protamine insulin.

## Pheochromocytoma

In 1927 Charles Mayo, during a laparotomy on a patient with paroxysmal hypertension, found a chromaffin tumor of the adrenal, the removal of which was followed by the disappearance of the patient's periodic episodes of tachycardia and hypertension.[34] A short time later, Maurice C. Pincoffs, a professor of medicine at the University of Maryland, encountered a patient with the same condition, from whom his surgical colleague, Arthur M. Shipley, had removed an adrenomedullary tumor and brought about complete relief of the patient's symptoms.[35] In the case of these two patients, epinephrine was isolated from the tumor. These were the first two patients with this disease to be treated successfully by surgery.

## Studies on the Adrenal Gland

In 1930 Rowntree and Greene reported a case of Addison's disease in crisis in whom "treatment with solutions of sodium chloride and glucose was instituted with only partial success."[36] Thirty-six hours after Swingle and Pfiffner's cortical extract[37] was started, however, the patient felt well. Rowntree, with Carl H. Greene, R. G. Ball, W. W. Swingle, and J. J. Pfiffner, soon reported similar benefit in most of twenty patients.[38] Greene reported on thirty-four cases of Addison's disease treated from 1930 to 1937.[39] In 1931 Rowntree and Snell published a monograph describing the clinical features of 109 patients with this relatively rare disorder.[40] This monograph is still used as a reference work.

In 1935 Robert F. Loeb, of Columbia, described the changes in plasma sodium and chloride concentration in adrenocortical insufficiency and pointed out the benefits of increasing the salt content of the diet of patients with Addison's disease. William D. Allers, of Kendall's group, confirmed these findings and showed that more base than acid was lost by adrenalectomized dogs. If base in the form of sodium bicarbonate was administered, the treatment was more satisfactory, and the survival of adrenalectomized dogs receiving sodium chloride was extended. Treatment was modified to include daily administration of ten grams of sodium chloride and five grams of sodium citrate. Allers, H. W. Nilson, and Kendall found that restriction of potassium intake further facilitated the maintenance of adrenalectomized dogs receiving salt and sodium citrate. This regimen was applied to patients, and the advantages reported in 1937 by Wilder, Kendall, Snell, Kepler,[41] Edward H. Rynearson,[42] and Mildred Adams.[43] Sodium and potassium seem, then, to have reciprocal effects. H. H. Cutler, M. H. Power, and R. M. Wilder later worked out a diagnostic test on the basis of the concentration of either chloride or sodium in the urine of patients with Addison's disease.[44] It was Robinson, Power, and Kepler who later developed the water excretion test for the diagnosis of Addison's disease.[45]

Rowntree and Snell had only the small amounts of extract that they received from Swingle and Pfiffner and appealed to Kendall for preparation of more liberal supplies. Although little progress was made in the first three years of the chemical investigation of the adrenal cortex, by 1933 potent extracts of beef adrenals were being made in Kendall's laboratory. The determination of their activity on adrenalectomized dogs, prepared by Frank C. Mann at the institute, became a routine process. The use of these extracts saved the life of many patients in Addisonian crisis, and patients no longer died of acute adrenal insufficiency following surgical removal of hyperfunctioning adrenal cortical tumors.

Kendall's real objective was, however, greater than the provision of relatively crude adrenal extracts for clinical use. His aim was the isolation, characterization, and eventual synthesis of the adrenal cortex's active principle, which is essential for life.

Kendall's interest in the adrenal cortex developed through a combination of circumstances. Late in 1926, after learning of Harington's synthesis of thyroxin, he focused his attention on glutathione and other biologically significant sulfhydryl compounds. Then, in the summer of 1929, Albert Szent-Gyorgyi came to Kendall's laboratory, where he worked on hexuronic acid, which he had previously found in high concentration in the adrenal cortex. He needed large quantities of fresh beef adrenal, which could be obtained from the large packing houses in St. Paul. During his eight-month stay, he was able to isolate some twenty grams of the compound, which later was shown to be identical with vitamin C. Kendall had his first contact with the adrenal gland while Szent-Gyorgyi was working in his [Kendall's] laboratory. From 1927 to 1930, several papers appeared describing the first successful attempt to prepare a physiologically active extract of the adrenal cortex. The project soon achieved top priority.[46]

In 1933 Kendall succeeded in isolating a "hormone" in crystalline form from the adrenal cortex. Evidence for the biological activity of this material was provided by a young biochemist who tested it on adrenalectomized dogs. Later, however, it was found that this report of activity was erroneous, because he had naïvely included salt in the diet of the dogs. When Dwight Ingle joined Kendall's group in 1934, he assayed the material in his muscle work test. It turned out to be inactive. Kendall continued with the chemical study of literally tons of adrenal glands

made available by Parke-Davis and Company, who paid for the adrenal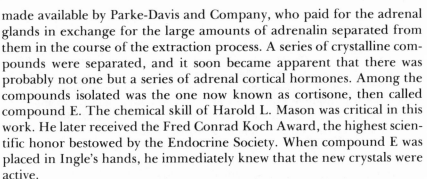
glands in exchange for the large amounts of adrenalin separated from
them in the course of the extraction process. A series of crystalline compounds were separated, and it soon became apparent that there was
probably not one but a series of adrenal cortical hormones. Among the
compounds isolated was the one now known as cortisone, then called
compound E. The chemical skill of Harold L. Mason was critical in this
work. He later received the Fred Conrad Koch Award, the highest scientific honor bestowed by the Endocrine Society. When compound E was
placed in Ingle's hands, he immediately knew that the new crystals were
active.

By 1940, some ten years after the initiation of his work on the adrenal
cortical hormones, Kendall decided to focus on compounds that have
activity on carbohydrate metabolism and in the work test, of which compound E was the prototype.[47]

The remainder of the story can best be told in Sprague's own words:

> It was not until December 1945, that chemists of Merck and Company
> completed the synthesis of a considerable amount of compound A, a close
> chemical relative of compound E, employing the methods which had been
> developed largely in Kendall's laboratory. Clinical studies with A here and
> elsewhere gave disappointing results. Our own studies of patients with
> Addison's disease indicated that 20 mg of naturally occurring compound E
> had more of the desired type of physiologic activity than 200 mg of syn-
> thetic compound A daily.
>
> In October 1946, a meeting of a group of steroid chemists, including
> Kendall, with officials of Merck and Company, led to the decision to push
> ahead with the synthesis of compound E. Dr. Lewis Sarett of Merck, in
> December 1944, had succeeded in preparing the first few milligrams of
> compound E, but the yield had been much too small to be of practical
> importance. In 1947, Sarett greatly improved the yield and in the same
> year our Dr. Vernon Mattox made the last necessary contribution for
> synthesis on a commercial scale when he discovered a new way to form a
> double bond in ring A of the hormone.
>
> At a meeting in New York on April 29, 1948, officials of Merck and
> Company announced that a total of nine grams of compound E had been
> prepared and was available for clinical investigation. Kendall and I were
> among the small group in attendance. We were asked to study its effects on
> a small group of patients with co-existing Addison's disease and diabetes
> mellitus because we had previously shown that such patients were excep-
> tionally sensitive subjects for demonstration of the carbohydrate effects of
> adrenal hormones. We were given two grams of compound E for this
> purpose. . . .
>
> One morning in June 1948, while I was making rounds on the endo-
> crine service at St. Mary's Hospital, I received a telephone call from Doctor
> Hench. He had heard, as he explained, that I had some synthetic com-
> pound E in my possession. He asked urgently if I would turn some of it
> over to him for administration to a patient with rheumatoid arthritis.[48]
> The thought went through my mind that this was, indeed, an absurd idea.

Then I recovered my composure and explained that Merck and Company had given us two grams of compound E for the specific purpose of studying its carbohydrate effects in patients with Addison's disease and diabetes, that such studies were already under way in the Nutrition Unit, and that I would not be acting in good faith if I were to relinquish some of this rare and costly compound for another purpose. Thus, I had the doubtful distinction of refusing to provide material for a clinical trial of compound E which was to culminate in the sharing of the Nobel Prize in Medicine and Physiology by Drs. Hench, Kendall and Reichstein.

The giving of the first dose of compound E to Mrs. G. on September 21, 1948, marked the beginning of the use of adrenal hormones as pharmacologic agents, in contrast to their seemingly more rational use as endocrine agents. Although Hench, Kendall and others for a time speculated that rheumatoid arthritis might in truth be an endocrine deficiency disease, we soon demonstrated that adrenal cortical function is quite normal in these patients. The principals in the great achievement were Drs. Hench, Kendall, Slocumb and Polley. Endocrinology benefited greatly from the ready availability of cortisone that resulted from their discovery, for it revolutionized the treatment of Addison's disease, pituitary insufficiency and the medical management of hyperfunctioning lesions of the adrenal cortex.[49]

## The Nutrition Unit

In the late 1930s, plans were undertaken for an additional medical pavilion at St. Mary's Hospital, which included a clinical research facility. It comprised two wards, one with two beds, the other with three beds; the wards shared a metabolic kitchen and a roomy laboratory. Plans for the unit were drawn with the aid of Eugene F. DuBois, who had organized such a unit at Bellevue Hospital in New York City. DuBois, an ardent sailor, planned the unit like a yacht so that "the helmsman would have all the sails within his range of vision all the time." In other words, the person in the metabolic kitchen should be able to overlook all that went on in the wards. It was Russell Wilder who was chiefly responsible for this development and who gave it the name *Nutrition Unit*.

## Clinical Science in Other Specialties of Internal Medicine

### Hematology

Herbert Z. Giffin[50] (M.D., Johns Hopkins, 1904) was one of the pioneer physicians at the Mayo Clinic (1906–45), and professor of medicine in the Mayo Graduate School of Medicine (1934–47). He interned at the Johns Hopkins Hospital (1904–5), following which he served another internship at the Children's Hospital of Philadelphia.

Giffin came to Rochester in 1906 as head of a section of medicine in what was then the partnership of the Drs. Mayo, Graham, Plummer, Judd, and Stinchfield. Giffin developed an interest in diseases of the blood and blood-forming organs. He became an authority on the various forms of anemia, leukemia, and particularly diseases of the spleen, playing an important role in establishing the value of removal of the spleen in the treatment of familial hemolytic jaundice. He was a member of the American Society for Clinical Investigation.

## Gastroenterology and Liver Disease

Albert M. Snell[51] received his M.D. degree from Minnesota in 1918. In 1923 Snell came to the Mayo Clinic as an assistant in Rowntree's section and at age thirty-three became head of a section in medicine. His great interest was in diseases of the adrenals and of the liver and biliary tract. He was the first to use vitamin K in jaundiced patients with prothrombin deficiency, work done in collaboration with his pupil Hugh R. Butt[52] and with Edgar V. Allen. He later became interested in intestinal absorption and contributed significantly to our understanding of the clinical aspects of sprue, nontropical sprue, and idiopathic steatorrhea.

Manfred Whitset Comfort[53] received his M.D. degree from the University of Texas. In 1923 he entered the Mayo Foundation as a fellow in neurology. In 1926 he transferred his interests to gastroenterology, and he became a professor in the graduate school in 1946. An interest in bilirubin metabolism led to the first American report on constitutional familial hyperbilirubinemia. In a study of gastric secretion in patients with gastric cancer, he demonstrated that the degree of anacidity was related to the area of tumor surface.

In 1935 he began, after observation of a patient with pancreatic lithiasis, a study of the physiological and pathological phenomena associated with progressive destruction of the pancreas. Comfort was instrumental in developing serum lipase determinations as a diagnostic aid. He also initiated a long series of studies on external pancreatic secretions in various diseases, developing new methods and correlating the findings with surgical and necropsy observations. In 1946 Comfort published, with E. E. Gambill and A. H. Baggenstoss, a paper on chronic relapsing pancreatitis that established the disease entity.[54]

Another staff member interested in gastroenterology was Walter C. Alvarez (M.D., Cooper Medical College, 1905), who joined the Mayo Foundation as an associate professor in 1926 and became head of a section of medicine at the Mayo Clinic, and professor of medicine.

Alvarez interned in San Francisco (1905–6), was an assistant in clinical pathology at Cooper Medical College (1906–7) and, from 1910 to 1926, practiced in Mexico and then in San Francisco. He was a postgraduate student in physiology at Harvard in 1913. He became a voluntary assistant in research medicine at the Hooper Foundation for Medical Research (see chapter 23) in 1915, assistant in 1916, instructor from 1916 to 1920, assistant professor from 1920 to 1924, and associate professor from 1924 to 1926. His interest was in gastroenterology, and he contributed to knowledge of the physiology of the digestive tract both in the experimental animal and in man by his studies, which extended over many years. He was a member of both the American Society for Clinical Investigation and the Central Society for Clinical Research.

## Cardiology

Electrocardiography was begun at the clinic in 1917, with Frederick A. Willius in charge. He later became head of a section on cardiology.

Clinical investigation was an important part of the activity of the section on cardiology. Willius,[55] in collaboration with others interested in heart disease, including Arlie Ray Barnes, George E. Brown, Julia Fitzpatrick, Samuel F. Haines, and Walter M. Boothby, published numerous articles that were concerned with the following subjects: the behavior of the heart in hyperthyroidism; electrocardiograms in relation to prognosis in heart disease; treatment of Stokes-Adams syndrome; metabolism in relation to cases of primary cardiac disease; clinical features of coronary sclerosis; study of clinical features of cases exhibiting electrocardiograms conforming to those of experimental complete bundle branch block; and many others.

Arlie Ray Barnes[56] came to the Mayo Graduate School from Indiana University in 1920. In 1929 he established the electrocardiographic concept of ventricular strain. He provided criteria for localization, electrocardiographically, of acute myocardial infarction to the anterior apical or posterior basal components of the left ventricular wall.[57] A later contribution was his description with Howard Burchell (1942) of the electrocardiographic changes that characterize acute nonspecific pericarditis.

The results of Barnes's clinical investigations were summarized in a monograph, *Electrocardiographic Patterns: Their Diagnostic and Clinical Significance.* That volume was a milestone in the progress of clinical electrocardiography from its established function in the analysis of cardiac arrhythmias to a new and substantial role in appraisal of the structural and functional integrity of the ventricular myocardium.

## Pulmonary Medicine

H. Corwin Hinshaw (M.D., Pennsylvania, 1933) entered the Mayo Foundation as a fellow in medicine in 1933 and soon developed an interest in pulmonary diseases. His most important work was done with William H. Feldman (D.V.M., Colorado Agricultural College, 1917). In 1927 he entered the Mayo Foundation as an instructor in comparative pathology. These two, working together, made important contributions to the antibiotic treatment of tuberculosis.

The discovery of streptomycin was reported in 1944. A fortunate circumstance made the testing of the drug easier than it might have been otherwise. In 1939, after Arnold R. Rich and Richard H. Follis, of Johns Hopkins, reported that sulfanilamide had a limited suppressive effect on experimental tuberculosis in the guinea pig, Hinshaw and Feldman, knowing the greater effect of sulfapyridine in pneumonia, explored its effectiveness against experimental tuberculosis. The results indicated that additional work with the sulfonamides would not be rewarding.

In 1940 Hinshaw learned of a new compound, promin, that was being tested against a variety of bacterial infections, but not against tuberculosis. He and Feldman observed a notable inhibition of a human-type tuberculous infection in guinea pigs. Hinshaw and Feldman, who published their findings in 1940, were convinced that tuberculosis was vulnerable to chemotherapy. Their observations on promin have great historical significance in that promin was the first antimicrobial substance proved unequivocally effective in an experimental infection induced by the human-type tubercle bacillus. The later use of promin against leprosy had a tremendous impact on the social and medical aspects of that disease. Hinshaw and Feldman's studies of sulfapyridine and promin resulted in the development of sound experimental procedures for the laboratory testing of antituberculous agents.

In 1943 they wrote to Waksman, at Rutger's, asking whether clavacin—a highly potent antibiotic that his group had recently discovered—might be available for experimental testing. They found that the drug was too toxic for use in animals. In November 1943, while visiting Waksman's laboratory, Feldman told him about the work that he and Hinshaw were doing in the treatment of experimental tuberculosis. In his studies of streptomycin, Waksman had found that *M. tuberculosis* was susceptible in vitro to the antagonistic action of this drug. Waksman wrote to Hinshaw, in March 1944, inquiring whether he and Feldman were prepared to undertake a test of streptomycin in the experimental tuberculosis of guinea pigs. Ten grams of the drug were sent, and the first experiment on only four guinea pigs was started on April 27, 1944, and terminated June 20. The results were promising. Additional studies were clearly indicated, but in wartime it was difficult to obtain supplies of any drug. In early July, Hinshaw and Feldman decided to inoculate a large group of guinea pigs with tubercle bacilli, hoping that if supplies were forthcoming, a more rapid answer could be obtained. Merck and Company did supply the drug on July 10. Experiment number two was highly successful and in every way confirmed the effect of streptomycin against tuberculous infection in guinea pigs. In December 1944, Hinshaw, in collaboration with Carl H. Pfuetze, then medical superintendent of the Mineral Springs Sanatorium in Cannon Falls, Minnesota, began a series of observations on the effect of the drug in clinical tuberculosis. In September 1945, a preliminary report on thirty-four cases was published.

Hinshaw and Feldman presented their findings at the forty-second annual meeting of the National Tuberculosis Association in June 1946. During the discussion that followed this paper, Walsh McDermott and Carl Muschenheim announced that they had fully confirmed Hinshaw and Feldman's observations. This was in marked contrast to the skepticism with which Hinshaw and Feldman's report on promin had been received at the annual meeting of the same organization four years previously. After the 1946 meeting, a conference with military and Veterans Administration authorities was held, and, soon thereafter, the initiative for large-scale control clinical studies was taken over by the Veterans Administration under the leadership of John Blair Barnwell and Arthur M. Walker.[58]

# 22

❦

# The Leland Stanford University School of Medicine

The Leland Stanford University School of Medicine had its beginning as the medical department of the University of the Pacific, chartered in 1858 as the Far West's first medical school.[1] Instruction began in 1859, in the top story of Dr. Elias Samuel Cooper's office in San Francisco. In 1872 the school became known as the Medical College of the Pacific, and, ten years later, its faculty formed the Cooper Medical College, under the guidance of Dr. Levi Cooper Lane.

George Blumer recalled his days as a student at the Cooper Medical College:[2] "Clinical medicine was taught by Joseph Oakland Hirschfelder,[3] who was an excellent clinician, and an investigator who worked for years to find a cure for tuberculosis."

In 1908 Stanford University accepted the Cooper Medical College as its school of medicine. For the next half-century (1909–59), preclinical instruction took place on the Stanford campus near Palo Alto, and the clinical years were housed in San Francisco. The first professors of medicine were William Fitch Cheney, Joseph O. Hirschfelder, and Ray Lyman Wilbur. Among the educational innovations during Wilbur's deanship (1911–16) was the provision of one-hundred hours for electives during the four years of the medical course. Wilbur was president of the American Medical Association in 1923, president of Stanford University from 1916 to 1943, and secretary of the interior from 1929 to 1933.[4]

William Ophüls, dean from 1916 to 1933, brought many outstanding teachers to Stanford, including George Barnett, A. L. Bloomfield, Leo Eloesser, Albion W. Hewlett, Emile Holman, and Frederick Reichert.

## Thomas Addis

Wilbur brought Thomas Addis[5] to Stanford in 1911 to supervise the clinical laboratory. Addis and Wilbur wrote one of the earlier papers on urobilin metabolism.[6] During World War I, Addis began his investigations into renal function, developing the widely used *Addis count*[7] and writing one of his first papers for the initial volume of the *Journal of Urology* (1917), in which he described the Addis "urea ratio."[8] As the more mathematically minded George Barnett pointed out to him, the Addis "urea ratio" represented that amount of blood freed of urea per unit of time and was thus the first of the modern tests of renal clearance.[9] Addis climaxed his studies in 1925 with an excellent paper on the natural history of Bright's disease. His book with Oliver, *The Renal Lesion in Bright's Disease,* is a classic, and *Glomerular Nephritis,* completed only a few months before his death, embodies his philosophy of disease and of science in general.[10]

## "Addis's Lab"

For many years, the main facility for research in the department of medicine at Stanford was referred to as "Addis's lab"—a high-ceilinged barn of a room that contained central stacks holding hoods in which Kjeldahl nitrogen determinations were performed; batteries of flasks for the urease method for urine and blood ureas; stills for water; a refrigerator room; a balance room; and a place for washing and drying laboratory beakers and other glassware.[11] The rat laboratories were outside of this main room. Chinese dieners helped in all phases of laboratory work (The names of Lew, Lee Poo, and other dieners appeared from time to time as coauthors of papers with Addis). In one corner cubicle of the "lab," Leona Bayer and Horace Gray studied growth and used formal statistical methods with the aid of a calculating machine, which was advanced for the time (the 1930s).

In another corner cubicle was Addis, his twenty-inch slide rule in hand, and his record player turning out classical music. Addis's cubicle also contained a simply constructed table for physical examinations. This is where Addis saw his patients with Bright's disease, hypertension, or conditions that simulated them. For example, at one time Addis had perhaps the area's largest group of patients with myxedema, who had been sent to him because of their puffiness, pallor, usually hypertension, and maybe a trace of proteinuria, all of which led the physician to diagnose erroneously some type of Bright's disease. The patients were composed of two groups—his own private patients, and patients of the Stanford University clinic service. They all sat in the waiting room, where they mixed comfortably. If there ever was any question over who was there first, Addis would take the clinic patient before he would take the private one. His wife, who had been a nurse-dietician, worked out their low-salt and adjusted protein intakes.

A succession of colleagues and students worked in this laboratory, which was supported mainly by the Rockefeller Fluid Research Fund. Perhaps the first were Douglas Drury and Eaton MacKay, Stanford graduate students who spent a year with Addis as an acceptable elective experience in lieu of Stanford's pre-1944 requirement for a year of internship prior to award of the M.D. degree. Later came William Dock, A. L. Bloomfield, B. O. Raulston,[12] Charles Barnett, David Rytand, Roy Cohn, Albert Snoke, David Karnofsky, Windsor Cutting, Richard Cutter, Marcus Krupp, Joseph Davis, Edward Persike, John Thayer, Richard Lippman, Eloise Jameson, and Florence Walter.

Belding Scribner, a Stanford medical student who was interested in Bright's disease and blood chemistry, worked in the laboratory. Addis had one of the early electric pH meters, perhaps the only one in the area in those days, and, in 1945, when Scribner went to the San Francisco County Hospital to intern, Addis presented him with this pH machine, which launched Scribner on what proved to be an outstanding career in the study and treatment of renal diseases.

Apart from the mainstream of studies in the laboratory, guest workers examined such things as specific dynamic action; hypoproteinemia; salmonellosis and reversible uremia in the rat; plasmapheresis; pulmonary compensatory hypertrophy after pneumonectomy; concentric and eccentric cardiac hypertrophy; renal blood flow after subtotal nephrectomy; the role of the kidney in hypertension with coarctation of the aorta; the number and size of glomeruli in the kidneys of elephants, rats and mice; the effect of thyroid on tadpole maturation; and electrophoresis of serum proteins.

John Luetscher, who was at Johns Hopkins, moved to Stanford in 1949, shortly after Addis's retirement. Luetscher inherited Addis's laboratory and was in charge of clinical chemistry. He installed the first flame photometer at Stanford and worked with a series of fellows, beginning with Quentin Deming,[13] demonstrating the presence of electrocortin, later called aldosterone, in the urine of nephrotic subjects.

## Albion Walter Hewlett[14]

In 1916 Hewlett was appointed professor of medicine at Stanford, having been at the University of Michigan since 1908 (see chapter 18). Hewlett and van Zwaluwenburg developed a plethysmographic method of determining blood flow in the arm. At Stanford, Hewlett maintained his interest in the physiology of the heart and the circulation.

During World War I, Hewlett served as a lieutenant commander in the Stanford Navy Base Hospital Unit. He was stationed for a time in

Scotland. Here he learned of the legendary reasoning powers of Dr. Joseph Bell, the man who gave rise in the mind of Sir Arthur Conan Doyle to that incomparable detective of fiction, Sherlock Holmes. Diagnosis, the supreme art of the physician, requires sound deductive reasoning, especially when not all of the information needed to solve the problem in question is at hand, and where every clue must be carefully weighed before a final conclusion can be reached. Hewlett possessed this gift to an extraordinary degree, accounting for his attraction to the story of Dr. Bell. The Stanford Navy Base Hospital Unit later served in France, and Hewlett and W. M. Alberty wrote an excellent description of their experience with influenza.[15]

In a paper published in 1918, Hewlett described the action of tyramin on the normal circulation of man, which resembled the changes that follow the intravenous injection of epinephrine in moderate doses. In a subsequent paper, Hewlett and W. E. Kay studied the effects of tyramin on the circulation during infections and during or after operations.[16] Repeated injections usually caused a transient rise of blood pressure and an increase in the volume of the pulse; effects less marked than those produced when the drug was given in similar doses to normal individuals.

In 1922 John K. Lewis and Hewlett studied the cause of increased vascular sounds after epinephrine injections.[17] They found a correlation between the changes in the sound and the changes in pulse pressure, which appeared to be better than the correlation between the changes in sounds and the changes in the pulse volume.

Hewlett carried out a series of studies on various phases of the response to exercise. In 1923 he and J. R. Nakada investigated the recovery from the hyperpnea of moderate exercise.[18] After muscular exercise, the excessive pulmonary ventilation lessens rapidly at first and then slower. They sought a numerical expression for the earlier and more rapid stages of recovery.

In 1923 Hewlett reported on the vital capacities of patients with cardiac complaints.[19] His paper was a statistical study of the vital capacity in a group of patients, most of whom complained of symptoms suggesting heart disease. Particular attention was paid to the association of diminished vital capacity with other objective evidences of cardiac disease. The vital capacity records utilized were obtained from patients referred to the electrocardiograph laboratory. Since May 1922, it had been customary in that laboratory to measure the vital capacities of all patients who were seen.[20] It was found that the vital capacity of college students based on a height standard was considerably greater than was the vital capacity of patients with cardiac complaints and without objective evidence of thoracic disease. The symptoms most commonly associated with low vital capacity were cough and dyspnea.

In 1925 the physiological mechanisms involved in dyspnea following exertion were largely obscure. In that year, Hewlett, Lewis, and Franklin studied the effect of artificial stenosis upon dyspnea produced by exercise.[21] Artificial obstruction to respiration was produced by having the subject breathe through two bored corks. During exercise, both bores reduced the respiratory rate and lessened the minute volume of respired air. With the smaller bore, a maximum minute volume of approximately thirty liters was attained, but the rapidly increasing distress indicated that this amount of ventilation was insufficient for the establishment of a steady state. With the larger bore, a steady state could be established with a minute volume of approximately forty-four liters. If a mixture rich in oxygen was breathed, the early distress was less marked, and exercise could be continued longer.

Hewlett's last paper (coauthored by George Barnett and Lewis), on the effect of breathing oxygen-enriched air during exercise upon pulmonary ventilation and upon the lactic acid content of blood and urine, was published posthumously.[22] They determined the increase, resulting from measured treadmill exercise, in lactic acid in blood and urine. A smaller rise of blood lactic acid and a smaller excretion of lactic acid were found when oxygen-enriched air was breathed. Earlier, this group had also studied the effect of training on lactic acid secretion.[23]

This sample of Hewlett's research demonstrates that he was first and foremost a clinical investigator, studying the effects of disease upon the function of the cardiovascular and pulmonary system in man. It was fitting that in 1925, the year of his death, he was president of the American Society for Clinical Investigation.

On May 3, 1926, at the eighteenth annual meeting of the society, in Atlantic City, New Jersey, the following resolution on the death of Hewlett was prepared by Rufus I. Cole and David M. Cowie:

> During the past year we have lost by death one of the small group of men to whom the foundation of this society was due and one who later became its president, Dr. Albion Walter Hewlett.
>
> While still a medical student his intellectual ability, his industry and his power of clear thinking and accurate expression marked him as one who was destined to become an important figure in his profession. He very early began to exhibit an interest in the fundamental processes concerned in disease and was not content merely to observe and describe the superficial and obvious. This interest led .him to the study of normal physiologic processes and to apply the methods of this study to the sick.
>
> These interests, which 20 years ago were not so common as they are now, led him and others of like mind to gravitate together, and as a result there came into being this organization of men bound together for searching out the underlying secrets of disease.
>
> But Dr. Hewlett was also interested in men, in sick individuals, in the classification of disease, in diagnosis and in treatment. He was a skillful clinician. These qualities were the ideal ones for the successful teacher and leader, and it was not surprising therefore that he was called while very young, to become the professor of medicine at one of the important universities, the University of Michigan. . . .
>
> Dr. Hewlett possessed not only an unusual intellectual equipment and

ability as an investigator, as teacher and physician, he was possessed of a most attractive personality. Quiet and thoughtful and giving the impression of much reserve power and force, yet he was a most interesting and agreeable companion. All the members of the early group comprising this society were his personal friends. He was always interested in the younger members of this society and many of them became greatly influenced in their later careers by his writings and by his personal influence.[24]

## Arthur Leonard Bloomfield[25]

Hewlett was succeeded in 1926 by Bloomfield. Bloomfield (M.D., Johns Hopkins, 1911) spent six years on the resident staff at Johns Hopkins. He then studied with Friedrich von Müller and returned to Baltimore, where he advanced to an associate professorship. Bloomfield was interested in infections and made significant studies of influenza, the common cold, and hemolytic streptococcal disease. His clinical and bacteriological studies of sore throat clearly established for the first time that streptococci were the only significant bacterial cause of this syndrome. He was also among the first to emphasize the importance of nonscarlatinal streptococcal respiratory infections.[26]

At Stanford, Bloomfield also did research on Addis's rats and worked on edema, which he produced in the rats by feeding them gels made of carrots. He wrote a series of papers on hypoproteinemia. In addition, he personally aspirated stomachs, while continuing his studies of gastric secretion and anacidity (begun in Baltimore with Chester S. Keefer[27]) and, with W. S. Polland, published a monograph on gastric anacidity.[28]

In later years, his interest turned to historical pursuits, which led to the publication of his two-volume work, *A Bibliography of Internal Medicine,* in which he outlined the development of the understanding of many infectious and other diseases by annotating the significant publications.[29] He was a president of the American Society for Clinical Investigation.

## Bloomfield's Associates

John K. Lewis trained under Hewlett, and together they worked, as noted earlier, on a variety of problems. When William Dock joined Lewis somewhat later, they continued his work on heart sounds. Lewis had the expertise to make very thin and tough membranes for recording heart sounds and, with Dock, used these in the study of the genesis of the first heart sound and the nature of gallop rhythms. This represented some of the earliest work in the field. Dock also studied heart sounds, hypertension, blood flow, digitalis,[30] specific dynamic action, and other problems. In 1932 Dock and Lewis published their study on the effect of thyroid feeding on the oxygen consumption of the heart and other tissues.[31] The increase in the oxygen consumption of the heart could be accounted for entirely by the increased rate and weight of the heart of thyroid-fed rats.

In 1938, in a paper that evoked a great deal of discussion, Lewis and Dock reported their thoughts on the origin of heart sounds and their variations in myocardial disease.[32] They felt that the heart sounds and the gallop sounds in diastole were due to tension of valve leaflets, with no appreciable muscular element.

## Other Members of the Faculty

Ernest Dickson, a professor of medicine, had a large laboratory and developed what was essentially a department of preventive medicine. His M.D. degree was obtained from Toronto, and he interned at Johns Hopkins. From 1908, he was on the faculty at Cooper Medical College and later at Stanford, first in pathology and medicine and later as professor of public health. He did early work on botulism and Valley fever,[33] as well as some studies on experimental uranium-induced nephritis. Dickson rose to fame by pointing out that Valley fever was actually the initial stage of coccidioidomycosis. He brought Charles E. Smith and then Rodney Beard to Stanford, both of whom contributed much to the understanding of this problem. Dickson had a large bacteriology laboratory. The routine urine and blood cultures were done on the medical wards, but the other routine bacteriology was sent to Dickson's laboratory. This laboratory was later directed by Lowell Addison Rantz.

Lowell Addison Rantz[34] (M.D., Stanford, 1936) spent three years as an intern and an assistant resident at the Stanford-Lane Hospital. He worked for two years as a research fellow for Keefer, then returned to Stanford and rapidly rose from instructor in 1939 to professor of medicine in 1955. Rantz became interested in the streptococcus and, more specifically, in rheumatic fever and glomerulonephritis.[35] He was a consultant to the secretary of war and a member of the Commission on Hemolytic Streptococcal Diseases, Army Epidemiological Board, from 1942 to 1946.

Robert S. Evans, who later went to Seattle, was interested in thrombocytopenic purpura and did much of his early work as an assistant and associate professor of medicine at Stanford. Herbert N. Hultgren, a Stanford alumnus, established the first catheter laboratory there.

During Bloomfield's reign, Lewis and David Rytand were in charge of basal metabolism studies and thyroid disease, as well as the EKG laboratory. Just as in many places, the technician did the basal metabolism estimations in the morning and then became the EKG technician; this was a matter of economics. The first cardiac catheterization laboratory was in the room previously housing the basal metabolism machines before these were supplanted by the protein-bound iodine determination.

This area was the forerunner of what later became Stanford's large empire of cardiology, which was directed by Donald Harrison.

David Rytand[36] was interested in cardiac hypertrophy; arterial hypertension; coarctation of the aorta; the number and size of glomeruli in various species; the nephrotic syndrome following poison oak dermatitis or reactions to bee stings; orthostatic proteinuria; obesity; murmurs with heart block in the elderly; and the circus movement hypothesis as related to atrial flutter. Rytand, who had first embarked on circus movement studies when Bloomfield retired in 1954, became chairman of the department and, later, Arthur L. Bloomfield Professor of Medicine—the first endowed chair in the Stanford University School of Medicine.

# 23

❦

# The University of California (San Francisco)

## Reorganization under Herbert Charles Moffitt

In 1912 Herbert Charles Moffitt[1] was appointed dean. Moffitt, after graduating from the University of California in 1889, entered the Harvard Medical School and received his M.D. degree four years later. During his period as a house pupil at the MGH, he came under the influence of Frederick C. Shattuck, Reginald Fitz, and other leading clinicians of the period. Moffitt then spent several years in Europe, visiting the medical centers at Munich, Berlin, Paris, Vienna, and London. In 1899 he was appointed lecturer in medicine and, in 1900, professor of medicine at the University of California Medical School.

As dean, Moffitt reorganized the school and recruited promising young investigators. Among those selected were such outstanding scientists as George Whipple, Karl F. Meyer, Frank W. Lynch, Herbert M. Evans, Frederick P. Gay, and William P. Lucas. Moffitt was largely responsible for the development of the clinical research facilities of the medical school. A three-hundred-bed teaching hospital, completed in 1917, was built through private donations. Moffitt served as a trustee of the Hooper Foundation for Medical Research. One of the first Cambridge electrocardiographs used in America, and many optical instruments of advanced design, were purchased by Moffitt and donated to the medical school. Moffitt also had an interest in pernicious anemia.[2]

Moffitt was active in teaching and administrative work until 1927, when he became clinical professor of medicine, serving in this capacity until 1937. He was the first to receive the Gold Headed Cane (1939), which was awarded annually by the department of medicine of the medical school. He was president of the Association of American Physicians in 1922.[3] Moffitt was enormously influential among all San Francisco

393

physicians as "dagen." He captured their imagination not only by his sound understanding of medicine and superb standards but also because of his great wit.

## George Hoyt Whipple and the Hooper Foundation

An influential figure in the development of medical research at the University of California, and Moffitt's successor as dean, was Whipple. He received his undergraduate training at Yale, where, in his senior year (1900), he studied under Lafayette B. Mendel and Russell H. Chittenden, who made biochemistry an exciting subject for him.[4] At the Johns Hopkins University School of Medicine, he was a student assistant to Walter Jones in the biochemistry course and in his research on nucleoproteins. Whipple also did special work in pathology for William G. MacCallum. After graduation, he obtained a position in pathology, with the expectation that he would continue clinical training. The year was very stimulating, and Welch provided a second year in the department, which served to anchor Whipple to a career in pathology. In 1907 he reported a case of "intestinal lipodystrophy," which later became known as Whipple's disease.[5] A year's leave of absence took him to Panama, where he gained valuable experience in tropical diseases. From 1908 to 1914, he was a member of the department of pathology at Johns Hopkins. After reading a paper by Howland and Richards (1908) on chloroform poisoning, he decided to produce similar lesions in dogs, with the expectation that cirrhosis of the liver would ensue. This did not occur, even after the repeated administrations of chloroform. Jaundice did develop in the chloroform-poisoned dogs, and Whipple and John King studied the excretion of bile pigment.

In the summer of 1909, Whipple worked with P. Morowitz in Heidelberg and, in 1911, studied pharmacology under Hans Meyer. On his return to Baltimore, he studied experimental icterus with Charles Hooper, using the Eck fistula, and described the rapid change of hemoglobin to bile pigment outside the liver.[6] The study of liver function led to collaboration with Leonard G. Rowntree in pharmacology.[7] Whipple also published a series of papers on experimental intestinal obstruction.[8]

In 1914 Whipple accepted an invitation to be director of the new Hooper Foundation for Medical Research[9] and Professor of Research Medicine at the University of California.

An old veterinary facility was assigned to the Hooper Foundation. It consisted of three floors in a building about ninety feet long, with large skylights in the roof over the third floor. The top floor, which was reconstituted with new partitions, had small rooms that served as laboratory space for research in experimental physiology, bacteriology, and parasitology. A chemical laboratory was located on the second floor; small animals were kept on the ground floor, and a new animal house for dogs was constructed behind the main building. Equipment and chemicals were in short supply, but Whipple received help from Gay, of the bacteriology department, and discovered some apparatus formerly used by Jacques Loeb.

Charles Hooper, from Johns Hopkins, came to San Francisco with Whipple. Two senior associates were appointed early in 1915. Ernest Walker, who had recently returned from the Philippines, continued his observations on amebic dysentery, leishmaniasis, and leprosy.[10] Karl F. Meyer, who had recently joined the department of pathology, worked with Whipple's group in investigations related to the infectious diseases.

Meyer and Walker surveyed the incidence of malaria in the Bay area while Meyer, along with several fellows, began studies on typhoid and paratyphoid fever as well as on brucellosis. In 1920 Meyer successfully traced an extensive outbreak of botulism to canned ripe olives. Walter C. Alvarez, who was later to become an outstanding gastroenterologist, carried out his observations on the smooth muscle of the intestinal tract in Whipple's laboratories and did his clinical work elsewhere (see chapter 21). A number of able part-time workers who were later outstanding clinicians with an interest in investigation, including Frank Hinman, Jean Cooke,[11] and William John Kerr, also joined the group. Frieda Robscheit-Robbins became a member of Whipple's research team in 1917. Through the help of George Corner, who was formerly at Johns Hopkins and was then in the department of anatomy in Berkeley, a number of students came to work in Whipple's laboratory. Several of them went on to distinguished careers, including Harry P. Smith, who became a professor of pathology at the College of Physicians and Surgeons in New York; Stafford Warren, radiologist, physicist, and later dean of the U.C.L.A. Medical School; Francis Scott Smyth, pediatrician and dean, University of California Medical School; Irvine McQuarrie, later professor of pediatrics at the University of Minnesota (see chapter 20); and Elmer Belt, the well-known urological surgeon at U.C.L.A.

Whipple resumed his study of intestinal obstruction in 1915 and, with Samuel H. Hurwitz, who had worked with him as a Johns Hopkins medical student, and William John Kerr, who came from Harvard on a Sheldon Traveling Fellowship, began to study the formation of the proteins of the blood plasma.[12] Most important, Whipple and Charles Hooper resumed their studies, begun in Baltimore, on the bile pigments.

When Whipple and Hooper first began their studies at Johns Hopkins in 1913, they encountered difficulty in keeping their bile fistula dogs in good health, because the loss of the bile led to emaciation and eventual death. When they fed them fresh pigs' liver, there was a marked improvement. Whipple and Hooper concluded that something formed in the liver facilitates the construction of body pigments from which the bile pigments are derived, including hemoglobin. In 1916 they stated that "there may be a prehemoglobin substance manufactured somewhere in the body, perhaps in the liver, which may be fixed by the bone marrow cells and appear as finished hemoglobin."[13] Hooper developed the idea that pernicious anemia might result from disturbance in the production of this hypothetical prehemoglobin substance. He made an alcoholic extract of liver, which he tried on six patients. The only evidence of this experiment is a letter from Whipple to Moffitt, dated July 25, 1916, stating that the results of the injections, though inconclusive, were hopeful. Hooper's extract probably did contain the $B_{12}$ factor; however, he was a shy young man, and, since the hospital physicians felt that what he was observing were spontaneous remissions, he became discouraged and stopped his investigations.

Whipple proceeded with his studies of anemic dogs by drawing off blood and then observing what diets and drugs would most effectively cause the depleted blood to regenerate.[14] He found that a diet of mixed table scraps would effect complete return of the normal blood picture in four to seven weeks. When the dogs were fed lean scrap meat, beef heart, or liver, regeneration was rapid, whereas on diets consisting mainly of carbohydrates, or carbohydrates and fat, it was slow. Iron, long a favored treatment for "secondary anemia," had no effect upon the rate of blood regeneration. These experiments were reported at a meeting of the American Physiological Society in late December 1917.

In order to calculate the rate of hemoglobin formation in the anemic dogs, it was necessary to know their blood volume. Drawing upon Herbert M. Evans's vast knowledge of analine dyes, Robscheit-Robbins tested various analogues and found one, with the necessary qualities of nontoxicity and very slow diffusion from the bloodstream, that enabled them successfully to estimate the blood volume in these dogs. Dawson, testing still other dyes supplied by Evans, later found one, the Toluidin derivative $T_{1824}$, known as *Evans blue dye*, that was better than any previously tested.[15]

Whipple recognized that the symptoms following x-ray exposure in man resembled those of the proteose intoxications that he had produced in his dogs.[16] He exposed dogs to intense x-radiation (with Charles C. Hall) and found that they did indeed develop such symptoms and showed changes in blood chemical abnormalities indicative of extensive breakdown of body protein. Pathological studies revealed, however, little injury beyond microscopically detectable damage of the lining epithelium of the intestine. Following up on this hint, Whipple and Stafford Warren exposed dogs to massive radiation over the thorax without producing any general reaction, but similar exposure of the abdomen was followed promptly by typical symptoms of intoxication. Microscopic study of the intestine revealed extensive destruction of the epithelial cells. This work was the beginning of Warren's professional career in radiology and of his lifetime interest in radiation disease, which fitted him to serve during World War II as chief advisor to the Manhattan Project on radiation risks and safety precautions in atomic energy research.[17]

## Student Fellowships

One of Whipple's innovations was his creation of student fellowships that provided time for scientific investigation. The first three were held by Elmer Belt, Charles C. Hall, and Harry P. Smith. In 1918 the fellows were Irvine McQuarrie,[18] Francis Scott Smyth, and Stafford Warren.[19]

The Hooper Foundation was a department in the medical school of the University of California. Moffitt was the dean of the school during the first six years of the operation of the foundation, of which he was also a trustee. In 1920 Whipple was invited to succeed Moffitt as dean of the school. His time in this position was short because, in the spring of 1921, he accepted the challenge of organizing a new medical school at the University of Rochester.

Karl F. Meyer remained a commanding figure after Whipple's departure. He isolated the virus of Western Equine Encephalitis, and, in the fields of psittacosis and plague, he held an undisputed position of world leadership. Meyer trained few successful investigators, however, William D. Hammon being a notable exception.

## William John Kerr as Professor of Medicine

In 1927 William John Kerr became chairman of the department of medicine, physician-in-chief to the University of California Hospital, and consulting physician to the San Francisco General Hospital. Kerr (M.D., Harvard, 1915) had completed six years of training in Boston, and had received a traveling fellowship in medical research while at Harvard. The following year he had worked with Whipple.

Kerr increased the staff of the department from three full-time men to a large, multidisciplined full-time department. His chief interest was in cardiovascular disease. From 1928 to 1929, he spent a sabbatical working with Sir Thomas Lewis in London. He wrote extensively on the pathophysiology and therapy of angina pectoris, other manifestations of coronary disease, peripheral vascular disease, and liver disease.[20] Kerr played a leading role in the establishment of the Herbert C. Moffitt Hospital and subsequently organized a metabolic unit and a cardiovascular research unit; however, his own research was not very productive. Kerr was a master and a president of the American College of Physicians, and president of the American Heart Association in 1937. He retired in 1952.

## Other Members of Kerr's Department

A prominent practicing physician and clinical investigator in endocrinology was Hans Lisser, who took his M.D. degree at Johns Hopkins in 1911.[21] He then served as house officer at the Johns Hopkins Hospital. From 1913 to 1914 he was assistant in medicine at Washington University and chief of the syphilis clinic. He entered private practice in San Francisco and became a member of the faculty of the university. He was chief of the ductless gland clinic from 1920 to 1958.

Beginning in 1919, he made contributions to endocrinology, writing numerous clinical papers as well as the section on diseases of ductless glands for George Blumer's *System of Bedside Diagnosis.* When Kerr stimulated Lisser to become an endocrinologist he gave up his interest in syphilis.

Lisser was a stimulating teacher, and soon a group of younger physicians were working under him in the endocrine clinic. He emphasized thorough workups and photographs of patients (an important technique in endocrinological research), and the reporting of new or unusual findings in endocrine diseases. In that era, many new endocrine preparations were made available for clinical trial and use, and these were carefully studied by Lisser and his associates. His monograph on the use of thyroid is a classic. Lisser and Minnie B. Goldberg published reports on early trials with the placental extract (Emmenin) in the treatment of acromegaly. Lisser was one of the first to emphasize the varied symptomatology of hypothyroidism. Lisser and Harry C. Shepardson first reported the treatment of a severe case of tetany resulting from accidental removal of the parathyroid, controlled by serum calcium determinations.[22]

Gilbert S. Gordon, who had served his internship and residency at the University of California Hospital in 1941 and 1942, became active in the endocrine clinic with Lisser. One of his early papers described the electrocardiographic changes in hyperthyroidism.[23] After military service in World War II, Gordan returned to the Clinic, where he worked with Evans and Miriam Simpson on nitrogen excretion with testosterone and later conducted a clinical appraisal with Escamilla on the sublingual administration of testosterone.[24]

Roberto Escamilla (M.D., Harvard, 1931), who had interned at the Peter Bent Brigham Hospital, did several studies with Lisser, including an exhaustive review of Simmonds's disease.[25] Later they coauthored *Atlas of Clinical Endocrinology,* published by the C. V. Mosby Company in 1957 and 1962, which was well accepted. Escamilla was the first to note carotinemia in myxedema and described, with Lisser and Shepardson, a patient with internal myxedema, which later was recognized in some quarters as the Escamilla-Lisser syndrome.[26] Early studies on the effects of testosterone were published with G. R. Biskind and then with L. E. Curtis.[27] Escamilla and Lisser studied the effects of estrogens in inducing menarche[28] and development and on testosterone therapy in Simmonds's disease.

Theodore L. Althausen (M.D., California, 1926) trained at the San Francisco and County hospitals and at the University of California Hospital in San Francisco. As a Guggenheim fellow, he studied in Leipzig,

Freiburg, and Paris from 1930 to 1931. His career was spent at the University of California, where he was promoted through the various grades until he became a full professor in 1947. He served as chairman of the department from 1951 to 1956. His research interests included the pathology of gestation in vitamin E deficiency; the role of the liver in the metabolism of carbohydrates; hepatic function in man; the thyroid gland and absorption in the intestine and kidneys; calcium balance in hyperthyroidism; hormonal and vitamin factors in intestinal absorption; and nutritional deficiencies in sprue.[29] Althausen was influenced in his research by Herbert M. Evans. He won the van Metre Prize of the American Association for the Study of Goitre in 1939. He was a member of the American Society for Clinical Investigation.

Stacy R. Mettier (M.D., University of California, 1926) trained at the Thorndike Laboratory, where he worked in hematology. After his return to San Francisco, he joined the faculty at California and became a professor of medicine and head of postgraduate instruction. He continued his investigation in hematology, with a special interest in hypersplenism.

In 1935, after serving as a house officer at the MGH, Mayo H. Soley came to the University of California as a graduate student in medicine. During the next thirteen years, he progressed to the rank of professor of medicine. For two years he served as chairman of the division of pharmacology, succeeding Chauncey D. Leake, and, from 1944 to 1948, he was assistant dean of the school. His scientific contributions were in the field of endocrinology, notably in diseases of the thyroid. With Joseph G. Hamilton, he made pioneer studies on the use of radioactive iodine in thyroid diseases. He also studied gas exchange in the hyperventilation syndrome. In 1948 he became dean and professor of experimental medicine at the University of Iowa College of Medicine.

Among other young men who began their work in the department under Kerr, before the end of World War II, were Paul Michael Aggeler (M.D., California, 1937) and Maurice Sokoloff. Aggeler served as a fellow in medicine (1939–41) and, in 1964, was promoted to full professor. In 1963 he became chief of the hematology division at the San Francisco General Hospital. He was an authority on the hemorrhagic diseases and the discoverer of a new thromboplastin component, whose isolation fostered understanding of the multiplicity of factors involved in coagulation of blood.[30] Salvatore P. Lucia was active in investigations in the field of hematology and, with Aggeler, was coauthor of a book on hemorrhagic disorders.[31] Sokoloff received his M.D. degree from California in 1936. He joined the department as a clinical instructor and became a full professor of medicine and chief of the cardiovascular service in the University Hospital in 1958. His particular interests in the cardiovascular field were rheumatic fever, hypertension, cardiac arrhythmias, and cardiac failure.

# Summary

    In this section, the development of clinical investigation at a variety of university-based medical schools and, in addition, at the Mayo Clinic, has been described. The various approaches to research in these institutions in terms of the techniques used, both observational and experimental, have been discussed. The careers of a number of important clinical scientists, with a description of their background, training, and fields of research, have been portrayed. It is of interest to trace the intellectual pedigree of the various clinical scientists, in terms of who they trained under and the influence this training had on the direction of their own research and also on the general pattern of clinical science in the school in which they did their work. One sees how the concept of full-time clinical professorships evolved in different universities, and how it in turn influenced the course of clinical science in the particular schools.

    These descriptions of individual schools document the history of clinical science in the United States and the emergence of the clinical scientist, whose accomplishments were primarily responsible for the creation of the scientific base of medical practice. Although it has not been possible to be all-inclusive, the examples selected illustrate the status of clinical science at each step from 1905 to 1945 and display the sequential advances that permitted medicine to gain its present prestige and permitted medical research to become established in the United States on a scale, and of a quality, that equalled the accomplishments in the best European centers.

    Most schools were slow to implement the type of change that Lewellys Franklin Barker initiated in 1905 when he established special full-time clinical research laboratories. Theodore Caldwell Janeway and Warfield Theobald Longcope, at Columbia's College of Physicians and Surgeons [P & S], were among those early appreciators of what was being accomplished in Germany by the application of the methods of the basic sciences to the study of disease in man. Their attempts at Columbia were, however, only partially successful, because it was not feasible to secure the facilities necessary for the best level of development. Longcope attracted a number of young men to the department, however, who were successful in conducting important clinical research, particularly in the fields of immunology and biochemistry, as represented by H. Rawle Geyelin and his pupils Eugene F. DuBois and John P. Peters. World War I interrupted these developments, however, and the flowering of clinical science at P & S did not come until 1921, when W. W. Palmer was appointed professor of medicine and brought to his full-time staff such young clinical investigators as Dana Atchley, Robert F. Loeb, and Alphonse Raymond Dochez.

At Cornell, the focus for the development of clinical science was the Russell Sage Institute of Pathology, where Graham Lusk was director and Eugene F. DuBois medical director. A metabolic research ward was established. Many young men trained in this institute later made important contributions to clinical science, including James H. Means, Joseph C. Aub, Ephraim Schorr, William S. McCann, David P. Barr, John P. Peters, and others.

The birth of modern clinical science in Boston came with the arrival of David Linn Edsall as Jackson Professor of Medicine at the MGH. Edsall promptly selected an outstanding group of young men who were sent to various centers to prepare themselves for careers in clinical science, including Means, Aub, Paul Dudley White, Oswald H. Robertson, and Carl A. L. Binger. Edsall created clinical research facilities and made plans for a clinical research ward, which were implemented by Means, leading to the establishment of the famous Ward 4. At the same time, the Peter Bent Brigham Hospital opened. Through the efforts of Henry A. Christian, professor of medicine, and Harvey Williams Cushing, professor of surgery, important advances in clinical investigation were made at that institution. A decade later (in 1923), the Thorndike Memorial Laboratory, with Francis W. Peabody as its first director, was established. This was the first clinical research facility to function in a public hospital, and many influential clinical scientists were trained there.

Shortly after full-time positions in medicine, surgery, and pediatrics were established at Johns Hopkins (1914), the Rockefeller Foundation gave financial support for the creation of similar positions at Washington University School of Medicine in St. Louis. The early developments in medicine there were hampered by administrative arrangements for the payment of laboratory and other services between the school of medicine and the hospital; and it was not until after World War II that clinical science in the department of medicine achieved excellence. Greater success came under Evarts A. Graham, of the department of surgery, and W. McKim Marriott, of pediatrics.

In the early 1920s, the Vanderbilt University School of Medicine underwent a major reorganization under George Canby Robinson, with the establishment of full-time clinical departments, the development of effective programs in clinical investigation, and the training of clinical scientists such as Tinsley R. Harrison in medicine and Alfred Blalock in surgery. Also at this time, a new school of medicine was founded, with support from the Rockefeller Foundation, at the University of Rochester. This school was under the leadership of George Whipple, the Nobel Laureate, who was its first dean. McCann, the first professor of medicine, had been trained at Cornell and Johns Hopkins.

In the early twenties, Milton C. Winternitz became dean at Yale, and, with the aid of a grant from the Rockefeller Foundation, full-time clinical chairs were established. The department of medicine, under Francis G. Blake, was highly successful. Blake recruited such outstanding young men as John P. Peters, William C. Stadie, and John R. Paul. The department of pediatrics was also successfully developed, first under Edwards A. Park and later under Grover Powers, both of whom were from Johns Hopkins, in terms of contributions to clinical research and the training of clinical investigators. Such outstanding clinical investigators as Daniel C. Darrow and James D. Trask did important work in pediatrics at Yale.

The University of Michigan was the first school in the Midwest to emphasize science. The preclinical sciences were developed early, and several members of the original faculty at Johns Hopkins had had their training at Michigan or had been members of the faculty there. George Dock was professor of medicine from 1891 to 1908 and was succeeded by Albion W. Hewlett, who was one of the first professors to take a functional, rather than an anatomical, approach to clinical medicine. He developed the method of plethysmography for the study of blood flow in man and had a very wide influence on clinical science, because he was a charter member of the American Society for Clinical Investigation. One of the brilliant clinical investigators at Michigan was Louis H. Newburgh, who had completed his early training at Harvard under William T. Porter in physiology. In addition to his research in the field of metabolism and nutrition, Newburgh trained many clinical investigators, including Alexander Leaf, of Boston, and Jerome Conn. Conn first delineated the clinical syndrome of primary aldosteronism.

The influence of clinical scientists, trained in the larger Eastern schools, who migrated to other institutions under reorganization is illustrated by the events at Western Reserve. The Cushing Laboratory of Experimental Medicine was established there, shortly after 1900, under George W. Stewart, but it never had much impact on research in the school's clinical departments. The situation changed after the arrival of Joseph T. Wearn as professor of medicine in 1927. Wearn had done excellent research on the coronary circulation and had been a member of the Thorndike Memorial Laboratory.

The outstanding clinical scientist to emerge in Chicago was Rollin T. Woodyatt, who had studied under Friedrich von Müller in Europe. Woodyatt was given financial aid by one of the first institutes created for the support of medical research in the United States, the Sprague Institute. He established one of America's first clinical research wards, whose eight beds were supported by a grant from the Sprague Institute. Another organization for research in Chicago, one of the earliest in the United States, was the John McCormick Institute for Infectious Diseases, where the Dicks did their important work on streptococcal infections and scarlet fever. Illustrative of the accomplishments of outstanding practitioners of medicine in clinical investigation is the story of James B. Herrick, of Chicago, who first described sickle cell disease and recognized that patients with coronary thrombosis could survive, and who was responsible for the delineation of the clinical syndrome of myocardial infarction. An important force in American medicine came in 1925, with the establishment of the University of Chicago School of Medicine, whose first dean was Franklin C. McLean. A superb full-time clinical faculty was recruited, with Oswald H. Robertson, C. Philip Miller, W. W. Palmer, and many others as leaders.

At the University of Minnesota, the development of an advanced degree program in the medical sciences provided an impetus for the advance of clinical science. Such outstanding individuals as Cecil J. Watson, in medicine, and Owen H. Wangensteen, in surgery, had their basic training here. At the Mayo Clinic, an unusual event took place in that, although there was no medical school, the Mayos recognized the importance of research and gave opportunity for its development under Henry Stanley Plummer, Edward C. Kendall, Russell Wilder, Leonard G. Rowntree (the first full-time professor at the University of Minnesota), and many other capable men.

Ray Lyman Wilbur played a significant role in the development of clinical science at Leland Stanford University School of Medicine when he brought Thomas Addis there. Addis did important work in relation to kidney disease and trained many outstanding young clinical scientists. In 1916 Hewlett became professor of medicine at Stanford, where he instilled a strong spirit of clinical investigation. In 1925 A. L. Bloomfield, who had done classic work in infectious disease at Johns Hopkins, succeeded Hewlett as professor of medicine and continued the emphasis on clinical science.

The story of clinical science at the University of California is the story of George Whipple's laboratory of experimental medicine in the Hooper Foundation. Here Whipple did much of the outstanding work that led to his receiving the Nobel Prize; in addition, he imbued many young investigators with a love for clinical science—Irvine McQuarrie, William John Kerr, and Shields Warren being among them. The full development of clinical investigation was not, however, reached at the school until after World War II, with the recruitment of Julius H. Comroe from Pennsylvania and the appointment of Lloyd H. Smith as professor of medicine.

# Epilogue

In this volume, an attempt has been made to follow the major pathways of the development of clinical science in the United States from 1869 to 1945. The training and accomplishments of the key clinical scientists have been presented; the facilities at their disposal have been described as well as the manner in which their results were made available to others; and the learned societies and other medical organizations that influenced the conduct and direction of clinical investigation have been discussed. A unique feature in the United States was the creation of full-time positions in clinical departments, which had a major impact both on medical education and on medical practice. How this professionalization of clinical investigation was handled in a variety of medical schools has been described. It is fully recognized that the story is far from complete. The selection of the specific university settings was designed to provide examples of the various ways in which these innovations were approached. A detailed account is presented of those schools who pioneered in the development of clinical science, and other settings were chosen for the purpose of showing how the interchange of individuals involved in clinical investigation occurred. Major emphasis has been placed on the events in departments of medicine and, to a lesser extent, the contributions in departments of pediatrics and surgery.

At the end of the Civil War, there were no clinical research laboratories in the United States, no training was provided in the research methods in the basic sciences that were being developed in Germany, and no career opportunities existed for a physician who might develop an interest in research. Perceptive medical statesmen, who became aware of the practical applications of the developments underway in Germany, and who realized how deficient medical education and medical science were in the United States, set out to change the situation. As the migration to the cities occurred and industry prospered, money became available for philanthropic purposes.

Steps were taken to provide training in physics, chemistry, and biology as preparation for the study of medicine and, by 1893, in some medical schools the basic sciences were taught by full-time professionals who not only did research, but in whose laboratories physicians interested in the study of disease in man could work.

The type of training available in German universities for a scientific career rapidly became available in the United States. The Land Grant Act of 1862 brought about a large increase in the number of American colleges, and in the 1870s there was a rise in the number of graduate schools, including the Johns Hopkins University, which was directly influenced by the German example.

Carl Ludwig, the physiologist in Leipzig, had a major influence on the men who trained under him, including William Henry Welch, Franklin Paine Mall, and Henry P. Bowditch. Ludwig instilled in these men the idea that medicine could not advance until the knowledge and methods of the basic sciences were applied to the study of human disease. Carl Voit was another German scientist who influenced the development of clinical investigation in the United States through the men he trained, notably Graham Lusk,

The United States provided a milieu similar to that in Germany, where competition within a decentralized system encouraged the establishment of specialized research roles and facilities. The importance of such developments in the clinical field was not generally recognized in the United States until the beginning of the twentieth century, and there was strong resistance against them. The problem of transforming the practitioner-amateur into a professional clinical investigator was to prove similar to the earlier problem of the professionalization of the basic scientists.

Thus, the rapid rise in America's accomplishments in clinical science starting in the early 1900s can be attributed to the effort of a small group of men who created specialized, rapidly expanding positions and facilities for clinical research. Competition determined many of the crucial decisions relating to these developments. Successful clinical scientists were rewarded with university chairs and facilities. Their success encouraged other universities to provide such facilities and to transform rapidly the pursuit of clinical science into a regular professional career. From the important beginnings in Baltimore, New York, and Boston, there soon emerged the middleman of medical science—the full-time clinical investigator—who formed the bridge between the basic scientist on the one side, and the practitioner of medicine on the other.

# Appendix A

# Brief Biographical Sketches of the Charter Members of the American Society for Clinical Investigation

### Colonel Bailey Kelly Ashford

Ashford received his M.D. degree from Georgetown University Medical School in 1896 and was an army medical officer from 1897 to 1927. He became a professor of tropical medicine and mycology at Columbia University College of Physicians and Surgeons. In 1900, while studying an epidemic of fatal anemia in an area of Puerto Rico, he noted a large number of eosinophils in the blood. Remembering a recent description of eosinophilia in trichinosis, Ashford looked for a parasitic infection and found hookworm infestation. Subsequently, hookworm infestation was found to be common in the southern United States by Charles W. Stiles. Ashford and Stiles devised effective means of prophylaxis among rural populations. Ashford's campaign against the disease in Puerto Rico (1903–4) reduced mortality by ninety percent.[1]

### Edwin R. Baldwin

Two years after graduation from Yale Medical School (1890), Baldwin found tubercle bacilli in his sputum and went to Saranac Lake. While there, he developed an interest in the study of tuberculosis and eventually became director of the Saranac Laboratory. In 1916, in collaboration with Walter Belknap James, he established the Edward Livingston Trudeau Foundation for research in tuberculosis. As director of the foundation's activities, he was largely responsible for its important scientific contributions. In 1936 he was awarded the Kober Medal of the Association of American Physicians.[2]

## William J. Calvert

Calvert received his M.D. degree from Johns Hopkins in 1898 and then interned at the Johns Hopkins Hospital. He entered the U.S. Army and, in 1902, served in the Philippines with Richard Pearson Strong. He was then an assistant professor of medicine and a professor of physical diagnosis and clinical pathology at the University of Missouri School of Medicine at Columbia. He later served as a professor of pathology at Washington University. His research was mostly clinical in nature, as evidenced by the titles of his papers.[3]

## David Murray Cowie

Cowie received his M.D. degree from Michigan in 1896 and studied in Heidelberg in 1908. At Michigan, he served as a clinical professor of medicine (1907–9) and a clinical professor of pediatrics and medicine (1909–19). He became a professor of medicine in 1919, and of pediatrics and infectious diseases in 1920. In 1920 he was vice-president of the American Society for Clinical Investigation. His interests were in immunity and infectious diseases and in digestion and metabolism.[4]

## Charles Phillips Emerson

Emerson received his M.D. degree from Johns Hopkins in 1899, interned at the Johns Hopkins Hospital, and was an assistant resident physician in charge of the clinical laboratory. During this period, he spent a part of each of three years in Strasbourg, Basel, and Paris. After three years as superintendent of the Clifton Springs (New York) Sanatorium and Clinic, he went to Indiana as a professor of medicine. Emerson wrote a comprehensive textbook on clinical pathology, the introduction of which was written by Osler. Although Emerson's most outstanding contributions were in the field of education and social service, he did report on clinical conditions and methods of treatment such as pneumothorax and the management of chronic arthritis.[5]

## Haven Emerson

Emerson graduated from Columbia's College of Physicians and Surgeons in 1899. He taught physiology and clinical medicine there while he carried on a general practice. In 1910 he developed tuberculosis and was sent to Saranac Lake, where he was treated by Edward Livingston Trudeau. This experience gave Emerson a lasting, intense interest in the disease and its dissemination. He found glaring defects in administrative health policy and decided to embrace public health as a career at a time when there were no full-time professionals in this field.

In New York City's Health Department, he exercised and developed his talent for organization and for vigorous, articulate, outspoken advocacy of the public welfare. In 1915 he became Commissioner of Health in New York City.

In 1922 Emerson found a permanent base in the newly constructed DeLamar Institute of Public Health at Columbia as a professor of administrative medicine. He was one of the first to see the relevance of the public health approach to the study and control of chronic disease.[6]

### Martin Henry Fischer

Fischer received his M.D. degree from Rush Medical College in 1901. He was an assistant in pathology (1898–1900) and in physiology (1900–1901) there, and was an associate in physiology (1901–2) at Chicago. He became an assistant professor at The College of Medicine at Cincinnati in 1902, and a professor of pathology at the Oakland College of Medicine and Surgery in 1905. In 1910 he was appointed a professor of physiology at Cincinnati. His principal interest was histopathology. He studied the toxic effects of formaldehyde and did work on edema, nephritis, glaucoma, and coma; on musuclar contraction and hemolysis; and on the absorption and secretion of water and dissolved substances by plants and animals.[7]

### Mark Wyman Richardson

After receiving his M.D. degree from Harvard in 1894, Richardson interned at the MGH. In 1895 he studied in Berlin and Vienna and, on his return, was made an assistant pathologist at the Harvard Medical School. He studied the bacteriology of typhoid fever, investigated immunity to the disease, and searched for a possible serum treatment.[8]

### Edward Carl Rosenow

Rosenow received his M.D. degree, in 1902, from the Rush Medical College. From 1902 to 1904 he was a fellow in pathology there. From 1904 to 1915 he was a member of the staff of the John McCormick

Memorial Institute for Infectious Diseases, where Ludwig Hektoen interested him in experimental bacteriology. His research work after 1903 was confined almost entirely to the study of bacteria and viruses, at first centering on the pneumococcus, but later embracing the streptococcus. A paper in 1913, on the transmutation of streptococci and pneumococci, was an early indication of his later work on the appearance of variants in certain pathogenic organisms. In July 1915, he joined the Mayo Graduate School of Medicine at Rochester, Minnesota, and, for the next twenty-eight years, worked there as a bacteriologist.[9]

## Joseph Sailer

Sailer received his M.D. degree from Pennsylvania in 1891. After an internship at the Philadelphia General Hospital, he studied in Zurich, Vienna, and Paris. Sailer became a demonstrator of morbid anatomy, an instructor in clinical medicine and, in 1912, a professor of clinical medicine. Most of his investigative work was related to diseases of the gastrointestinal tract. After World War I, his interest shifted to cardiology. He was an organizer and a president of the American Heart Association.[10]

## Charles E. Simon

Simon was a student in the chemical-biological course (the premedical course) at Johns Hopkins in 1876. He received his M.D. degree from the University of Maryland in 1890. Following this, he was a resident under Osler. In 1891 he went to Paris for special work in physiological chemistry. He entered private practice, specializing in gastrointestinal diseases and, in 1896, published his manual of clinical diagnosis. He became a professor of clinical pathology at the University of Maryland. He published a book on infection and immunity in 1912 and another on human infection carriers in 1919. He was a pioneer in the field of virology.[11]

## John Dutton Steele

After obtaining an M.D. degree from Pennsylvania in 1893, Steele studied internal medicine and pathology at Heidelberg. He served his internship at Philadelphia General Hospital. He was an assistant director in gross anatomy, and an instructor and then an associate in medicine at Pennsylvania. The majority of Steele's publications pertained to the gastrointestinal tract.[12]

## Richard Pearson Strong

Strong was a member of the first class to receive the M.D. degree from Johns Hopkins (1897). After interning at the Johns Hopkins Hospital, he was commissioned in the U.S. Army as a first lieutenant during the Spanish-American War and, after its termination, was assigned to the Philippine Islands as organizer and first president of the army's Medical Research Board for the Investigation of Tropical Diseases. He resigned from the army in 1902 and became director of the biological laboratories (located in the Bureau of Science in Manila) of the government of the Philippine Islands. He was also chief of medicine in the Philippine General Hospital and a professor of tropical medicine at the medical school of the University of the Philippines. In 1913 Strong was called to Harvard University, where he became the first professor of tropical medicine.[13]

## Wilder Tileston

Tileston received his M.D. degree from Harvard in 1899 and served his internship at the MGH. At the Harvard Medical School he was an assistant in chemistry (1902–3), an assistant in clinical medicine (1906–9), and an instructor in pathology (1908–9). In 1908–9 he was a Dalton Fellow at the MGH. He reported the effects on the digestion and absorption of fat in cases in which there was complete absence of pancreatic secretion from the intestines, and he also studied the administration of pancreatic preparations. In 1909 Tileston became an assistant professor of medicine at Yale and, in 1919, a professor of clinical medicine. He was secretary of the American Society for Clinical Investigation from 1909 to 1912 and vice-president in 1913.[14]

## George Barclay Wallace

Wallace received his M.D. degree from Michigan in 1897. He studied in Vienna and Strasbourg. He was an instructor in pharmacology at Michigan from 1897 to 1900. He then served as an instructor (1901–3), a lecturer (1903–5), an associate professor (1905–7), and a professor (1907 to retirement) at the University and Bellevue Hospital Medical College. His interests were in a variety of fields, including saline cathartics, volatile oils, cyanide, nitrite, diuretics, and bile pigment.

# Appendix B

❧

# Interview with Joseph T. Wearn,
## March 25, 1976

"If I go back to my medical school days ... I think the first sparks ignited were by Walter Cannon and Otto Folin. Both were involved in rugged contests with others in their field; Cannon was working on adrenalin at the time and was engaged in an argument with Stewart at Western Reserve; Folin was engaged in research on the amino acids in the blood and also in his development of new chemical methods for urinary and blood substances. This was in 1913. Folin recounted to us his trips to the meetings on biological chemistry, and Cannon his to the Physiological Society. They gave us a pretty good picture of both sides of the argument. This showed me how difficult it is to establish a fact and to arrive at a conclusion. [In 1917], in fourth year medicine, I was sitting in the student's laboratory, looking at a blood smear. Francis Peabody came in and sat down beside me. He asked what I was doing, and I told him that I was counting the cells in a patient with myelogeneous leukemia. It turned out that he knew, because he was on duty in the wards at that time, and he had come to see the smear. He looked at it, and then he said, 'How would you like to follow this patient? We are going to take him over to the Huntington Hospital and put radium over his spleen.' This was in the early days of radiation for leukemia. I said, 'I'd love it.' He said, 'All right, that's your job. I want daily blood counts, smears, etc., right down the line, beginning today, and after doing this for three or four days and establishing a baseline, we will radiate him.' I remember to this day that the count was 1,016,000, and after radiation it dropped to somewhere in the neighborhood of 22,000, but the blood smear still showed everything in the way of blasts, nucleated red cells, many of which I could not identify. To my surprise, Peabody said, 'I can't tell what those are.' It impressed me that this man would say, 'I don't know.' That was my first real contact with clinical research.

411

"Chandler Walker was doing research in asthma and was doing skin tests on one of my patients [in 1913]. Noon had just introduced the skin test in 1911; a couple of years later Cooke did the dermal test and put it on a more quantitative basis. At that time, Samuel Levine was in charge of the electrocardiographic laboratory. Christian was making observations on the vital capacity in heart failure. His chief interest was in nephritis, and he and James O'Hare were studying the effects of various diets on renal function tests. That will give a little picture of the research atmosphere in the Brigham as it existed in the beginning. The only other department then was surgery with Harvey Cushing, who had the Arthur Tracy Cabot Fellowships. Lewis Weed came from Baltimore with Cushing, and that's where all the work on the cerebrospinal fluid began, which was important for the development of neurosurgery.

"I had a course in fourth year medicine at the Boston City Hospital, and my visiting physicians there were George Sears and Edwin Locke. At the time, there was no investigative program on the Harvard Service at the City Hospital. Edsall had only been at the MGH for a few years. He was getting things started then and had, as a resident at the time, Arlie Bock, who later did such important investigations with L. J. Henderson. It was an uphill chore there, too, to get research started. J. Homer Wright, in pathology, was doing some original work in blood stains. Wright was the developer of the reticulocyte stain. Wright came from Hopkins. He interested me so much that I took a one-month course with him in pathology in my fourth year. Shortly after I got there, he was doing some 'Wright stains' at the sink and I said, 'How do you time this, how long does it take?' He said, 'Well, look out that window there, and you'll see a clock on the Charles Street jail. I go by that clock.' In other words, he just knew when to take it off without any timing at all. He had a nice sense of humor, rather dry type, but would sit down with you and criticize the smear and your staining of it and then put you through a course of staining ten slides. Minot used to drop into the laboratory, and he picked the staining technique up from Wright. The reticulocyte count was the key technique in Minot's evaluation of liver in the treatment of pernicious anemia.

"After graduation I went to the Brigham Hospital as an intern in medicine. Then I went into the army and was asked by Peabody to join his group at Lakewood, New Jersey. William S. Thayer had requested Peabody to set it up and was instrumental in having research physicians assigned to the Lakewood Hospital. All of the cases of the so-called 'irritable heart' syndrome were sent to Lakewood. You'd be surprised at the patients that came in labeled 'irritable heart.' There was hyperthyroidism, tachycardias of every kind, paroxysmal and otherwise, and there were patients that were labeled by Thomas Lewis as having 'effort syndrome.' Peabody recognized that this was really a scrap basket for any patient that had a rapid pulse rate or perspired freely. He asked Macfie Campbell, who was professor of psychiatry at Harvard, to come down.

Campbell said that there was every branch of neurosis that he'd ever encountered anywhere in this group of patients. We found, and I think quite by accident, that a small dose of epinephrine given to these patients produced a striking rise in blood pressure and pulse rate, profuse sweating, and a reaction of fear and trembling. I was then sent to Fort Dix with Cyrus Sturgis, where we were able to get thirty to forty men in a division who had gone through training and were ready to go overseas. These were selected as normal because they had stood all of the regular training. All of these but two, as I recall, got no reaction in the sense of rising blood pressure or pulse rate over 8 or 10 beats, in contrast to the so-called 'irritable heart' patients that got a rise from 120 to 180. We published this—first paper I ever put my name on.[1] Later some of these were examined while in training, where the sound of gunfire would produce the same reaction as epinephrine. Walter Cannon was quite impressed with our observations and felt that this was a 'fear response.'

"After the war I went back to the Brigham Hospital for two years as assistant resident. I made some observations on myocardial infarcts and coronary thrombosis, because I had a patient come into the hospital critically ill, in shock, with a blood pressure almost unattainable. I got the patient on the electrocardiogram machine, and Sam Levine looked at the record with me. It showed almost everything—bundle branch block, complete heart block, and the amplitude of the complexes was almost zero. Autopsy revealed a left anterior descending occlusion and a large, well-demarcated infarct. I found nineteen other infarcts in the autopsy records, none of which had been recognized during life. Herrick had already published his paper on the EKG findings. Christian invited him to give a clinic at the Brigham, and he reviewed my paper with me, etc. I had the advantage of a good critic.

"Ashby had just published her method of recognizing transfused erythrocytes, and I studied the transfused red cells in pernicious anemia and found that they lived a normal span. I then thought of trying to transfuse some pernicious anemia red cells into another patient, but found that it was a little precarious and gave it up. I had some offers, rather nice ones; one to go with Van Slyke, another to stay at the Brigham, and another to go to Washington University. Peabody said, 'Before you make any decisions on this I want you to go to Philadelphia and visit A. N. Richards.' I was interviewed by A. N. Richards, and before I left I knew exactly where I wanted to go. He showed me a frog's kidney, in a living frog, which he transilluminated, and through the binocular microscope you could watch the entire circulation through the glomeruli. So I accepted the job as instructor in pharmacology at the University of Pennsylvania. I did no clinical work, just straight physiology.

"After that [1921–23], I went back to Boston to join Peabody at the Thorndike Laboratory, where he had been made director. There were some broad-minded trustees in the BCH then, including George Sears, who had been professor of medicine; a man by the name of Dreyfuss; and an Irish physician from Brighton, Dr. Rowen. With Sears's urging and the support of those two, they decided to build a research laboratory, and the Thorndike was the result. Henry Jackson, Jr., who had worked in biochemistry, and Robert Nye, the first one to study viruses in tissue culture, in charge of bacteriology, were two of the original members. Jackson and I were assigned duties on the ward, because I had specified that I wanted clinical duty, and Peabody was delighted.

"At that time, Peabody was doing the pathology of the bone marrow in pernicious anemia and had actually started giving special diets to these patients. I had a visitor who was a physician for the United Fruit Company, who told him about giving a special soup to patients in Central America with sprue anemia; a mixture of 'soup' which had everything in it, including livers and kidney. He actually preceded George Minot in the dietary approach. George Whipple had done his work. Peabody was getting some remission with this 'soup' and was just getting ready to start dissecting it apart to identify what its active material was. George Minot was at the Brigham at that time. William Murphy was the one who sat by the bed and said to the patient, 'Open your mouth,' and put the liver in the mouth.

"One of the exceptional people who came to the Thorndike was William B. Castle. I think I can take credit for having gotten him there. I was living in Brookline with Philip Drinker, William B. Castle, and Allen Butler. I found Bill Castle an extremely interesting person to talk to about physiology. He and I both held instructorships in the department of physiology in the School of Public Health. I saw him there because I was working on lung capillaries and Bill was interested in blood. Peabody, who had then become ill [with what proved to be a fatal malignancy], was told about Castle. He said to bring him over, interveiwed him, and told me to get him if I could. Castle was offered a job and accepted. Later Soma Weiss came—Gene DuBois sent him up from New York. One of the other outstanding ones was Herrman Blumgart. Herrman and I had been interns at the Brigham together. He was responsible for the method of blood flow with radioactive material; the first use of a radioisotope in clinical medicine. Soma Weiss worked with him, but Herrman was well underway before Weiss came.

"I was working then on the capillaries of the heart and in the lung. It was in an attempt to inject human heart capillaries that I found that there was a shortcut from the arteries to the chambers of the heart. Injecting a gelatin mass, you could see the little spurts of gelatin rising out of openings in the chambers of the heart. We did serial sections on those areas and found that there was a direct lumen. That was the first description of collaterals in the coronary circulation and arteries. I wanted to get these capillaries showing in the heart in order to put to test an idea that I had; namely, that a hypertrophied heart didn't have as much capillary circulation as a normal heart. I started by getting human hearts to beat after death. First, I got some hearts from the Children's Hospital. If you got them within three or four hours after death and perfused them through the coronary circulation with a modified Ringer's solution, they would beat well. Our studies immediately revealed something that was quite puzzling. The child's heart had about one capillary to five or six fibers. The normal adult heart had one capillary per fiber. The five or six fibers in the child's heart occupied the same area in cross section that the one fiber in the adult heart did. We perfused some hypertrophied hearts (500–600 g), and there was still one capillary per fiber, but the fiber occupied some three times as much area.

"Joe Aub's best work was done while he was in the department of physiology [Drinker's department] in the School of Public Health. Aub overlapped Castle and me there. Aub was a good clinician and a good investigator. His lead work created an interest in calcium and from there influenced Fuller Albright at the General.

"The two choice appointments in the Harvard school were the Boston City and Jim Mean's place [MGH], to the detriment of the Brigham at the time, until Soma [Weiss] got there. Edsall had a steady favorable influence on building the investigative spirit at the MGH. He was ably assisted by Means and Bock. Edsall was responsible for getting [W. W.] Palmer into research. Henderson had a lot of influence on Palmer and Bock and also on Gamble and Dick Richards. L. J. Henderson was one of the best influences on research in medicine of anybody in the picture. I came out of the School of Public Health one day, and he was just outside the medical school on his way to Cambridge. I said, 'I'm going to Cambridge, can I take you?' He said, 'Yes, I've got a meeting.' We got to Cambridge before two o'clock, and he asked what I was doing. I told him about lung capillaries and how we were finding that the flow alternated just as in the kidney. He said, 'That interests me terribly.' We sat down and talked until four o'clock. He missed his meeting; he said, 'It's unimportant, this is very important.' He called me later. He had gotten the aid of Wilson, who was the mathematician in the School of Public Health, to calculate the area of the air sacs in the lung from my findings on the blood flow in those air sacs. He came back saying, 'This is not a formula for anything but discussion. We may tear it up later after we finish, but I want you to know that my calculations and Wilson's agree with your area of the lung sacs.' After that he would stop by or call up (I had switched from the School of Public Health to the Thorndike Laboratory) and have lunch with me and ask what was going on with the lung. That was an unusual stimulus for a young fellow.

"Joe Pratt sort of stimulated Peabody's interest originally. When I was an assistant resident at Brigham, he turned up there. He didn't have an appointment there, but Christian was very fond of him, and he could roam the wards. Joe Pratt carried a vital capacity outfit in the back of his car; he'd rather use his own. He was the most absent-minded individual I ever knew. I had the opportunity twice to be at the front door when he came. He said, 'I would like to see "so and so" down on Ward E. Would you take me down?' He'd come out and the question would be, 'Where is my car?' He couldn't remember, and twice he had to call a cab. Charming individual."

# Appendix C

## Interview with Nolan Kaltreider
## August 12, 1978

At Swathmore College (1923–27), Kaltreider was interested in physiology by Dr. Detlev Bronk. During medical school at Johns Hopkins, Kaltreider spent his elective time at the Johnson Foundation for Medical Physics at Pennsylvania with Bronk. He also worked with Charles Snyder, associate professor of physiology at Johns Hopkins, on heat production of smooth muscle, publishing a paper in the *Journal of Pharmacology and Experimental Therapeutics* (1930), entitled "A Study of the Innervation of the Pylorus of the Terrapin." At David Rioch's suggestion, he applied for and received an internship at Rochester. McCann knew of Kaltreider's interest in research and suggested the problem to which he dedicated himself:

"I've forgotten what it was now, skin temperatures, I believe, during my internship. At the time, W. J. Merle Scott[1] of the department of surgery was interested in peripheral vascular disease. When I became assistant resident, McCann asked me if I didn't want to work with Alberto Hurtado from Lima, Peru, who came to Rochester in 1931. We got to be great friends, and he told me that Francis Peabody got him interested in coming back to the states for further study. (Hurtado was a graduate of Harvard Medical School.) He got a Rockefeller grant, stopped off in New York City, and saw Mr. Hanson. He was all set to go to Harvard, and Mr. Hanson said, 'Why don't you go up to Rochester (Hanson was in charge of the fellows at the Rockefeller Foundation at that time), there's a new school there, and see what it's all about?' So he arrived here, and Dr. McCann gave him facilities. He was interested in the function of the lung, and we started making determinations of the various subdivisions of the pulmonary capacity. We used to call it *lung*

417

*volume,* but, when we sent our papers in to the *Journal of Clinical Investigation,* Alfred Cohn said, 'You can't call it lung volume; you can't have two nouns together.' So we had to change all our illustrations, and we finally decided on *pulmonary capacity.* During my second year here as an assistant resident, I spent all of my free time with Alberto. We had no technicians at that time, so I did a lot of the technical work; so did he. As chief resident (1933–34), I also spent time with him. During that year, McCann, Hurtado, and I spent a number of days at the Naval Base in Washington, D.C., where we used the low pressure chamber—to study the effects of low atmospheric pressure on the cardiorespiratory system. . . . Hurtado felt it was time to return to Lima. He was interested in his high-altitude research laboratory, and I continued on as instructor in medicine in charge of what we called the 'chest laboratory.' At that time there was very little interest (elsewhere) in the function of the lung. There were only two other groups that I recall: Ronald Christie, of The Royal Victoria Hospital, Montreal, who measured the elasticity of the lung in emphysema; and Eleanor Baldwin, Dickinson Richards, and André Cournand, at Bellevue. I think that these three groups really got people interested in the function of the lung. In about 1931, there were a lot of cases of silicosis in Rochester, and the industry wanted to have some idea about rating these people as far as disability was concerned. Our work was directed toward trying to determine the degree of disability in silicosis and various other types of lung disease. Because industry was having trouble, our 'chest laboratory' was almost entirely supported by money from industry.

"While I was in the laboratory (I continued there until 1946), we had fellows who were second year medical students or residents in medicine who worked there. W. D. W. Brooks, from London, spent a year with us and went back as a chest consultant on Harley Street and at St. Mary's Hospital. We had Fasciolo, from Argentina, who had previously worked with Houssay and was interested in hypertension.

"I think we got the most advice about research problems during that period of time (in the thirties) from Samuel H. Bassett, who was a very critical worker. You could take any problem to Sam and in a few days or a week he'd come back and give you a lot of help. We always felt that he should have been made professor of medicine in charge of research. Bassett went to Cornell Medical College, came here as resident, then was appointed to the staff. He was in charge of our metabolic ward for many years. Henry Keutmann went through our residency here, worked with Sam in the metabolic ward, and then became interested in nephritis. Later on he switched to endocrinology. I guess he and Robert Burton were among the first to do paper electrophoresis. H. B. Slavin, after his residency, became interested in infectious disease and the herpes virus. At that time, George P. Berry was here, and Slavin was associated with him and in charge of our infectious disease unit. We had two people who came up from the Veterinary School at Cornell—Bock and

Carpenter—who were interested in the brucella infections. During the thirties, many of the psychoneurotics were thought to have chronic brucellosis. If they had a positive skin test and a certain group of neurotic symptoms, they were labeled *chronic brucellosis*. I don't know whether hypoglycemia came after that or before that, but there was also a period when all the neurotics were hypoglycemic.

"George Meneely, who had many ideas, was with us for three or four years. He and I developed the helium method for the determination of the residual air or the functional residual air, and we also investigated the extracellular fluids of the body with radioactive sodium. We measured the extracellular and the plasma volume in various disease conditions. We were mainly interested in congestive heart disease at a time when there was so much discussion about forward failure and backward failure. We were trying to relate plasma volume, cell volume, and venous pressure.

"When the war [World War II] began, most of the research ceased here. Dr. McCann went in as captain of the navy, and I thought that was a bit unfortunate. It was a vital time, when national grants were available for war research, and we had little direction. Dr. Lawrence did get us some money from the Manhattan project. Our staff was depleted during the war, and most of us made rounds or taught nine months of the year, so we had little chance to do research. I think about the only thing we did in the 'chest laboratory' was service work.

"When Hurtado arrived here in 1931, there was nothing in the laboratory. Most of the apparatus was made here in Rochester; we had an excellent glass blower who used to work for Bausch and Lomb, and we had another man in town who made all our spirometers and the Van Slyke machine and Haldane equipment we used for the analysis of blood, air, even carbon monoxide. We used the carbon monoxide method (Harrop's method) for determination of the cell volume, and Gibson's method for plasma volume. Doran Stephens was here for about seven or eight years. He had his residency at Barnes Hospital and then returned to Rochester as an instructor. He was a bright chap, who developed an overwhelming pneumonitis following a viral infection and died in the late thirties. He and I were among the first, I believe, to study a series of people with polycythemia vera. At that time chemicals were being used to destroy the red cell. We used venesection and found that it was a very excellent method of controlling polycythemia. After we got rid of the iron stores, we got very low reticulocyte counts, and it proved to be a very successful way of treating these people, preventing thromboses.

"We all had to work out the techniques ourselves and set them up from scratch. No one in that group, in the beginning, had any basic investigative training in respiration, and I think it was the same with all the men that started here: Sam Bassett didn't have any special training in metabolism. In other words, they weren't imported from some place else where they had had training in a special field of research. (There were places like the Russell Sage, where Dr. McCann himself was trained.) Once you got here, you stayed here or you didn't have a job. Dr. McCann didn't have the resources to take young promising residents and send them off for special training and then bring them back to try to develop the various areas of research.

"We tried what Dr. Whipple did originally in California. He would select two or three students at the end of the second year, and they would work in his department for a year doing research. Dr. McCann did that to some extent; usually after the third year. We had one or two in our section. They would drop out and then finish medical school a year late."

# Appendix D

⌒⅊⌒

# Interview with Joseph T. Wearn,
# March 25, 1976

"I went to Cleveland in 1929 after making arrangements with them [the administrative authorities at Western Reserve and the Lakeside Hospital] to include the Cushing Laboratory of Experimental Medicine in the department of medicine of the new Lakeside Hospital. I found that there were no laboratories connected with the department of medicine; or, for that matter, with the department of surgery in the new hospital. . . . I had an interview with Samuel Mather, who was president of the university hospital, and pointed out to him that there were no laboratories in connection with the new department of medicine in the Lakeside Hospital. He said, 'Why don't you draw the plans for them? We will hold up building, and include them in it.' Despite the fact that it was 1929, and there were ominous signs on the horizon financially, they held up building and built two floors, or rather one wing and one central portion of a floor, including about thirty-odd rooms for laboratories, which I thought was a very broad-minded approach. We housed the Cushing Laboratory in one wing. It gave us ample laboratory space for experimental work in medicine. When I went there, there was practically no research in the department of medicine. C. F. Hoover, who had preceded me, was a clinician, and his emphasis was largely in clinical signs, and he had his name attached to one related to the diaphragm.[1] His pupils were not interested primarily in research, so that one had to start from scratch in building not only a research team, but in getting the whole atmosphere changed. The research in the Cushing Laboratory of Experimental Medicine had practically come to a standstill when Stewart died. I took Joe Hayman, who had been working with Richards, and Gerald Shibley, who was with Dochez, as a starter. We then got younger people, almost breeding our own. Berryhill, who had been with Peabody

421

and me at the City Hospital, came as my first resident physician and made a great contribution in stimulating the house staff to take an interest in investigation, which they had not been accustomed to before.

"Elliott Cutler was professor of surgery and had introduced a dog laboratory for experimental work, but at the time there wasn't too much going on in it; it was mostly used as a training laboratory for students. The departments of pediatrics and obstetrics had no investigations going on. So it meant not only establishing a program of investigation but also getting the spirit moving in the place. We had two or three rooms in the medical school for work on dogs. The really active person in the place was Carl Wiggers in physiology. He did have things going on, and that represented about the main thing in the preclinical laboratories.

"We started something in medicine there and in our laboratories. They were referred to as the twenty-four empty rooms by some of the faculty. We finally filled them up; Hayman with his renal work; Shibley contributed largely to the vaccine for whooping cough. The battle was an uphill one because with the collapse of the financial market, the medical school had a very rugged time. The budget, which had been $100,000 in the department of medicine, dropped to $25,000, and the school budget, which had been as high as $1 million, dropped to about $300,000—that's total. I found that I had to go out and raise money for the department of medicine first and the school second. I found that the local people in Cleveland were extremely generous, despite the fact that the market was not a favorable one.

"Torald Sollman was dean. I went to Alan Gregg at the Rockefeller Foundation, who had been a schoolmate of mine, and spoke of the needs of the school. He said to tell the dean to at least present a program. I told Sollman about this, and a week later he showed me his proposal, which was for $10,000. The president of the university then went to see Gregg, who told him to send me to talk about the medical school, but not about the university. Gregg said to me, 'I'll give you $90,000 as a board to slide down on so when you hit a certain part of your anatomy at the bottom it won't be too hard of a bump.' The university promptly removed $90,000 from the medical school budget. It made it difficult to get anything out of the Rockefeller from then on.

"Hayman's publications in nephritis and in his renal function studies, as well as Shibley's in bacteriology, stimulated some of our younger men in training. I got one or two chemists to come in, including Hans Hirschman. Among our younger faculty were Brauer, who came from Philadelphia; Shipley, a graduate of Western Reserve; and several others of the resident grade. We had no money to pull outsiders in. Through the thirties and up to the beginning of the war, we were just beginning to get the place back to two-thirds of its original budget—about $60,000. Christian offered me a job back at the Brigham. I found that it was a difficult task, but having got in it, I decided to stick with it. I carried on with my injections of human hearts, and it was there that we eventually demonstrated the connections in the chamber. In the meantime, we got enough of a clinical department going, so that we began to get some interns from other schools, where before all interns had come from Western Reserve.

"With the onset of World War II, I went to Washington three days a week to work with the Committee on Medical Research, headed by A. N. Richards in the Office of Scientific Research and Development. It turned out to be a valuable experience, meeting a number of investigators from medical schools all over the country, having a chance to see the work of their various departments, and a chance to size up men of ability in these departments. I was made chairman of the Committee on Blood Substitutes, which also broadened my contacts; that and being in charge of the section of physiology and clinical medicine and the Committee on Medical Research. It was educational, to say the least. The people I spent weekends with there were Det Bronk, Baird Hastings, Dochez, and visitors from almost every department of medicine in the country.

"It was after the war that I was able to make a major turnover in the department heads at Western Reserve and, therefore, to start the new educational program. When I got back to Cleveland in 1945, Sollman, the dean, was ready to retire. I put in some names to get them to approach. They announced very clandestinely to the trustees that the new dean was to be Wiggers. They considered making it a two-year school instead of a four-year one, because of the financial state. I went straight to two or three trustees without consulting the president or anybody else, and said if you do this the whole school is dead and that is it. I gave them the names of Hugh Long, Dick Richards, Chester Keefer, and Alan Moritz as possible candidates for dean. They invited all of them for interviews. Wiggers, Karsner, and all the others advised them not to come. They said, 'You don't want to come to this place. You wouldn't be welcome.' Then the trustees asked Alan Gregg to come out, to take a look, and to give some advice. He said they were in a pretty bad way, suggesting that they try those people again, 'if not you'd better make Joe Wearn dean. It is either that or have the place collapse on its ears.' That's when Christian came and said he had a job for me when the place [broke] up. I took the deanship with the proviso that I could raise money myself without going through the president—he fought it, but the trustees approved it—and that I would have an absolutely free hand in the reappraisal of the curriculum. The university administration backed that, and we started. There were eleven vacancies within a year in heads of departments. We recruited Bill Wallace in pediatrics, and Rammelkamp and John Dingle's group in preventive medicine. We got an obstetrician who was a good one, but not too much of a researcher— Alan Barnes. I had to raise money for all of these departments. I went to the trustees and told them about this team of Dingle and Rammelkamp[2]—the president asked how much we needed. I said we would need $75,000 a year as a starter, and it ought to be $150,000 shortly after that. He said, 'Go ahead, we'll lend the money and you use it as you see fit.' That's the university hospital lending the medical school money. Then I went to the Prentiss Foundation, which is a local one in Cleveland, and said we needed a biochemist. They said, 'How much do you need?' I told them, and they gave us the budget for ten years. By that time we had started trying to change the curriculum, and we were voted down every time until we got seven new professors out of thirteen heads of the departments. When we got seven, it went through over the opposition of Wiggers, Karsner, and others.

"Thus the groundwork for the new curriculum was worked out. In its design, it was hoped that it would meet effectively what was becoming rather widespread; complaints by students, residents, and young physicians that medical education had not been providing what they needed and that changes were required. After the plan had been outlined, Hale Ham was brought to Cleveland [in 1952], with the assignment to put it into action."

# Appendix E

❦

## Interview with Cecil J. Watson
## May 3, 1976

"Before going to medical school, I had a conflict in my mind between English literature and biology. I had a superb teacher in English literature and an equally outstanding and stimulating one in zoology, a man named Sigerfoos. . . . He did stimulate my early thinking about investigation in the broad sense. . . . About that time I took a course in physiology given by Lund. . . . This was an elective course mostly devoted to the effects of light on behavior; rather curious that I got interested in that, in terms of my later interest in the photodynamic activity of porphyrins. This no doubt added to my tendency toward biology. . . .

"The next step was medical school. I got a tremendous stimulus from Tommy Bell, professor of pathology. He was eventually to give me a fellowship, which started me on the road to academic medicine and research. I was doing autopsies in Tommy's laboratory as a medical student . . . the bodies were often embalmed before the autopsy was done; which in this particular instance turned out to be extremely unfortunate. . . . The patient had a peculiar type of pneumonia with pulmonary nodules of various sizes on x-ray, fever, enlargement of the liver and spleen. At autopsy there were many areas of 'unresolved' pneumonia, patchy in various parts of both lungs. There was extensive lymphadenopathy . . . microscopically there were numerous peculiar granulomata which were different from tubercles. We tried for a long time to stain something in these areas and failed. . . . Finally we put on a Gram-Weigert stain and in large phagocytes saw myriads of round organisms that obviously had a capsule. This illustrates the value of a university. I took these sections over to Henrici, the great mycologist. He studied [them] for awhile and said, 'I think that's kala azar.' I was set back; I said, 'This woman was born near Minnetonka, she's never been out of Minnesota.' I then walked over to the other side of the pathology building to Professor Riley, the famous parasitologist. He said, 'I don't know what that is, but let me keep this for a day or two, and then I will call you.' He called, and when I went over he had the *American Journal of Parasitology* opened to the article by Darling describing the first three cases of histoplasmosis he discovered in the Panama Canal Zone. Ours was the first of histoplasmosis in the United States, and the fourth in toto. Later on, the area where this woman lived proved to be rich in histoplasmosis. This stimulated my interest in pathology, and I stayed five years with Bell, the last two years as pathologist in charge of laboratories at the Minneapolis General Hospital. . . .

"During the time that I was at the General I got hepatitis, which stimulated my interest in the bile pigments, and I started doing some work on urobilinogen . . . I had a chemist with me, and we naïvely hoped to crystallize urobilinogen . . . I decided that I would like to go abroad and really work for a time on bile pigments and pyrrol chemistry. I had at that time very little interest in the porphyrins. It was obvious that the man to work with was Hans Fischer in Munich. George Fahr knew Friedrich von Müller, the senior professor of medicine in Munich. He wrote to Müller and paved the way for me to visit his clinics, but more importantly, to get an entree to Hans Fischer. Hans Fischer was an M.D., as well as a Ph.D. in chemistry, and he had been the chemist in von Müller's research unit years before.

"I went regularly to von Müller's clinics during the two years that I was in Munich. He had several research laboratories in his clinic; one of the major ones was the one that had been Hans Fischer's. When I was there, Kurt Felix, who was a professor of biochemistry, was in charge of the old Fischer laboratories. These were research laboratories but they also did . . . consultative work in relation to patient's problems. Von Müller introduced me to Hans Fischer and told him what I had in mind to try to crystallize urobilinogen, urobilin or stercobilin. Fischer had crystallized urobilinogen from urine, but nobody had crystallized stercobilinogen from feces. There was a basic question—whether they were different, whether they had the same significance in relation to disease. From the pure chemical standpoint, Fischer was very much interested in this, and that was the chief reason he took me. At first he made no promises at all. A couple of months elapsed, and then he suggested that I come over and see him again. When I did, he said, 'I'll take you on and give you whatever help I can in terms of crystallizing stercobilinogen.' That's what I went to work on in his laboratory. That was a great experience; Fischer was a superb chemist, both theoretical and in terms of his own handiwork. He'd come into the laboratory and say, 'Where's that solution that you showed me last week? I'd like to see how that behaves.' He was very keen at crystallizing compounds by taking a concentrate, putting it in a watch glass, and scratching it as the solution evaporated; or, as an example, making a picrate, or another complex which might crystallize more readily than the compound itself. That didn't happen with stercobilin, the crystallization of which was pure serendipity. Trying to isolate stercobilin I had partially purified a solution which was a beautiful violet color. . . . This violet solution turned out to be important, but we didn't know quite what to do with it as I was trying to crystallize stercobilin, which we had reason to believe was yellow orange. So I set this solution on a shelf in the laboratory, and a couple of weeks later I noticed, to my amazement, that beautiful orange crystals had separated out of the violet solution. This was the first crystallization of stercobilin. I worked on that for years afterwards, observing that while stercobilin differs chemically from urobilin, they may both be found in urine or feces, either alone or as a mixture. From a clinical standpoint, there is no difference in significance; they are the same. This led to various researches, and later on I was very pleased when Irving London came out to our laboratory and learned how to crystallize stercobilin so that he could go back and use $N_{15}$ glycine to show that the $N_{15}$ turned up in the stercobilin. He first noted the 'early' and 'late' labeling, which later became of such great interest.

"I had relatively little interest in the porphyrins during my time in Fischer's laboratory. I couldn't help but hear about them of course, and inevitably became involved in some porphyrin research, crystallizing a deutero- and a coproporphyrin from feces, in the course of my work on stercobilin.

"Fischer had 90 'mitarbeiters,' graduate students in his cavernous laboratories. He had generous support from the Rockefeller Foundation. I used to translate his English letters for him, so I couldn't help but gain information about his extensive research support.

"In the spring of 1933, Fischer asked me if I planned to stay on another year. I replied that I would certainly like to, if I could get some financial support. A short time later, he called me into his office and introduced me to Alan Gregg, whom I had not met before. He asked if I would be interested in a National Research Council Fellowship and, of course, I was. About two months later I received the appointment. In later years, Alan Gregg was always a good friend.

"In 1932 I went back to the Minneapolis General, as a resident in medicine. After six months, I was appointed instructor at the University Hospital and given modest research laboratory facilities to continue work on the bile pigments and porphyrins, insofar as my clinical and teaching responsibilities permitted. Charnley McKinley was then head of the department; he was a neurologist. Neurology was then, and for several years thereafter, in the department of medicine; it was later taken out, which I have always thought personally was a great mistake. Hobart Reimann was the director of the division of internal medicine. He was always very helpful to me, and I enjoyed his friendship. The division of internal medicine was very small during the transition period 1933–36. In 1934 I became an assistant professor . . . I was teaching the whole course in clinical chemistry and microscopy for two quarters per year.... I had a research laboratory going and was able to attract the interest of several young men, including Sam Schwartz and I. J. Pass. In 1936 I was made associate professor and director of the division, and, in 1940, I was promoted to full professorship. Hobart Reimann was there until 1936, when he accepted the professorship at Jefferson. For a number of years we kept the old Berglund laboratory, a monstrosity, with a great central bench. Berglund had active clinical-chemical research going on prior to 1932. He came here as head of medicine from China—the Peking Union Medical College—in 1925. Berglund had a big kidney symposium in 1930, undoubtedly the high point of his Minnesota period. He antagonized practically everybody.

"I had very pleasant contacts with the Mayo Clinic. Al Snell was one of my dear friends who showed keen interest in my work. Jess Bollman was a fine friend. I felt quite close to Russell Wilder then and in after years.... I must also mention Arlie Barnes, Ed Allen, Eddie Rynearson, among many others. Lou Brunsting, in dermatology, was also a good friend, interested in porphyria cutanea tarda, which has been an increasing interest of mine these many years. Others there of whom I think with pleasure are Charlie Code and Hugh Butt. All gave me stimulus in terms of research, particularly on jaundice, liver disease, and other problems in that general sphere. Bollman was Frank Mann's right-hand man, interested to a certain extent in clinical research in the area of liver disease. Magath had a great deal to do with total hepatectomy in dogs; he and Mann proved the extrahepatic formation of bilirubin.

"Russell Wilder was the director of the division of medicine at the Mayo Clinic during those early years. Russell at one point, I know with Al Snell's proposing, offered me a job at the Mayo Clinic. I was flattered and asked what I'd be doing. He said to take my choice—research entirely or clinical medicine entirely. I said no thanks, I wanted them together, and some of each. I may have been unwise, but I have no regrets.

"I should mention my occupation with the Manhattan project, which brought me in contact with many people around the country. I was the associate director for health of that project. Bob Stone, a radiologist, was the director. Our philosophies about our program were not in very good agreement. He strongly favored long-term rat-radiation studies, while I thought we ought to push hard to find out all we could about early detection of radiation and chemical injury. We had a very fine laboratory there. They invited me to come to Chicago as professor of medicine and head of the department. I said that I didn't want to make up my mind about it yet. If they wanted me on a part-time basis, to supervise the above type of research on the Manhattan project, I would. We would consider the rest later. They gave me a fine laboratory, and Leon Jacobson was my right-hand man, my executive officer, a great help, and a valued friend ever since. I took Sam Schwartz to Chicago with me, full-time, as my laboratory director, although he was also under Jacobson. Jacobson was the administrative man, and Sam handled laboratory problems, although Leon was also well started in his research, ultimately to prove so fruitful. We hoped that we could predict, or at least say with some feeling of certainty, that in a given individual there had been radiation injury on the one hand or chemical toxicity on the other. We didn't get very far actually. When the bomb fell on Hiroshima, we asked the army specifically to send us a few injured Japanese, in order to study them, chiefly from a biochemical standpoint. The army wouldn't consider it. Although by no means on that account, I decided not to go to Chicago; I did not like their system of supporting their hospital enterprise, and the staff salary structure. They had to engage rather heavily in private practice, with too little time for research.

"Over a whole decade, the Macy Foundation supported very generously a Liver Injury Conference, which met once or twice a year. It was started during the war, in relation to chemical injury to the liver. It branched out into hepatitis, and cirrhosis of the liver, and it was an excellent conference, with a number of men who were all keenly interested, such as Paul Gyorgy, Charles Davidson, Jess Bollman, Frank Hanger. Fred Hoffbauer was the permanent secretary of the group and did a marvelous job. Fred was one of my staunch supporters and helpers, and he did excellent work on liver disease. That led into the Commission on Liver Disease of the Armed Forces Epidemiological Board. I had charge of the commission for a number of years. Those two responsibilities provided the greatest stimulus to intercommunication on the problems of liver disease, including the porphyrins. The agencies were extremely helpful and made quite a contribution. The Commission on Liver Diseases was finally abolished, somewhat unhappily, through the machinations of one Tom Rivers, president of the board. The commission had worked for a long time on war problems. Tom said that there was just too much money being spent on it, and that ended the Commission on Liver Disease. It was wonderful while it lasted."

# Notes and References

## Preface

1. Chambers, T. K. On corpulence. *Lancet* 1: 523, 1850.

## Introduction

1. Osler, W. The evolution of the idea of experiment in medicine. *Trans. Cong. Am. Phys. Surg.* 7: 1, 1907.

2. Shryock, R. H. *American Medical Research—Past and Present,* pp. 1-7. New York: Commonwealth Fund, 1947.

3. Ibid., p. 6.

4. Smith, T. to E. B. Krumbhaar, October 11, 1933, in The influence of research in bringing into closer relationship the practice of medicine and public health activities. *Am. J. Med. Sci.* 178: 741, 1929.

5. Osler, W. *Man's Redemption of Man,* p. 22. London: Constable, 1910.

6. Morgan, T. H. The relation of biology to physics. *Science* 65: 213, 1927.

7. Shryock, *American Medical Research,* pp. 1-7.

8. Osler, The evolution of the idea of experiment in medicine.

9. Conklin, E. G. The twenty-fifth anniversary of initiation of research in the Carnegie Institution of Washington. *Science* 69: 588, 1929.

10. Rosen, G. Critical levels in historical process: A theoretical exploration dedicated to Henry Ernest Sigerist. *J. Hist. Med.* 13: 179, 1958.

## Chapter 1

1. Shryock, R. H. *American Medical Research—Past and Present.* New York: Commonwealth Fund, 1947.

2. Ibid., pp. 1-7.

3. Fox, D. R. The transit of culture. *Am. Historical Rev.* 32: 753, 1927.

Underwood, E. A. *Boerhaave's Men at Leyden and After,* pp. 120–21. Edinburgh: Edinburgh University Press, 1977.

4. Wilson, J. G. The influence of Edinburgh on American medicine in the eighteenth century. *Proc. Inst. Med. Chicago* 7: 129, 1929.

5. Ibid.

6. Ibid.

7. Morgan, J. *A Discourse upon the Institution of Medical Schools in America.* Philadelphia: William, Bradford, 1765. (Reprint ed., Baltimore: Johns Hopkins Press, 1937.)

8. Williams, W. H. *America's First Hospital: The Pennsylvania Hospital, 1751–1841.* Wayne, Pa.: Haverford House, 1976.

9. Bollet, A. J. Pierre Louis: The numerical method and the foundation of quantitative medicine. *Am. J. Med. Sci.* 266: 93, 1973.

Greenwood, M. *The Medical Dictator and Other Biographical Studies.* London: Williams & Norgate, 1936.

Klebs, A. C. Osler at the tomb of Louis. *J.A.M.A.* 46: 1716, 1906.

Osler, W. Influence of Louis on American medicine. *Bull. Johns Hopkins Hosp.* 8: 161, 1897.

Osler, W. The influence of Louis on American medicine. In *An Alabama Student and Other Biographical Essays.* New York: Oxford University Press, 1908.

Woillez, E. J. *Le Docteur P.C.A. Louis; Sa Vie, Ses Oeuvres (1787–1872).* Paris: P. Dupont, 1873.

10. Klebs, Osler at the tomb of Louis.

11. Ackernecht, E. H. *Medicine at the Paris Hospital, 1794–1848.* Baltimore: Johns Hopkins Press, 1967.

12. Greenwood, Louis and the numerical method. In *The Medical Dictator and Other Biographical Studies.*

Louis, P. Anatomic, pathologic, and therapeutic research on the disease known by the name of gastroenteritis, putrid fever, adynamic, atoxic typhoid, etc. *Am. J. Med. Sci.* 4: 403, 1829.

Louis, P. Pathological researches on phthisis. *Am. J. Med. Sci.* 18: 445, 1836.

Louis, P. Anatomical, pathological and therapeutic researches on the yellow fever of Gibraltar, 1828. *Am. J. Med. Sci.* 25: 378, 1839.

Louis, P. Anatomical, pathological and therapeutic researches concerning the disease known by the name of typhoid fever, etc. *Am. J. Med. Sci.* 2: 150, 1841.

Means, J. H. *The Association of American Physicians: Its First Seventy-Five Years.* New York: McGraw-Hill, 1961.

Osler, Influence of Louis on American medicine.

Sewall, H. The influence of Louis on American medicine. *Colorado Med.* 23: 269, 1926.

13. Stewart, F. C. *The Hospitals and Surgeons of Paris.* New York and Philadelphia: J. & H. G. Langley and Carey & Hart, 1843.

14. Flexner, S. *The Evolution and Organization of the University Clinic.* Oxford: Clarenden Press, 1939. (Two lectures given at the Nuffield Institute in 1938.)

15. Peisse, L. *La mèdecine et les mèdecins.* 2 vols. Paris: J. B. Baillière, 1857.

16. Louis, P. C. A. *Researches on the Effects of Blood Letting in Some Inflammatory Disorders.* Trans. G. C. Putnam, with preface and appendix by James Jackson, M.D. [physician of the Massachusetts General Hospital]. Boston, 1836.

17. Osler, W. The natural method of teaching clinical medicine. *J.A.M.A.* 36: 1673, 1901.

18. Obituary: Louis, P. C. A. *Lancet* 2: 355, 1872.

19. Jackson, J. *Memoir of James Jackson, Jr.* Boston: Hilliard Gray, 1836. (Written by his father, with extracts from letters.)

20. Bowditch, H. I. *Brief Memories of Louis and Some of His Contemporaries in the Parisian School of Medicine of Forty Years Ago.* Boston: John Wiley & Son, 1872.

21. *Boston Society for Medical Observation, Constitution and By-Laws.* Boston: David Clapp & Son, 1872.

22. Jarcho, S. The young stethoscopist (H. I. Bowditch, 1846). *Am. J. Cardiol.* 13: 808, 1964.

Jarcho, S. Henry I. Bowditch on pleuritic effusions and thoracentesis (1852). *Am. J. Cardiol.* 15: 832, 1965.

Kelly, H. A., and Burrage, W. C. *Dictionary of American Medical Biographies.* New York and Boston: D. Appleton, 1928.

Wilson, J. C. The President's Address. *Trans. Assoc. Am. Physicians* 17: 1, 1902.

23. Osler, W. Oliver Wendell Holmes. *Bull. Johns Hopkins Hosp.* 5: 85, 1894.

24. Holmes, O. W. *Medical Essays, 1842–1882.* Boston: Houghton Mifflin, 1891.

25. Kelly and Burrage, *Dictionary of American Medical Biographies.*

26. Ibid.

27. Ibid.

28. Kiebber, J. C. William Wood Gerhardt, M.D., 1809–1872, clinical teacher. *Penn. Health* 1: 26, 1940.

Rogers, F. William Wood Gerhardt: Pioneer in nosography. *Phila. Med.* October 15, 1957, p. 1239.

29. Gerhardt, W. W. On the typhus fever, which occurred at Philadelphia in the spring and summer of 1836; showing the distinction between this form of disease and typhoid fever with alteration of the follicles of the small intestine. *Am. J. Med. Sci.* 19: 289, 1837.

30. Stillé, A. Biographical Memoir. *Univ. Penn. Med. Bull.* June 1902, p. 232. (This memoir was read at a meeting of College of Physicians of Philadelphia, April 2, 1902. In addition to details of Stillé's career, it contains much information about Louis and his other pupils, especially those from Philadelphia.)

31. See *Dictionary of American Medical Biographies,* s.v. Stillé, Alfred.

32. Stillé, Biographical Memoir.

33. Physiology as a systematic discipline emerged at the beginning of the nineteenth century. François Magendie, considered to be the founder of experimental physiology, was a professor of medicine and could follow his new specialty (though practically unsupported) at the Collège de France because of the prevailing degree of academic freedom. His disciple Claude Bernard, had, however, to use his private laboratory and private means to pursue his research for many years. Finally, against the opposition of those who looked upon physiology as merely a branch of anatomy, a special chair was created for Bernard at the Sorbonne in 1854.

34. Ben-David, J. Scientific productivity and academic organization in nineteenth century medicine. *Am. Sociol. Rev.* 25: 828, 1960.

35. The developments within the German universities which led to the integration of teaching and research occurred at a time of political and economic upheaval in Germany. It is not possible to discuss the various forces that impacted on German education and science in the nineteenth century, but their complexity and significance must be appreciated. The French Revolution and its impact on Germany was important in the restructuring of the German universities. The major figure in this reorganization was Wilhelm von Humboldt (1767–1835), who served as minister of education during the years of reform. Both teaching and research were implemented in the University of Berlin, founded in 1809, which was to serve as the model for a number of new German universities. Social, political, and philosophical instability characterized the German states throughout the first half of the nineteenth century. All aspects of German culture, including medicine and science, were strongly influenced by *Naturphilosophie,* which had been formulated at the turn of the century, largely by Friedrich von Schelling (1775–1854) and Georg Wilhelm Friedrich Hegel (1770–1831). This philosophy, which placed romantic speculation and mysticism before objective analysis, led to a period of relative stagnation in German science and medicine. The movement peaked around 1810–15, after which it gradually declined in importance, to be replaced in the 1830s and 1840s by a spirit of scientific inquiry accompanied by a return to rational investigation. The "Revolution of 1848" was the culmination of this period of philosophical and political instability, and it was then that the growing influence of German science and higher education began to be felt.

Paul Cranefield has written several papers on the individuals most instrumental in promoting the new experimentalism; he terms their activities "the biophysics movement of 1847" and considers Emil DuBois-Reymond, Carl Ludwig, Hermann von Helmholtz, and Ernst Brücke the main figures in this "movement." See:

Ackerknecht, E. Beitrage zur Geschichte der Medizinalreform von 1848. *Sudhoff's Arch. Gesch. Med.* 25: 61–109, 113–83, 1932. (A comprehensive study of the events of 1848.)

Cranefield, P. The philosophical and cultural interests of the biophysics movement of 1847. *J. Hist. Med.* 21: 7, 1966.

Fye, B. Henry Pickering Bowditch: A case study of the Harvard physiologist and his impact on the professionalization of physiology in America. Ph.D. dissertation, Johns Hopkins University, 1978.

Temkin, O. Materialism in French and German physiology. *Bull. Hist. Med.* 20: 322, 1946.

36. Haberling, W. *Johannes Müller; das Leben des Naturforschers*, p. 176. Leipzig: Akad. Verlagsgesellschaft b. D. H., 1924.

37. Faber, K. *Nosography in Modern Internal Medicine*. New York: Paul B. Hoeber, 1923.

38. Virchow, R. Über die standpunkte in der wissenschaftlichen medicin. *Virchow's Archiv für Pathol. Anat. und Pathol. Physiol.* 1: 3, 1847.

39. Flexner, S. *Evolution and Organization of the University Clinic.*

40. Faber, *Nosography in Modern Internal Medicine.*

Magnus-Levy, A.: The heroic age of German medicine. *Bull. Hist. Med.* 16: 331, 1944.

Naunyn, B. *Erinnerungen, Gedanken, und Meinungen*, pp. 125, 132, and 134. München: J. F. Bergmann, Verlag, 1925.

Temkin, O. The era of Paul Ehrlich. *Bull. NY Acad. Sci.* 30: 958, 1954.

41. Naunyn, *Erinnerungen, Gedanken, und Meinungen.*

42. Ibid.

43. Cushing, H. *The Life of William Osler.* Vol. 1, p. 225. Oxford: Clarenden Press, 1925.

44. Osler, W. *Aequanimitas, With Other Addresses to Medical Students, Nurses, and Practitioners of Medicine*, 2nd ed., p. 472. Philadelphia: Blakiston's Son, 1925.

45. Faber, *Nosography in Modern Internal Medicine,* p. 182.

46. Naunyn, *Erinnerungen, Gedanken, und Meinungen.*

47. Magnus-Levy, The heroic age of German medicine.

48. Mall to Barker, May 20, 1901. Alan M. Chesney Archives, The Johns Hopkins Medical Institutions.

49. Burdon-Sanderson, J. Ludwig and modern physiology. *Sci. Prog.* 5: 1, 1896.

Lombard, W. P. The life and work of Carl Ludwig. *Science* 4: 363, 1916.

Rosen, G. Carl Ludwig and his American students. *Bull. Hist. Med.* 4: 609, 1936.

Rosen, G. Carl Friederich Wilhelm Ludwig. *Dict. Sci. Biog.* 8: 540, 1973.

Sterling, W. Carl Ludwig—Professor of physiology in the University of Leipzig. *Sci. Prog.* 4: 155, 1895.

50. Fishman, A. P., and Richards, D. W. *Circulation of the Blood—Men and Ideas*, pp. 85–90. Oxford: Oxford University Press, 1964. This article contains a discussion of the significance of this invention and the steps leading to its development.

51. Cranefield, P. The organic physics of 1847 and the biophysics of today. *J. Hist. Med.* 12: 407, 1957.

Frank, M. H., and Weiss, J. J. The "Introduction" to Carl Ludwig's *Textbook of Human Physiology. Med. Hist.* 10: 76, 1966. (In this introduction, Ludwig's commitment to the physicochemical approach in physiology is dramatically displayed.)

Rothschuh, K. *History of Physiology*, pp. 195–263. New York: Robert E. Krieger, 1973. This article is a thorough and well-documented discussion of these men and their impact on German physiology.

52. Lombard, The life and work of Carl Ludwig.

53. Osler, W. Letter from abroad to the editor. *Can. Med. Surg. J.* 13: 18, 1884.

54. Sabin, F. R. *Franklin Paine Mall: The Story of a Mind.* Baltimore: Johns Hopkins Press, 1934.

55. Rosen, G. Carl Ludwig and his American students.

56. Lusk, G. Carl von Voit, master and friend. *Ann. Med. Hist.* 3: 583, 1931.

57. Just as one can construct a family pedigree in order to display the basic data for genetic analysis, one can trace the scientific descent of those who have contributed to the advancement of clinical science. Such a pedigree of the Voit School was published by Graham Lusk in *The Elements of the Science of Nutrition,* 4th ed. Philadelphia and London: W. B. Saunders, 1931:

SCIENTIFIC DESCENT OF THE VOIT SCHOOL

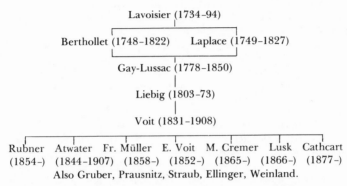

Lavoisier (1734–94)

Berthollet (1748–1822)    Laplace (1749–1827)

Gay-Lussac (1778–1850)

Liebig (1803–73)

Voit (1831–1908)

| Rubner | Atwater | Fr. Müller | E. Voit | M. Cremer | Lusk | Cathcart |
|--------|---------|-----------|---------|-----------|------|----------|
| (1854–) | (1844–1907) | (1858–) | (1852–) | (1865–) | (1866–) | (1877–) |

Also Gruber, Prausnitz, Straub, Ellinger, Weinland.

58. Talbott, J. H. Max von Rubner (1854–1932). In *A Bibliographical History of Medicine; Excerpts and Essays on the Men and Their Work.* New York and London: Grune & Stratton, 1970.

59. Robinson, G. C. *Adventures in Medical Education.* Cambridge, Mass.: Harvard University Press, 1957.

60. Barker, L. F. *Time and the Physician.* New York: G. P. Putnam's Sons, 1942.

61. Ibid.

62. Lusk, G. Medical education: A plan for the development of leaders. *J.A.M.A.* 52: 1229, 1909.

63. Meltzer, S. J. The science of clinical medicine. What it ought to be and the men to uphold it. *J.A.M.A.* 53: 508, 1909.

64. Lusk, G. On the proposed reorganization of departments of clinical medicine in the United States. *Science* 41: 531, 1915.

# Chapter 2

1. Chittenden, R. H. *History of the Sheffield Scientific School.* 2 vols. New Haven: Yale University Press, 1928.

2. Prudden, L., ed. *Biographical Sketches and Letters of T. Mitchell Prudden, M.D.* New Haven: Yale University Press, 1927.

3. Chittenden, *History of the Sheffield Scientific School.*

4. Ibid.

5. Ibid.

6. Franklin, F. *The Life of Daniel Coit Gilman.* New York: Dodd, Mead, 1910.

7. Brieger, G. H. The California origins of the Johns Hopkins Medical School. *Bull. Hist. Med.* 51: 339, 1977.

8. Gilman, D. C. The Johns Hopkins University in its beginning. An inaugural address.

Baltimore, February 22, 1876. In *University Problems in the United States,* pp. 22–23. New York: Century, 1898.

9. *Johns Hopkins University Circular #9:* March 1881.

10. Ibid.

11. Adami, J. G. *The Art of Healing and the Science of Medicine: Ceremonies at the Opening of the New Medical Building,* p. 47. Ann Arbor: University of Michigan, 1901.

# Chapter 3

1. Meek, W. J. The beginnings of American physiology. *Ann. Hist. Med.* 10: 111, 1928.

2. For a more extensive discussion of early physiological studies in the United States, see Atwater, E. C. Squeezing mother nature: Experimental physiology in the United States before 1870. *Bull. Hist. Med.* 52: 313, 1978, and Bylebyl, J. J. William Beaumont, Robley Dunglison and the "Philadelphia physiologists." *J. Hist. Med.* 25: 3, 1970.

3. Burr, A. R. *Weir Mitchell—His Life and Letters.* New York: Duffield, 1930.

4. Ellis, F. W. Henry Bowditch and the development of the Harvard laboratory of physiology. *N. Engl. J. Med.* 219: 819, 1938.

Minot, C. S. Henry Pickering Bowditch. *Science* 33: 598, 1911.

5. Fye, B. Personal communication, 1978.

6. William Henry Welch to his sister, April 21, 1878. In Flexner, S., and Flexner, J. T. *William Henry Welch and the Heroic Age of American Medicine,* pp. 112–13. New York: Viking Press, 1941.

7. *The Harvard University Catalog, 1872–1873,* pp. 119 and 125. Cambridge, Mass., 1873.

Cohn, T. E. Dr. Henry Pickering Bowditch on the growth of children: An unappreciated classic study. *Trans. Stud. Coll. Physicians Phila.* 42: 67, 1974.

For a discussion of the first laboratory of experimental physiology at the University of Pennsylvania, which was established in 1875 by Francis Gurney Smith, see:

Nancrede, C. D. Francis Gurney Smith. *Med. Soc. State Penn. Trans.* 6: 404, 1878.

Osler, W. Harvard School of Medicine. *Can. J. Med. Sci.* 2: 274, 1877.

8. Warren, J. W. Description of the physiological laboratory of the Harvard Medical School. *Science* 4: 128, 1884.

9. Bowditch, H. P. Letter to the editor. *Boston Med. Surg. J.* 82: 305, 1870.

Bowditch, H. P. The physiological laboratory at Leipzig. *Nature* 3: 142, 1870.

Bowditch, H. P. The advancement of medicine by research. *Science* 4: 85, 1884.

Bowers, J. Z. The influence of Charles W. Eliot on medical education. *Pharos* 35: 156, 1972.

Cannon, W. B. President Eliot's relations to medicine. *N. Engl. J. Med.* 210: 730, 1934.

Cohn, Dr. Henry Pickering Bowditch on the growth of children.

Hawkins, H. *Pioneer: A History of the Johns Hopkins University, 1874–1899.* Ithaca: Cornell University Press, 1960.

Lusk, G. Physiology at the Harvard Medical School, 1870–1871—A part of the introductory lecture and synopsis of the experimental demonstrations given by William T. Lusk. *Boston Med. Surg. J.* 167: 921, 1912.

Osler, Harvard School of Medicine.

For a discussion of the importance of Bowditch's contributions to cardiovascular physiology, see Mommaerts, W.F.H.M. Heart muscle. In *Circulation of the Blood—Men and Ideas,* ed. Fishman, A. P., and Richards, D. W., pp. 127–98. New York: Oxford University Press, 1964.

10. Davenport, H. W. Walter B. Cannon's contribution to gastroenterology. *Gastroenterology* 63: 878, 1972.

11. Kronecker, H., and Meltzer, S. J. Ueber die Schluckmechanisms und dessen ner-

vöse Hemmungen. Monatsbericht der Königl Akademic der Wissenschaften zu Berlin. January 24, 1881.

12. Davenport, H. W. The first Walter Bradford Cannon lecture before the Society of Gastrointestinal Radiologists. *Am. J. Roentgenol. Rad. Ther. Nucl. Med.* 119 (2): 235, 1973.

13. Members of the Staff, Research Fellows, and Graduate Students in the Department of Physiology, Harvard Medical School, 1871–1971. Compiled from publications, old catalogs, and old memories. (Courtesy, S. Benison.)

14. Garrison, F. H. Sir Michael Foster and the Cambridge School of Physiologists. *Md. Med. J.* 58: 106, 1915.

15. Rothschuh, K. E. *History of Physiology.* New York: Robert E. Krieger, 1973.

16. Howell, W. H. The American Physiological Society during its first twenty-five years. In *History of the American Physiological Society, 1887–1937*, p. 1. Baltimore: n.p., 1938.

Howell, W. H. Celebration of the sixtieth anniversary of William H. Howell's graduation from Johns Hopkins University. *Bull. Johns Hopkins Hosp.* 68: 291, 1941.

17. Sewall, H. The beginnings of physiological research in America. *Science* 58: 187, 1923.

18. Harvey, A. McG. *Adventures in Medical Research: A Century of Discovery at Johns Hopkins,* p. 84. Baltimore: Johns Hopkins University Press, 1976.

19. Howell, W. H. Vagus inhibition of the heart and its relation to the inorganic salts of the blood. *Am. J. Physiol.* 15: 289, 1906.

20. Folin, O. Chemical problems in hospital practice. *Harvey Lectures* 3: 187, 1908.

21. Liebow, A. A. Medical research at Yale in the twentieth century. *Yale J. Biol. Med.* 33: 193, 1960.

22. Chittenden, R. H. *The Development of Physiological Chemistry in the United States.* American Chemical Society, Monograph Series, pp. 94, 163, New York: Chemical Catalog Co., 1930.

23. Harvey, *Adventures in Medical Research,* p. 114.

24. Chittenden, *Development of Physiological Chemistry,* p. 138.

McCollum, E. V. Stanley Rossiter Benedict (1884–1936). *Biog. Mem. Natl. Acad. Sci.* 27: 155, 1952. (Contains Benedict's complete bibliography.)

25. Chittenden, *Development of Physiological Chemistry,* pp. 54–65.

26. Ibid., pp. 79–82.

Shaffer, P. A. Otto Folin (1867–1934). *Biog. Mem. Natl. Acad. Sci.* 27: 47, 1952. (Contains Folin's complete bibliography.)

27. Ibid.

28. Shaffer, P. A. Otto Folin. *Science* 81: 35, 1935.

29. McCollum, Stanley Rossiter Benedict.

30. Christian, H. A. Tribute to Professor Folin. *Science* 81: 37, 1935.

31. Shaffer, Otto Folin (1867–1934).

32. Bock, A. V. Lawrence Joseph Henderson, 1878–1942. *Trans. Assoc. Am. Physicians* 57: 17, 1942.

Cannon, W. B. Lawrence Joseph Henderson (1878–1942). *Biog. Mem. Natl. Acad. Sci.* 23: 31, 1943. (Contains Henderson's complete bibliography.)

33. Chittenden, *Development of Physiological Chemistry,* pp. 103–5, 153–58.

34. Edmunds, C. W. Presentation of the Kober Medal to J. J. Abel. *Trans. Assoc. Am. Physicians* 49: 5, 1934.

Harvey, *Adventures in Medical Research,* p. 49.

35. Clark, W. M. Walter Jones. *Science* 81: 307, 1935.

Clark, W. M. Walter (Jennings) Jones (1865–1935). *Biog. Mem. Natl. Acad. Sci.* 20: 79, 1938. (Contains Jones's complete bibliography.)

36. Chittenden, *Development of Physiological Chemistry,* pp. 275–284, 399–400.

Hench, P. S. Presentation of the Kober Medal to Edward Calvin Kendall. *Trans. Assoc. Am. Physicians* 65: 42, 1952.

37. Chittenden, *Development of Physiological Chemistry,* pp. 116–24, 133–37, 220–24.

38. Ibid., pp. 99–101, 195–262.

39. Dole, V. P. Donald Dexter Van Slyke. *Trans. Assoc. Am. Physicians* 85: 49, 1972.

Hastings, A. B. Donald Dexter Van Slyke (1883–1971). *Biog. Mem. Natl. Acad. Sci.* 48: 309, 1976. (Contains Van Slyke's complete bibliography of scientific papers.)

40. Keefer, C. S. A. Baird Hastings: The man—the scientist—the cosmopolite. *Fed. Proc.* 25: 822, 1966.

41. Van Slyke, D. D. Reminiscences of life and work with A. Baird Hastings. *Fed. Proc.* 25: 820, 1966.

42. Flexner, A. William Henry Welch. *Johns Hopkins Hosp. Bull.* 87: 39, 1950.

43. Temkin, O. The European background of the young Dr. Welch. *Bull. Hist. Med.* 24: 308, 1950.

44. Flexner and Flexner, *William Henry Welch.*

# Chapter 4

1. Osler, W. The natural method of teaching medicine. *J.A.M.A.* 36: 1673, 1901.

2. Evarts Graham, professor of surgery at the Washington University School of Medicine, evaluated this contribution in this Report of The Surgical Service, 1928–29 (to the director of the Barnes Hospital):

> The graded system of appointments of the house staff, which is now in vogue in many of the best hospitals in this country, is an American contribution to the methods of medical education. From Germany we acquired the laboratory methods of instruction, from England we obtained the idea of permitting medical students to go to the bedsides of the patients and actually to see and observe their condition, and from America has come the third great contribution of giving intensive postgraduate training over a period of a few years to a carefully selected group of young men.

This type of training was, of course, essential to the creation of a clinically expert group of young men, many of whom chose academic careers and became outstanding clinical investigators.

3. Osler, W. L'Envoi. Remarks at a farewell dinner given by the Medical Profession of the United States and Canada, New York, May 2, 1905. *Med. News* 136: 859, 1905.

4. Sabin, F. *Franklin Paine Mall, The Story of a Mind.* Baltimore: Johns Hopkins Press, 1934.

5. Means, J. H. Experiences and opinions of a full-time medical teacher. *Perspect. Biol. Med.* 2: 127, 1958.

> From the modern point of view, the third year then was dreadful. Five afternoons a week we had to attend three, sometimes four, hour-long lectures, one after another.... No patients were shown at these lectures.... The mornings were better—then we saw patients. For an hour each day they were shown to the whole class in hospital amphitheaters by the great men of the clinical staff. These were worthwhile exercises. The first time one saw a patient with a disease previously known only through lecture or textbook, it made a deep impression. We also had the opportunity in these third year mornings to visit outpatient clinics in small groups under the direction of younger instructors and talk with and actually get our hands on patients. In the afternoon lectures the emphasis was on diseases, but in the mornings we were concerned with history-taking, examination, and diagnosis; in other words, at last we got to the problems of the individual patient. Usually there was very little time left over for the discussion of treatment....
>
> The fourth year curriculum in those days at Harvard was entirely elective. A wide choice of clinical and preclinical subjects was offered. The fourth-year student could walk the wards of hospitals but not in any such responsible role as that enjoyed by the clinical ward clerk of later years. We were taken around as if on a Cook's tour by an instructor who showed us interesting patients and quizzed us on them a bit, but we were actually observers, not participants in the casework process.... I can recall practically nothing being said to us about research or research centers in the third and fourth years at Harvard Medical School. The whole current was flowing strongly toward the practice of medicine and nearly all of us got caught up in it.

6. Bondy, P. K., and Brainard, E. R. The American Society for Clinical Investigation, 1909–1959 and the *Journal of Clinical Investigation, 1924–59. J. Clin. Invest.* 38: 1783, 1959.

7. Harvey, A., McG. *The Interurban Clinical Club, 1905–1976. A Record of Achievement in Clinical Science,* p. 52. Philadelphia: W. B. Saunders, 1978.

8. Barker, L. F. A case of circumscribed unilateral, and elective sensory paralysis. *J. Exp. Med.* 1: 348, 1896.

9. Barker, L. F. Medicine and the universities. *Am. Med.* 4: 143, 1902.

10. The following letters are in the Alan M. Chesney Archives, Johns Hopkins Medical Institutions:

Mall to Barker, Feb. 2, 1902:

I think that a far greater task is to develop leadership in scientific medicine, as it is in Europe.... It is of the greatest satisfaction to see that the strategic point is realized by John D., Jr. in founding the new Institute ... Philanthropists ... will finally see that research is the thing. We need in this country a Medical School for research ... which will take the lead in what Medicine next needs.... It will be a difficult task to reform the practical chairs, for the idea is firmly implanted that they are the prizes of the local professor. Maybe when we have real University Schools we can look to see freedom in the choice of the professors in medicine, surgery, etc."

In a letter to Barker dated July 26, 1902 Welch stated:

That is a capital address of yours on "Medicine and Universities." Of course there is no university medical school, not even in Germany.... The clinical professors there engage in private practice ... and pocket their fees.... We now have admirable opportunities for ... everything which leads up to the study of diseased human beings, but very inadequate ones for the latter. I believe I told you something about my views on this subject when you went to Chicago, and you have expressed much better and more fully just what I had in mind.

Barker to Flexner, Aug. 6, 1902:·

I am glad you will write a letter. The points to be emphasized are, it seems to me, as follows:
1. No true Univ. Med. Sch. exists in America or elsewhere.
2. Medicine advances as far as med. ed. is concerned *pari passu* with the extension of Univ. methods.
3. We have now excellent facilities for study up to the time we undertake the study of diseased *human beings.* Then the bottom drops out.
4. The characters of a true Univ. professor in a clinical branch.
5. The money required.
6. Universities, like the U.S. Steel Corporation, should control for itself the whole time and energies of the best men—if only as a business proposition.
7. The tremendous opportunities at the moment for clinical research. Clinical research now almost unknown.

Barker to Flexner, Aug. 26, 1902:

I have just gotten hold of a copy of American Medicine for Aug. 9. You picked out just the right points ... I believe that we are really at a crucial period in medical education. We are at the point where, if ever, undergraduate teaching must be made an appendage and investigation the main work of the University departments in medicine. May we strike the right path.... P.S. One drawback ... is that clinicians think they have what we are striving for. As long as they have the title of Univ. professors they think they are such. The detail of private practice they do not consider from the Univ. standpoint. They are incapable of imagining anything that does not lend to aggrandizement of practice. That is what they are here for—"what we are all after." To them, what would be the good of Research Hospitals if the professors could not profit by the reputations which they gained through them?

Again, they confuse publication in medical journals with research. Writers of pot-boilers out here speak disparagingly of men who do not write pot-boilers saying "So-and-so does not do much research work" or "He is not very productive." They have caught the lingo and use it with nonchalance. You talk to them about the real thing and they agree with you but say, "Yes, but don't you think the seed is pretty well planted now. Johns Hopkins and Harvard insist on this sort of thing and we are doing it here. The others will have to fall into line!" They have an opacity of the crystalline lens which will take much needling of the sort we are giving them to cure.

11. Barker, L. F. The laboratories of the medical clinic. *Bull. Johns Hopkins Hosp.* 18: 193, 1907. In this same issue of the *Bulletin,* a series of research papers from the three laboratories appeared.

12. Longcope, W. T. Thomas Richard Boggs. *Trans. Assoc. Am. Physicians* 54: 9, 1939.

13. Hurd, H. *Eighteenth Annual Report of the Johns Hopkins Hospital,* p. 11. Baltimore: Johns Hopkins Press, 1907.

14. Cole, R. I. Remarks made at the dinner in honor of Doctor Cole on the occasion of his retirement as Director of the Hospital of the Rockefeller Institute held at the Institute, Saturday, April 30, 1938. The addresses at this dinner are available in the Archives of the Hospital of the Rockefeller Institute.

15. Firor, W. M. The story of the Hunterian Laboratory. *Surgery* 32: 485, 1952.

16. Halsted to Welch, 1922. Alan M. Chesney Archives, Johns Hopkins Medical Institutions.

17. Cushing to Jay McLean, January 24, 1920, in which Cushing details the beginning of the laboratory and its history during his period as director. Alan M. Chesney Archives, Johns Hopkins Medical Institutions.

18. MacCallum, W. G. On the relation of the parathyroid to calcium metabolism and the nature of tetany. *Bull. Johns Hopkins Hosp.* 19: 91, 1908.
MacCallum, W. G., and Voegtlin, C. Relation of tetany to calcium metabolism. *Bull. Johns Hopkins Hosp.* 18: 244, 1908.

19. Cushing, H., and Branch, J. R. B. Experimental and clinical notes on chronic valvular lesions in the dog and their possible relation to a future surgery of the cardiac valve. *J. Med. Res.* 17: 471, 1908.

20. *Bull. Johns Hopkins Hosp.* Vol. 18, 1907.

21. Barker, L. F. On some methods of investigating cardiovascular conditions. The Jerome Cochran Lecture, Alabama State Medical Association, 1909. *Bull. Johns Hopkins Hosp.* 20: 297, 1909.

22. Harvey, A. McG. Creators of clinical medicine's scientific base: Franklin Paine Mall, Lewellys Franklin Barker, and Rufus Cole. *Johns Hopkins Med. J.* 136: 168, 1975.

23. MacCallum, W. G., and Voegtlin, C. On the relation of tetany to the parathyroid glands and to calcium metabolism. *J. Exp. Med.* 11: 118, 1909.

24. Cole, R. I. Frequency of typhoid bacilli in the blood. *Bull. Johns Hopkins Hosp.* 12: 203, 1902.

25. Harvey, A. McG. Applying the methods of science to the study of tropical diseases—The story of Andrew Watson Sellards. *Johns Hopkins Med. J.* 144: 45, 1979.

26. The Reminiscences of Dana Atchley, found in the Columbia Oral History Collection, is copyrighted by The Trustees of Columbia University in the City of New York, 1975, and is used with permission.

27. Austrian, C. R. Lewellys Franklin Barker. *Johns Hopkins Hosp. Bull.* 73: 401, 1943.

28. Cole, R. Lewellys Franklin Barker, 1867–1943. *Trans Assoc. Am. Physicians* 58: 13, 1944.

29. Crowe, S. J. *Halsted of Johns Hopkins. The Man and His Men.* Springfield, Ill.: Charles C Thomas, 1957.
Halsted, W. S. *Surgical Papers.* 2 vols. Baltimore: Johns Hopkins Press, 1924.
Harvey, A. McG. *Adventures in Medical Research: A Century of Discovery at Johns Hopkins,* p. 70. Baltimore: Johns Hopkins University Press, 1976.
Heuer, G. J. Dr. Halsted. *Johns Hopkins Hosp. Bull.* 90: 1, 1952.
MacCallum, W. G. *William Stewart Halsted.* Baltimore: Johns Hopkins Press, 1930.

30. Councilman, W. T. Franklin Paine Mall, 1862–1917. *Proc. Am. Acad. Arts Sci.* 57: 495, 1922.

31. Sabin, *Franklin Paine Mall,* p. 77.

32. Councilman, Franklin Paine Mall.

33. Halsted, W. S. Ligature and suture material. The employment of fine silk in preference to cat gut and the advantages of transfixation of tissues and vessels in control of

hemorrhage. Also an account of the introduction of gloves, gutta percha tissue and silver foil. *J.A.M.A.* 40: 1119, 1913.

34. Halsted, *Surgical Papers.*

35. Sabin, *Franklin Paine Mall*, p. 77.

36. Fulton, J. F. *Harvey Cushing. A Biography*, p. 95. Springfield, Ill.: Charles C Thomas, 1946.

37. Ibid., p. 122.

38. Ibid., p. 120.

39. Cushing, H. Concerning the poisonous effect of pure sodium chloride on nerve muscle preparations. *Am. J. Physiol.* 6: 77, 1901.

40. Cushing, H. The hypophysis cerebri—clinical aspects of hyperpituitarism and of hypopituitarism. *J.A.M.A.* 53: 249, 1909.

41. Cushing, H. The basophil adenomas of the pituitary body and their clinical manifestations (pituitary basophilism). *Johns Hopkins Hosp. Bull.* 50: 137, 1932.

42. Cushing, H. The special field of neurological surgery. *Cleve. Med. J.* 4: 1, 1905.

43. Dandy, W. E., and Blackfan, K. D. An experimental and clinical study of internal hydrocephalus. *J.A.M.A.* 61: 2216, 1913.

44. Crowe, *Halsted of Johns Hopkins.*

Dandy, W. E. Fluoroscopy of the cerebral ventricle. *Bull. Johns Hopkins Hosp.* 30: 29, 1916.

Dandy, W. E. Ventriculography following the injection of air into the cerebral ventricles. *Ann. Surg.* 68: 5, 1918.

45. Harvey, *Adventures in Medical Research*, p. 60.

46. Harvey, A. McG. Halsted's innovative ventures in the surgical specialties: Samuel J. Crowe and the development of otolaryngology at Johns Hopkins. *Johns Hopkins Med. J.* 140: 101, 1977.

47. Crowe, S. J., and Burnam, C. F. Recognition, treatment and prevention of hearing impairment in children. *Ann. Otol. Rhinol. Laryngol.* 50: 15, 1941.

Park, E. A. Dr. Crowe, the man. Memorial program for Samuel James Crowe, 1883–1955. On the occasion of the biannual meetings, The Johns Hopkins Medical and Surgical Association, March 1, 1957. Alan M. Chesney Archives, Johns Hopkins Medical Institutions.

# Chapter 5

1. Duffus, R. L., and Holt, L. E., Jr. *L. Emmett Holt: Pioneer of a Children's Century.* New York: D. Appleton-Century, 1940.

Holt, L. E. The formal opening of the laboratory of the Rockefeller Institute for Medical Research. A sketch of the development of the Rockefeller Institute for Medical Research. *Science* 24: 1, 1906.

2. On February 29, 1902, Flexner wrote to Barker as follows:

> It seems that Mr. Rockefeller is now about ready to go forward with the foundation of the Institute in New York that bears his name....
>
> The proposition has been made to me tentatively to assume charge of the first department and become the central head.... This would give me more or less dictation of the first organization of the Institute and of its policies although all will be done under the direction of the Board of Directors....
>
> The undertaking is so important for the future medical progress of this country and so vast in itself that I cannot but view it with some misgiving . . . if I should follow my inclinations there is no doubt of my accepting. But is it best that I rather than another make this important start? You know me better than any other person, even, perhaps, better than I do myself. Tell me what your advice is—freely and without reserve and "from the heart."

Barker's reply was written on March 5, 1902:

The only three men who could be considered for the position are Theobald Smith, Herter and yourself and in my opinion you have more of the desirable qualities than either of the other two. You know enough to get the strongest men available around you and to give them a free hand and all the credit. Your love for scientific work is so great that there will be no danger of the prostitution of the fund and the opportunities to unworthy objects; your position in science is such that young and clever minds will be attracted to you, will have confidence in you and will work enthusiastically under you.

My own opinion is that such a research institution ought to be in the medical faculty of a university. It is the fault of university presidents and Boards of Trustees that we are having research institutions endowed independently. It is because university authorities, though they talk of research and ask in a way for money for research, are not really convinced of its paramount necessity.... The rapid springing up of endowed research institutions should teach a salutary lesson; if it does not, the universities will become colleges and the research institutions will become the universities, though perhaps not under that name.... I should take it and I shall hope to see you develop in New York not only a Pasteur Institute or an Ehrlich Institute ... but also a research hospital.

Flexner's letter is from the Alan M. Chesney Archives, Johns Hopkins Medical Institutions. Barker's letter is from the Flexner Papers, American Philosophical Society. Both letters were published in *Trends in Biomedical Research, 1901–1976*. Proceedings of the Second Rockefeller Archive Center Conference, Dec. 10, 1976, p. 13. New York: Rockefeller Archive Center Publication, 1977.

3. Work of practical value to the practicing physician was done in these temporary laboratories of the institute. In the spring of 1905, the New York City Board of Health asked Flexner to serve on a commission formed to investigate an epidemic of meningococcal meningitis. Flexner knew the disease, for, in 1893, he and Barker had been given a similar assignment by the governor of Maryland during an epidemic in that state. A small bacterium, the *Micrococcus meningiditis* (first isolated by Weichselbaum in 1887) was correctly suspected of being the causative agent, and the two young men, Flexner and Barker, had been able to find this organism in the brain and spinal cord of persons who had died from the Maryland epidemic. By 1905, when Flexner was again confronted with this disease, he had the advantage of knowing that the micrococcus had been proved fully responsible and could thus be cultivated without much difficulty. Using cultures obtained from New York victims of the fever, he quickly succeeded in infecting monkeys and in passing the disease, by inoculation, from monkey to monkey. Flexner had the brilliant idea of placing serum directly at the seat of the disease—the inflamed meningeal membranes—by injecting it into the spinal canal. Thus administered to monkeys, soon after they had been inoculated with the bacteria, the serum made in Flexner's laboratory was very effective. It was tried with success in an epidemic in Ohio in April 1907.

According to George W. Corner, the modest Mr. Rockefeller may have winced when, on August 6, 1907, the *New York World* published the story, under the caption "Cure Is Found for Meningitis with John D's Aid." In May 1908, John D. Rockefeller, Jr., wrote to Holt that his father would give the money needed for a hospital at the institute: "My father thus enlarges the scope and the possibilities of the Institute in grateful recognition of the services of Dr. Simon Flexner, as Director, rendered in those orderly and progressive scientific investigations, which sanctioned and encouraged by your Board, and aided by his learned associates and assistants, led him at length to the discovery of a cure for epidemic cerebrospinal meningitis." John D. Rockefeller, Jr., to L. Emmett Holt, May 26, 1908, entered in Minutes, May 30, 1908. In Corner, G. *History of the Rockefeller Institute, 1901–1953; Origins and Growth,* p. 61. New York: Rockefeller Institute Press, 1964.

4. Hawthorne. R. M., Jr. Christian Archibald Herter, M.D. (1865–1910). *Perspect. Biol. Med.* 18: 24, 1974.

5. Herter, C. A. An experimental study of fat starvation with especial reference to the production of serous atrophy of fat. *J. Exp. Med.* 3: 293, 1898.

Herter, C. A. The acid intoxication of diabetes and its relation to prognosis. *J. Exp. Med.* 5: 617, 1901.

Herter, C. A., and Wakeman, A. J. On alterations in the composition of the blood resulting from experimental double nephrectomy. *J. Exp. Med.* 4: 117, 1899.

6. Hawthorne, Christian Archibald Herter.

7. Means, J. H. *The Association of American Physicians: Its First Seventy-Five Years*, p. 71. New York: McGraw-Hill, 1961.

8. Harvey, A. McG. *Trends in Biomedical Research*, p. 13.

9. Flexner to Herter, January 6, 1902. Rockefeller Institute Files. See also Corner, *History of the Rockefeller Institute*, p. 88.

10. See Corner, *History of the Rockefeller Institute.*

11. Ibid.

12. For a more detailed biographical sketch of Cole, see Harvey, A. McG. Rufus Cole and the Hospital of the Rockefeller Institute; and Harvey, A. McG. *Adventures in Medical Research: A Century of Discovery at Johns Hopkins*, p. 124. Baltimore: Johns Hopkins University Press, 1976.

13. Outline of Plan for the Organization of a Research Hospital (Tentatively approved by the Board of Directors at the meeting, June 13, 1907 [Herter Plan]). Archives, Hospital of the Rockefeller Institute, New York.

14. Harvey, *Trends in Biomedical Research (1901–1976)*, p. 13.

15. Cole's concept of what a university department of medicine should be was clearly presented in an article entitled "The University Department of Medicine," which was published in *Science* in 1920 (Cole, R. I. *Science* 51: 329, 1920). He emphasized that medicine should be generally recognized as an independent science, just as physiology and anatomy are independent sciences. "Medicine may then be defined as the science dealing with the phenomena of disease."

16. Suggestions in Regard to the Organization of the Rockefeller Hospital for Medical Research—R. I. Cole, December 1908. Archives, HRI, New York.

17. Cole, R. Address made at the dinner in honor of Doctor Cole on the occasion of his retirement as director of the Hospital of the Rockefeller Institute at the Rockefeller Institute. New York, April 30, 1938, pp. 59–61. Archives, HRI.

18. Harvey, A. McG. George Canby Robinson: Peripatetic medical educator. *Johns Hopkins Med. J.* 143: 84, 1978. (Contains a bibliography of Robinson's research contributions.)

Robinson, G. C. *Adventures in Medical Education.* Cambridge, Mass.: Harvard University Press, 1957. (In a chapter in this autobiographical account of his career, Robinson discusses his period as Cole's resident physician.)

19. For a biographical sketch of Draper, see Kneeland, Y., Jr. George Draper, 1880–1950. *Trans. Assoc. Am. Physicians* 73: 9, 1960.

20. McCrudden, F. H., and Fales, H. L. Chemical studies on intestinal infantilism. II. The relation of endogenous to exogenous metabolism: nitrogen and sulphur distribution, and calorimeter experiments. *J. Exp. Med.* 15: 113, 1912.

The HRI supported a laboratory for biochemical research in children at the Babies Hospital. This laboratory, where McCrudden and Fales did most of their work, was established by Holt, a member of the institute's Board of Scientific Directors. The work of this laboratory was summarized in each of Cole's annual reports to the trustees.

21. Medigreceanu, F. On the composition of urinary albumin. *J. Exp. Med.* 14: 298, 1911.

Medigreceanu, F. On the mechanism of chloride retention in pneumonia. *J. Exp. Med.* 14: 289, 1911.

22. Archives, HRI.

23. Robinson, *Adventures in Medical Education*, p. 99.

24. In 1930 Cole summarized this early work in The Hospital of the Rockefeller Institute. *Forschungs Institut, ehre Geschicte, Organization und Ziele.* Vol. 2. Ed. Brauer, L., Mendelssohn-Bartoldy, A., and Meyer, A., p. 491. Hamburg: Paul Hartung, Verlag, 1930. Also available for information regarding the details of the work as it progressed are Cole's reports to the Board of Scientific Advisors of the Rockefeller Institute. They were pre-

pared annually from the time of the first report on January 20, 1911. The copies sent to Welch, chairman of the board, are available in the Welch Medical Library, Johns Hopkins University School of Medicine. See also Cole, R. Pneumococcus infection and lobar pneumonia. *Harvey Lectures* 9: 85, 1913.

25. For a biographical sketch of Dochez, see Kneeland, Y., Jr. Alphonse Raymond Dochez. *Trans. Assoc. Am. Physicians* 78: 21, 1965.

26. Dubos, R. *The Professor, the Institute, and DNA.* New York: Rockefeller University Press, 1976. (Contains a complete list of references to Avery's research.)

27. Dochez, A. R. Etiology of scarlet fever. *Harvey Lectures,* 20: 131, 1925.

28. Marks, H. K. Complementoid and the resistance of the mid-piece of complement. *J. Exp. Med.* 13: 590, 1911.

Marks, H. K. The resistance of the end-piece and mid-piece of complement inactivated by distilled water. *J. Exp. Med.* 13: 652, 1911.

29. For biographical material on Peabody see:

Butterfield, E. E., and Peabody, F. W. The action of pneumococcus on blood. *J. Exp. Med.* 17: 587, 1913.

Memorial Note: Francis Weld Peabody. *J. Clin. Invest.* 5: 1, 1927.

Peabody, F. W. The carbon dioxide content of the blood in pneumonia. *J. Exp. Med.* 16: 701, 1912.

Peabody, F. W. The oxygen content of the blood in lobar pneumonia. *J. Exp. Med.* 18: 7, 1913.

Peabody, F. W. The soul of the clinic. *J.A.M.A.* 90: 1193, 1928. (During the last days of his life, Peabody wrote a letter to his friend Warfield Theobald Longcope, explaining his conception of the relationships and responsibilities of the medical chief to his clinic.)

Williams, T. F. Cabot, Peabody and the care of the patient. *Bull. Inst. Hist. Med.* 24: 462, 1950.

30. Dochez, A. R., and Avery, O. T. Varieties of pneumococcus and their relation to lobar pneumonia. *J. Exp. Med.* 21: 114, 1915.

Dochez, A. R., and Gillespie, L. J. A biological classification of pneumococci by means of immunity reactions. *J.A.M.A.* 61: 727, 1913.

31. For the description of the work in Avery's laboratory, extensive use has been made of *The Professor, the Institute, and DNA,* by René Dubos.

32. See Ibid.

For further biographical data on Avery, see:

Dubos, R. J. Oswald Theodore Avery, 1877–1955. *Biog. Mem. Fell. Royal Soc.* (London) 2: 35, 1956.

MacLeod, C. Oswald Theodore Avery, 1877–1955. *J. Gen. Microbiol.* 17: 539, 1957.

For further references to the pneumonia studies, see the bibliography of Oswald T. Avery in *Biog. Mem. Natl. Acad. Sci.* 32: 31, 1958.

For the publications after 1920, see *Investigations and Other Publications by the Members of the Staff of the Hospital of the Rockefeller Institute for Medical Research, 1920–1930.* New York: Hospital of the Rockefeller Institute for Medical Research, October 1930.

33. Avery, O. T., and Heidelberger, M. Immunological relationships of cell constituents of pneumococcus. [Second paper.] *J. Exp. Med.* 42: 367, 1925.

Heidelberger, M. A "pure" organic chemist's downward path. *Ann. Rev. Microbiol.* 31: 1, 1977.

Heidelberger tells the story of his training with Richard Willstatter, his work with W. A. Jacobs at the Rockefeller Institute in synthesizing drugs for the cure of poliomyelitis, then their conquest of trypanosomiasis with Tryparsamide. After World War I, Flexner assigned Heidelberger and Jacobs to study chemotherapy in pneumonia. They worked with sulfanilamide, but it never occurred to them that so simple a substance could cure bacterial infections by a mechanism other than direct killing of the microorganisms. If they had, they might have saved hundreds of thousands of lives in the twenty years before Gerhard Domagk, Jacques and Thérèse Tréfonels, François Nitti, and Daniel Bovet made their discoveries. In 1921 Heidelberger joined Van Slyke when he first worked on oxyhemoglobin; during this work the first refrigerated centrifuge was invented.

When Karl Landsteiner joined the institute, he was interested in the immunological properties of hemoglobin and collaborated with Heidelberger. It was during this period that Heidelberger met W. W. Palmer, later to become a professor of medicine at Columbia. When the oxyhemoglobin work was finished, Heidelberger joined the pneumonia team and worked on the immunochemistry of the specific soluble substance. Flexner encouraged Heidelberger to get a job on his own, so that he would be better recognized as an independent worker. He succeeded Samuel Bookman as chemist at Mount Sinai Hospital. Soon he was recruited by Palmer to become a full-time chemist in a department of medicine, as Voegtlin had done with Barker.

Heidelberger, M., and Avery, O. T. The soluble specific substance of pneumococcus. *J. Exp. Med.* 38: 73, 1923.

For a brief authoritative summary, see Avery, O. T. The role of specific carbohydrates in pneumococcus infection and immunity. *Ann. Intern. Med.* 6: 1, 1932.

Heidelberger, M., and Avery, O. T. The soluble specific substance of the pneumococcus. *J. Exp. Med.* 40: 301, 1924.

Heidelberger, M., Goebel, W. F., and Avery, O. T. The soluble specific substance of pneumococcus. [Third paper.] *J. Exp. Med.* 42: 727, 1925.

Kabat, E. A. Michael Heidelberger as a carbohydrate chemist. *Carbohydr. Res.* 40: 1, 1975.

Kallos, P., and Westphal, O. Michael Heidelberger. *Int. Arch. Allergy Appl. Immunol.* 57: 97, 1978.

34. In 1900 K. Landsteiner examined the workers in his Vienna laboratory and found, by agglutination tests on their red blood cells, that they could be divided into three groups. This discovery of the blood groups solved the riddle as to why some transfusions were successful whereas others provoked serious and sometimes fatal reactions.

Landsteiner accepted an invitation to join the staff of the Rockefeller Institute in 1922. In 1930, for this discovery of the blood groups, he became the first U.S. citizen to receive the Nobel Prize. (Carrel, who received the prize in 1912, had not become a U.S. citizen, though he had been on the institute staff since 1902.)

In 1927 Landsteiner discovered the minor blood groups, designated $M$ and $N$, which are of significance for establishment of paternity and in studies of racial differences. In 1940, working with A. S. Wiener, Landsteiner discovered the Rh factor. In addition to his work on the blood, Landsteiner made monumental contributions to immunochemistry and to the study of the mechanisms of allergy and the nature of antibody reactions. (Hutchins, P. History of blood transfusion. *Surgery* 64: 685, 1968; Bordley, J., III, and Harvey, A. McG. *Two Centuries of American Medicine, 1776–1976,* p. 312. Philadelphia: W. B. Saunders, 1976.)

35. Avery, O. T., Chickering, H. T., Cole, R., and Dochez, A. R. Acute lobar pneumonia, prevention and serum treatment. *Monogr. Rockefeller Inst. Med. Res.,* no. 7, 1917.

36. Opie, E. L., Blake, F. G., and Small, J. C. *Epidemic Respiratory Disease: The Pneumonias and Other Infections of the Respiratory Tract Accompanying Influenza and Measles.* St. Louis: C. V. Mosby, 1921.

37. Julianelle, L. A. A biological classification of *Encapsulatus pneumoniae* (Friedlander's bacillus). *J. Exp. Med.* 44: 113, 1926.

38. Stillman, E. G. Further studies on the epidemiology of lobar pneumonia. *J. Exp. Med.* 26: 513, 1917.

Stillman, E. G. Production of immunity in mice by inhalation of pneumococci. *J. Exp. Med.* 40: 567, 1924.

39. Levy, R. L. The size of the heart in pneumonia. A teleroentgenographic study, with observations on the effect of digitalis therapy. *Arch. Intern. Med.* 32: 359, 1923.

Wright, I. S. Robert L. Levy, 1888–1974. *Trans. Assoc. Am. Physicians* 88: 27, 1975.

40. Stadie, W. C. The oxygen of the arterial and venous blood in pneumonia and its relation to cyanosis. *J. Exp. Med.* 30: 215, 1919.

41. Harvey, A. McG. Classics in clinical science: Anoxemia in pneumonia and its successful treatment by oxygen. *Am. J. Med.* 66: 193, 1979.

Stadie, W. C. Construction of an oxygen chamber for the treatment of pneumonia. *J. Exp. Med.* 35: 323, 1922.

Stadie, W. C. The treatment of anoxemia in pneumonia in an oxygen chamber. *J. Exp. Med.* 35: 337, 1922.

42. Van Slyke, D. D. Presentation of the Kober Medal for 1955 to William C. Stadie. *Trans. Assoc. Am. Physicians* 68: 25, 1955.

43. Stadie, W. C. Acceptance of the Kober Medal. *Trans. Assoc. Am. Physicians* 68: 29, 1955.

44. Binger, C. A. L. Therapeutic value of oxygen in pneumonia. *NY State J. Med.* 25: 953, 1925.

Binger, C. A. L. Oxygen therapy in pneumonia. *Bull. NY Acad. Med.* 1 (series 2): 17, 1925.

Binger, C. A. L. Anoxemia in pneumonia and its relief by oxygen inhalation. *J. Clin. Invest.* 6: 203, 1928.

45. Avery, O. T., and Tillett, W. S. Anaphylaxis with the type-specific carbohydrates of pneumococcus. *J. Exp. Med.* 49: 251, 1929.

Cole, R. Acute pulmonary infections. *De Lamar Lectures* 1: 103, 1927-28.

Davis, J. S., Jr. The effect of morphine on the respiration in pneumonia. *J. Clin. Invest.* 6: 187, 1928.

Davis, J. S., Jr., and Binger, C. A. L. A body plethysmograph for the study of respiratory movements in human beings. *Proc. Soc. Exp. Biol. Med.* 25: 607, 1928.

Dawson, M. H. The interconvertibility of "R" and "S" forms of pneumococcus. *J. Exp. Med.* 47: 577, 1928.

Heidelberger, I. M., Goebel, W. F., and Avery, O. T. The soluble specific substance of a strain of Friedlander's bacillus. *J. Exp. Med.* 42: 701, 1925.

Robertson, O. H., Woo, S., Cheer, S. N., and Sia, R. H. P. The occurrence of antipneumococcus substances in the blood serum in lobar pneumonia. *Proc. Soc. Exp. Biol. Med.* 22: 406, 1925.

Thjötta, T. Studies on bacterial nutrition. I. Growth of *Bacillus influenzae* in hemoglobin-free media. *J. Exp. Med.* 33: 763, 1921.

Tillett, W. S. Studies on immunity to *Pneumococcus mucosus* (Type III). I. Antibody response of rabbits immunized with Type III pneumococcus. *J. Exp. Med.* 45: 713, 1927.

Tillett, W. S., and Francis, T., Jr. Cutaneous reactions to the polysaccharides and proteins of pneumococcus in lobar pneumonia. *J. Exp. Med.* 50: 687, 1930.

46. Swift, H. F. The absorption of arsenic following intramuscular injections of Salvarsan and Neosalvarsan. *J. Exp. Med.* 16: 83, 1912.

47. Ellis, A. W. M., and Swift, H. F. The cerebrospinal fluid in syphilis. *J. Exp. Med.* 18: 162, 1913.

Swift, H. F., and Ellis, A. W. M. The direct treatment of syphilitic diseases of the central nervous system. *NY Med. J.* 96: 53, 1912.

Swift and Ellis, stimulated by Flexner's direct application of serum to the subarachnoid space in meningitis, conceived the idea of a similar procedure in neurosyphilis. In preliminary experiments with monkeys (Ellis, A. W. M., and Swift, H. F. The effect of intraspinous injections of Salvarsan and Neosalvarsan in monkeys. *J. Exp. Med.* 18: 428, 1913) they found that even small amounts of Salvarsan were excessively irritating. They resorted, therefore, to intravenous injection of Salvarsan, following which the patient was bled, and serum diluted with saline was injected intraspinally.

48. Dochez, A. R. Homer Fordyce Swift. *Trans. Assoc. Am. Physicians* 67: 25, 1954.

49. *Investigations and Other Publications by the Members of the Staff of the Hospital of tne Rockefeller Institute, 1920-1930.* (Contains curriculum vitae of Ellis and other early members of the staff.)

50. Robinson, *Adventures in Medical Education,* p. 95.

51. Hastings, A. B. Donald Dexter Van Slyke, 1883-1971. *Biog. Mem. Natl. Acad. Sci.* 48: 309, 1976. (Contains Van Slyke's complete bibliography.)

52. McLean, F. C. The numerical laws governing the rate of excretion of urea and

chlorides in man. II. The influence of pathological conditions and of drugs on excretion. *J. Exp. Med.* 22: 366, 1915.

Palmer, W. W. Acidosis and acid excretion in pneumonia. *J. Exp. Med.* 26: 495, 1917.

Van Slyke, D. D. An apparatus for determination of the gases in blood and other solutions. *Proc. Natl. Acad. Sci.* 7: 299, 1921. This article was important because this method was widely used in clinical research.

Van Slyke, D. D., and Palmer W. W. Studies of acidosis. IX. Relationship between alkali retention and alkali reserve in normal and pathological individuals. *J. Biol. Chem.* 32: 499, 1917. (There were eighteen articles in this series, Studies of Acidosis, which were all published in the *Journal of Biological Chemistry*.)

Van Slyke, D. D., Stillman, E., and Cullen, G. E. The nature and detection of diabetic acidosis. *Proc. Soc. Exp. Biol. Med.* 12: 165, 1915.

53. See Hastings, Donald D. Van Slyke, pp. 343–346.

54. Garvin, A., Lundsgaard, C., and Van Slyke, D. D. Studies of lung volume. III.Tuberculous women. *J. Exp. Med.* 27: 129, 1918.

Hiller, A., Linder, G. C., Lundsgaard, C., and Van Slyke, D. D. Fat metabolism in nephritis. *J. Exp. Med.* 39: 931, 1924.

Linder, G. C., Lundsgaard, C., Van Slyke, D. D., and Stillman, E. Changes in the volume of plasma and absolute amount of plasma proteins in nephritis. *J. Exp. Med.* 39: 921, 1924.

Lundsgaard, C. Studies of oxygen in the venous blood. IV. Determinations on five patients with incompensated circulatory disturbances. *J. Exp. Med.* 27: 219, 1918.

Lundsgaard, C. Studies on cyanosis. II. Secondary causes of cyanosis. *J. Exp. Med.* 30: 271, 1919.

55. Edsall, D. Presentation of the George M. Kober Medal to Dr. Donald D. Van Slyke. *Trans. Assoc. Am. Physicians* 57: 39, 1942.

For other references see Hastings, Donald D. Van Slyke.

56. Van Slyke, D. D., et al. Observations on the courses of different types of Bright's disease and the resultant changes in renal anatomy. *Medicine* 9: 257, 1930.

57. Van Slyke, D. D., Austin, J. H., and Stillman, E. Factors governing the excretion rate of urea. *J. Biol. Chem.* 46: 91, 1921.

58. Alving, A. S., and Van Slyke, D. D. The significance of concentration and dilution tests in Bright's disease. *J. Clin. Invest.* 13: 969, 1934.

Van Slyke, D. D., and Cullen, G. E. A permanent preparation of urease and its use in the determination of urea. *J. Biol. Chem.* 19: 211, 1914.

Van Slyke, D. D., Linder, G. C., Hiller, A., Leiter, L., and McIntosh, J. F. The excretion of ammonia and titratable acid in nephritis. *J. Clin. Invest.* 2: 255, 1925.

Van Slyke, D. D., Page, I. H., Hiller, A., and Kirk, E. Studies of urea excretion. IX. Comparison of urea clearances calculated from the excretion of urea, of urea plus ammonia, and of nitrogen determinable by hypobromite. *J. Clin. Invest.* 14: 901, 1935.

59. Edsall, Presentation of the Kober Medal to Van Slyke.

Van Slyke, D. D. Acceptance of the Kober Medal Award. *Trans. Assoc. Am. Physicians* 57: 42, 1942.

60. Harvey, George Canby Robinson.

61. Robinson, *Adventures in Medical Education,* p. 101. This chapter deals with Robinson's period at Washington University.

62. Duncan, G. G. Frederick Madison Allen, 1879–1964. *Trans. Assoc. Am. Physicians* 79: 13, 1966.

63. Allen, F. M. *Studies Concerning Glycosuria and Diabetes.* Boston: W. M. Leonard, 1913.

Allen, F. M. Experimental studies on diabetes. Series I. Production and control of diabetes in the dog. 4. Control of experimental diabetes by fasting and total dietary restriction. *J. Exp. Med.* 31: 575, 1920.

64. Peabody, F., Dochez, A., and Draper, G. A clinical study of acute poliomyelitis. *Monog. Rockefeller Inst. Med. Res.,* no. 4: 1–187, 1912.

65. Paul, J. R. *The History of Poliomyelitis.* New Haven: Yale University Press, 1971.

66. Corner, *History of the Rockefeller Institute,* p. 107. Corner refers in his bibliography to two letters: first, a letter from Cole to Flexner, October 30, 1911. Flexner Papers, American Philosophical Society; and two, an undated letter from Cole to Flexner. Archives, HRI.

67. Paul, *History of Poliomyelitis.*

68. Steele, J. M. Alfred Einstein Cohn, 1879–1957. *Trans. Assoc. Am. Physicians* 71: 17, 1958.

69. Cohn, A. E. Auricular tachycardia with a consideration of certain differences between the two vagi. *J. Exp. Med.* 15: 49, 1912.

Cohn, A. E., and Crawford, J. H. Studies on human capillaries. I. An apparatus for cinematographic observation of human capillaries. *J. Clin. Invest.* 2: 343, 1926.

Cohn, A. E., Fraser, F. R., and Jamieson, R. A. The influence of digitalis on the T wave of the human electrocardiogram. *J. Exp. Med.* 21: 593, 1915.

Cohn, A. E., and Levy, R. L. A modification of Van Leersum's bloodless method for recording blood pressures in animals. *J. Exp. Med.* 32: 351, 1920.

Cohn, A. E., and Lundsgaard, C. The peripheral blood pressure in fibrillation of the auricles. *J. Exp. Med.* 27: 505, 1918.

Cohn, A. E., and Murray, H. A., Jr. Physiological ontogeny. A. Chicken embryos. IV. The negative acceleration of growth with age as demonstrated by tissue cultures. *J. Exp. Med.* 42: 275, 1925.

70. Anson, M. L., and Mirsky, A. E. A description of the glass electrode and its use in measuring hydrogen ion concentration. *J. Biol. Chem.* 81: 581, 1929.

Mirsky, A. E., and Cohn, E. A. The pH of the blood of chicken embryos. *Proc. Soc. Exp. Biol. Med.* 25: 562, 1928.

71. MacLeod, C. M. J. Murray Steele, 1900–1969. *Trans. Assoc. Am. Physicians* 84: 41, 1971.

72. Barondess, J. A. Harold J. Stewart, 1896–1975. *Trans. Assoc. Am. Physicians* 89: 82, 1976.

Stewart, H. J., and Cohn, A. E. Evidence that digitalis influences contraction of the heart in man. *J. Clin. Invest.* 1: 97, 1924.

Stewart, H. J., and Cohn, A. E. Studies on the effect of the action of digitalis on the output of blood from the heart. III. Part 1, The effect on the output in normal human hearts; Part 2, The effect on the output of hearts in heart failure with congestion, in human beings. *J. Clin. Invest.* 11: 917, 1932.

Stewart, H. J., Crawford, J. H., and Gilchrist, A. R. Studies on the effect of cardiac irregularity on the circulation. I. The relation of pulse deficit to rate of blood flow in dogs subject to artificial auricular fibrillation and to regular tachycardia. *J. Clin. Invest.* 5: 317, 1927–28.

Stewart, H. J., Crawford, J. H., and Hastings, A. B. The effect of tachycardia on the blood flow in dogs. I. The effect of rapid irregular rhythms as seen in auricular fibrillation. *J. Clin. Invest.* 3: 435, 1926–27.

73. Annual Reports of the Director of the Hospital to the Board of Trustees of the Rockefeller Institute for Medical Research (William Henry Welch, chairman). Welch's copies of these reports are in the Welch Medical Library, Johns Hopkins University School of Medicine.

74. Dochez, A. R. Homer Fordyce Swift, 1881–1953. *Trans. Assoc. Am. Physicians* 67: 25, 1954.

75. Kinsella, R. A. The relation between hemolytic and non-hemolytic streptococci, and its possible significance. *J. Exp. Med.* 28: 181, 1918.

Kinsella, R. A., and Swift, H. F. A classification of non-hemolytic streptococci. *J. Exp. Med.* 25: 877, 1917.

Kinsella, R. A., and Swift, H. F. The classification of hemolytic streptococci. *J. Exp. Med.* 28: 169, 1918.

76. Cohn, A. E., and Swift, H. F. Electrocardiographic evidence of myocardial involvement in rheumatic fever. *J. Exp. Med.* 39: 1, 1924.

77. Swift, H. F. The pathogenesis of rheumatic fever. *J. Exp. Med.* 39: 497, 1924.

Swift, H. F. Rheumatic fever. *J.A.M.A.* 92: 2071, 1929. In this masterly lecture, Swift brought every phase of acute rheumatic fever—clinical variations, pathology, etiology—up to date.

78. Dochez, A. R., Avery, O. T., and Lancefield, R. C. Studies on the biology of streptococcus. I. Antigenic relationships between strains of *Streptococcus haemolyticus. J. Exp. Med.* 30: 179, 1919.

Lancefield, R. C. The immunological relationships of *Streptococcus viridans* and certain of its chemical fractions. II. Serological reactions obtained with antinucleoprotein sera. *J. Exp. Med.* 42: 397, 1925.

79. Lancefield, R. C. A serological differentiation of human and other groups of hemolytic streptococci. *J. Exp. Med.* 57: 571, 1933. In this extremely important paper, Lancefield showed that immune sera satisfactory for precipitin tests with extracts of streptococci could be readily prepared. By this method, practically all hemolytic streptococci fell into five groups, "which bear a definite relationship to the sources of the cultures." Most pathogenic strains from human disease, including scarlet fever, fall into group A, which can be further subdivided by appropriate methods. This work made possible the final conclusion that the only feature that scarlatinal streptococci necessarily have in common is the ability to produce erythrogenic toxin and that such toxin may be produced by serologically distinct types.

80. Derick, C. L., and Andrewes, C. H. The skin response of rabbits to non-hemolytic streptococci. II. Attempts to determine whether the secondary reaction is of the nature of an Arthus phenomenon. *J. Exp. Med.* 44: 55, 1926.

Derick, C. L., Andrewes, C. H., and Swift, H. F. A study of hemolytic streptococci in acute rheumatic fever, with an analysis of the antigenic relationships existing among certain strains. *J. Exp. Med.* 43: 13, 1926.

Derick, C. L., Hitchcock, C. H., and Swift, H. F. Reactions of rabbits to nonhemolytic streptococci. III. A study of modes of sensitization. *J. Exp. Med.* 52, 1, 1930.

Faber (Faber, H. K. Experimental arthritis in the rabbit: A contribution to the pathogenesis of arthritis in rheumatic fever. *J. Exp. Med.* 22: 615, 1915) deserves credit for opposing the idea that rheumatic fever was a simple, direct infection with streptococci and for promoting the concept of altered reactivity (allergy) in the mechanism of production of the clinical phenomena of the disease. Nevertheless, Swift's work dominated the stage for many years. He regarded hypersensitivity as implicit in the reaction of rheumatic fever and, with his associates, developed a hypothesis that they formulated as follows: "The theory is advanced that the pathogenesis of rheumatic fever can be explained by the existence in certain individuals of a condition of hypersensitiveness (allergy or hypergy) to streptococci resulting from repeated low grade infections or from the persistence of foci of infection in the body. When under suitable circumstances streptococci or products of streptococci are disseminated to the tissues, those tissues over-react and the characteristic picture of the disease results." (Swift, H. F., Derick, C. L., and Hitchcock, C. H. Rheumatic fever as a manifestation of hypersensitiveness [allergy or hypergy] to streptococci. *Trans. Assoc. Am. Physicians* 43: 192, 1928.) Swift's hypothesis was based on analogies with syphilis and tuberculosis.

81. Blake, F. G., and Trask, J. D., Jr. Experimental measles. *J.A.M.A.* 77: 192, 1921.

Blake, F. G., and Trask, J. D., Jr. Studies on measles. III. Acquired immunity following experimental measles. *J. Exp. Med.* 33: 621, 1921.

82. See Harvey, A. McG. *The Interurban Clinical Club, 1905–1976. A Record of Achievement in Clinical Science.* Philadelphia: W. B. Saunders, 1978, for biographical sketches of Blake (p. 126) and Trask (p. 184).

83. Annual Report of the Director of the Hospital to the Board of Trustees of the Rockefeller Institute for Medical Research, 1930.

84. Other biographical notes on those who worked at the HRI may be found in Harvey, *Interurban Clinical Club:* Rufus I. Cole, p. 47; Francis G. Blake, p. 126; George H. Draper, p. 128; John P. Peters, p. 138; James D. Trask, p. 184; Thomas M. Rivers, p. 193;

William S. Tillett, p. 201; Harold Amoss, p. 175; Reginald Fitz, p. 131; Colin M. MacLeod, p. 326; Cornelius P. Rhoads, p. 238.

85. Horsfall, F. L., Jr. Thomas Milton Rivers, Sept. 3, 1888–May 12, 1962. *Biog. Mem. Natl. Acad. Sci.* 38: 263, 1964. (Contains Rivers's complete bibliography.)

86. Harvey, A. McG. Pioneer American virologist—Charles E. Simon. *Johns Hopkins Med. J.* 142: 161, 1978.

87. Harvey, *Interurban Clinical Club,* p. 201.

88. Rivers, T. M., and Tillett, W. S. Studies on varicella. The susceptibility of rabbits to the virus of varicella. *J. Exp. Med.* 38: 673, 1923.

Rivers, T. M., and Tillett, W. S. The lesions in rabbits experimentally infected by a virus encountered in the attempted transmission of varicella. *J. Exp. Med.* 39: 281, 1924.

89. Andrewes, C. H. Nature, the scientist and the pitfall. *St. Bartholomew's Hosp. J.* 32: 20, 1924. Andrewes describes the isolation of the mouse virus.

90. Harvey, *Interurban Clinical Club,* pp. 296, 307.

91. Woodward, T. E. Joseph E. Smadel, 1907–1963. *Trans. Assoc. Am. Physicians* 77: 29, 1964.

92. Harvey, *Interurban Clinical Club,* p. 305.

93. Francis, T., Jr. A new type of virus from epidemic influenza. *Science* 92: 405, 1940.

Francis, T., Jr., and Magill, T. P. Immunological studies with the virus of influenza. *J. Exp. Med.* 62: 505, 1935. Francis and Magill made the important observation that subcutaneous inoculation of rabbits and mice with influenza virus did not cause clinical disease, but produced active immunity, with the appearance of antibodies in the blood. Studies of this sort later furnished the basis for attempts to immunize human beings actively.

Francis, T., Jr., and Magill, T. P. The incidence of neutralizing antibodies for human influenza virus in the serum of human individuals of different ages. *J. Exp. Med.* 63: 665, 1936. Francis and Magill found that about 50 percent of the sera of individuals of various ages with no history of influenza contained sufficient antibody *after* the first year of life to furnish complete protection to mice. These observations suggested, of course, a high degree of unrecognized infection with influenza virus.

Francis, T., Jr., and Magill, T. P. The antibody response of human subjects vaccinated with the virus of human influenza. *J. Exp. Med.* 65: 251, 1937. Francis and Magill vaccinated human volunteers by the subcutaneous or intradermal routes with virus grown in tissue culture medium. A "good titer" of circulating antibodies effective against mouse passage virus developed. The antibodies persisted for at least five months. A preliminary note of this work appeared in 1936 (Vaccination of human subjects with virus of human influenza. *Proc. Soc. Exp. Biol. Med.* 33: 604). These experiments furnished the basis for the attempts at systematic vaccination against influenza which were later made.

Early reports of clinical experiences are to be found in the *American Journal of Hygiene* for 1945, where the entire July issue is devoted to the subject. T. Francis, Jr., J. Salk, and their associates also made important observations (Protective effect of vaccination against induced influenza. *J. Clin. Invest.* 24: 536, 1945).

McDermott, W. Thomas Francis, Jr., 1900–1969. *Trans. Assoc. Am. Physicians* 83: 16, 1970.

94. See Paul, *History of Poliomyelitis.* Chapter forty relates the important contributions to the development of influenza vaccine and the field trials in the study of poliomyelitis vaccine. Biographical material on Francis may be found there. For additional material see McDermott, Thomas Francis, Jr.

95. Harvey, Pioneer American virologist—Charles E. Simon.

96. Harvey, *Interurban Clinical Club,* p. 406.

97. Castle, W. B. Cornelius Packard Rhoads. *Trans. Assoc. Am. Physicians* 73: 25, 1960.

98. Castle, W. B., Rhoads, C. P., Lawson, H. A., and Pagne, G. C. Etiology and treatment of sprue. Observations on patients in Puerto Rico and subsequent experiments in animals. *Arch. Intern. Med.* 56: 627, 1935.

Rhoads, C. P., Castle, W. B., Pagne, G. C., and Lawson, H. A. Observations on the etiology and treatment of anemia associated with hookworm infection in Puerto Rico. *Medicine* 13: 317, 1934.

# Chapter 6

1. Bylebyl, J. J. Personal communication, 1980.

Cole, R. Medical societies and progress in medical research. *J. Michigan State Med. Soc.* 40: 19, 1941.

2. Delafield, F. Presidential address. *Trans. Assoc. Am. Physicians* 1: 1, 1886.

3. Means, J. H. *The Association of American Physicians: Its First Seventy-Five Years.* New York: McGraw-Hill, 1961.

4. Ibid., pp. 1–8.

5. Councilman, W. T. Certain elements found in the blood in cases of malarial fever. *Trans. Assoc. Am. Physicians* 1: 89, 1886.

6. Fitz, R. H. Perforating inflammation of the vermiform appendix. *Trans. Assoc. Am. Physicians* 1: 107, 1886.

7. Welch, W. H. An experimental study of glomerulonephritis. *Trans. Assoc. Am. Physicians* 1: 171, 1886.

8. Mitchell, S. W. The tendon-jerk and muscle-jerk in disease. *Trans. Assoc. Am. Physicians* 1: 11, 1886.

9. Osler, W. The coming of age of internal medicine. *Int. Clin.* 4 (series 25): 1, 1915.

10. Herter, C. On the origin of oxaluria from fermentation in the gastroenteric tract. *Trans. Assoc. Am. Physicians* 15: 48, 1900.

11. Herter, C. The pathology of acid intoxication. *Trans. Assoc. Am. Physicians* 15: 236, 1900.

12. Welch, W. H. Presidential address. *Trans. Assoc. Am. Physicians* 16: xvi, 1901.

13. Kinnicutt, F. P. Presidential address. *Trans. Assoc. Am. Physicians* 22: 1, 1907.

14. Harvey, A. McG. *The Interurban Clinical Club, 1905–1976. A Record of Achievement in Clinical Science.* Philadelphia: W. B. Saunders, 1978.

15. Ibid., p. 4.

16. Ibid.

17. Fordtran, J. S. An ASCI tradition. (Presidential address before the sixty-ninth annual meeting of the American Society for Clinical Investigation, Washington, D.C., 1 May 1977.) *J. Clin. Invest.* 60: 271, 1977.

Harvey, A. McG. Samuel J. Meltzer: Pioneer catalyst in the evolution of clinical science in America. *Perspect. Biol. Med.* 21: 431, 1978.

18. Howell, W. H. Samuel James Meltzer, 1851–1920. *Biog. Mem. Natl. Acad. Sci.* 21: 1, 1927. (Contains Meltzer's complete bibliography.)

19. Ibid.

20. Meltzer, S. J. Bronchial asthma as a phenomenon of anaphylaxis. *J.A.M.A.* 55: 1021, 1910.

21. Brainard, E. R. History of the American Society for Clinical Investigation, 1909–1959. *J. Clin. Invest.* 38: 1784, 1959.

22. This list was either expanded by the addition of three names prior to the organizational meeting, or the list given in the minutes of the November committee meeting is incomplete, for the records of the charter meeting (May 11, 1908) contain the names of twenty-five men (in addition to the nine committee members) who had been invited to be present. (Through the courtesy of Dr. John S. Fordtran, the author has had access to the original minutes books of the society.)

23. Brainard, History of the American Society for Clinical Investigation, p. 1785.

24. The details of this meeting are recorded in the original minutes book of the society, which is in the possession of its current secretary.

25. John T. Edsall recalls an entertaining childhood incident relating to the American

Society for Clinical Investigation. His father, David Linn Edsall, on returning from a dinner meeting of the society in 1912, told him of the songs sung there, which were based on some of the current hits of the day.

One was inspired by the then popular song "Everybody's doing it. Doing what? Turkey Trot," which went:

> Think up something never done before,
> Write it up and make an awful roar,
> That's the way they do in Baltimore,
> It's a bore, it's a bore, it's a bore, it's a bore,
> But everybody's doing it, doing it, doing it.

Another was inspired by the song "Anybody here seen Kelly? Kelly with the green necktie," which went:

> Anybody here seen Flexner?
> What, Simon? No. Abie.
> He is a great man, maybe,
> But you can't prove it by me.

(Edsall, J. T. Personal communication, August 10, 1978.)

26. The members of the new society were called "Young Turks" after the real "Young Turks," who, in 1908, startled the world by revolting against Sultan Abdul Hamid II, deposing him the following year, and, with nationalistic fervor, setting about to establish a constitutional regime and to institute sweeping reforms in the decrepit Ottoman empire.

27. The young clinical scientists who were stimulated by Meltzer to form the American Society for Clinical Investigation were all members of the Interurban Clinical Club.

28. Brainard, History of the American Society for Clinical Investigation, p. 1793.

29. Austin, J. H. A brief sketch of the history of the American Society for Clinical Investigation. *J. Clin. Invest.* 28: 401, 1949.

30. Brainard, History of the American Society for Clinical Investigation, p. 1794.

31. Among the seven honorary members of the Association of American Physicians when it was founded, were the following five physicians, who had studied under Louis in Paris: Henry I. Bowditch, Alonzo Clark, Meredith Clymer, John T. Metcalfe, and Alfred Stillé.

32. More details concerning the research activities of many of these founding members may be found elsewhere in this volume: Joseph A. Capps (p. 349); Henry A. Christian (p. 260); Rufus I. Cole (p. 80); David Linn Edsall (p. 207); Nellis Barnes Foster (p. 237); Albion W. Hewlett (p. 331); John F. Howland (p. 159); Theodore Caldwell Janeway (p. 153); Warfield Theobald Longcope (p. 172); and Joseph Hersey Pratt (p. 261). A brief biographical sketch of the others will be found in Appendix A.

33. Meltzer, S. J. The science of clinical medicine; what it ought to be and the men to uphold it. *J.A.M.A.* 53: 508, 1909.

34. The following is a list of the fourteen papers, in the order in which they were presented: "Some Observations on the Effect of the Vasodilators on Blood Pressure," by Joseph L. Miller (Chicago); "Blood Pressure in Tuberculosis," by Haven Emerson (New York); "A Modification of the Riva-Rocci Method of Determining the Blood Pressure for Use in the Dog," by Theodore C. Janeway (New York); "The Effect of Compression of the Splanchnic Arteries upon the Systemic Blood Pressure," by W. T. Longcope (Philadelphia); "Blood Pressure Changes Following Reduction of the Renal Artery Circulation," by Theodore C. Janeway (New York); "The Advantages of Intermittent Positive Pressure in Resuscitation with Some Experimental Observations," by Joseph A. Capps and Dean D. Lewis (Chicago); "Miliary Tuberculosis of the Skin," by Wilder Tileston (Boston); "The Sensory Symptomatology of the Facial Nerve," by J. Ramsay Hunt (New York); "A Study of Experimental Anaemia," by Joseph H. Pratt (Boston); "Observations on Metabolism in Cases of Muscle Spasms due to Heat," by D. L. Edsall (Philadelphia); "The Relation of Atrophy of the Pancreas to Glycosuria," by Joseph H. Pratt (Boston); "Some Further Observations on Experimental Nephritis," by H. A. Christian (Boston); "Respiration by

Continuous Intra-Pulmonary Pressure without the Aid of Muscular Action," by S. J. Meltzer and John Auer (New York); "Some Experiments upon the Possibility of Catheterizing the Pylorus in Dogs," by Joseph Sailer and R. G. Torrey (Philadelphia).

35. Blake, F. G. Clinical investigation. *Science* 74: 27, 1931.

36. From the official minutes book of the society, kindly made available to me by Dr. John S. Fordtran.

37. Cohn, A. E. Purposes in medical research. *J. Clin. Invest.* 1: 1, 1924.

38. Starr, I. Functions and dysfunctions of learned societies. *J. Clin. Invest.* 19: 765, 1940.

39. Austin, J. H. A brief sketch of the history of the American Society for Clinical Investigation. *J. Clin. Invest.* 28: 401, 1949.

40. Thompson, L. D. Early history of the Central Society for Clinical Research. *J. Lab. Clin. Med.* 41: 3, 1953.

41. Colwell, A. R., Sr. Catalyst of midwestern medicine: A history of the Central Interurban Clinical Club. Privately printed, March 1969.

42. The discussion of the formation of the Central Interurban Club and the Central Society for Clinical Research is based on study of the original minutes book of the Central Interurban Club, which is in the library of the Northwestern University School of Medicine.

43. Copy of a letter kindly furnished me by Maurice A. Schnitker.

44. Schnitker, M. A. President's Address: First Annual Meeting of the American Federation for Clinical Research. Minneapolis, Minnesota, April 20, 1942.

# Chapter 7

1. Welch, W. H. Presidential address. *Trans. Assoc. Am. Physicians* 16: xvi, 1901.

2. Barker, L. F. Medicine and the universities. An address delivered at the meeting of the Western Alumni of the Johns Hopkins University held at Chicago, February 28, 1902. *Am. Med.* 4: 143, 1902. Reprinted in *Medical Education and Research.* Ed. Cattell, J. McKeen, p. 223. New York: Science Press, 1913.

3. Editorial: The university medical school. *J.A.M.A.* 39: 989, 1902.

4. Dobson, J. M. The modern university school—its purposes and methods. *J.A.M.A.* 39: 521, 1902.

5. Billings, F. Medical education in the United States. *J.A.M.A.* 40: 1271, 1903.

6. Bevan, A. D. Medical education in the United States. The need of a uniform standard. *J.A.M.A.* 51: 566, 1908.

7. Flexner, A. The history of full-time clinical teaching. Unpublished manuscript. See Flexner, S., and Flexner, J. T. *William Henry Welch and the Heroic Age of American Medicine,* p. 303. New York: Viking Press, 1941.

8. Welch, W. H. The unity of the medical sciences. *Boston Med. Surg. J.* 155: 367, 1906.

9. Welch, W. H. Medicine and the university (Address delivered at the University of Chicago, December 17, 1907). *J.A.M.A.* 50: 1, 1908; Papers and addresses, vol. 3, p. 89.

10. Howell, W. H. The medical school as part of the university. *Science* 30: 129, 1909.

11. Mall to Minot. See Sabin, F. R. *Franklin Paine Mall: The Story of a Mind,* p. 260. Baltimore: Johns Hopkins Press, 1934.

12. Thayer, rather than Barker, was Osler's choice as his successor, as indicated by the following letter from Osler to Barker, March 4, 1905 (Alan M. Chesney Archives, Johns Hopkins Medical Institutions):

> The faculty seems to be unanimous in favor of you as my successor. You may have heard something from Welch about this, as I was not at the meeting and only heard last eve of the action. Naturally I was placed in a most awkward position. Thayer has done so much 1st class work and is such a good fellow that it seemed cruel to pass him by; but the general feeling was not towards him in the faculty or on the Hospital board and while I might have perhaps forced

it, had I felt more strongly, everything came round to a choice between you and Dock. I suppose the governors will act shortly. The important thing will be to make Thayer comfortable and you can help in this. He has behaved splendidly and we must do everything possible for him. This is only a preliminary note—there will be hosts of things to confer about. . . . I am taking Plato's advice and sitting under a wall until the storm is over.

13. Robinson, G. C. *Adventures in Medical Education.* Cambridge, Mass.: Harvard University Press, 1957.

14. William Osler to Ira Remsen, September 1, 1911. See McGovern, J. P., and Roland, C. G. *William Osler, The Continuing Education,* p. 291. Springfield, Ill.: Charles C Thomas, 1969.

15. Flexner and Flexner, *William Henry Welch,* p. 305.

16. F. T. Gates to William Henry Welch, January 6, 1911. In ibid., p. 305.

17. Flexner, A. Medical education in the United States and Canada. Bull. No. 4. New York: Carnegie Foundation for the Advancement of Teaching, 1910.

18. Flexner and Flexner, *William Henry Welch,* p. 308.

19. Ibid., p. 309.

20. Ibid., p. 310.

21. Ibid.

22. Ibid., p. 311.

23. Ibid.

24. Ibid., p. 312.

25. Ibid.

26. Ibid., p. 314.

27. Cushing, H. *The Life of Sir William Osler.* Vol. 1, p. 270. Oxford: Clarendon Press, 1925.

28. Flexner and Flexner, *William Henry Welch,* p. 318.

29. Ibid., p. 320.

30. Ibid., p. 321.

31. Stedman, T. L. Full-time professors. *Med. Record* 85: 850, 1914.

32. Editorial: Full-time salaried professors. *J.A.M.A.* 61: 1906, 1913.

33. Editorial: A new departure in clinical teaching. *J.A.M.A.* 62: 853, 1914.

34. Vaughan, V. C. Reorganization of clinical teaching. *J.A.M.A.* 64: 785, 1915.

35. Flexner and Flexner, *William Henry Welch,* p. 324.

36. Barker, L. F. Some tendencies in medical education in the United States. In *Medical Education and Research,* p. 241.

37. Meltzer, S. J. Headship and organization of clinical departments of first class medical schools. *Science* 40: 620, 1914.

38. Flexner, S. The full-time teacher of medicine. *Trans. Assoc. Am. Physicians* 29: 1, 1914.

39. Pearce, R. M. The work and opportunities of a department of research medicine in the university. *Science* 43: 53, 1916.

40. Pearce's selected publications include:

Pearce, R. M. Concerning the depressor substance of dog's urine and its disappearance in certain forms of experimental acute nephritis. *J. Exp. Med.* 12: 128, 1910.

Pearce, R. M. The retention of foreign protein by the kidney. A study in anaphylaxis. *J. Exp. Med.* 16: 349, 1912.

Pearce, R. M., Austin, J. H., and Pepper, O. H. P. The relation of the spleen to blood destruction and regeneration and to hemolytic jaundice. XIII. The influence of diet upon the anemia following splenectomy. *J. Exp. Med.* 22: 682, 1915.

Pearce, R. M., Hill, M. C., and Eisenbrey, A. B. Experimental acute nephritis: The vascular reactions and the elimination of nitrogen. *J. Exp. Med.* 12: 196, 1910.

Pearce, R. M., Karsner, H. T., and Eisenbrey, A. B. Studies in immunity and anaphylaxis. The proteins of the kidney and liver. *J. Exp. Med.* 14: 44, 1911.

41. Lee, F. S., Cannon, W. B., and Pearce, R. M. Medical research and its relation to medical schools. *Proc. Assoc. Am. Med. Coll.* 27: 19, 1917.

42. Robinson, G. C. The use of full-time teachers in clinical medicine. *South. Med. J.* 15: 1009, 1922.

43. Marriott, W. McK. See discussion at the end of reference forty-two.

44. McCann, W. S. Unpublished memoirs. MS. Library. University of Rochester School of Medicine. (McCann was on the faculty at Johns Hopkins [1921–24] before assuming the chairmanship of medicine at the University of Rochester.)

45. Castle, W. B. Presidential address. *Trans. Assoc. Am. Physicians* 73: 1, 1960.

46. Burnet, F. M. Autoimmune disease. I. Modern immunological concepts. *Br. Med. J.* 2: 645, 1959.

47. Albright, F. Some of the "do's" and "do-not's" in clinical investigation. *J. Clin. Invest.* 23: 921, 1944.

48. See also Strauss, M. B. The climate for the cultivation of clinical research. *N. Engl. J. Med.* 262: 805, 1960.

# Chapter 8

1. Barker, L. F. Theodore Caldwell Janeway. *Science* 47: 273, 1918.

2. Atchley, D. W. The uses of elegance. *Ann. Intern. Med.* 52: 881, 1960.

Flaxman, N. Janeway on hypertension. Theodore Caldwell Janeway (1872–1917). *Bull. Hist. Med.* 9: 505, 1941.

Harvey, A. McG. *The Interurban Clinical Club, 1905–1976. A Record of Achievement in Clinical Science,* p. 30. Philadelphia: W. B. Saunders, 1978.

Janeway, T. C. Important contributions to clinical medicine during the past thirty years from the study of human blood pressure. *Bull. Johns Hopkins Hosp.* 26: 341, 1915. (Contains references to Janeway's many important contributions.)

3. Janeway, T. C. The use and abuse of digitalis. *Am. J. Med. Sci.* 135: 781, 1908.

Janeway, T. C. The comparative value of cardiac remedies. *Arch. Intern. Med.* 13: 361, 1914.

4. Mosenthal, H. O. Nitrogen metabolism and the significance of the non-protein nitrogen of the blood in experimental uranium nephritis. *Arch. Intern. Med.* 14: 844, 1914.

Mosenthal, H. O. Renal function as measured by the elimination of fluids, salt and nitrogen and the specific gravity of the urine. *Arch. Intern. Med.* 16: 733, 1915.

Mosenthal, H. O., and Barker, L. F. On the control of the symptoms of diabetes insipidus by subcutaneous injections of extracts of the hypophysis cerebri (pars posterior and pars intermedia). *J. Urol.* 1: 449, 1917.

Mosenthal, H. O., and Harrop, G. A. The comparative food value of protein, fat and alcohol in diabetes mellitus as measured by the nitrogen equilibrium. *Arch. Intern. Med.* 22: 750, 1918.

Mosenthal, H. O., and Lewis, D. S. The D:N ratio in diabetes mellitus. *Bull. Johns Hopkins Hosp.* 28: 187, 1917.

5. Keith, N. M., and Hench, P. S. Leonard George Rowntree, 1883–1959. *Trans. Assoc. Am. Physicians* 73: 29, 1960.

Rowntree, L. G., Abel, J. J., and Turner, B. B. On the removal of diffusible substances from the circulating blood of living animals by dialysis. *J. Pharmacol. Exp. Ther.* 5: 275, 1914.

Rowntree, L. G., Chesney, A. M., and Marshall, E. K., Jr. Studies in liver function. *J.A.M.A.* 63: 1533, 1914.

Rowntree, L. G., and Geraghty, J. T. An experimental and clinical study of the functional activity of the kidneys by means of phenolsulphonephthalein. *J. Pharmacol. Exp. Ther.* 1: 579, 1909–10.

Abel and Rowntree (On the pharmacological action of some phthaleins and their derivatives, with especial reference to their behavior as purgatives. I. *J. Pharmacol. Exp. Ther.* 1: 231, 1909), in the course of studies of certain phthaleins as subcutaneous purgatives, noted excretion of phenolsulphonephthalein in the urine. It occurred to Rowntree that excretion of phthalein could be used quantitatively as a measure of renal function. His paper, with Geraghty, opened a new era in the study of renal function. (See Rowntree, L. G., and Geraghty, J. T. The phthalein test, an experimental and clinical study of phenolsulphonephthalein in relation to renal function in health and disease. *Arch. Intern. Med.* 9: 284, 1912; and Fitz, R. Studies of renal function in renal, cardiorenal and cardiac disease. *Arch. Intern. Med.* 11: 121, 1913.)

The entire position of renal-function tests at this time was well summarized in the symposium in which Christian, Janeway, and Rowntree participated (On the study of renal function. *Trans. Cong. Am. Physicians Surg.* 9: 1, 1913).

Rowntree, L. G., and Levy, R. L. A study of the buffer action of the blood. *Arch. Intern. Med.* 17: 525, 1916.

6. Baetjer, W. A. Paul W. Clough, 1882–1970. *Trans. Assoc. Am. Physicians* 85: 11, 1972.

7. Rantz, L. A. Arthur Leonard Bloomfield, 1888–1962. *Trans. Assoc. Am. Physicians* 76: 12, 1963.

8. Austrian, C. R. The viscosity of the blood in health and disease. *Bull. Johns Hopkins Hosp.* 22: 1, 1911.

Austrian, C. R. The effect of hypersensitiveness to a tuberculoprotein upon subsequent infection with bacillus tuberculosis. *Bull. Johns Hopkins Hosp.* 24: 11, 1913.

Austrian, C. R. Experimental tuberculous meningitis. *Bull. Johns Hopkins Hosp.* 27: 237, 1916.

Chesney, A. M. Charles Robert Austrian, 1885–1956. *Trans. Assoc. Am. Physicians* 70: 11, 1957.

9. Krause, A. K. Experimental studies on the cutaneous reaction to tuberculo-protein. I. Factors governing the reaction. *J. Med. Res.* 35: 1, 1916.

Krause, A. K. The anaphylactic state in its relation to resistance to tuberculous infection and tuberculous disease. *J. Med. Res.* 35: 25, 1916.

Krause, A. K. Nature of resistance to tuberculosis. *Bull. Johns Hopkins Hosp.* 28: 191, 1917.

Long, E. R. Allen Kramer Krause, 1881–1941. *Trans. Assoc. Am. Physicians* 57: 22, 1942.

10. Clough, P. W. Some observations on hypersensitiveness to pneumococcus protein, with special reference to its relation to immunity. *Bull. Johns Hopkins Hosp.* 26: 37, 1915.

Ireland, R. A., Baetjer, W. A., and Ruhrah, J. A case of lymphatic leukemia with apparent cure. *J.A.M.A.* 65: 948, 1915. An early description of infectious mononucleosis in an adult.

Keith, N. M., and Lamson, P. D. The relation of plasma volume to the number of erythrocytes per unit volume of blood. *J. Pharmacol. Exp. Ther.* 18: 247, 1916.

Moss, W. L. A simplified method for determining the isoagglutinin group in the selection of donors for blood transfusion. *J.A.M.A.* 68: 1905, 1917.

Sellards, A. W. A clinical method for studying titratable alkalinity of the blood and its application to acidosis. *Bull. Johns Hopkins Hosp.* 25: 101, 1914.

Sellards, A. W. The relationship of the renal lesions of Asiatic cholera to the ordinary nephritides with especial reference to acidosis. *Am. J. Trop. Dis.* 2: 104, 1914.

Sellards, A. W., and Baetjer, W. A. The experimental production of amebic dysentery by direct inoculation into the caecum. *Bull. Johns Hopkins Hosp.* 25: 323, 1914.

11. Harvey, A. McG. Tuberculosis: The study of a specific disease at Johns Hopkins. *Johns Hopkins Med. J.* 141: 198, 1977.

12. Mosenthal, H. O. Theodore Caldwell Janeway, A. M., M.D. *Johns Hopkins Alumni Mag.* 2: 264, 1918.

13. Levy, R. L. Studies on the conditions of activity in endocrine glands. IV. The effect of thyroid secretion on the pressor action of adrenalin. *Am. J. Physiol.* 41: 492, 1916.

Levy, R. L. The effects of thyroid secretion on the excitability of the endings of the cardiac vagus. *Arch. Intern. Med.* 21: 263, 1918.

Levy, R. L., Rowntree, L. G., and Marriott, W. McK. A simple method for determining variations in the hydrogen-ion circulation of blood. *Arch. Intern. Med.* 16: 389, 1915.

14. Barker, L. F., and Richardson, H. B. An unusual combination of cardiac ar-

rhythmias of atrial origin occurring in a patient with focal infections and thyroid adenomata. *Arch. Intern. Med.* 23: 158, 1919.

Janeway, T. C., and Richardson, H. B. Experiments on the vasoconstrictor action of blood serum. *Arch. Intern. Med.* 21: 565, 1918.

15. Denny, G. P., and Minot, G. R. The origin of antithrombin. *Am. J. Physiol.* 38: 233, 1915.

Denny, G. P., and Minot, G. R. The coagulation of blood in the pleural cavity. *Am. J. Physiol.* 39: 455, 1916.

Minot, G. R. Nitrogen metabolism before and after splenectomy in a case of pernicious anemia. *Bull. Johns Hopkins Hosp.* 25: 1, 1914.

Minot, G. R., and Denny, G. P. Prothrombin and antithrombin factors in the coagulation of blood. *Arch. Intern. Med.* 17: 103, 1916.

16. Evans, F. A. An oxydase reaction on blood smears: A valuable test in the identification of white blood cells of uncertain origin. *Arch. Intern. Med.* 16: 1067, 1915. Evans was a resident medical house officer when he wrote this paper.

Evans, F. A. Observations on the origin and status of the so-called "transitional white blood cell." *Arch. Intern. Med.* 17: 1, 1916.

Sprunt, T. P., and Evans, F. A. Mononuclear leukocytosis in reaction to acute infections (infectious mononucleosis). *Bull. Johns Hopkins Hosp.* 31: 410, 1920.

17. For additional biographical data on various members of the department of medicine during the tenure of Janeway, see the following memorial tributes in the *Transactions of the Association of American Physicians:* W. A. Baetjer—88: 12, 1975; T. R. Boggs—54: 9, 1939; T. R. Brown—64: 5, 1951; Alan M. Chesney—78: 17, 1965; Frank A. Evans—70: 13, 1957; R. L. Haden—65: 18, 1952; Louis Hamman—59: 17, 1946; George A. Harrop, Jr.—59: 21, 1946; N. M. Keith—89: 23, 1976; Robert L. Levy—88: 27, 1975; Verne R. Mason—79: 62, 1966; George R. Minot—63: 11, 1950; Herman O. Mosenthal—68: 15, 1955; W. L. Moss—71: 34, 1958; M. C. Pincoffs—74: 33, 1961; Henry Barber Richardson—79: 74, 1966; Thomas M. Rivers—76: 16, 1963; Leonard G. Rowntree—73: 29, 1960; Andrew Watson Sellards—59: 34, 1946; Thomas P. Sprunt—69: 30: 1956; Harold J. Stewart—89: 32, 1976; V. P. Sydenstricker—79: 79, 1966.

18. The Reminiscences of Dana Atchley, 1956, found in the Columbia Oral History Collection, is copyrighted by The Trustees of Columbia University in the City of New York, 1975, and is used with permission.

19. Atchley, D. W. Nuclear digestion and uric acid excretion in cases of total occlusion of the pancreatic duct. *Arch. Intern. Med.* 15: 5, 1915.

20. Atchley, The uses of elegance.

21. Lusk, G. Theodore Caldwell Janeway. *Am. J. Med. Sci.* 155: 1918.

22. Janeway, T. C. Outside professional engagements by members of professional faculties. *J.A.M.A.* 90: 1315, 1928; idem, *Educ. Rev.* 55: 207, 1918.

23. Davidson, W. C. Pediatric profiles: John Howland (1873–1926). *J. Pediatr.* 46: 473, 1955.

Faber, H. K., and McIntosh, R. *History of the Pediatric Society, 1887–1965.* New York: McGraw-Hill, 1966.

Harvey, A. McG. *Adventures in Medical Research: A Century of Discovery at Johns Hopkins,* p. 195. Baltimore: Johns Hopkins University Press, 1976.

Harvey, A. McG. *Interurban Clinical Club,* p. 88.

Park, E. A. John Howland. *Science* 64: 80, 1926.

24. Williams, O. T. In memory of Christian Herter, 1865–1910. *Biochem. J.* 5: xxi, 1911. Delivered at the opening of the medical school of College of Physicians and Surgeons in September 1909.

25. Duffus, R. L., and Holt, L. E., Jr. *L. Emmett Holt: Pioneer of a Children's Century.* New York: D. Appleton-Century, 1940.

26. See Annual Reports. Director of the Hospital of the Rockefeller Institute to Board of Trustees; also, Corner, G. W. *History of the Rockefeller Institute, 1901–1953; Origins and Growth,* p. 129. New York: Rockefeller Institute Press, 1964.

27. Duffus and Holt, *L. Emmett Holt,* p. 112.

28. Harvey, *Interurban Clinical Club:* Kenneth Blackfan, p. 176; Edwards A. Park, p. 173; Grover Powers, p. 188; Oscar Schloss, p. 202.

29. Harrison, H. E. Edwards A. Park: An appreciation of the man. *Johns Hopkins Med. J.* 132: 361, 1973.

Howard, J. E. Edwards A. Park, 1877–1969. *Trans. Assoc. Am. Physicians* 89: 28, 1976.

30. Park, E. A. Kenneth Blackfan, 1883–1941. *Trans. Assoc. Am. Physicians* 57: 7, 1942.

31. Park, E. A. John Howland, 1873–1926. *Science* 64: 80, 1926.

32. Howland, J., and Marriott, W. M. Acidosis occurring with diarrhea. *Am. J. Dis. Child.* 11: 309, 1916.

Howland, J., and Marriott, W. M. A study of acidosis occurring in the nutritional diseases of infancy. *Trans. Assoc. Am. Physicians* 30: 330, 1915, and *Bull. Johns Hopkins Hosp.* 27: 63, 1916.

33. Utheim, K. A study of the blood and its circulation in normal infants and in infants suffering from chronic nutritional disturbances. *Am. J. Dis. Child.* 20: 366, 1920.

34. Blackfan, K., and Maxcy, K. F. Intraperitoneal injection of saline solution. *Am. J. Dis. Child.* 15: 19, 1918.

Gamble, J. L. The early history of fluid replacement therapy. *Pediatrics* 11: 554, 1953.

35. Marriott, W. M., and Howland, J. Use of a new reagent for microcolorimetric analysis, as applied to the determination of calcium and of inorganic phosphates in the blood serum. *J. Biol. Chem.* 32: 233, 1917.

Veeder, B. Pediatric profiles. William McKim Marriott (1885–1936). *J. Pediatr.* 47: 791, 1955.

36. Marriott, W. M., and Haessler, F. H. A micromethod for determination of inorganic phosphates in blood serum. *J. Biol. Chem.* 32: 241, 1917.

37. Marriott, W. M., and Howland, J. The calcium content of blood in rickets and tetany. *Am. J. Obstet.* 74: 541, 1916; also, *Trans. Assoc. Am. Physicians* 30: 102, 1915; and *Trans. Am. Pediatr. Soc.* 28: 202, 1916.

38. Howland, J., and Marriott, W. M. Observations upon the calcium content of the blood in infantile tetany and upon the effect of treatment by calcium. *Q. J. Med.* 11: 289, 1918.

Marriott, W. M., and Howland, J. Observation upon calcium in rickets and tetany. *Trans. Assoc. Am. Physicians* 32: 307, 1917.

Marriott devised other important methods for the study of the blood and its components: The determination of acetone bodies in blood and tissues by micromethods. (Abstract) *Proc. Soc. Biol. Chem.* 14: xxvii, 1912–13. Marriott and Shaffer, P. A. The determination of oxybutyric acid. *J. Biol. Chem.* 16: 265, 1913–14; idem, The determination of acetone. *J. Biol. Chem.* 16: 281, 1913; idem, *J. Biol. Chem.* 16: 289, 1913–14. Marriott, Levy, R. L., and Rowntree, L. G. A simple method for determining variations in the hydrogen-ion concentration of the blood. *Arch. Intern. Med.* 16: 389, 1915; idem, The determination of alveolar $CO_2$ tension by a simple method. *J.A.M.A.* 66: 1594, 1916.

39. Howland, J., and Kramer, B. Calcium and phosphorus in the blood in relation to rickets. *Am. J. Dis. Child.* 22: 105, 1921.

Howard, J., and Kramer, B. Factors concerned in the calcification of bone. *Trans. Am. Pediatr. Soc.* 34: 204, 1922.

Kramer, B., and Howland, J. Factors which determine the concentration of calcium and inorganic phosphorus in the blood of rats. *Bull. Johns Hopkins Hosp.* 33: 313, 1922.

40. Gamble, J. L. Presentation of the Kober Medal to Dr. E. A. Park. *Trans. Assoc. Am. Physicians* 63: 21, 1950.

McCollum, E. V., Simmonds, N., Parsons, H. T., Shipley, P. G., and Park, E. A. Studies on experimental rickets. I. The production of rickets and similar diseases in the rat by deficient diets. *J. Biol. Chem.* 45: 333, 1921.

McCollum, E. V., Simmonds, N., Parsons, H. T., Shipley, P. G., and Park, E. A. II. The effect of cod liver oil administered to rats with experimental rickets. *J. Biol. Chem.* 45: 343, 1921.

McCollum, E. V., Simmonds, N., Parsons, H. T., Shipley, P. G., and Park, E. A. VIII.

The production of rickets by diets low in phosphorus and fat soluble A. *J. Biol. Chem.* 47: 507, 1921; idem, *Am. J. Hygiene* 1: 492, 1921.

McCollum, E. V., Simmonds, N., Parsons, H. T., Shipley, P. G., and Park, E. A. XII. Is there a substance other than fat soluble A associated with certain fats which plays an important role in bone development? *J. Biol. Chem.* 50: 5, 1922.

Park, E. A. Acceptance of the Kober Medal. *Trans. Assoc. Am. Physicians* 63: 26, 1950.

Taussig, H. B. Dr. Edwards A. Park: Physician, teacher, investigator, friend. *Johns Hopkins Med. J.* 132: 370, 1973.

41. Butler, A. M. James Lawder Gamble, 1883–1959. *Trans Assoc. Am. Physicians* 73: 13, 1960.

Janeway, C. A. Pediatric profiles. James Lawder Gamble (1883–1959). *J. Pediatr.* 56: 701, 1960.

42. Butler, A. M. Presentation of the John Howland Medal and Award of the American Pediatric Society to James L. Gamble. *Am. J. Dis. Child.* 90: 483, 1955.

Gamble, J. L. Acceptance of the Kober Medal Award. *Trans. Assoc. Am. Physicians* 64: 36, 1951.

Janeway, Pediatric profiles. James Lawder Gamble, p. 702.

Loeb, R. F. Presentation of the Kober Medal Award to James Lawder Gamble. *Trans. Assoc. Am. Physicians* 64: 29, 1951.

43. Loeb, R. F. James Lawder Gamble (July 18, 1883–May 28, 1959). *Biog. Mem. Natl. Acad. Sci.* 36: 146, 1962. (Contains Gamble's complete bibliography.)

44. Gamble, J. L., Ross, G., and Tisdall, F. F. A study of acidosis due to ketone acids. *Trans. Am. Pediatr. Soc.* 34: 289, 1922.

45. Ibid.

46. Loeb, James Lawder Gamble, p. 152.

47. Gamble, Acceptance of the Kober Medal Award.

Loeb, Presentation of the Kober Medal Award to James Lawder Gamble.

Wallace, W. M. An account of the origins of the investigations of James L. Gamble and an analysis of his contributions to physiology and medicine. *Pediatrics,* 26: 899, 1960.

48. Wallace, W. M. An account of the origins of the investigations of James L. Gamble and an analysis of his contributions to physiology and medicine.

49. Peters, J. P., and Van Slyke, D. D. *Quantitative Clinical Chemistry.* Vol. 1, *Interpretations.* Baltimore: Williams & Wilkins, 1931.

50. Janeway, Pediatric profiles: James Lawder Gamble, p. 704.

51. Gamble, Acceptance of the Kober Medal Award.

52. Carter, E. P. William Sydney Thayer (June 23, 1864–December 10, 1932). *Johns Hopkins Hosp. Bull.* 52: 1, 1933.

Reid, E. A. The Life and Convictions of William Sydney Thayer—Physician. London: Oxford University Press, 1936.

53. Harvey, *Adventures in Medical Research,* p. 139.

Harvey, *Interurban Clinical Club,* pp. 94, 287.

Harvey, J. C. The writings of Louis Hamman. *Johns Hopkins Hosp. Bull.* 101: 13, 1957.

54. Flexner, S. The Thayer Memorial Exercises held in the Hurd Memorial Amphitheater, February 24, 1934. *Johns Hopkins Hosp. Bull.* 55: 201, 1934.

55. Ibid.

56. Thayer, W. S. *Lectures on Malarial Fever.* New York: D. Appleton, 1897.

57. Thayer, W. S. On the early diastolic sound (the so-called third heart sound). *Bost. Med. Surg. J.* 158: 713, 1908; idem, *Arch. Intern. Med.* 4: 297, 1909; idem, *Trans. Assoc. Am. Physicians* 23: 326, 1908, and 24: 81, 1909.

58. Thayer, W. S. On the presence of a venous hum in the epigastrium in cirrhosis of the liver. *Am. J. Med. Sci.* 141: 313, 1911.

59. Thayer, W. S., and MacCallum, W. G. Experimental studies of cardiac murmurs. *Am. J. Med. Sci.* 133: 249, 1907.

60. Thayer, W. S., and Blumer, G. Ulcerating endocarditis due to gonococcus, gonorrheal septicemia. *Bull. Johns Hopkins Hosp.* 3: 57, 1896.

61. Thayer, W. S. The Medical Education of Jones, by Smith. (First published anonymously in the Harvard Graduates' Magazine for March 1927 and again in *Physician and Patient, etc.* Ed. Emerson, L. E. Cambridge, Mass.: Harvard University Press, 1929.)

Thayer, W. S. *Osler and Other Papers,* p. 51. Baltimore: Johns Hopkins Press, 1931.

62. Thayer, W. S. Teaching and practice. *Science* 43: 691, 1916.

63. Selected references from the Department of Medicine, 1917–1922, include:

Atchley, D. W. Studies in the regulation of osmotic pressure. I. Effect of increasing concentrations of gelatin on the conductivity of sodium chloride solution. *J. Gen. Physiol.* 3: 801, 1921.

Atchley, D. W., Loeb, R. F., Palmer, W. W., and Benedict, E. M. On the equilibrium condition between blood serum and serous cavity fluids. *J. Gen. Physiol.* 5: 591, 1922.

Bliss, W. P. A biological study of hemolytic streptococci from throats of patients suffering from scarlet fever: Preliminary report. *Bull. Johns Hopkins Hosp.* 31: 173, 1920.

Bloomfield, A. L. The fate of bacteria introduced into the upper air passage. *Bull. Johns Hopkins Hosp.* 30: 317, 1919.

Bloomfield, A. L., and Harrop, G. A., Jr. Clinical observations on epidemic influenza. *Bull. Johns Hopkins Hosp.* 30: 1, 1919. This was a clinical study based on three hundred cases from the hospital's physicians, nurses, and service staff who were admitted during the epidemic.

Clough, M. C., and Richter, I. M. A study of an autoagglutinin occurring in a human serum. *Bull. Johns Hopkins Hosp.* 29: 86, 1918.

Guthrie, C. G., Marshall, B. C., and Moss, W. L. Experimental inoculation of human throats with avirulent diphtheria bacilli. *Bull. Johns Hopkins Hosp.* 31: 381, 1920.

Hamman, L., and Hirschman, I. I. Studies on blood sugar. *Arch. Intern. Med.* 20: 761, 1917.

Harrop, G. A., Jr. The oxygen consumption of human erythrocytes. *Arch. Intern. Med.* 23: 745, 1919.

Harrop, G. A., Jr. The production of tetany by the intravenous infusion of sodium bicarbonate. *Bull. Johns Hopkins Hosp.* 30: 62, 1919.

Palmer, W. W. Studies of acidosis. XVI. The titration of organic acids in urine. *J. Biol. Chem.* 41: 567, 1920.

64. Andrus, E. C. Edward Perkins Carter. *Trans. Assoc. Am. Physicians* 69: 9, 1956; see also Harvey, *Interurban Clinical Club,* p. 135; and Harvey, *Adventures in Medical Research,* pp. 272–75.

Carter, E. P. A note upon the technique and accuracy of the method of Douglas and Haldane for calculating the dead space in breathing. *J. Exp. Med.* 20: 81, 1914.

Carter, E. P. The effect upon the cold blooded heart of changes in the ionic content of the perfusate. *Am. J. Physiol.* 59: 227, 1921.

Carter, E. P., and Greene, C. H. The electrocardiogram and ventricular preponderance. *Arch. Intern. Med.* 24: 638, 1919.

65. Hastings, A. B. Francis Raymond Dieuaide, 1892–1977. *Trans. Assoc. Am. Physicians* 91: 25, 1978.

66. Henderson, L. J., and Palmer, W. W. On the intensity of urinary acidity in normal and pathological conditions. *J. Biol. Chem.* 13: 393, 1912–13.

Loeb, R. F. Walter Walker Palmer (1882–1950). *Dict. Am. Biog.* (suppl. 4): 642, 1946–50; idem, Atchley, D. W. *Trans. Assoc. Am. Physicians* 64: 19, 1951.

Palmer, W. W., and Henderson, L. J. Clinical studies on acid base equilibrium and the nature of acidosis. *Arch. Intern. Med.* 12: 153, 1913.

Palmer, W. W., and Jackson, H., Jr. A modification of Folin's uric acid method. *Proc. Soc. Exp. Biol. Med.* 18: 126, 1920–21.

Palmer, W. W., and Ladd, W. S. The carbohydrate-fat ratio in relation to the production of ketone bodies in diabetes mellitus. *Proc. Soc. Exp. Biol. Med.* 18: 109, 1920–21.

Palmer, W. W., Salvesen, H., and Jackson, H., Jr. Relationship between the plasma bicarbonate and urinary acidity following the administration of sodium bicarbonates. *J. Biol. Chem.* 45: 101, 1920–21.

67. See Bloomfield, A. L. *A Bibliography of Internal Medicine: Communicable Diseases,* pp. 117–25. Chicago: University of Chicago Press, 1958.

68. Baetjer, Paul W. Clough.

69. Levine, S. A., and Ladd, W. S. Pernicious anemia. A clinical study of 150 consecutive cases with special reference to gastric anacidity. *Bull. Johns Hopkins Hosp.* 32: 254, 1921.

70. Atchley, D. W. Walter Walker Palmer. *Trans. Assoc. Am. Physicians* 64: 19, 1951.

Burwell, C. S. Hugh Jackson Morgan. *Trans. Assoc. Am. Physicians* 75: 33, 1962.

Castle, W. B. Henry Jackson, Jr., 1892–1968. *Trans. Assoc. Am. Physicians* 82: 37, 1969.

Chesney, A. M. George Argale Harrop, Jr. *Trans. Assoc. Am. Physicians* 59: 21, 1946.

King, J. T. Henry M. Thomas, Jr., 1891–1966. *Trans. Assoc. Am. Physicians* 80: 27, 1967.

Kneeland, Y., Jr. Alphonse R. Dochez, 1882–1964. *Trans. Assoc. Am. Physicians* 78: 21, 1965.

Ragan, C. A., Jr. Robert Frederick Loeb, 1895–1973. *Trans. Assoc. Am. Physicians* 87: 29, 1974.

Rantz, L. Arthur Leonard Bloomfield. *Trans. Assoc. Am. Physicians* 76: 12, 1963.

71. Brem, T. H. Verne Rheem Mason. *Trans. Assoc. Am. Physicians* 79: 62, 1966. Mason graduated from the Johns Hopkins University School of Medicine in 1915 and remained on the staff for the next six years as an intern, assistant resident, resident, and instructor in medicine. In 1921 he returned to the Los Angeles County Hospital, where, for the next twelve years, he had a major role in the instruction of the resident staff. When the University of Southern California School of Medicine was opened in 1930, he was named professor of clinical medicine and contributed in many ways to the development of that school.

The name *sickle cell anemia* was first coined by Mason (Sickle cell anemia. *J.A.M.A.* 79: 1318, 1922). His was apparently the fourth case of this disease to be described. In his discussion, Mason pointed out a number of facts that indicated that a sickle cell anemia was an hereditary or congenital anomaly.

72. The Reminiscences of Dana Atchley.

73. Robinson, G. C. *Adventures in Medical Education.* Cambridge, Mass.: Harvard University Press, 1967.

74. Bloomfield, A. L. The dissemination of bacteria in the upper air passages to the circulation of bacteria in the mouth. *Bull. Johns Hopkins Hosp.* 33: 145, 1922.

Bloomfield, A. L. The mechanisms of elimination of bacteria from the respiratory tract. *Am. J. Med. Sci.* 164: 854, 1922.

Bloomfield, A. L., and Felty, A. R. On the dissemination of hemolytic streptococci among a group of healthy people. *Bull. Johns Hopkins Hosp.* 34: 414, 1923.

75. Guthrie, C. G., and Huck, J. G. On the existence of more than four isoagglutinin groups in human blood. Part III. *Bull. Johns Hopkins Hosp.* 34: 128, 1923.

76. Huck, J. G. Sickle cell anemia. *Bull: Johns Hopkins Hosp.* 34: 335, 1923.

77. Barondess, J. A. Harold J. Stewart, 1896–1975. *Trans. Assoc. Am. Physicians* 89: 32, 1976.

78. Youmans, J. B., and Kolls, A. C. Quantitative studies with arsphenamine. II. Distribution and excretion after intravenous injection. *Bull. Johns Hopkins Hosp.* 34: 181, 1923.

79. The syphilis clinic was organized in 1914 by George Walker. After a few years, Albert Keidel became the principal architect in this fruitful program of clinical investigation; he was succeeded by Joseph Earle Moore. After the advent of penicillin, the unique epidemiological and other study techniques that had been developed were applied to the investigation of a variety of chronic diseases. In 1955, the clinic became the focal point of the medical genetics program under Victor McKusick. It was the first outpatient clinical research facility supported by the National Institutes of Health and is still a successful outpatient research clinic, after seventy-five years of productive work. (Harvey, A. McG. Clinical investigation of chronic diseases: Its successful pursuit in an outpatient setting. *J. Chronic Dis.* 33: 529, 1980.)

Chesney, A. M. Immunity in syphilis. *Medicine* 5: 375, 1926. Chesney's summary of the whole question of immunity in syphilis.

Chesney, A. M. Joseph Earle Moore, 1892–1957. *Trans. Assoc. Am. Physicians* 71: 31, 1958.

Moore, J. E. *The Modern Treatment of Syphilis,* p. 535. Springfield, Ill.: Charles C Thomas, 1933.

Turner, T. B. Alan Mason Chesney, 1888–1964. *Trans Assoc. Am. Physicians* 78: 17, 1965.

80. Eppinger, E. C. C. Sidney Burwell, 1893–1967. *Trans. Assoc. Am. Physicians* 81: 9, 1968.

81. McCann, W. S. Unpublished memoirs. MS. Library. University of Rochester School of Medicine.

Young, L. E. William Sharp McCann, 1889–1971. *Trans. Assoc. Am. Physicians* 85: 35, 1972.

82. Hannon, R. R., and McCann, W. S. A graphic method for the calculation of diabetic diets in the proper ketogenic-antiketogenic ratio. *Bull. Johns Hopkins Hosp.* 33: 128, 1922.

Hannon, R. R., McCann, W. S., and Dodd, K. Studies of diabetes mellitus. III. The use of pancreatic extract insulin in the treatment of diabetes. *Bull. Johns Hopkins Hosp.* 34: 205, 1923.

Hannon, R. R., McCann, W. S., Robinson, G. C., and Perlzweig, W. A. Behavior of certain phosphorus compounds in normal and diabetic metabolism. *J.A.M.A.* 78: 1753, 1922.

83. Bordley, J., III. Warfield Theobald Longcope, 1877–1953. *Trans. Assoc. Am. Physicians* 66: 9, 1953.

Harvey, *Interurban Clinical Club,* p. 42.

84. Tillett, W. S. Warfield Theobald Longcope (March 29, 1877–April 25, 1953). *Biog. Mem. Natl. Acad. Sci.* 33: 205, 1959. (Contains Longcope's complete bibliography.)

85. W. T. Longcope. The pathogenesis of glomerular nephritis. *Johns Hopkins Hosp. Bull.* 45: 335, 1929. Longcope developed the view that hypersensitivity to streptococcal products was part of the mechanism by which glomerular nephritis was produced; when streptococci were later shown to fall into antigenically different groups, it was found that certain types predominated in the infections that were followed by nephritis. This was convincingly demonstrated by C. A. Stetson, C. H. Rammelkamp, Jr., R. M. Krause, R. J. Kohen, and W. D. Perry (Epidemic acute nephritis: Studies on etiology, natural history and prevention. *Medicine* 34: 431, 1955), who showed that, during convalescence, acute nephritis occurred from Type 12 pharyngitis, but in no one convalescent from other types such as Types 3, 6 and 19. Certain strains are "nephritogenic."

86. Longcope, W. T., and Winkenwerder, W. L. Clinical features of the contracted kidney due to pyelonephritis. *Johns Hopkins Hosp. Bull.* 53: 255, 1933.

87. Longcope, W. T., and Pierson, J. W. Boeck's sarcoid (sarcoidosis). *Johns Hopkins Hosp. Bull.* 60: 223, 1937.

88. Longcope, W. T. Bronchopneumonia of unknown etiology (variety X): A report of thirty-two cases with two deaths. *Johns Hopkins Hosp. Bull.* 67: 268, 1940.

89. Richter, I., and Clough, M. A study of an autoagglutinin occurring in a human serum. *Bull. Johns Hopkins Hosp.* 29: 86, 1918.

90. Longcope, W. T. Acceptance of the Kober Medal. *Trans. Assoc. Am. Physicians* 61: 25, 1948.

91. Harvey, *Adventures in Medical Research,* p. 158.

Harvey, *Interurban Clinical Club,* p. 42.

Mackenzie, G. M. Presentation of the Kober Medal to Dr. Warfield T. Longcope. *Trans. Assoc. Am. Physicians* 61: 22, 1948.

92. Longcope, W. T. *Methods and Problems in Medical Education,* 11th series, p. 67. New York: Rockefeller Foundation, 1928.

93. Harvey, A. McG. Tuberculosis: The study of a specific disease at Johns Hopkins. *Johns Hopkins Med. J.* 141: 198, 1977.

94. Longcope, *Methods and Problems in Medical Education,* p. 67.

Longcope, W. T. Description of the Osler clinic; its organization. *Johns Hopkins Hosp. Bull.* 52: 255, 1933.

95. McCann, in his unpublished memoirs, made an interesting comment about the composition of the faculty:

At the end of the first World War the great medical centers in Germany lay prostrate. The English situation was not much better, in view of the tremendous toll the war had taken of her best young men, and the terrific cost of the struggle to her economy. The United States stood on the threshold of its great post-war development. Its medical household had been put in order; first by the Flexner report of 1910, which had weeded out the inferior half of its 160 medical schools. The remaining 80 were ready for development into true university centers.

British and European physicians and scientists began to appear in our midst in Baltimore. Leonore Michaelis of Kiel found a temporary place in our Chemical Division [at Johns Hopkins] during my last six months. This distinguished physical chemist and authority on the hydrogen ion had been an "ausserordentlich" professor at Kiel, which meant that he received little or no financial support from the university, so that he was obliged to earn his daily bread by his services as bacteriologist to a hospital nearby. From Michaelis I learned the story of the development of his career, which is illustrative of the way in which German scholars developed. He had originally gone to study under Ehrlich, who had assigned him a problem to work on. He soon found that he would need to learn physical chemistry before he could carry out the assignment. On delving into physical chemistry he soon found that he must first master higher mathematics. He set about this himself, and as he progressed he wrote a little book entitled *Einfuhrung in die Mathematik,* which records his progress as a pilgrim in the field of mathematics. Prepared in this way he went on with physical chemistry and became an authority on the measurement of the hydrogen ion concentration, using the bacteriology he learned from Ehrlich as a means of livelihood.

96. Chang, H. C., and Harrop, G. A., Jr. The determination of the circulating blood volume with carbon monoxide. *J. Clin. Invest.* 4: 393, 1927–28.

Harrop, G. A., Jr., and Barron, E. S. G. The excretion of intravenously injected bilirubin as a test of liver function. *J. Clin. Invest.* 9: 577, 1931.

Harrop, G. A., Jr., and Heath, E. H. (with the technical assistance of B. M. Schaub). Pulmonary gas diffusion in polycythemia vera. *J. Clin. Invest.* 4:. 53, 1927.

Harrop, G. A., Jr., Soffer, L. J., Ellsworth, R., and Trescher, J. H. Studies on the suprarenal cortex. III. Plasma electrolytes and electrolyte excretion during suprarenal insufficiency in the dog. *J. Exp. Med.* 58: 17, 1933.

Harrop, G. A., Jr., Soffer, L. J., Nicholson, W. M., and Strauss, M. IV. The effect of sodium salts in sustaining the suprarenalectomized dog. *J. Exp. Med.* 61: 839, 1935. In this study, the authors undertook the problem of "whether this regulation of salt and water is the primary function of the cortical hormone . . . or, whether there are other physiological derangements produced by removal of the suprarenal glands in the dog." On the basis of a study of adrenalectomized dogs, which were kept in apparently good health up to five or six months, by the administration of sodium chloride and bicarbonate alone, Harrop was inclined to the former view, as were many investigators at the time. In another paper, Harrop, Nicholson, and Strauss (V. The influence of the cortical hormone upon the excretion of water and electrolytes in the suprarenalectomized dog. *J. Exp. Med.* 64: 233, 1936) studied the effect of cortical extracts upon the electrolyte balance in dogs, showing again that administration of extract promoted sodium retention and potassium excretion and that the reverse changes took place when the extract was withheld. Pursuing this phase of the subject, Harrop (The influence of the adrenal cortex upon the distribution of body water. *Johns Hopkins Hosp. Bull.* 59: 11, 1936) concluded that "an actual shrinkage of interstitial fluid volume occurs during insufficiency, and that this volume is restored as a result of reinjection of the hormone"; and, finally, Harrop showed (The salt and water hormone of the adrenal cortex. *Johns Hopkins Hosp. Bull.* 59: 25, 1936) that "the adrenalectomized animal in the absence of the salt and water hormone is peculiarly sensitive to the proportions of ingested potassium and sodium salts; increased amounts of one tend to drive out the other."

97. Albright, F., and Ellsworth, R. Studies on the physiology of the parathyroid glands.

I. Calcium and phosphorus studies on a case of idiopathic hypoparathyroidism. *J. Clin. Invest.* 7: 183, 1929. Albright and Ellsworth suggested that the fundamental difficulty in parathyroid tetany is an inability to excrete phosphorus, which is corrected by parathyroid extract, and that the changes in calcium are secondary to this.

Ellsworth (Observations upon a case of postoperative hypoparathyroidism. *Johns Hopkins Hosp. Bull.* 52: 131, 1933) also reported similar careful studies on a case of postoperative hypoparathyroidism.

Ellsworth, R. Secondary alterations in total serum calcium after the administration of glucose and insulin. *J. Clin. Invest.* 8: 139, 1929–30.

Ellsworth, R., and Howard, J. E. Studies on the physiology of the parathyroid glands. VII. Some responses of normal human kidneys and blood to intravenous parathyroid extract. *Johns Hopkins Hosp. Bull.* 55: 296, 1934.

98. Howard, J. E., and Barker, W. H. Paroxysmal hypertension and other clinical manifestations associated with benign chromaffin cell tumors (pheochromocytoma). *Johns Hopkins Hosp. Bull.* 61: 371, 1937.

99. Harvey, *Adventures in Medical Research,* pp. 331, 355.

Howard, J. E. Adventures in clinical research on bones and stones. *J. Clin. Endocrinol. Metab.* 21: 1254, 1961.

Howard, J. E. The recognition and isolation from urine and serum of a peptide inhibitor to calcification. *Johns Hopkins Med. J.* 120: 119, 1967.

Howard, J. E. Serendipity in clinical investigation. (On the occasion of the presentation of the Passano Award, June 17, 1965.) *J.A.M.A.* 207: 38, 1969.

Howard, J. E. Hypertension due to ischemia of one kidney: A survey of twenty years experience. *Yale J. Biol. Med.* 41: 363, 1969.

Howard, J. E., Berthrong, M., Sloan, R. D., and Yendt, E. R. Relief of hypertension by nephrectomy in four patients with unilateral renal vascular disease. *Trans. Assoc. Am. Physicians* 66: 164, 1953.

Howard, J. E., and Cary, R. A. Potassium as a therapeutic agent. *Trans. Am. Clin. Climatol. Assoc.* 61: 145, 1948.

Howard, J. E., Duncan, L. E., Jr., and Meyer, R. J. Cellular needs and capability during various types of starvation. *Trans. Conf. Metab. Aspects of Convalescence.* Seventeenth meeting, sponsored by the Josiah Macy, Jr., Foundation. New York, March 20–30, 1938.

100. Osler, W. Six cases of Addison's disease with the report of a case greatly benefited by the use of suprarenal extract. *Intern. Med. Mag.* 5: 3, 1896.

101. Harrop, G. A., Jr., and Thorn, G. W. The influence of sex hormones on salt and water metabolism. *Trans. Assoc. Am. Physicians* 52: 164, 1937.

Thorn, G. W., Nelson, K., and Thorn, D. W. A study of the mechanism of edema associated with menstruation. *Endocrinology* 22: 155, 1938.

102. Thorn, G. W., Engel, L. L., and Eisenberg, H. The effect of corticosterone and related compounds on the renal excretion of electrolytes. *J. Exp. Med.* 68: 161, 1938.

Thorn, G. W., Koepf, G. F., Lewis, R. A., and Olsen, E. T. Carbohydrate metabolism in Addison's disease. *J. Clin. Invest.* 19: 813, 1940.

103. Harvey, *Adventures in Medical Research,* p. 347.

104. Cahill, G. F., Jr. Presentation of the George M. Kober Medal to George W. Thorn. *Trans. Assoc. Am. Physicians* 89: 39, 1976.

Thorn, G. W. Acceptance of the George M. Kober Medal for 1976. *Trans. Assoc. Am. Physicians* 89: 50, 1976.

105. Andrus, E. C., and Carter, E. P. Q-T interval in human electrocardiogram in absence of cardiac disease. *J.A.M.A.* 27: 1921, 1922.

Andrus, E. C., and Carter, E. P. The genesis of normal and abnormal cardiac rhythm. *Science* 58: 376, 1923.

Andrus, E. C., and Carter, E. P. The mechanism of the action of the hydrogen ion upon the cardiac rhythm. *J. Clin. Invest.* 3: 555, 1926–27.

Harvey, *Adventures in Medical Research,* p. 277.

Harvey, *Interurban Clinical Club,* p. 208.

Hill, W. H. P., and Andrus, E. C. Effects of renin and of angiotonin upon the isolated perfused heart. *Proc. Soc. Exp. Biol. Med.* 44: 213, 1940.

Ross, R. S. E. Cowles Andrus, 1896–1978. *Trans. Assoc. Am. Physicians* 91: 10, 1978.

Wilcox, H. B., Jr., and Andrus, E. C. The effects of anaphylaxis and of histamine upon the coronary arteries in the isolated heart. *J. Exp. Med.* 67: 169, 1938.

106. Harvey, *Adventures in Medical Research*, p. 272.

107. Lewis, J. K., and McEachern, D. Persistence of an accelerated rate in the isolated hearts and isolated auricles of thyrotoxic rabbits: response to iodides, thyroxine and epinephrine. *Johns Hopkins Hosp. Bull.* 48: 228, 1931.

McEachern, D., and Rake, G. Experimental hyperthyroidism and its effect upon the myocardium in guinea pigs and rabbits. *J. Exp. Med.* 54: 23, 1931.

108. Baker, B. M. The effect of cardiac rate and inhalation of oxygen on transient bundle branch block. *Arch. Intern. Med.* 45: 814, 1930.

Baker, B. M., Thomas, C. B., and Penick, R. M., Jr. Experimental carditis. Changes in the myocardium and pericardium of rabbits sensitized to streptococci. *J. Clin. Invest.* 14: 465, 1935.

Thomas, C. B., and France, R. A preliminary report of a prophylactic use of sulfanilamide in patients susceptible to rheumatic fever. *Johns Hopkins Hosp. Bull.* 64: 67, 1939.

109. Harvey, *Adventures in Medical Research*, p. 288. (For references see p. 441.)

Watson, C. J. Presentation of the George M. Kober Medal to Maxwell M. Wintrobe. *Trans. Assoc. Am. Physicians* 87: 45, 1974.

Wintrobe, M. M. Diseases of the blood (with J. H. Musser). *Tice Practice of Medicine* 6: 739, 1931.

Wintrobe, M. M. Macroscopic examination of the blood. Discussion of its value and description of the use of a single instrument for the determination of sedimentation rate, volume of packed red cells, leukocytes and platelets and of icterus index. *Am. J. Med. Sci.* 185: 58, 1933.

Wintrobe, M. M. Relations of variations in mean corpuscular volume to number of reticulocytes in pernicious anemia. *J. Clin. Invest.* 13: 669, 1934.

Wintrobe, M. M. Anemia: Classification and treatment on the basis of differences in the average volume and hemoglobin content of the red corpuscles. *Arch. Intern. Med.* 54: 256, 1934.

Wintrobe, M. M. Acceptance of the Kober Medal for 1974. *Trans. Assoc. Am. Physicians* 87: 58, 1974.

Wintrobe, M. M., and Buell, M. V. Hyperproteinemia associated with multiple myeloma with report of a case in which an extraordinary hyperproteinemia was associated with thrombosis of the retinal veins and symptoms suggesting Raynaud's disease. *Johns Hopkins Hosp. Bull.* 52: 156, 1933.

Wintrobe, M. M., and Shumacker, H. B., Jr. Comparisons of hematopoiesis in the fetus and during recovery during pernicious anemia (together with a consideration of the relationship of fetal hematopoiesis to macrocytic anemia of pregnancy and anemia in infants). *J. Clin. Invest.* 14: 837, 1935.

110. Bloomfield, A. L., and Felty, A. R. Quantitative factors in "test-tube infection." *J. Exp. Med.* 39: 367, 1924.

Bloomfield, A. L., and Felty, A. R. The relation of dose of bacteria to group infection. *J. Exp. Med.* 40: 679, 1924.

Bloomfield, A. L., and Keefer, C. S. The rate of gastric secretion in man. *J. Clin. Invest.* 4: 485, 1927.

111. Harvey, Tuberculosis: The study of a specific disease at Johns Hopkins.

Krause, A. K. The dissemination of tubercle bacilli in the immune guinea pig, with a discussion of the probable factors involved in tuberculo-immunity. *Am. Rev. Tuberc.* 14: 211, 1926.

During the early decades of the twentieth century, an immense amount of work was done on the problem of immunity to tuberculosis. Krause dominated this field in America.

He sustained the thesis that the allergic reaction associated with reinfection fixed bacilli at their portal of entry and largely prevented invasion and spread. This he considered the essence of immunity, and, in his conclusions to this paper, he said: "It is believed more probable that, upon being re-infected, the tissues of the immune guinea pig react promptly with some process that serves to impede the further passage of bacilli. It is submitted that this process is the allergic exudative or inflammatory reaction which invariably sets in upon re-infection of the tuberculous immune guinea pig which is otherwise normal." Innumerable papers by Krause and his associates dealing with this subject are to be found in the *American Review of Tuberculosis* from 1918 to 1928.

Krause dominated tuberculosis research in America for a good many years, and his views were widely accepted. The objective quality of his experiments leaves them unimpaired, although his main thesis, first questioned by Arnold Rich, has been weakened.

112. Amoss, H. L., and Poston, M. A. Cultivation of Brucella from the stools and bile. *J.A.M.A.* 95: 482, 1930.

Morgan, H. J. H. L. Amoss, 1886–1956. *Trans. Assoc. Am. Physicians* 70: 9, 1957.

113. Garner, R. L., and Tillett, W. S. Biochemical studies on the fibrinolytic activity of hemolytic streptococci. I. Isolation and characterization of fibrinolysin; II. Nature of the reaction. *J. Exp. Med.* 60: 239, 1934.

Harvey, *Interurban Clinical Club,* p. 201.

Sherry, S. William Smith Tillett, 1892–1974. *Trans. Assoc. Am. Physicians* 88: 32, 1975.

Tillett, W. S. The bactericidal action of human serum on hemolytic streptococci. II. Factors which influence the phenomenon in vitro. *J. Exp. Med.* 65: 163, 1937.

Tillett, W. S., Edwards, L. B., and Garner, R. L. Fibrinolytic activity of hemolytic streptococci. The development of resistance to fibrinolysis following acute hemolytic streptococcus infections. *J. Clin. Invest.* 13: 47, 1934.

114. Long, P. H. *The Clinical and Experimental Use of Sulfanilamide, Sulfapyridine and Allied Compounds.* New York: Macmillan, 1939.

Long, P. H., Bliss, E. A., and Carpenter, H. Etiology of influenza. *J.A.M.A.* 97: 1122, 1931.

Long, P. H., Bliss, E. A., and Carpenter, H. Studies upon the nasal secretions. I. The cellular content of the nasal secretions in acute disease of the respiratory tract. *J. Clin. Invest.* 12: 1127, 1933.

Long, P. H., and Doull, J. A. Etiology of acute upper respiratory infections (common cold). *Proc. Soc. Exp. Biol. Med.* 28: 53, 1930.

Rich, A. R., Long, P. H., Brown, J. H., Bliss, E. A., and Holt, L. E., Jr. Experiments upon the cause of whooping cough. *Science* 76: 330, 1932.

115. Tillett, W. S. Perrin Hamilton Long, 1889–1966. *Trans. Assoc. Am. Physicians* 79: 59, 1966.

116. Harvey, *Adventures in Medical Research,* p. 390. (See p. 447 for references to the work of Long and Bliss and for biographical sketches.)

117. Harvey, *Interurban Clinical Club,* p. 254.

Harvey, *Adventures in Medical Research,* p. 168.

Keefer worked closely with Resnik, who was an assistant in medicine from 1923 to 1925. In addition to important papers on the pathogenesis of jaundice in pulmonary infarction, they published a classical paper on the pathogenesis of angina pectoris, in which they advanced the theory that it was due to anoxemia of the heart.

Keefer, C. S. Report of a case of Malta fever originating in Baltimore, Maryland. *Johns Hopkins Hosp. Bull.* 35: 6, 1924. Keefer reported the first case of "a disease in man corresponding to Malta fever due to an organism belonging to the abortus group." Keefer's patient, a laboratory worker, ran a typical undulating fever. Over a period of three and one-half months, there were thirteen positive blood cultures for Brucella. The infection was probably due to cow's milk, and, by appropriate serologic tests, Keefer showed that the organism was of the abortus type.

Keefer, C. S., and Resnik, W. H. Angina pectoris; a syndrome caused by anoxemia of the myocardium. *Arch. Intern. Med.* 41: 769, 1928.

Resnik, W. H. Observations on the effect of anoxemia on the heart. II. Intraventricular conduction. *J. Clin. Invest.* 2: 117, 1925.

Resnik, W. H., and Keefer, C. L. Jaundice following pulmonary infarction in patients with myocardial insufficiency. II. An experimental study. *J. Clin. Invest.* 2: 389, 1925–26.

Wilkins, R. W. Chester Scott Keefer, 1897–1972. *Trans. Assoc. Am. Physicians* 85: 24, 1972.

118. Bordley, J. Reactions following transfusion of blood with urinary suppression and uremia. *Arch. Intern. Med.* 47: 288, 1931.

Chesney, A. M., Clawson, T. A., and Webster, B. Endocrine goitre in rabbits. I. Incidence and characteristics. *Johns Hopkins Hosp. Bull.* 43: 261, 1928.

Eagle, H. Studies in the serology of syphilis. III. Explanation of the fortifying effect of cholesterin upon the antigen as used in the Wassermann and flocculation test. *J. Exp. Med.* 52: 747, 1930.

Eagle, H., Arbesman, C. E., and Winkenwerder, W. The production in experimental animals of antibodies to short ragweed pollen. *J. Immunol.* 36: 425, 1939.

Eichna, L. W., and Bordley, J. Capillary blood pressure in man. Comparison of direct and indirect methods of measurement. *J. Clin. Invest.* 18: 695, 1939.

Harvey, A. M., and Masland, R. L. A method for the study of neuromuscular transmission in human subjects. *Johns Hopkins Hosp. Bull.* 68: 81, 1941.

Harvey, A. M., and Masland, R. L. The electromyogram in myasthenia gravis. *Johns Hopkins Hosp. Bull.* 69: 1, 1941.

Harvey, A. M., and Whitehill, M. R. Prostigmin as an aid in the diagnosis of myasthenia gravis. *J.A.M.A.* 108: 1329, 1937.

# Chapter 9

1. Lamb, A. R. *The Presbyterian Hospital and the Columbia Presbyterian Medical Center, 1868–1943.* New York: Columbia University Press, 1955.

2. Harvey, A. McG. *The Interurban Clinical Club, 1905–1976. A Record of Achievement in Clinical Science,* p. 24. Philadelphia: W. B. Saunders, 1978.

Shrady, J., ed. *The College of Physicians and Surgeons of New York.* 2 volumes. p. 426. New York and Chicago: Lewis, n.d.

3. Harvey, *Interurban Clinical Club,* p. 28.

4. Barker, L. F. Theodore Caldwell Janeway. *Science* 47: 273, 1918.

Flaxman, N. Janeway on hypertension. Theodore Caldwell Janeway (1872–1917). *Bull. Hist. Med.* 9: 505, 1941.

Harvey, *Interurban Clinical Club,* p. 30.

Mosenthal, H. O. Theodore Caldwell Janeway, A.M., M.D. *Johns Hopkins Alumni Mag.* 6: 264, 1918.

5. The annual reports of the dean give a picture of the development of the school and hospital from 1912 to 1917. Columbia University, College of Physicians and Surgeons. Report of the Dean for the Academic Years 1912–1917.

In his report for 1913, the dean noted that there were new laboratories for the medical clinic. In these laboratories, not only was the routine work of the hospital's medical service carried on but, in addition, research work on clinical cases in the hospital wards was done. (Reprints of the papers stemming from this work are in the Department of Medicine at Columbia University College of Physicians and Surgeons. They are bound together as volume one of department reprints for 1914–21.)

In the report of 1914 it was noted that, at Presbyterian Hospital, both the medical and surgical divisions were placed under the single control of the heads of those departments in the school. The organization of the personnel of each clinic was placed on a "university basis." Each clinic was a thoroughly equipped hospital unit and had clinical record rooms, a teaching laboratory, a departmental library, research laboratories, teaching lecture rooms, and an intimate connection—through mutual assistants—with the pathological department. The alliance between Presbyterian Hospital and Columbia University was an attempt to solve one of the most important problems in medical education confronting the medical schools of the United States at that time. (College of Physicians and Surgeons. Report of the dean for the academic year ending June 30, 1913.)

6. Perera, G. A. Herman Otto Mosenthal, 1878–1954. *Trans. Assoc. Am. Physicians* 68: 15, 1955.

7. Janeway, T. C., and Mosenthal, H. O. An unusual paroxysmal syndrome, probably allied to recurrent vomiting, with a study of the nitrogen metabolism. *Trans. Assoc. Am. Physicians* 23: 504, 1908.

8. Howland, J., and Richards, A. N. Some possible etiological factors in the recurrent vomiting of children. *Arch. Pediatr.* 24: 401, 1907.

9. Bordley, J., III. Warfield Theobald Longcope, 1877–1953. *Trans. Assoc. Am. Physicians* 66: 9, 1953.

Harvey, A. McG. Classical descriptions of disease. *Johns Hopkins Med. J.* 136: 254, 1975.

Harvey, *Interurban Clinical Club*, p. 42.

Longcope, W. T. Acceptance of the Kober Medal Award. *Trans. Assoc. Am. Physicians* 61: 25, 1948.

Mackenzie, G. M. Presentation of the George M. Kober Medal to Dr. Warfield T. Longcope. *Trans. Assoc. Am. Physicians* 61: 22, 1948.

Tillett, W. S. Warfield Theobald Longcope (March 29, 1877–April 25, 1953). *Biog. Mem. Natl. Acad. Sci.* 33: 205, 1959. (Contains Longcope's complete bibliography.)

10. Levy, R. L. Theodore Stuart Hart, 1869–1951. *Trans. Assoc. Am. Physicians* 64: 10, 1951.

11. Dochez, A. R. Homer Fordyce Swift, 1881–1953. *Trans. Assoc. Am. Physicians* 67: 25, 1954.

12. Geyelin, H. R. A clinical study of amylase in the urine. *Arch. Intern. Med.* 13: 96, 1914.

Geyelin, H. R. The significance of glycosuria. *Med. Clin. North Am.* 4: 1375, 1920–21.

Geyelin, H. R., and DuBois, E. F. A case of diabetes of maximum severity with marked improvement. *J.A.M.A.* 66: 1532, 1916.

Peters, J. P. and Geyelin, H. R. The relation of adrenalin hyperglycemia to decreased alkali reserve of the blood. *J. Biol. Chem.* 31: 471, 1917.

13. Rhoads, C. P. Francis Carter Wood, 1869–1951. *Trans. Assoc. Am. Physicians* 64: 27, 1951.

14. Harvey, *Interurban Clinical Club*, p. 29.

15. Ibid., p. 24.

16. Brill, N. E. An acute infectious disease of unknown origin. *Am. J. Med. Sci.* 139: 484, 1910.

Strong, R. P. Nathan Brill. *Trans. Assoc. Am. Physicians* 41: 5, 1926.

17. Baehr, G. Emanuel Libman, 1872–1946. *Trans. Assoc. Am. Physicians* 60: 7, 1947. (For further details of his work, see p. 115.)

18. Amberson, J. B. James Alexander Miller. *Dict. Am. Biog.* (suppl. 4): 577, 1946–50; idem, *Trans. Assoc. Am. Physicians* 62: 9, 1949.

19. Harvey, *Interurban Clinical Club*, p. 25.

20. Ibid., pp. 91, 398.

21. Ibid., pp. 197, 228.

22. Stewart, H. J. Harold Ensign Bennett Pardee, 1886–1973. *Trans. Assoc. Am. Physicians* 87: 34, 1974.

23. Gutman, A. B. Bernard Sutro Oppenheimer, 1876–1958. *Trans. Assoc. Am. Physicians* 72: 31, 1959.

24. Bordley, J., III. George Miner Mackenzie. *Trans. Assoc. Am. Physicians* 65: 26, 1952.

Harvey, *Interurban Clinical Club*, p. 74.

Mackenzie, G. M. The relation of antibody to the rate of disappearance of circulating antigen. *J. Exp. Med.* 37: 491, 1923.

Mackenzie, G. M. The significance of anaphylaxis in pneumococcus immunity. *J. Exp. Med.* 41: 53, 1925.

Mackenzie, G. M., and Leake, W. H. Relation of antibody and antigen to serum disease susceptibility. *J. Exp. Med.* 33: 601, 1921.

Mackenzie, G. M., and Woo, S. T. The production and significance of cutaneous allergy to pneumococcus protein. *J. Exp. Med.* 41: 65, 1925.

25. Frawley, T. F. Ralph A. Kinsella, Sr., 1886–1966. *Trans. Assoc. Am. Physicians* 80: 13, 1967.

26. Atchley, D. W., Loeb, R. F., Benedict, E. M., and Palmer, W. W. Physical and chemical studies of the human blood serum. III. A study of miscellaneous disease conditions. *Arch. Intern. Med.* 31: 616, 1923.

Loeb, R. F. Walter Walker Palmer, 1882–1950. *Dict. Am. Biog.* (suppl. 4): 642, 1946–50; idem, Atchley, D. W. *Trans. Assoc. Am. Physicians* 64: 19, 1951.

Palmer, W. W. The Department of Medicine, 1921–1947. Columbia Presbyterian Medical Center, New York. The fourth of a series of reports for friends of the hospital. Separately printed.

Palmer, W. W., Carson, D. A., and Sloan, L. W. The influence of iodine on the excretion of creatine in exophthalmic goiter. *J. Clin. Invest.* 6: 597, 1928–29.

27. Avery, O. T. Presentation of the Kober Medal to Dr. Alphonse R. Dochez. *Trans. Assoc. Am. Physicians* 62: 24, 1949.

Dochez, A. R. Acceptance of the Kober Medal Award. *Trans. Assoc. Am. Physicians* 62: 30, 1949.

Kneeland, Y., Jr. Alphonse Raymond Dochez, 1882–1964. *Trans. Assoc. Am. Physicians* 78: 21, 1965.

28. Chesney, A. M. George Argale Harrop, Jr., 1890–1945. *Trans. Assoc. Am. Physicians* 59: 21, 1946.

29. Harvey, *Interurban Clinical Club,* pp. 198, 288.

30. Hunter, T. H. Alvin Frederick Coburn, 1899–1975. *Trans. Assoc. Am. Physicians* 90: 30, 1977.

31. Ragan, C. A., Jr. David Seegal, 1899–1972. *Trans. Assoc. Am. Physicians* 86: 42, 1973.

32. W. W. Palmer and Henry D. Dakin, an English-born chemist of "chloramine T" and Dakin pad fame, had collaborated in a study of thyroid function. Palmer was determined, partly as a result of Dakin's influence and accomplishments, to have a chemist in his newly expanded department. He succeeded in obtaining $500,000 for that purpose from Edward Harkness. Palmer chose Heidelberger, whom he had known when he worked with Van Slyke at the HRI. Heidelberger produced a classical work on the estimation of antibodies in units of weight as a prerequisite to determining their nature. He also collaborated with Palmer on a study of thyroglobulin; with Dochez on fractionation of the antigens of hemolytic streptococci; and with a variety of other colleagues who needed help in overcoming unforeseen difficulties of one type or another in their investigations. (Heidelberger, M. A "pure" organic chemist's downward path. *Ann. Rev. Biochem.* 48: 1, 1979. See also chapter 2, *The Years at P & S.*

33. The Reminiscences of Dana Atchley, found in the Columbia Oral History Collection, is copyrighted by the Trustees of Columbia University in the City of New York, 1975, and is used with permission.

34. Atchley, D. W. Franklin M. Hanger, 1894–1971. *Trans. Assoc. Am. Physicians* 85: 15, 1972.

Hanger, F. M. Flocculation of cephalin-cholesterol emulsions by pathological sera. *Trans. Assoc. Am. Physicians* 53: 148, 1938.

Hanger, F. M., and Gutman, A. B. Obstructive type of jaundice caused by arsphenamine. *Trans. Assoc. Am. Physicians* 55: 179, 1940.

Hanger, F. M., and Patek, A. J. The prognostic value of the cephalin flocculation test in cirrhosis of the liver. *Trans. Assoc. Am. Physicians* 56: 372, 1941.

35. Ragan, C. A., Jr. Ralph Henderson Boots, 1891–1968. *Trans. Assoc. Am. Physicians* 82: 26, 1969.

36. West, R. Martin Henry Dawson. *Trans. Assoc. Am. Physicians* 59: 7, 1946.

37. Dochez, A. R., Shibley, G. S., and Mills, K. C. Studies in the common cold. IV. Experimental transmission of the common cold to anthropoid apes and human beings by means of a filtrable agent. *J. Exp. Med.* 52: 701, 1930.

38. Dochez, A. R., Mills, K. C., and Kneeland, Y., Jr. Studies of the etiology of influenza. *Proc. Soc. Exp. Biol. Med.* 30: 1017, 1933.

Smith, W., Andrewes, C. H., and Laidlaw, P. P. A virus obtained from influenza patients. *Lancet* 2: 66, 1933.

39. Wasserman, L. R. Alexander Benjamin Gutman, 1902–1973. *Trans. Assoc. Am. Physicians* 87: 26, 1974.

40. Coburn, A. F. *The Factor of Infection in the Rheumatic State.* Baltimore: Williams & Wilkins, 1931.

Coburn, A. F., and Moore, L. V. The prophylactic use of sulfanilamide in streptococcal respiratory infections, with special reference to rheumatic fever. *J. Clin. Invest.* 18: 147, 1939.

41. Atchley, D., and Benedict, E. Serum electrolyte studies in normal and pathological conditions: Pneumonia, renal edema, cardiac edema, uremic and diabetic acidosis. *J. Clin. Invest.* 9: 265, 1929–30.

Atchley, D., Richards, D. W., Jr., and Benedict, E. M. Blood electrolyte studies during histamine shock in dogs. *J. Clin. Invest.* 10: 1, 1931.

42. Reminiscences of Dana Atchley.

43. Loeb, R. F., Atchley, D. W., et al. On diabetic acidosis. A detailed study of electrolyte balances following the withdrawal and reestablishment of insulin therapy. *J. Clin. Invest.* 12: 297, 1933.

44. Loeb, R. F., Atchley, D. W., et al. On the mechanism of sodium depletion in Addison's disease. *Proc. Soc. Exp. Biol. Med.* 31: 130, 1933.

45. Harvey, *Interurban Clinical Club,* p. 186.

46. Bearn, A. Robert Frederick Loeb (1895–1973). *Biog. Mem. Natl. Acad. Sci.* 49: 149, 1978. (Contains Loeb's complete bibliography.)

47. Loeb, R. F. Effect of sodium chloride in treatment of a patient with Addison's disease. *Proc. Soc. Exp. Biol. Med.* 30: 808, 1932–33.

Loeb, R. F. Chemical changes in the blood in Addison's disease. *Science* 76: 420, 1932. Loeb was impressed by the resemblance between the clinical picture of adrenal insufficiency and "medical shock," which he knew was often associated with loss of sodium and with nitrogen retention. He made careful electrolyte measurements of the blood in several patients with Addison's disease. He made the important observation in Addisonians that the total base of the blood was low at the expense of sodium, although potassium was high. Loeb stated that "the mechanism of base loss in Addison's disease is not clear," but one patient treated with daily intravenous injection of 12–15 gm of NaCl "became almost entirely symptom free," and "simultaneously the abnormalities of her blood practically disappeared." When she was placed on a salt-poor diet, her blood sodium fell and she deteriorated. Loeb concluded that "this fact associated with the evidence that adrenalectomy in dogs causes a striking loss of sodium through the kidney makes it reasonable to assume that the beneficial effects of NaCl upon the symptoms of adrenal insufficiency in this patient were due to the replacement of sodium lost from the body."

48. Loeb, R. F., Kuhlmann, D., et al. Toxic effects of desoxycorticosterone esters in dogs. *Science* 90: 496, 1939.

Loeb, R. F., Ragan, C., et al. A syndrome of polydipsia and polyuria induced in normal animals by desoxycorticosterone acetate. *Am. J. Physiol.* 131: 73, 1940.

49. Loeb, R. F. Acceptance of the Kober Medal for 1959. *Trans. Assoc. Am. Physicians* 72: 38, 1959.

50. Barach, A. L. A new type of oxygen chamber. *J. Clin. Invest.* 2: 463, 1925–26.

Barach, A. L. Methods and results of oxygen treatment of pneumonia. *Arch. Intern. Med.* 37: 186, 1926.

Barach, A. L. *Principles and Practice of Inhalational Therapy.* Philadelphia: J. B. Lippincott, 1944. This work contains a full description of the technique of oxygen administration.

51. Harvey, *Interurban Clinical Club,* p. 233.

52. Cournand, A., Bryan, N. A., and Richards, D. W., Jr. Cardiac output in relation to unilateral pneumothorax in man. *J. Clin. Invest.* 14: 181, 1935.

Cournand, A., and Ranges, H. A. Catheterization of the right auricle in man. *Proc. Soc. Exp. Biol. Med.* 46: 462, 1941.

Richards, D. W. The contributions of right heart catheterization to physiology and medicine with some observations on the physiopathology of pulmonary heart disease [Nobel Prize Lecture]. *Am. Heart J.* 54: 161, 1957.

Richards, D. W., Jr., Cournand, A., and Bryan, N. A. Applicability of rebreathing method for determining mixed venous $CO_2$ in cases of chronic pulmonary disease. *J. Clin. Invest.* 14: 173, 1935.

Richards, D. W., Jr., and Strauss, M. L. Oxy-hemoglobin dissociation curves of whole blood in anemia. *J. Clin. Invest.* 4: 105, 1927.

Richards, D. W., Jr., and Strauss, M. L. Circulatory adjustment in anemia. *J. Clin. Invest.* 5: 161, 1927–28.

Richards, D. W., Jr., and Strauss, M. L. Carbon dioxide and oxygen tensions of the mixed venous blood of man at rest. I. The problem of equilibration of lung gases with incoming venous blood. II. Experimental. *J. Clin. Invest.* 9: 475, 1929–30.

53. Cournand, A. Presentation of Kober Medal for 1970 to Dickinson W. Richards. *Trans. Assoc. Am. Physicians* 83: 36, 1970.

Cournand, A. Dickinson Woodruff Richards, 1895–1973. *Trans. Assoc. Am. Physicians* 86: 33, 1973.

Cournand, A. Dickinson Woodruff Richards, 1895–1973: A survey of his contributions to the physiology and physiopathology of respiration in man. *Am. J. Med.* 57: 312, 1974.

54. Richards, D. W. Acceptance of the Kober Medal for 1970. *Trans. Assoc. Am. Physicians* 83: 43, 1970.

55. Cournand, A. Dickinson Woodruff Richards, p. 36.

56. Wright, I. S. Robert L. Levy, 1888–1974. *Trans. Assoc. Am. Physicians* 88: 27, 1975.

57. Levy, R. L. Mild forms of coronary thrombosis. *Trans. Assoc. Am. Physicians* 45: 417, 1930.

Levy, R. L., Bruenn, H. G., and Williams, N. E. Effects of induced anoxemia in patients with coronary sclerosis as modified by certain drugs. *Trans. Assoc. Am. Physicians* 54: 244, 1939.

Levy, R. L., and von Glahn, W. C. Further observations on cardiac hypertrophy of unknown etiology in adults. *Trans. Assoc. Am. Physicians* 52: 259, 1937.

58. Benedict, E. M., and Turner, K. B. The serum calcium in polycythemia vera. *J. Clin. Invest.* 9: 263, 1930–31.

Turner, K. B., and Benedict, E. M. Thyroid hyperplasia produced in chickens by ultraviolet light deficiency. *J. Clin. Invest.* 11: 761, 1932.

59. Harvey, *Interurban Clinical Club,* p. 128.

60. Ibid., p. 140.

61. West, R., and Moore, D. H. Electrophoretic pattern of hematopoietic liver extract. *Trans. Assoc. Am. Physicians* 57: 259, 1942.

West, R., and Reisner, E. H., Jr. Treatment of Addisonian pernicious anemia with vitamin B 12. *Trans. Assoc. Am. Physicians* 62: 186, 1949.

62. Wasserman, L. R. Alexander Benjamin Gutman, 1902–1973. *Trans. Assoc. Am. Physicians* 87: 26, 1974.

# Chapter 10

1. Welch, W. H. The evolution of modern scientific laboratories (An address delivered at the opening of the William Pepper Laboratory of Clinical Medicine, Philadelphia, December 4, 1895.) *Bull. Johns Hopkins Hosp.* 7: 19, 1896.

2. Cowgill, D. B: A Brief History of the William Pepper Laboratory of Clinical Medicine, March 3, 1969. Unpublished MS.

3. Miller, T. G. Alfred Stengel, 1868–1939. *Trans. Assoc. Am. Physicians* 54: 15, 1939.

4. Cowgill, A Brief History of the William Pepper Laboratory.

5. Aub, J. C., and Hapgood, R. K. *Pioneer in Modern Medicine: David Linn Edsall,* p. 9. Boston: Harvard Medical Alumni Association, 1970.

6. Edsall, D. L. The Trend of Medical Research. Speech at Thirty-Fourth Annual Conference, Association of American Universities, Iowa City, Iowa. November 11, 1932. Unpublished MS.

7. Mitchell, J. K., Flexner, S., and Edsall, D. L. A brief report of the clinical, physiological and chemical study of three cases of family periodic paralysis. *Brain* 25: 109, 1902.

8. Edsall, D. L., and Miller, C. W. A contribution to the chemical pathology of acromegaly. *Univ. Penn. Med. Bull.* 16: 143, 1903.

9. Edsall, D. L. Two cases of violent but transitory myokymia and myotonia apparently due to excessive hot weather. *Am. J. Med. Sci.* 28: 1003, 1904.

10. Edsall, D. L. Further studies of the muscular spasms produced by exposure to great heat. *Trans. Assoc. Am. Physicians* 24: 625, 1909.

11. Edsall, D. L. Diseases due to chemical agents. In *Modern Medicine: Its Theory and Practice in Original Contributions by American and Foreign Authors,* ed. Osler, W., pp. 84, 114, 124, and 141. Philadelphia: Lea Brothers, 1907.

12. Aub and Hapgood, *Pioneer in Modern Medicine,* p. 69.

13. Ibid., p. 103.

14. Edsall, D. L. Some of the relations of occupation to medicine. Address to the Wisconsin State Medical Society. *J.A.M.A.* 53: 1873, 1909.

15. Starr, I. Personal recollections. Interview with A. McGehee Harvey, April 1976.

16. Miller, Alfred Stengel.

17. Joseph T. Wearn, who was at Pennsylvania during Stengel's tenure, commented as follows in a personal interview (April 1976):

> Stengel insisted that everybody in his department had to earn his living by the practice of medicine and had no sympathy whatever for anybody who wanted to be a full-time person with a limited amount of practice. Despite all that Richards tried to do, Stengel resisted having people in his department who were not earning their living by the practice of medicine. The result was that Jack Starr didn't go into Stengel's department but had a separate division and maintained a relationship with Richards. The only real research work in the picture at that time was Grier Miller's in gastroenterology which was carried on under some difficulty. Stengel had a chance to get Starr, Hayman and several other young fellows there at the time. Stengel offered me a job but it was on the condition that I set up an office and earn my living by practice.

18. Harvey, A. McG. *The Interurban Clinical Club, 1905–1976. A Record of Achievement in Clinical Science,* p. 234. Philadelphia: W. B. Saunders, 1978.

Henderson, L. J. Presentation of the Kober Medal to A. N. Richards. *Trans. Assoc. Am. Physicians* 48: 8, 1933.

Keefer, C. S. Dr. Richards as chairman of the committee on medical research. *Ann. Intern. Med.* 71: 64, 1969.

Richards, A. N. Acceptance of the Kober Medal. *Trans. Assoc. Am. Physicians* 48: 10, 1933.

Schmidt, C. F. Alfred Newton Richards. *Biog. Mem. Natl. Acad. Sci.* 42: 271, 1971. (Contains Richards's complete bibliography.)

Starr, I., et al. Alfred Newton Richards, scientist and man. *Ann. Intern. Med.* 71: 7, 1969.

19. Wearn, J. T. Interview with A. McGehee Harvey, April 1976.

Wearn described the events:

> Shortly after I got there Richards handed me Cushney's volume on the kidney and said: "I wish you'd take this, go away and read it, think about it, and come back and talk to me." I did and went back to report. Richards was planning to inject some epinephrin into the glomerulus . . . I said:

"If you don't mind I'd like to approach this whole thing in a different way . . . I would like to withdraw some fluid from the glomerulus; that is, glomerular urine . . . and do chemical tests on it." He patted me on the back. We devised a pipette (about the diameter of a red blood cell) that would go into the glomerulus. By surrounding the pipette with cork and by putting it in a mechanical manipulator you could move it down to the kidney. We eventually succeeded in inserting the tip into the glomerular capsule and withdrawing some fluid. I found it necessary to work at night because the vibration of people walking in the laboratory would shake the pipette so much that we couldn't use it. I also gave up alcohol and cigarettes because of the very small but definite tremor they caused. We finally got a little spot of light in this pipette and pulled it out. It proved to be an infinitesmally small drop of glomerular fluid. We transferred it to a capillary tube, sealed it, and put it in the refrigerator. The next day we added Benedict's solution to it, put it in boiling water, and found no sugar which was puzzling. Then we tested the blood of the frogs. They were fasting frogs and had been in distilled water. They had no sugar to put through the glomerulus so we gave the next frog some dextrose and then found a positive test in the glomerular urine but none in the bladder urine. That was exciting, of course, because it meant reabsorption. There was so much dust that it was difficult to work because two or three pieces of dust hitting a glomerular cup would cloud the whole thing. So we rigged up a little closet about four by four with a nephalometer in it, sprayed the entire closet with water, put a 100 lb. cube of ice on the floor which created a fog, and as the fog settled the atmosphere was dust free. We each wore a laboratory coat and sprayed one another with water so that we didn't shed dust, and that became part of the technique of microphysiology. We demonstrated this at the International Physiological Congress in Edinburgh in 1921. We took frogs over but the frogs perished en route and we got Scotch frogs. The Scotch frogs had smaller glomeruli. In attempting to put this pipette into a glomerulus I was assigned a little room where I would not be interrupted. It was a difficult job to do there because I was very excited at the idea of demonstrating it in such distinguished company. I heard a door open, Richards was in the room, I finally looked up and with him were Bayliss, Starling, Dale, Laidlaw, and Krogh. It was useless for me to try anything after that illustrious invasion. They all took a look at it and then about the fifth one knocked the pipette out; but we put it back on the glomerulus and none of them knew the difference.

20. Richards, A. N. *Methods and Results of Direct Investigations of the Function of the Kidneys.* (Beaumont Foundation Lecture No. 8) Baltimore: Williams & Wilkins, 1929.

21. See Starr et al., Alfred Newton Richards.

22. Wearn, J. T. Acceptance of the Kober Medal for 1965. *Trans. Assoc. Am. Physicians* 78: 48, 1965.

23. Harvey, *Interurban Clinical Club,* p. 205.

24. Stadie, W. C. William Osler Abbott, 1902–1943. *Trans. Assoc. Am. Physicians* 58: 7, 1944.

25. For information on Bordley, see Harvey, *Interurban Clinical Club,* p. 230.

26. For a full description of this department, see chapter 7.

27. McCrae, T. Richard Mills Pearce. *Trans. Assoc. Am. Physicians* 45: 6, 1930.

28. Stadie, W. C. James Harold Austin. *Trans. Assoc. Am. Physicians* 65: 7, 1952.

29. Lukens, F. D. W. William Christopher Stadie. *Trans. Assoc. Am. Physicians* 73: 39, 1960.

30. Stadie (Fat metabolism in diabetes mellitus. *J. Clin. Invest.* 19: 843, 1940) questioned both the theory that fatty acids were broken down by beta-oxidation and the view that combustion of fatty-acids was dependent on glucose in the metabolic mixture. He showed that "the diabetic animal utilizes ketone bodies in the periphery abundantly and independently of carbohydrate oxidation," and he concluded that, if too little carbohydrate is burned, the body must obtain its calories from fat. But since there is a limit to the amount of fatty acid that can be burned daily, the excess then appears as ketone bodies. Stadie (Fat metabolism in diabetes mellitus. *Ann. Intern. Med.* 15: 783, 1941) later stated his views precisely:

The diabetic who . . . is unable to utilize carbohydrate . . . must fall back on fat for his energy requirements. Part of this need is met by the initiation and complete fat oxidation in the muscles themselves. However, a considerable fraction . . . of the total caloric needs from fat is obtained by preliminary oxidation of fats in the liver to ketone bodies only. . . . These hepatic ketone bodies are freely utilized for energy by the periphery without insulin and without the necessity of simultaneous carbohydrate oxidation. . . . When the demand for fat calories exceeds a certain level, approximately 2.5 gm. of fat/kg/day for the resting state, ketone bodies in excess of needs are formed by the liver. The excess is excreted as ketones in the urine. If this excessive fat catabolism continues unchecked ketosis and coma follow.

31. Starr, Personal recollections.

32. Stadie, W. C. Acceptance of the Kober Medal for 1955. *Trans. Assoc. Am. Physicians* 68: 29, 1955.

33. Harvey, *Interurban Clinical Club,* p. 303.

Starr, I. Acceptance of the Kober Medal. *Trans. Assoc. Am. Physicians* 80: 42, 1967.

Stokes, J., Jr. Presentation of the Kober Medal to Dr. Isaac Starr. *Trans. Assoc. Am. Physicians* 80: 32, 1967.

34. Hayman, J. M., Jr., and Starr, I. Experiments on the glomerular distribution of blood in the mammalian kidney. *J. Exp. Med.* 42: 641, 1925.

35. Starr, I., Collins, L. H., Jr., and Wood, F. C. Studies of the basal work and output of the heart in clinical conditions. *J. Clin. Invest.* 12: 13, 1933.

36. Starr, I. Studies made by simulating systole at necropsy. XI. On the higher dynamic functions of the heart and their reflections in the pulse wave. *Circulation* 17: 589, 1958.

Starr, Collins, and Wood, Studies of the basal work and output of the heart in clinical conditions.

Starr, I., and Luchi, R. J. Blind study on the action of digitoxin on elderly women. *Am. Heart J.* 78: 740, 1969.

Starr, I., and Noordergraaf, A. *Ballistocardiography in Cardiovascular Research.* Philadelphia: Lippincott, 1967.

Starr, I., Verdouw, P. D., and Noordergraaf, A. Clinical evidence of cardiac weakness and coordination secured by simultaneous records of the force BCG and the carotid pulse derivative, and interpreted by an electrical analogue. *Am. Heart J.* 85: 341, 1973.

Starr, I., and Wood, F. C. Twenty-year studies with the ballistocardiograph. *Circulation* 23: 714, 1961.

37. This summary of Starr's work is based on a personal interview with him in April 1976.

38. Miller, T. G. A consideration of the clinical value of ephedrin. *Am. J. Med. Sci.* 170: 157, 1925.

K. K. Chen and Carl F. Schmidt (The action of ephedrine, the active principle of the Chinese drug Ma Huang. *J. Pharmacol. Exp. Ther.* 24: 339, 1924) first studied the pharmacology of ephedrine and pointed out the relationship to epinephrine. They demonstrated bronchodilation after physostigmine had produced marked bronchial spasm, but they did not try the drug in patients. Miller felt that ephedrine had "distinct practical advantages over epinephrine because of its more prolonged action" and because it could "be administered effectively by mouth." It gave relief in the paroxysmal attacks of certain cases of asthma. With S. S. Leopold (The use of ephedrine in bronchial asthma and hay fever. *J.A.M.A.* 88: 1782, 1927), he reported more extensively on the subject.

39. Abbott, W. O. Intubation of the human small intestine. XII. The treatment of intestinal obstruction in a procedure for identifying the lesion. *Arch. Intern. Med.* 63: 453, 1939.

Harvey, *Interurban Clinical Club,* p. 251.

Karr, W. G., and Abbott, W. O., with the technical assistance of Albert B. Sample: Intubation studies of the human small intestine. IV. Chemical characteristics of the intestinal contents in the fasting state and as influenced by the administration of acids, of alkalies and of water. *J. Clin. Invest.* 14: 893, 1935.

Miller, T. G. William Osler Abbott. *Trans. Am. Clin. Climatol. Assoc.* 58: lxxxiv, 1946.

Miller, T. G., and Abbott, W. O. Intestinal intubation, a practical technique. *Am. J. Med. Sci.* 167: 595, 1934.

40. Harvey, *Interurban Clinical Club,* p. 170.

Palmer, W. L. Presentation of the Julius Friedenwald Medal to T. Grier Miller. *Gastroenterology* 33: 7, 1957.

41. Harvey, *Interurban Clinical Club,* pp. 246, 333.

Lukens, F. D. W. Cyril Norman Hugh Long, 1901-1970. *Trans. Assoc. Am. Physicians* 84: 27, 1971.

Smith, O. L. K., and Hardy, J. D. Cyril Norman Hugh Long (1901-1970). *Biog. Mem. Natl. Acad. Sci.* 46: 265, 1975. (Contains Long's complete bibliography.)

42. Winegrad, A. I. Francis D. W. Lukens. *Trans. Assoc. Am. Physicians* 92: 35, 1979.

43. Gibbon, J. H., Jr., and Landis, E. M. Vasodilatation in the lower extremities in response to immersing the forearms in warm water. *J. Clin. Invest.* 11: 1019, 1932.

Harvey, *Interurban Clinical Club,* p. 205.

Landis, E. M., Elsom, K. A., Bott, P. A., and Shiels, E. Observations on sodium chloride restriction and urea clearance in renal insufficiency. *J. Clin. Invest.* 14: 525, 1935.

Landis, E. M., and Gibbon, J. H., Jr. The effects of temperature and of tissue pressure on the movement of fluid through the human capillary wall. *J. Clin. Invest.* 12: 105, 1933.

Landis, E. M., and Gibbon, J. H., Jr. The effects of alternate suction and pressure on blood flow to the lower extremities. *J. Clin. Invest.* 12: 925, 1933.

Landis, E. M., Jonas, L., Angevine, M., and Erb, W. The passage of fluid and protein through the human capillary wall during venous congestion. *J. Clin. Invest.* 11: 717, 1932.

44. Harvey, *Interurban Clinical Club,* pp. 187, 256.

45. Starr, Collins, and Wood. Studies of the basal work and output of the heart in clinical conditions.

Wolferth, C. C., and Wood, F. C. The electrocardiographic diagnosis of coronary occlusion by the use of chest leads. *Am. J. Med. Sci.* 183: 30, 1932.

Wood, F. C. The diastolic heart beat. *Trans. Assoc. Am. Physicians* 64: 95, 1951.

Wood, F. C., and Wolferth, C. C. Angina pectoris: The clinical and electrocardiographic phenomena of the attack and their comparison with the effects of experimental temporary coronary occlusion. *Arch. Intern. Med.* 47: 339, 1931.

# Chapter 11

1. Lusk, G. Medical education. A plea for the development of leaders. *J.A.M.A.* 52: 1229, 1909.

Lusk, G. On the proposed reorganization of departments of clinical medicine in the United States. *Science* 41: 431, 1915.

2. Lusk, Medical education.

3. Lusk, On the proposed reorganization of departments of clinical medicine.

4. DuBois, E. F. Graham Lusk (1866-1932). *Biog. Mem. Natl. Acad. Sci.* 21: 95, 1940. (Contains Lusk's complete bibliography.)

5. Murlin, J. R. Graham Lusk: A brief review of his work. *J. Nutr.* 5: 527, 1932.

6. Lusk, G. Scientific medicine—Yesterday and tomorrow. *J.A.M.A.* 73: 181, 1919.

7. One of Lusk's contemporaries pointed out that Lusk was impatient in his efforts to reform clinical medicine. He tried at times to push men, when their teachings were so far above the heads of the students that they could not be appreciated. There were probably a good many factors in this protest from the faculty.

8. McCann, W. S. The influence of Graham Lusk upon his students. In Addresses given at a Memorial Meeting for Graham Lusk at the N.Y. Academy of Medicine on December 10, 1932. (Held under the auspices of the Harvey Society.), p. 10. Baltimore, 1933.

9. Light, A. Graham Lusk. *Yale J. Biol. Med.* 6: 487, 1933-34.

Lusk, G. Carl von Voit, master and friend. *Ann. Med. Hist.* 3: 583, 1931.

10. Collaborators in Clinical Calorimetry Series. Papers 1 to 50, 1915 to 1932. Clinical Calorimetry papers 1-32 published in the *Arch. Intern. Med.* 1915 to 1922; papers 33-48

published in the *J. Biol. Chem.* 1923 to 1932; papers 49–53 published in *J. Nutr.* 1938. J. A. Riche, G. F. Soderstrom, F. C. Gephart, E. F. DuBois, W. Coleman, Margaret Sawyer, R. H. Stone, D. DuBois, A. L. Meyer, F. W. Peabody, F. M. Allen, J. C. Aub, J. H. Means, J. B. Murphy, D. P. Barr, W. S. McCann, R. L. Cecil, H. B. Richardson, E. H. Mason, W. S. Ladd, A. M. Michaelis, S. Z. Levine, W. S. McClellan, A. Biasotti, R. R. Hannon, H. J. Spencer, E. A. Falk, V. Toscani, V. R. Rupp.

11. Murlin, Graham Lusk: A brief review of his work.

12. Aub, J. C. Eugene Floyd DuBois. *Biog. Mem. Natl. Acad. Sci.* 36: 125, 1962.

Means, J. H. Eugene Floyd DuBois. *Trans. Assoc. Am. Physicians* 72: 23, 1959.

13. Peters, J. P., and Barr, D. P. Studies of the respiratory mechanism in cardiac dyspnea. *Am. J. Physiol.* 54: 307, 335, 345, 1920.

Peters, J. P., and Barr, D. P. III. The carbon dioxide absorption curve and carbon dioxide tension of the blood in severe anemia. *J. Biol. Chem.* 45: 571, 1921.

14. Hannon, R. R., Shorr, E., McClellan, W. S., and DuBois, E. F. A case of osteitis fibrosa cystica (osteomalacia?) with evidence of hyperactivity of the parathyroid bodies: Metabolic study. *J. Clin. Invest.* 8: 215, 1930.

The authors described a man of thirty, who for eight years had suffered from aches and pains, fractures, shortening of his body height, and the passage of urinary gravel. X-rays showed diffuse atrophy, fractures, and cyst formation of bones. The serum calcium was 14.5 mg/dl, the phosphorus 3.3. Careful balance studies showed hypercalcemia, low blood phosphorus, and increased urinary excretion of calcium and phosphorus.

W. Bauer, F. Albright, and J. C. Aub (Metabolic Study II. *J. Clin. Invest.* 8: 229, 1930) reported further studies on this patient. His negative calcium balance on a low-calcium diet was markedly increased over that found in normal controls, and the findings were practically identical with those of a man receiving one hundred units of parathormone a day. Two of the parathyroid glands were removed on this entry without affecting the calcium abnormalities. A second exploratory operation revealed no abnormal parathyroid tissue. Still further studies of this patient were reported by McClellan and Hannon (Metabolic Study III. *J. Clin. Invest.* 8: 249, 1930); his condition remained essentially unchanged, the serum calcium remained above 14 mg/dl.

Further explorations were done in the attempt to find a parathyroid tumor. Finally, on the seventh attempt, a tumor was found, extending behind the esophagus into the posterior medastinum (Churchill, E. D. The operative treatment of hyperparathyroidism. *Ann. Surg.* 100: 606, 1934).

Hannon's paper was presented first before the Interurban Clinical Club in New York City in April 1927.

15. DuBois, E. F. *Basal Metabolism in Health and Disease.* 3rd ed. Philadelphia: Lea & Febiger, 1936.

16. Means, J. H. Eugene Floyd DuBois, 1882–1959. *Trans. Assoc. Am. Physicians* 72: 23, 1959.

17. DuBois, E. F. Fifty years of physiology in America—A letter to the editor. *Ann. Rev. Physiol.* 12: 1, 1950.

18. Barr, D. Presentation of the Kober Medal to Dr. Eugene F. DuBois. *Trans. Assoc. Am. Physicians* 60: 9, 1947.

19. After Aub completed his internship at the MGH, Edsall sent him to work with Eugene DuBois:

> The person who really concerned me at Cornell was Gene DuBois, who was superb....
>
> DuBois made it mandatory for me to become acquainted with the German literature on physiology and metabolism and . . . I spent . . . the rest of my time being accurate in my work. DuBois was a fantastically methodical and accurate investigator and I'm afraid when I came to New York I was more than a little sloppy in my work habits; to put it another way I was undisciplined compared to what DuBois wanted . . . I think that he basically wanted a docile and methodical assistant, instead he got somebody volatile. For instance, when I first came to New York I thought myself a kingpin. I was very cocky and I suppose insufferable—after all I had been a house officer at the MGH. DuBois set to work disabusing me of those notions and

molding me to the shape and form he thought an investigator should have; the first job he gave me when I came to work in the laboratory was to clean out the calorimeter with dustpan and broom. I didn't recognize then it was just DuBois' way of getting me in line.

The second job he gave me was even worse, at least it was more tedious. He gave me reams of coordinate graph paper and made me write 1, 2, 3, 4, 5, 6, 7, 8, 9, 0 over and over again until there was no question that my 7's were not 9's and that my 5's were not 3's. I thought that was dreadful. However the funny thing is when I took my first assistant to work on respiratory metabolism I met him with the same chore. Gene obviously felt that task was necessary in order to produce letter perfect work. I now agree with him. He just couldn't run an enormous experiment, spend days and hours on it and then come back to me and say, "Aub is this a 7 or a 1?" Everything had to be done with infinite caution, and I should add that it was. There was nothing sloppy about the work that went on in DuBois' metabolism unit.

I'd like now to say something of the unit itself. In a way it was an anomaly. Here was a beautiful little metabolism unit consisting of the calorimeter, four beds for patients, the investigation unit of researchers and three very devoted and competent nurses. I say it was an anomaly because it was set in the hustle and bustle of Bellevue's enormous wards and the tumult of patients and visitors constant coming and going. At all times we worked as a team, and it took DuBois, myself and Soderstrom to run any given metabolic experiment. At most we could run 2 or 3 experiments a week because it took us a great deal of time to weigh bottles and do calculations. Much time for example was also taken for testing the calorimeter for leaks. All of this took infinite patience. The nurses played an equally important role. They saw to it that the patients ate what they were told to eat; I can't stress too much the fact that everything was done with infinite accuracy. The metabolism unit, for example, was the only place in Bellevue where one could get a 24 hour sample urine and be sure it was right. Again when a patient was weighed on the table that Eugene DuBois had invented it was correct to a few grams. . . .

We did much work on hyperthyroids . . . I remember one day DuBois sent me to the ward and asked me to bring back a hyperthyroid. An easy enough chore I thought for a man from the MGH. I looked carefully until I found a patient who I thought was a moderate hyperthyroid and brought her triumphantly back to the metabolism ward. DuBois took one look and politely informed me that the patient was hypertensive not hyperthyroid. Although I was extremely embarrassed, I learned a great deal from that experience because I hadn't previously known that many hypertensives look a great deal like hyperthyroids. . . .

DuBois was a superb instructor and a dedicated investigator. He was probably a greater physiologist than he was a clinician. His clinical work was not without criticism at Cornell but for my taste he was a very good clinician . . . DuBois always loved to encourage independent investigation and although we were always more than busy in the laboratory he always gave me time off when I got a flight of ideas.

The Reminiscences of Joseph C. Aub, found in the Columbia Oral History Collection, is copyright by The Trustees of Columbia University in the City of New York, 1975, and is used by permission.

20. DuBois, E. F. Acceptance of the Kober Medal. *Trans. Assoc. Am. Physicians* 60: 12, 1947.

21. McCann, W. S. Unpublished memoirs. MS. Library. University of Rochester School of Medicine.

22. Bishop, M. *A History of Cornell.* Ithaca: Cornell University Press, 1962. (Most of these notes were taken from the original minutes book of the Trustees of the Loomis Laboratory, which is in the Cornell–New York Hospital Archives.)

23. Warthin, A. S. Presidential address. *Trans. Assoc. Am. Physicians* 43: 7, 1928.

24. Harvey, A. McG. *The Interurban Clinical Club 1905–1976. A Record of Achievement in Clinical Science,* p. 25. Philadelphia: W. B. Saunders, 1978.

25. DuBois, E. F. Walter Lindsay Niles, 1898–1941. *Trans. Assoc. Am. Physicians* 57: 32, 1942.

26. Hastings, T. W., and Niles, W. L. The bacteriology of the sputum in common non-tuberculous infections of the upper and lower respiratory tracts with special reference to lobar and bronchopneumonia. *J. Exp. Med.* 13: 638, 1911.

Niles, W. L., and Wiggers, C. J. The details of the photographically recorded venous pulse in auricular fibrillation. *J. Exp. Med.* 25: 1, 1917.

Wiggers, C. J., and Niles, W. L. The significance of the diastolic waves of the venous pulse in auricular fibrillation. *J. Exp. Med.* 25: 21, 1917.

27. Harvey, *The Interurban Clinical Club*, p. 27.

28. Ibid., p. 30.

29. Crehore, A. C., and Meara, F. S. The micrograph. An instrument which records the microscopic movements of the diaphragm by means of light interference and some records of physiological events showing the registration of sound waves including the human voice. *J. Exp. Med.* 13: 616, 1911.

Meara, F. S., Coffen, T. H., and Crehore, A. C. A comparison of simultaneous polygraph and micrograph tracings. *J. Exp. Med.* 16: 280, 1912.

30. Palmer, W. W. Alexander Lambert, 1861–1939. *Trans. Assoc. Am. Physicians* 55: 19, 1940.

31. Harvey, *Interurban Clinical Club*, p. 118.

32. Thompson, W. G. Clinical experiments with homologous vaccines in the treatment of septic endocarditis and pyemia. *Am. J. Med. Sci.* 138: 169, 1909.

33. Conner, L. A., and Roper, J. C. The relations existing between bilirubinemia, urobilinuria and urobilinemia. *Arch. Intern. Med.* 2: 532, 1909.

34. Hoobler, E. R. The standardization of blood pressure readings by means of an automatic device for indicating systolic and diastolic pressures in children. *Am. J. Dis. Child.* 4: 46, 1912.

35. Harvey, *Interurban Clinical Club*, p. 132.

36. While working in pathology at Presbyterian Hospital, Cecil made a notable contribution to the pathology of diabetes mellitus (Cecil, R. L. A study of the pathological anatomy of the pancreas in ninety cases of diabetes mellitus. *J. Exp. Med.* 11: 266, 1909). He concluded that anatomical lesions of the pancreas occur in more than seven-eighths of all cases of diabetes mellitus and that in diabetes associated with lesions of the pancreas, the islets constantly showed changes (sclerosis, hyaline degeneration, infiltration with leukocytes, and hypertrophy).

See also Cecil, R. L. On hypertrophy and regeneration of the Islands of Langerhans. *J. Exp. Med.* 14: 500, 1911; and Cecil, R. L. The effect of certain experimental procedures on the Islands of Langerhans. *J. Exp. Med.* 16: 1, 1912.

37. Cecil, R. L. A study of experimental non-hemolytic streptococcus lesions in vitally stained rabbits. *J. Exp. Med.* 24: 739, 1916.

Cecil, R. L., and Austin, J. H. Results of prophylactic inoculation against pneumococcus in 12,519 men. *J. Exp. Med.* 28: 19, 1918.

Cecil, R. L., and Blake, F. G. Studies on experimental pneumonia. VII. Treatment of experimental pneumococcus Type I pneumonia in monkeys with Type I antipneumococcus serum. *J. Exp. Med.* 32: 1, 1920.

Cecil, R. L., and Steffen, G. I. Studies on pneumococcus immunity. II. Active immunization of monkeys against pneumococcus Types II, III and IV pneumonia with the homologous pneumococcus vaccine. *J. Exp. Med.* 38: 149, 1923.

38. Rackemann, F. M. Robert Anderson Cooke, 1880–1960. *Trans. Assoc. Am. Physicians* 74: 11, 1961.

39. Stewart, H. J. Harold Ensign Bennett Pardee, 1886–1973. *Trans. Assoc. Am. Physicians* 87: 34, 1974.

40. Young, L. E. William Sharp McCann, 1889–1971. *Trans. Assoc. Am. Physicians* 85: 35, 1972.

41. Moore, C. V. Harry L. Alexander. *Trans. Assoc. Am. Physicians* 82: 24, 1969.

42. Reznikoff, P. Henry Barber Richardson. *Trans. Assoc. Am. Physicians* 77: 27, 1964.

43. Castle, W. B. Soma Weiss, 1899–1942. *Trans. Assoc. Am. Physicians* 57: 36, 1942.

44. Weiss, S., Morris, R. M., and Witter, M. S. An unusual sensitizing action of thyroid on the effect of epinephrine in man. *Proc. Soc. Exp. Biol. Med.* 21: 149, 1923.

45. Rogers, D. E. David Preswick Barr, 1889–1977. *Trans. Assoc. Am. Physicians* 91: 15, 1978.

46. Barr, D. P. Ephraim Shorr, 1897–1956. *Trans. Assoc. Am. Physicians* 69: 28, 1956.

47. Master, A. M., and Oppenheimer, E. T. A simple exercise tolerance test for circulatory efficiency with standard tables for normal individuals. *Am. J. Med. Sci.* 177: 223, 1929.

48. Barondess, J. A. Harold J. Stewart, 1896–1975. *Trans. Assoc. Am. Physicians* 89: 32, 1976.

49. Almy, T. P. Harold George Wolff, 1898–1962. *Trans. Assoc. Am. Physicians* 75: 45, 1962.

50. Wolf, S. G. *The Stomach,* pp. 29–35. New York: Oxford University Press, 1965.

51. Wolf, S. Personal communication, 1978.

52. DuBois, E. F. Annual Report of the Physician-in-Chief, New York Hospital, dated June 6, 1935. Archives, Cornell University School of Medicine.

# Chapter 12

1. See Appendix B for a description of clinical science in Boston by Joseph T. Wearn.

2. Bowditch, H. P. The medical school of the future. *Phila. Med. J.* 5: 1011, 1900.
For further information about Eliot, see:
Bowers, J. Z. The influence of Charles W. Eliot on medical education. *Pharos* 35: 156, 1972.
Cannon, W. B. President Eliot's relations to medicine. *N. Engl. J. Med.* 210: 730, 1934.

3. Eliot, C. W. The future of medicine. *Science* 24: 449, 1906.

4. Edward Cowles (M.D., P & S, 1863) interned in the Hartford Retreat for the Insane at Hartford, Connecticut, and then entered the Medical Corps of the United States Army, resigning in 1872. He settled in South Boston and was appointed visiting physician to the Carney Hospital. In a few months, he was elected medical superintendent of the Boston City Hospital. This was one of the first big hospitals in the United States to have a medical, rather than a lay, superintendent. He established a training school for nurses, among the first of such schools, and made it an integral part of the hospital. He inaugurated the plan of having patients admitted to the hospital by the executive or his representative, rather than by an outside physician. His successes as an administrator were so great that he was called, in 1879, to the superintendency of the McLean Hospital.

5. Cowles, E. The advancement of psychiatry in America. *Am. J. Insanity* 52: 36, 1895.
Hall, G. S. Laboratory of the McLean Hospital. Somerville, Massachusetts. *Am. J. Insanity* 51: 358, 1894.
Washburn, F. C. *The Massachusetts General Hospital: Its Development, 1900–1935,* p. 279. Boston: Houghton Mifflin, 1939.
Whitehorn, J. C. A century of psychiatric research in America. In *One Hundred Years of American Psychiatry,* ed. Zilboorg, G., p. 167. New York: Columbia University Press, 1944.

6. Ricketts, H. T. Joseph Almarin Capps, 1872–1964. *Trans. Assoc. Am. Physicians* 78: 15, 1965.

7. Cowles, The advancement of psychiatry in America.

8. See *Fiftieth Year Reports,* Graduating Class of 1921, Harvard Medical School.

9. DuBois, E. F., and Riddle, O. Francis Gano Benedict (1870–1957). *Biog. Mem. Natl. Acad. Sci.* 32: 67, 1958. (Contains Benedict's complete bibliography.)

10. Ibid.

11. Benedict, F. G., and Joslin, E. P. Metabolism in diabetes mellitus. Washington, D.C.: Carnegie Institution Publications, No. 136.
This is a lengthy report of the observations on the metabolism of diabetes, measured with the help of a respiration chamber. These classical experiments showed no *qualitative* differences in the metabolism in diabetics as contrasted against normal individuals, with allowances for the type of food burned. Such matters as the respiratory quotient, the influence on the respiratory exchange, the total catabolism, and the influence of muscular work upon metabolism in diabetes are discussed. In another monograph by these authors

(A Study of Metabolism in Severe Diabetes. Carnegie Institution Publications, No. 176), the observations were amplified.

12. Marble, A. Elliott Proctor Joslin, 1869–1962. *Trans. Assoc. Am. Physicians* 75: 25, 1962.

13. Joslin, E. P. Acceptance of the Kober Medal. *Trans. Assoc. Am. Physicians* 47: 11, 1932.

Woodyatt, R. T. Presentation of the Kober Medal to E. P. Joslin. *Trans. Assoc. Am. Physicians* 47: 8, 1932.

14. Harvey, A. McG. *The Interurban Clinical Club, 1905–1976. A Record of Achievement in Clinical Science,* p. 125. Philadelphia: W. B. Saunders, 1978.

15. Warthin, A. S. James Homer Wright, 1869–1928. *Trans. Assoc. Am. Physicians* 43: 9, 1928.

16. Washburn, *The Massachusetts General Hospital,* p. 112.

17. Harvey, *Interurban Clinical Club,* p. 19.

18. Washburn, *The Massachusetts General Hospital,* p. 117.

19. In 1891 Charles H. Dalton and Henry R. Dalton gave to the MGH, in memory of two other brothers who had been associated with that hospital, a fund in the amount of $10,000. The fund was "to be permanent and the income to be used to promote investigations in any branch of the science of medicine by pecuniary aid either to a 'house pupil' [intern] of the hospital or a graduate of any regular medical college, engaged in scientific work as above described and deemed worthy of and requiring assistance."

In the MGH–Harvard Medical School affiliation, a true full-time clinical investigator was first appointed in 1910, when Frederick C. Shattuck gave to the university the sum of $25,000, the income of which was to pay the salary of a research fellow in medicine. Shattuck named the fellowship in honor of his friend Henry P. Walcott, a long-time trustee of the hospital.

20. Means, J. H. *Ward 4: The Mallinckrodt Research Ward of the Massachusetts General Hospital,* p. 13. Cambridge, Mass.: Harvard University Press, 1958.

21. Harvey, *The Interurban Clinical Club,* p. 11.

22. Warthin, James Homer Wright, p. 9.

23. Hamburger, M. Oswald Hope Robertson, 1886–1966. *Trans. Assoc. Am. Physicians* 79: 76, 1966.

24. Harvey, A. McG. Applying the methods of science to the study of tropical diseases—The story of Andrew Watson Sellards. *Johns Hopkins Med. J.* 144: 45, 1979.

Rackemann, F. M. Andrew Watson Sellards, 1884–1942. *Trans. Assoc. Am. Physicians* 59: 34, 1946.

25. Harvey, *Interurban Clinical Club,* p. 16.

26. Aub, J. C., and Hapgood, R. K. *Pioneer in Modern Medicine: David Linn Edsall,* p. 61. Boston: Harvard Medical Alumni Association, 1970.

27. Cabot, R. C. *Boston Transcript,* May 11, 1912.

28. Means, J. H. Cecil Kent Drinker, 1887–1956. *Trans. Assoc. Am. Physicians* 69: 11, 1956.

29. Bland, E. F. Paul Dudley White, 1886–1973. *Trans. Assoc. Am. Physicians* 87: 41, 1974.

30. Burrage, W. S. Francis Minot Rackemann, M.D. *Trans. Am. Clin. Climatol. Assoc.* 85: xl, 1973.

31. Hamburger, Oswald Hope Robertson.

Robertson, O. H. Acceptance of the Kober Medal for 1961. *Trans. Assoc. Am. Physicians* 74: 57, 1961.

Rous, P. Presentation of the Kober Medal for 1961 to O. H. Robertson. *Trans. Assoc. Am. Physicians* 74: 49, 1961.

32. Adams, R. D. Stanley Cobb. *Trans. Assoc. Am. Physicians* 82: 28, 1969.

Cobb, S. Acceptance of the Kober Medal for 1956. *Trans. Assoc. Am. Physicians* 69: 41, 1956.

Harvey, *Interurban Clinical Club,* p. 196.

Kubie, L. S. Stanley Cobb, 1887–1968. *Psychosom. Med.* 31: 97, 1969.

Wolff, H. G. Presentation of the Kober Medal (1956) to Stanley Cobb. *Trans. Assoc. Am. Physicians* 69: 34, 1956.

33. Edsall, D. L. Medical-industrial relations of the war. *Bull. Johns Hopkins Hosp.* 29: 197, 1918.

34. Aub and Hapgood, *Pioneer in Modern Medicine*, p. 170.

35. Means, J. H. The medical laboratory. In *The Massachusetts General Hospital Memorial and Historical Volume, Together with the Proceedings of the Centennial of the Opening of the Hospital,* p. 182, Boston: Griffith-Stillings, 1921.

36. W. W. Palmer was the second Walcott fellow. He worked under Henderson on the hydrogen-ion concentration of human urine in health and disease and on related problems of acid-base balance.

Arlie Bock returned from World War I with an interest in hemodynamic problems, stimulated by his experience with wounded soldiers with hemorrhagic shock. Bock collected data on blood gases and chlorides, from which Henderson constructed his celebrated nomogram (1924). Over a period of years, associates of Henderson and Bock included Henry L. Field, Jr., Lewis M. Hurxthal, David B. Dill, and John H. Talbott. See:

Bock, A. V., Dill, D. B., and Edwards, H. T. On the relation of changes in blood velocity and volume flow of blood to change of posture. *J. Clin. Invest.* 8: 533, 1929.

Bock, A. V., Dill, D. B., and Edwards, H. T. Lactic acid in the blood of resting man. *J. Clin. Invest.* 11: 775, 1932.

Denning, H., Talbott, J. H., Edwards, H. T., and Dill, D. B. Effect of acidosis and alkalosis upon capacity for work. *J. Clin. Invest.* 9: 601, 1930–31.

Field, H., Jr., and Bock, A. V. Orthopnoea and the effect of posture upon the rate of blood flow. *J. Clin. Invest.* 2: 67, 1925–26.

Field, H., Jr., Bock, A. V., Gildea, E. F., and Lathrop, F. L. The rate of the circulation of the blood in normal resting individuals. *J. Clin. Invest.* 1: 65, 1924.

Lawrence, J. S., Hurxthal, L. M., and Bock, A. V. Variations in blood flow with changes in position in normal and pathologic subjects. *J. Clin. Invest.* 2: 613, 1925–26.

Talbott, J. H., and Michelsen, J. Heat cramps. A clinical and chemical study. *J. Clin. Invest.* 12: 533, 1933.

37. Palmer, W. L. Chester Morse Jones, 1891–1972. *Trans. Assoc. Am. Physicians* 86: 19, 1973.

38. Means, J. H., and Aub, J. C. The basal metabolism in exophthalmic goitre. *Arch. Intern. Med.* 24: 645, 1919.

39. Means, J. H. Experiences and opinions of a full-time teacher. *Perspect. Biol. Med.* 2: 127, 1958.

40. Ibid.

41. Ibid.

42. Castle, W. B. James Howard Means, 1885–1967. *Trans. Assoc. Am. Physicians* 81: 16, 1968.

Means, J. H. Acceptance of the Kober Medal. *Trans. Assoc. Am. Physicians* 77: 41, 1964.

Sprague, H. B. Presentation of the Kober Medal for 1964 to James Howard Means. *Trans. Assoc. Am. Physicians* 77: 37, 1964.

43. Means, *Ward 4.*

44. Means, J. H. *The Thyroid and Its Diseases.* Philadelphia: J. B. Lippincott, 1937.

Means, J. H. and Lerman, J.: Symptomatology of myxedema: Its relation to metabolic levels, time intervals, and rations of thyroid. *Arch. Intern. Med.* 55: 11, 1935.

A. Magnus-Levy (Untersuchungen zur Schildrüsenfrage. *Ztschr. f. klin. Med.* 33: 269, 1897) had already measured the gas exchange in a cretin and found it to be very low. He predicted that with spontaneous myxedema one would find a marked lowering only in cases with marked degeneration. A. E. Epstein (The reciprocal functions of the thyroid gland and iodine: Their relation to the fundamental metabolism of the body. In *Contributions in Honor of Dr. Emanuel Libman.* New York: International Press, 1: 365, 1932) emphasized that there was a low level of oxygen consumption below which the body could not drop. This he designated as the fundamental metabolism in distinction to basal metabolism. Means and Lerman developed this concept further and pointed out that, even with complete athyrosis, the metabolic rate does not fall below approximately 40 percent of the basal ("fundamental") level.

Salter, W. T., and Lerman, J. The metabolic effects of human·thyroglobulin and its proteolytic cleavage products. *J. Clin. Invest.* 14: 691, 1935.

Salter, W. T., Lerman, J., and Means, J. H. The calorigenic action of thyroxin polypeptide. *J. Clin. Invest.* 12: 327, 1933.

45. Means, J. H. Some new approaches to the physiology of the thyroid. *Ann. Intern. Med.* 19: 567, 1943.

Some of the early work on the thyrotropic hormone of the pituitary was summarized by J. B. Collip and E. M. Anderson (Studies on the thyrotropic hormone of the anterior-pituitary. *J.A.M.A.* 104: 965, 1935); see also Evans, H. M. Clinical manifestations of dysfunction of the anterior pituitary. *J.A.M.A.* 104: 464, 1935; and Smith, P. E. General physiology of the anterior hypophysis. *J.A.M.A.* 104: 438, 1935. A little later, W. O. Thompson, S. G. Taylor III, P. K. Thomson, S. B. Nadler, and L. F. N. Dickie (The calorigenic action of extracts of the anterior lobe of the pituitary in man. *Endocrinology* 20: 55, 1936) demonstrated an increase in basal metabolism during administration of pituitary extracts containing thyrotropic principle. In six of eleven patients with exophthalmic goiter, the severity of the disease was increased. The authors concluded that "these observations show that in disorders of thyroid function, the possible role of the pituitary should be considered." But it was Means who integrated, in clinical terms, the relations between pituitary and thyroid glands and coined the term *pituitary-thyroid axis* to indicate the reciprocal action of the hormones of the two glands. Means (The nature of Graves' disease with special reference to its ophthalmic component. *Am. J. Med. Sci.* 207: 1, 1944) further developed his views on the relation of the anterior pituitary to Graves's disease, especially the ophthalmopathic form. "Considerable evidence supports the view that an excess of thyrotropic hormone has something to do with the ophthalmic pathogenesis." (Bloomfield, A. L. *A Bibliography of Internal Medicine: Selected Diseases,* p. 178. Chicago: University of Chicago Press, 1960.)

When radioactive isotopes became available for medical research, iodine could be traced, not only through the thyroid, but throughout the entire body. Means and Carl T. Compton organized a joint research enterprise between MIT and the thyroid clinic of the MGH and did fundamental work on the thyroid gland and its function in health and disease. Among the important members of this research group were Rulon W. Rawson, John B. Stanbury, Saul Hertz, and Robley Evans.

Hertz, S., and Roberts, A. Radioactive iodine in the study of thyroid physiology. *J.A.M.A.* 131: 81, 1946.

The story of the development of use of radioactive isotopes in the diagnosis and treatment of thyroid disease is told by Means (Historical background of the use of radioactive iodine in medicine. *N. Engl. J. Med.* 252: 936, 1955). The treatment of hyperthyroidism by means of radioactive iodine was based on the fact that overactive glands took up iodine in excessive amounts, so that enough radiant energy could be delivered to the gland to impair or destroy its activity. (Hertz, S., Roberts, A., and Evans, R. D. Radioactive iodine as an indicator in the study of thyroid physiology. *Proc. Soc. Exp. Biol. Med.* 38: 510, 1938; Hertz, S., Roberts, A., Means, J. H., and Evans, R. D. Radioactive iodine as an indicator in thyroid physiology. II. Iodine collection by normal and hyperplastic thyroids in rabbits. *Am. J. Physiol.* 128: 565, 1940; Hamilton, J. G., and Soley, M. H. Studies in iodine metabolism of the thyroid gland in situ by the use of radioiodine in normal subjects and in patients with various types of goiter. *Am. J. Physiol.* 131: 135, 1940). Hertz and Roberts (Application of radioactive iodine in therapy of Graves' disease. *J. Clin. Invest.* 21: 624, 1942) first made a brief note on the treatment of Graves's disease in man, but later gave a fuller report on twenty-nine cases. The details of the procedure were told, and it was concluded that the treatment was highly effective in about 80 percent of the cases. Similar results were reported at the same time by E.. M. Chapman and R. D. Evans (The treatment of hyperthyroidism with radioactive iodine. *J.A.M.A.* 131: 86, 1946). See also Bloomfield, *A Bibliography of Internal Medicine: Selected Diseases,* p. 178.

46. Beecher, H. K., and Altschule, M. D. *Medicine at Harvard: The First Three Hundred Years,* p. 299. Hanover, N.H.: University Press of New England, 1977.

47. Zamecnik, P. Presentation of the Kober Medal to Joseph Charles Aub. *Trans. Assoc. Am. Physicians* 79: 84, 1966.

Joseph C. Aub graduated from the Harvard Medical School in 1915. His contact with Walter B. Cannon in the physiology course (1911) introduced him to research. Cannon was interested in the effect of epinephrine on the gastrointestinal tract. Aub and Binger studied the influence of smoking on the flow of epinephrine. It was shown that nicotine stimulated the flow of epinephrine. Aub (with Cannon and Binger) published his first research paper in the *Journal of Pharmacology and Experimental Therapeutics* (3: 379, 1912).

After graduation, Aub interned at the MGH, where he met Edsall and Means. He worked with DuBois from 1915 to 1916, a period when the concepts of basal metabolism and calorimetry were being applied to human problems. An important study, The Basal Metabolism of Dwarfs and Legless Men with Observations on the Specific Dynamic Action of Protein (*Arch. Intern. Med.* 19: 865, 1917) and another, written with Means, Studies of Exophthalmic Goiter from the Point of View of the Basal Metabolism (*J.A.M.A.* 69: 33, 1917), forecasted Aub's growing interest in the metabolism of all the organs of internal secretion.

48. Means, *Ward 4,* p. 23.

49. Aub, J. C., Minot, A. S., Fairhall, L. T., and Resnikoff, P. *Lead Poisoning.* Medicine Monographs, Volume 7. Baltimore: Williams & Wilkins, 1925.

Means, *Ward 4,* p. 23.

50. Albright, F., Bauer, W., Ropes, M., and Aub, J. C. Studies of calcium and phosphorus metabolism. IV. The effects of the parathyroid hormone. *J. Clin. Invest.* 7: 139, 1929.

Albright, F., Burnett, C. H., Parson, W., Reifenstein, E. C., Jr., and Roos, A. Osteomalacia and late rickets. The various etiologies met in the United States with emphasis on that resulting from a specific form of renal acidosis, the therapeutic indications for each etiological sub-group, and the relationship between osteomalacia and Milkman's syndrome. *Medicine* 25: 399, 1946.

Aub, J. C., and Farquharson, R. F. Studies of calcium and phosphorus metabolism. XV. In various metabolic and bone diseases. *J. Clin. Invest.* 11: 235, 1932.

Bauer, W., Albright, F., and Aub, J. C. Metabolic study II. A case of osteitis fibrosa cystica (osteomalacia?) with evidence of hyperactivity of the parathyroid bodies. *J. Clin. Invest.* 8: 229, 1929.

Bauer, W., and Marble, A. Studies on the mode of action of irradiated ergosterol. II. Its effect on the calcium and phosphorus metabolism of individuals with calcium deficiency diseases. *J. Clin. Invest.* 11: 21, 1932.

51. Albright, F. A page out of the history of hyperparathyroidism. *J. Clin. Endocrinol.* 8: 637, 1948.

Bauer, W., and Federman, D. D. Hyperparathyroidism epitomized: The case of Captain Charles E. Martell. *Metabolism* 11: 21, 1962.

Means, *Ward 4,* p. 32.

52. Farquharson, R. F., Salter, W. T., Tibbetts, D. M., and Aub, J. C. Studies of calcium and phosphorus metabolism. XII. The effect of the ingestion of acid-producing substances. *J. Clin. Invest.* 10: 221, 1931.

53. Forbes, A. P. In appreciation, Fuller Albright. *Metabolism* 11: 1, 1962.

Harvey, *Interurban Clinical Club,* p. 248.

Howard, J. E. Fuller Albright, 1900–1969. *Trans. Assoc. Am. Physicians* 85: 10, 1972.

54. Albright, F., Aub, J. C., and Bauer, W. Hyperparathyroidism. A common and polymorphic condition as illustrated by seventeen proved cases from one clinic. *J.A.M.A.* 102: 1276, 1934.

Albright, F., Baird, P. C., Cope, O., and Bloomberg, E. Studies on the physiology of the parathyroid glands. IV. Renal complications of hyperparathyroidism. *Am. J. Med. Sci.* 187: 49, 1934.

55. Albright, F., and Ellsworth, R. Studies on the physiology of the parathyroid glands. I. Calcium and phosphorus studies on a case of idiopathic hypoparathyroidism. *J. Clin. Invest.* 7: 183, 1929.

56. Reifenstein, E. C., Jr., and Albright, F. The metabolic effect of steroid hormones in osteoporosis. *J. Clin. Invest.* 26: 24, 1947.

57. Albright, F. Cushing's syndrome: Its pathological physiology; its relationship to the adreno-genital syndrome and its connection with the problem of the reaction of the body to injurious agents ("Alarm reaction" of Selye). *Harvey Lecture Series* 38: 123, 1942–43.

58. Faxon, N. W. *The Massachusetts General Hospital: Its Development, 1935–1955.* Cambridge, Mass.: Harvard University Press, 1959.

Richards, D. W., Jr. Walter Bauer. *Trans. Assoc. Am. Physicians* 77: 9, 1964.

59. Churchill, E. D., *The Reminiscences of J. Collins Warren, 1842–1927*, p. 229. Cambridge, Mass.: Harvard University Press, 1958.

60. Ibid.

61. Ibid., p. 232.

62. Ibid, p. 235.

63. With Robley Evans (a physicist from MIT), Aub initiated a study of radium excretion in 1936. This involved some patients who had ingested radium salts in the course of "pointing" their brushes while painting luminous watch dials, and others who had taken radium salts for arthritis. An effort was made to promote radium excretion, based on its close metabolic resemblance to lead and calcium. These studies were not successful, because radium ingested so long before had become fixed in the metabolically inert bone cortex. In a physicist who had inhaled radium salt in a recent laboratory explosion, however, the excretion-promoting program was more effective. These investigations lit the first therapeutic candle for the atomic era, and, at a meeting at the Argonne Laboratories twenty years later, Aub was hailed as the father of all of the subsequent work on the elimination of radioactive substances. (Zamecnik, P. Presentation of the Kober Medal for 1966 to Joseph Charles Aub. *Trans. Assoc. Am. Physicians* 79: 84, 1966.)

64. McCord, D. *The Fabrick of Man. Fifty Years of the Peter Bent Brigham Hospital, 1913–1963.* Portland: Anthaenson Press, 1963.

When the Harvard Medical School moved to its new quarters on Boylston Street, it was no longer in close proximity to the MGH. The move emphasized the interdigitation of the two institutions; this recognition became more evident in 1886, when Robert T. Edes resigned from the Jackson Professorship of Clinical Medicine. At that time the question arose as to the advisability of selecting his successor from another clinical center. After some discussion among the trustees, it was generally agreed that such a selection was not practicable, owing to the inability to provide clinical facilities for a teacher who was not already a member of a local hospital staff. Shortly before, the University of Pennsylvania, which had a hospital of its own, had been able to appoint William Osler to a professorship of medicine, calling him from McGill University. A few years later, when the faculty of the new Johns Hopkins University School of Medicine was being organized, the availability of a university-controlled hospital enabled that institution to select the most able talent, wherever it happened to be found. At Harvard, the necessity for a more intimate understanding between school and hospital was felt more strongly by the medical faculty as time went on. President Eliot, in his report for 1888–89, recommended a more intimate union of school and hospital:

> The question before the Governing Board of the University is—not who is the best man for the place in Boston or elsewhere—but who is the most available man as a teacher among the Boston practitioners already holding cognate appointments given by other Boards of Trustees, who in making their selection had teaching not at all in mind. More than once this limitation of choice has proved unfortunate. More than once the school and community have lost an important

medical reinforcement because the school was not in a position to offer to the desired person an adequate hospital appointment as well as a professorship.

A committee was appointed to find a way of accomplishing this end. Negotiations were opened with the trustees of the MGH early in 1890. It was pointed out that the hospital had had its origin in a demand both for the relief of the sick poor and for the advance of medical knowledge. It was suggested that the university donate the old building at the head of Grove Street to the hospital, in exchange for the privilege of a nomination for a hospital appointment in connection with the organization of the academic departments of medicine and surgery. After a lengthy deliberation, the trustees were unable to come to a favorable decision on the matter.

The faculty committee then considered the feasibility of establishing a hospital under complete control of the school. In November 1890, the committee reported favorably upon the project, but the magnitude of the undertaking made it seem advisable to consider other possibilities. About this time, Bowditch, then dean of the faculty, discovered a possible solution in the will of Peter Bent Brigham, who had died in 1877. Money had been left by him for a hospital for the sick poor of the city of Boston. The will provided that this money should be held by his executors for twenty-five years, at which time the funds would be sufficiently large to carry out the intention of the testator. The expiration of this twenty-five year period seemed far distant but, inasmuch as any scheme would involve preparation of an entirely new plan, the element of time did not constitute a serious obstacle. After careful consideration, the faculty became convinced that there was nothing impracticable about the plan, and, during the following decade, they kept constantly in mind the possibility of taking an ambitious forward step. Meanwhile, the expansion of the school's laboratory work had gone on rapidly, and a new generation was identifying itself with scientific medicine. The medical department needed a more elaborate system of laboratory accommodations and, most important of all, an association with hospital facilities of a varied character. Fortunately, the date for the employment of this bequest for the building of a hospital was growing near. By the time the Peter Bent Brigham Hospital was finally completed, William Henry Welch was able to say, in his address on Founder's Day (November 12, 1914), that "the time has gone by when the great clinicians, those who stand before the community as the great consultants, can at the same time be the heads of departments in schools and hospitals. Theirs is a different career." The readjustments occasioned during this change caused many heartaches and led to bitter misunderstandings. (Churchill, ed., *The Reminiscences of J. Collins Warren,* p. 193.)

65. Harvey, *Interurban Clinical Club,* p. 79.

66. Fulton, J. F. *Harvey Cushing, a Biography.* Springfield, Ill.: Charles C Thomas, 1946.

67. McCord, *The Fabrick of Man,* p. 32.

68. For Christian's biography, see Harvey, *Interurban Clinical Club,* p. 79.

69. McCord, *The Fabrick of Man,* p. 34. See also:

Blake, F. G. The etiology of rat-bite fever. *J. Exp. Med.* 23: 39, 1916.

Blake, F. G. The formation of methemoglobin by streptococcus viridans. *J. Exp. Med.* 24: 315, 1916.

Blumgart, H. L. The antidiuretic effect of pituitary extract applied intranasally in a case of diabetes insipidus. *Arch. Intern. Med.* 29: 508, 1922.

Bryan, A. H., Evans, W. A., Jr., Fulton, M. N., and Stead, E. A., Jr. Diuresis following the administration of salyrgan. Its effect on the specific gravity, the total nitrogen and the colloid osmotic pressure of the plasma of normal and of edematous dogs. *Arch. Intern. Med.* 55: 735, 1935.

Dock, W., and Harrison, T. R. The blood-flow through the lungs in experimental pneumothorax. *Am. Rev. Tuberc.* 10: 534, 1924–25.

Evans, W. A., Jr., and Gibson, J. G., II. The blood volume in diuresis. A study employing the colloidal blue dye T-1824 in dogs rendered edematous by plasmapheresis. *Am. J. Physiol.* 118: 251, 1937.

Folin, O., Berglund, H., and Derick, C. The uric acid problems: An experimental study on animals and man, including gouty subjects. *J. Biol. Chem.* 60: 351, 1924.

Gibson, J. G., II, and Evans, W. A., Jr. Clinical studies of the blood volume. III. Changes in blood volume, venous pressure and blood velocity rate in chronic congestive heart failure. *J. Clin. Invest.* 16: 851, 1937.

Grant, S. B. Tetany. A report of cases with acid-base disturbance. *Arch. Intern. Med.* 30: 355, 1922.

Grant, S. B. The role of anoxemia in the causation of tetany during hyperpnea. *Am. J. Physiol.* 66: 274, 1923.

Grant, S. B. A study of the blood oxygen in diabetes mellitus. *Arch. Intern. Med.* 32: 764, 1923.

Grant, S. B., and Goldman, A. A study of forced respiration: experimental production of tetany. *Am. J. Physiol.* 52: 209, 1920.

Harrison, T. R., Dock, W., and Holman, E. Experimental studies in arteriovenous fistulae: Cardiac output. *Heart* 11: 337, 1924.

Isaacs, R. Properties of young erythrocytes in relation to agglutination and their behavior in hemorrhage and transfusion. *Arch. Intern. Med.* 33: 193, 1924.

Lyons, R. H., Kennedy, J. A., and Burwell, C. S. The measurement of venous pressure by the direct method. *Am. Heart J.* 16: 675, 1938.

Massie, E., Ethridge, C. B., and O'Hare, J. P. Thiocyanate therapy in vascular hypertension. *N. Engl. J. Med.* 219: 736, 1938.

Starr, P., and Fitz, R. The excretion of organic acids in the urine of patients with diabetes mellitus. *Arch. Intern. Med.* 33: 97, 1924.

Sturgis, C. C., and Greene, J. A. Nutritional changes in exophthalmic goiter: The effect of Lugol's solution. *Arch. Intern. Med.* 36: 561, 1925.

Sturgis, C. C., and Tompkins, E. H. A study of the correlation of the basal metabolism and pulse rate in patients with exophthalmic goiter. *Med. Rec.* 98: 165, 1920.

Sturgis, C. C., Wearn, J. T., and Tompkins, E. H. Effects of the injection of atropin on the pulse rate, blood pressure and basal metabolism in cases of "effort syndrome." *Am. J. Med. Sci.* 158: 496, 1919.

Tompkins, E. H., Sturgis, C. C., and Wearn, J. T. Studies on epinephrin. II. The effects of epinephrin on the basal metabolism in soldiers with "irritable heart" in hyperthyroidism and in normal men. *Arch. Intern. Med.* 24: 269, 1919.

Wearn, J. T. Thrombosis of the coronary arteries with infarction of the heart. *Am. J. Med. Sci.* 165: 250, 1923.

Wearn, J. T., Warren, S., and Ames, O. The length of life of transfused erythrocytes in patients with primary and secondary anemia. *Arch. Intern. Med.* 29: 527, 1922.

70. McCord, *The Fabrick of Man.*

71. Peabody, F. W. *J. Clin. Invest.* 5: 1, 1927.

Warthin, A. S. Francis Weld Peabody. *Trans. Assoc. Am. Physicians* 48: 12, 1928.

Williams, T. F. Cabot, Peabody and the care of the patient. *Bull. Hist. Med.* 24: 462, 1950.

72. Cabot, R. C. Joseph H. Pratt, an appreciation. Anniversary volume. Scientific contributions in honor of Joseph Hersey Pratt on his sixty-fifth birthday. Lancaster, Pa.: Lancaster Press, 1937.

Ceremony in honor of Joseph Hersey Pratt, M.D. on the occasion of his sixty-fifth birthday. December 5, 1937. Brochure with portrait. Privately printed.

Harvey, *Interurban Clinical Club,* p. 20.

Proger, S. Dr. Joseph Hersey Pratt. *N. Engl. J. Med.* 254: 920, 1956.

Rackemann, F. M. Joseph Hersey Pratt, M.D. *Trans. Am. Clin. Climatol. Assoc.* 68: xlviii, 1956.

Spector, B. Joseph Hersey Pratt, M.D., Sc.D. *Bull. Hist. Med.* 30: 473, 1956.

73. Pratt, J. H. The personality of the physician. *N. Engl. J. Med.* 214: 364, 1936.

74. Peabody, F. W. The bacteriologic diagnosis of typhoid fever. *J.A.M.A.* 51: 978, 1908. (This paper was read at the joint meeting of the Section on Practice of Medicine and

the Section on Pathology and Physiology of the AMA at the fifty-ninth Annual Session at Chicago, June 1908.)

75. Pratt, The personality of the physician.

76. Boothby, W. M. and Peabody, F. W. A comparison of methods of obtaining alveolar air. *Arch. Intern. Med.* 13: 497, 1914.

Drinker, C. K., Peabody, F. W., and Blumgart, H. L. The effect of pulmonary congestion on the ventilation of the lungs. *J. Exp. Med.* 35: 77, 1922.

Peabody, F. W. Studies on acidosis and dyspnea in renal and cardiac disease. *Arch. Intern. Med.* 14: 236, 1914.

Peabody, F. W. Some aspects of the clinical study of the respiration: The significance of alveolar air analyses. *Am. J. Med. Sci.* 151: 184, 1916.

Peabody, F. W., Meyer, A. L., DuBois, E. F., and Soderstrom, G. F. Clinical calorimetry: The basal metabolism of patients with cardiac and renal disease. *Arch. Intern. Med.* 17: 980, 1916.

Peabody, F. W., Sturgis, C. C., Barker, B. I., and Read, M. N. Clinical studies on the respiration. IX. The effect of normal subjects and patients with heart disease. *Arch. Intern. Med.* 29: 277, 1922.

Peabody, F. W., and Wentworth, J. A. The vital capacity of the lungs, and its relation to dyspnea in heart disease. *Trans. Assoc. Am. Physicians* 31: 433, 1916.

77. Rackemann, F. R. Isaac Chandler Walker. *Trans. Assoc. Am. Physicians* 64: 23, 1951.

78. Walker, I. C. Studies on the cause and the treatment of bronchial asthma. *J.A.M.A.* 69: 363, 1917.

Following the brilliant suggestion of Meltzer, numerous workers developed the idea of an allergic reaction as the cause of asthmatic attacks. Walker developed the skin test as a means of detecting the cause of an attack. He found that attacks of asthma could be produced by proteins to which the patient was sensitive. He obtained good results by "desensitization" with repeated small injections of the offending agent.

Walker, I. C., and Adkinson, J. Study XIII. The relationship between the cutaneous reaction, serum agglutination tests and bacterial examination of the sputum and nasal secretions in determining the part staphylococcus pyogenes aureus and albus play in the cause of bronchial asthma. *J. Med. Res.* 36: 295, 1917.

79. Levine, S. A. Channing Frothingham, 1881–1959. *Trans. Assoc. Am. Physicians* 73: 11, 1960.

80. Composed of the medical chiefs of the Massachusetts General, Peter Bent Brigham, Boston City, and Beth Israel hospitals.

81. Denny, G. P., and Frothingham, C., Jr. Experimental arterial disease in rabbits. *J. Med. Res.* 31: 277, 1914–15.

Frothingham, C., Jr. A glomerular and arterial lesion produced in rabbits' kidneys by diphtheria toxin. *J. Med. Res.* 30: 365, 1914.

Frothingham, C., Jr., and Smillie, W. G. The relation between the phenolsulphonephthalein excretion in the urine and the non-protein nitrogen content of the blood in human cases. *Arch. Intern. Med.* 14: 541, 1914.

82. Eppinger, E. C. Clifford Lambie Derick, 1894–1972. *Trans. Assoc. Am. Physicians* 86: 10, 1973.

83. Derick, C. L., and Fulton, M. N. Skin reactions of patients and normal individuals to protein extracts of streptococci. *J. Clin. Invest.* 10: 121, 1931.

Swift, H. F., Derick, C. L., and Hitchcock, C. H. Bacterial allergy (hyperergy) to nonhemolytic streptococci and its relation to rheumatic fever. *J.A.M.A.* 90: 906, 1928.

84. Thorn, G. W. James P. O'Hare, 1886–1974. *Trans. Assoc. Am. Physicians* 91: 44, 1978.

85. Massie, E., Ethridge, C. B., and O'Hare, J. P. Thiocyanate therapy in vascular hypertension. *N. Engl. J. Med.* 219: 736, 1938.

O'Hare, J. P. Study XXIV. The effect of theobromin sodium salicylate in acute chromate nephritis. *Arch. Intern. Med.* 15: 1053, 1915.

Shelburne, S. A., Blain, D., and O'Hare, J. P. The spinal fluid in hypertension. *J. Clin. Invest.* 11: 489, 1932.

86. Cutler, E. C., Levine, S. A., and Beck, C. S. The surgical treatment of mitral stenosis. Experimental and clinical studies. *Arch. Surg.* 9: 689, 1924.

The appearance of fibrillating auricles experimentally induced had been familiar to experimenters for a long time. No one knew whether fibrillation in humans presented the same characteristics. In 1924 these authors gave a graphic description of human auricles in a state of fibrillation in a patient with mitral stenosis, in whom they attempted valvulotomy: "The right auricle was enormously dilated, blue in color, and in complete rest, without even fibrillary motions running across it. The right auricular appendage from time to time showed irregular convulsive contractions." The left auricle was similarly immobile. Now, of course, with open heart surgery, fibrillating auricles are seen every day. (Bloomfield, *A Bibliography of Internal Medicine: Selected Diseases,* p. 12.)

Levine, S. A. Observations on sino-auricular heart block. *Arch. Intern. Med.* 17: 153, 1916.

Levine, S. A., Cutler, E. C., and Eppinger, E. C. Thyroidectomy in the treatment of advanced congestive heart failure and angina pectoris. *N. Engl. J. Med.* 209: 667, 1933.

Levine, S. A., and Wilson, F. N. Observations on the vital capacity of the lungs in cases of "irritable heart." *Heart* 7: 53, 1918-19.

87. Derick, C. L. Gustave Philip Grabfield, 1892-1965. *Trans. Assoc. Am. Physicians* 79: 47, 1966.

Grabfield, G. P. *American Men of Science,* 11th ed., p. 1901.

88. Grabfield, G. P. II. Observations on the nitrogen and sulphur excretion in patients without renal edema. *J. Clin. Invest.* 10: 309, 1931.

Grabfield, G. P. Experimental observations on function of the renal nerves. *Trans. Assoc. Am. Physicians* 51: 331, 1936.

Grabfield, G. P. Effect of certain polyhydric alcohols and sugars on purine excretion. *Trans. Assoc. Am. Physicians* 54: 91, 1939.

89. Burwell, C. S. Reginald Fitz, 1885-1953. *Trans. Assoc. Am. Physicians* 67: 12, 1954.

Fitz, R. The value of tests for renal function in early and advanced Bright's disease. *Med. Rec.* 85: 682, 1914.

Fitz, R. Study XXIII. The relation between amylase retention and excretion and non-protein nitrogen retention in experimental uranium nephritis. *Arch. Intern. Med.* 15: 524, 1915.

Harvey, *Interurban Clinical Club,* p. 131.

Quinby, W. C., and Fitz, R. Observations on renal function in acute experimental unilateral nephritis. *Arch. Intern. Med.* 15: 303, 1915.

90. Minot, G. R., and Murphy, W. P. Treatment of pernicious anemia by a special diet. *J.A.M.A.* 87: 470, 1926.

Minot, G. R., Murphy, W. P., and Stetson, R. P. The response of the reticulocytes to liver therapy, particularly in pernicious anemia. *Am. J. Med. Sci.* 175: 581, 1928.

Murphy, W. P., Fitz, R., and Monroe, R. D. Physiological aspects of patients with pernicious anemia partaking of a special diet. *Trans. Assoc. Am. Physicians* 41: 73, 1926.

Murphy, W. P. *American Men of Science,* 8th ed, p. 1785.

91. Castle, W. B. Soma Weiss, *Trans. Assoc. Am. Physicians* 57: 36, 1942.

92. Weiss, S., and Hatcher, R. A. The mechanism of the vomiting induced by antimony and potassium tartrate (tartar emetic). *J. Exp. Med.* 37: 97, 1923.

93. Warren, J. V. The legacy of Soma Weiss. *N. Engl. J. Med.* 286: 658, 1972.

Warren, J. V. Personal communication, 1979.

94. Byrne, J. J., ed., *A History of the Boston City Hospital, 1905-1964,* pp. 57-89, 91-92. Boston: Sheldon Press, 1964.

95. Means, J. H. George Gray Sears, 1859-1940. *Trans. Assoc. Am. Physicians* 56: 26, 1941.

96. King, J. T., Jr. Henry M. Thomas, Jr., 1891-1966. *Trans. Assoc. Am. Physicians* 80: 27, 1967.

97. Peabody, F. W. Thorndike Memorial Laboratory. In *Methods and Problems of Medical Education,* vol. 1, p. 113, Chicago: Rockefeller Foundation, 1924.

98. Castle, W. B. Henry Jackson, Jr. *Trans. Assoc. Am. Physicians* 82: 37, 1969.

99. Blumgart, H. L., and Weiss, S. II. The velocity of blood flow in normal resting individuals, and a critique of the method used. *J. Clin. Invest.* 4: 15, 1927.

Broun, G. O., Ames, O., Warren, S., and Peabody, F. W. Blood pigments in pernicious anemia. *J. Clin. Invest.* 1: 295, 1924.

Jackson, H., Jr., and Moore, O. J. The effect of high protein diets on the remaining kidney of rats. *J. Clin. Invest.* 5: 415, 1927–28.

Long, P. H. Effect of phenylhydrazine derivatives in the treatment of polycythemia. *J. Clin. Invest.* 2: 315, 1925–26.

Muller, G. L. The influence of a diet, high in butter fat, on growth, blood formation and blood destruction. *J. Clin. Invest.* 5: 521, 1927–28.

Weiss, S., and Blumgart, H. L. The effect of the digitalis bodies on the velocity of blood flow through the lungs and on other aspects of the circulation. A study of normal subjects and patients with cardiovascular disease. *J. Clin. Invest.* 7: 11, 1929.

100. Peabody, F. W. The pathology of the bone marrow in pernicious anemia. *Am. J. Pathol.* 3: 179, 1927.

I. Zadek (Blut- und Knochenmark befunde am Lebenden bei Kryptogenetischer perniciöser Anämie, insbesondere im Stadium der Remission. *Ztschr. f. klin. Med.* 95: 66, 1922) studied the bone marrow in relapse and during spontaneous remission. He concluded that "the change from (physiological) fatty marrow into (pathological) megaloblastic marrow during relapse and its return to fatty marrow during the period of remission is demonstrated." With the advent of liver therapy, Peabody showed the same to hold in the controlled induced remission. "The essential lesion . . . which dominates the histological picture during clinical relapse is an hyperplasia of the myeloid cells in which the megaloblasts play the chief part."

After his initial paper, Minot modified his thoughts as to the rationale of liver therapy and emphasized Peabody's recent studies: "Apparently the masses of megaloblasts found in the marrow in pernicious anemia during a relapse are unable to mature properly and it is a logical deduction to assume that they lack some factor on which this maturation depends." (Bloomfield, *A Bibliography of Internal Medicine: Selected Diseases,* pp. 65, 75.)

101. This was the first use of a radioisotope (radon C) in medical research, for which Blumgart later was honored by the American Society of Nuclear Medicine.

102. Castle, W. B. Presentation of the Kober Medal for 1965 to Joseph Treloar Wearn. *Trans. Assoc. Am. Physicians* 78: 39, 1965.

Harvey, *Interurban Clinical Club,* p. 179.

Wearn, J. T. The role of the Thebesian vessels in the circulation of the heart. *J. Exp. Med.* 47: 493, 1928.

Wearn, J. T. Acceptance of the Kober Medal for 1965. *Trans. Assoc. Am. Physicians* 78: 48, 1965.

103. Peabody, F. W. *Doctor and Patient.* New York: Macmillan, 1930.

104. Castle, W. B. Functional stresses within full-time departments of medicine. Presidential address. *Trans. Assoc. Am. Physicians* 73: 1, 1960.

105. Alfred E. Cohn to Simon Flexner, August 1, 1928. (Flexner papers, American Philosophical Society, Philadelphia.)

This letter is reproduced, as is that of Peabody to Longcope, in Benison, S. *Tom Rivers: Reflections on a Life in Medicine and Science: An Oral History Memoir,* pp. 102–7. Cambridge, Mass.: M.I.T. Press, 1967.

106. Castle, W. B. George Richards Minot, 1885–1950. *Trans. Assoc. Am. Physicians* 63: 11, 1950.

Castle, W. B. Contributions of George Richards Minot to experimental medicine. *N. Engl. J. Med.* 247: 585, 1952.

Harvey, *Interurban Clinical Club,* p. 122.

Kober, G. Presentation of the Kober Medal to George Richards Minot. *Trans. Assoc. Am. Physicians* 44: 7, 1929.

Minot, G. R. Remarks on accepting the Kober Medal. *Trans. Assoc. Am. Physicians* 44: 11, 1929.

Minot, G. R. Development of liver treatment in pernicious anemia. *Lancet* 1: 361, 1935. (Nobel Lecture.)

Minot, G. R., and Murphy, W. P. Treatment of pernicious anemia by a special diet. *J.A.M.A.* 87: 470, 1926.

Minot's first papers did not deal strictly with liver, but with a diet rich in liver. The diet (Murphy, W. P., and Minot, G. R. A special diet for patients with pernicious anemia. *Boston Med. Surg. J.* 195: 410, 1926) included much more than liver, although it turned out that only liver contained the specific effective substance.

By the time Minot and Murphy's second paper (A diet rich in liver in the treatment of pernicious anemia. *J.A.M.A.* 89: 759, 1927) appeared, there were already confirmatory reports. E. J. Cohn and his associates (I. The nature of the material in liver effective in pernicious anemia. *J. Biol. Chem.* 74: lxix, 1927) had reported that the potent fraction was not a protein, and that it was effective in minute amounts.

> Liver was chosen as a food in the hope that it might contain ingredients that would promote the growth of red blood cells, because it had been shown that liver feeding could profoundly affect the growth of animals, and that substances within it could enhance cell division.
>
> Another reason for its choice was the demonstration by Whipple and his associates that liver exerted a striking effect on the regeneration of hemoglobin. In pernicious anemia, however, it has appeared to us [Minot and Murphy] that what the patients needed was something to permit the growth of red blood cells, or, as Whipple has suggested, to supply their stroma, rather than something that particularly caused regeneration of hemoglobin.
>
> Thus, it may be that pernicious anemia is a disease that arises in a predisposed person because of a lack of unavailability in the body of something that permits the proper growth of blood cells. The lack of this, which may be a rather specific substance, is perhaps responsible for other lesions than those in the bone marrow, for example, degeneration of the spinal cord. (Bloomfield, *A Bibliography of Internal Medicine: Selected Diseases,* p. 74)

Rackemann, F. M. George Richards Minot. *Trans. Am. Clin. Climatol. Assoc.* 62: xlix, 1950.

107. Weiss, S., Dexter, L., Parker, F., Jr., and Tenney, B., Jr. Arterial hypertension in pregnancy and the hypertensive toxemia syndrome of pregnancy (preëclampsia and eclampsia). *Trans. Assoc. Am. Physicians* 55: 282, 1940.

Weiss, S., Ferris, E. B., Jr., and Capps, R. B. Influence of reflexes in induction of intracardiac disturbances. *Trans. Assoc. Am. Physicians* 49: 177, 1934.

Weiss, S., and Parker, F., Jr. Vascular changes in pyelonephritis and their relation to arterial hypertension. *Trans. Assoc. Am. Physicians* 53: 60, 1938.

Weiss, S., and Wilkins, R. W. Nature of cardiovascular disturbances in vitamin deficiency states. *Trans. Assoc. Am. Physicians* 51: 341, 1936.

108. Jackson, H., Jr., and Parker, F., Jr. *Hodgkin's Disease and Allied Disorders.* New York: Oxford University Press, 1947.

109. Castle, W. B. Curriculum vitae and bibliography. *Arch. Intern. Med.* 101: 175, 1928.

Castle, W. B. The aetiological relationship of achylia gastrica to pernicious anemia. *Proc. R. Soc. Med.* 22: 1214, 1929.

Castle, W. B. Acceptance of the Kober Medal. *Trans. Assoc. Am. Physicians* 75: 54, 1962.

Castle, W. B. Achylia gastrica in retrospect. *Am. J. Med. Sci.* 267: 25, 1974.

Castle, W. B. Maurice B. Strauss, 1904-1974. *Trans. Assoc. Am. Physicians* 87: 36, 1974.

Castle, W. B. The Story behind the Story. Personal communication to A. McGehee Harvey from William B. Castle. February 25, 1976.

Castle, W. B., and Rhoads, C. P. Observations on etiology and treatment of sprue in Puerto Rico. *Trans. Assoc. Am. Physicians* 47: 245, 1932.

Ham, T. H., and Castle, W. B. Relation of increased hypotonic fragility and of erythrostasis to the mechanisms of hemolysis in certain anemias. *Trans. Assoc. Am. Physicians* 55: 127, 1940.

Harvey, *Interurban Clinical Club,* p. 199.

Heath, C. W., Strauss, M. B., and Castle, W. B. Quantitative aspects of iron deficiency in hypochromic anemia (the parenteral administration of iron). *J. Clin. Invest.* 11: 1293, 1932.

Means, J. H. Presentation of the Kober Medal for 1962 to William Bosworth Castle. *Trans. Assoc. Am. Physicians* 75: 48, 1962.

Strauss, M. B. Of medicine, men and molecules: Wedlock or divorce. *Medicine* 43: 619, 1964.

110. Davidson, C. S. Presentation of the Kober Medal for 1978 to Maxwell Finland. *Trans. Assoc. Am. Physicians* 91: 51, 1978.

Finland's long-term studies of pneumonia illustrate the importance of careful clinical studies in the critical evaluation of the various therapeutic agents. While "pneumonia resident," Finland worked with Milton Rosenau in the department of preventive medicine and hygiene at Harvard, where concentrated antipneumococcus serum was being produced by Lloyd D. Felton. During these studies, Rosenau trained many physicians who later became successful clinical scientists. The successes in diagnosis of pneumococcal pneumonia by typing, and its treatment by antisera, was followed by studies of the sulfonamides. Finland and his coworkers also studied primary atypical pneumonia due to the Eaton agent (*Mycoplasma pneumoniae*). The observation by Oscar Peterson of red cell agglutination in the cold by serum of patients with this disease led to a classic series of papers by Finland and T. Hale Ham on this subject, beginning in 1943.

Finland's contributions continued with the study of new sulfonamides and then of penicillin and the tetracyclines, with data not only on their clinical efficacy but also on their clinical pharmacology. Finland was among the first to recognize the emergence of hospital-acquired staphylococcal infections and their increasing antibiotic resistance in the 1950s. Later, the age of the gram negative infections was also recognized. The value of long-continued observations is illustrated by Finland's description of the cyclical change in the prevalence and virulence of staphylococcal disease. Finland had kept data, and preserved specimens in the deep freeze, for more than thirty-five years. This remarkable story has emerged from more than fifty years of continuous, careful study of community and hospital infections, their cause, their treatment with antibacterial drugs, and the effects of these drugs upon the prevalence of the infections seen. See *Journal of Infectious Diseases,* Vol. 135: March 1977.

Finland, M. Acceptance of the Kober Medal for 1978. *Trans. Assoc. Am. Physicians* 91: 63, 1978.

Finland, M., and Ruegsegger, J. M. Immunization of human subjects with the specific carbohydrates of type III and the related type VIII pneumococcus. *J. Clin. Invest.* 14: 829, 1935.

Finland, M., and Winkler, A. W. Antibody response to infections with type III and the related type VIII pneumococcus. *J. Clin. Invest.* 13: 79, 1934.

Winkler, A. W., and Finland, M. Antibody response to infections with the newly classified types of pneumococci (Cooper). *J. Clin. Invest.* 13: 109, 1934.

111. Harvey, *Interurban Clinical Club,* p. 254.

Wainwright, C. W. Chester Scott Keefer, 1897–1972. *Trans. Am. Clin. Climatol. Assoc.* 84: xxxiii, 1972.

Wilkins, R. W. Chester Scott Keefer, 1897–1972. *Trans. Assoc. Am. Physicians* 85: 24, 1972.

112. Keefer, C. S., Holmes, W. F., Jr., and Myers, W. K. The inhibition of tryptic digestion of cartilage by synovial fluid from patients with various types of arthritis. *J. Clin. Invest.* 14: 131, 1935.

Keefer, C. S. and Spink, W. W. Gonococcic arthritis: Pathogenesis, mechanism of recovery and treatment. *J.A.M.A.* 109: 1448, 1937.

Myers, W. K., and Keefer, C. S. Antistreptolysin content of the blood serum in rheumatic fever and rheumatoid arthritis. *J. Clin. Invest.* 13: 155, 1934.

Myers, W. K., Keefer, C. S., and Oppel, T. W. Skin reactions to nucleoprotein of streptococcus scarlatinae in patients with rheumatoid arthritis and rheumatic fever. *J. Clin. Invest.* 12: 279, 1933.

Oppel, T. W., Myers, W. K., and Keefer, C. S. The sedimentation rate of the red blood cells in various types of arthritis. *J. Clin. Invest.* 12: 291, 1933.

113. Vilter, R. Eugene Beverly Ferris, 1905–1957. *Trans. Assoc. Am. Physicians* 71: 25, 1958.

114. Rammelkamp, C. H., Jr. Richard B. Capps, 1906–1976. *Trans. Assoc. Am. Physicians* 91: 21, 1978.

115. Castle, W. B. Maurice B. Strauss, 1904–1974. *Trans. Assoc. Am. Physicians* 87: 36, 1974.

116. Kimmelstiel, P., and Wilson, C. Intracapillary lesions in glomeruli of the kidney. *Am. J. Pathol.* 12: 83, 1936.

117. Ham, T. H. *American Men of Science,* 11th ed., p. 2061.

118. Kass, L. William B. Castle and intrinsic factor. *Ann. Intern. Med.* 89: 983, 1978.

119. Castle, The Story behind the Story.

120. Strauss, Of medicine, men and molecules.

121. Flint, A. A clinical lecture on anaemia. *Am. Med. Times* 1: 181, 1860.

122. Castle, W. B. A century of curiosity about pernicious anemia. *Trans. Am. Clin. Climatol. Assoc.* 73: 54, 1961; idem, Achylia gastrica in retrospect.

123. Finland, M. The Harvard Medical Unit of the Boston City Hospital. *Harvard Med. Alumni Bull.* 39: no. 1, Fall 1964.

124. Harvey, *Interurban Clinical Club,* p. 196.

125. Adams, R. D., Binger, C. A., Castle, W. B., et al. Memorial minute adopted by the faculty of medicine of Harvard University. May 23, 1969.

Cobb, S. Electromyographic studies of clonus. *Bull. Johns Hopkins Hosp.* 29: 247, 1918.

Harvey, *Interurban Clinical Club,* p. 196.

126. Lennox, W., and Lennox, M. *Epilepsy.* Boston: Little, Brown, 1960.

127. Cobb, S. Acceptance of the Kober Medal for 1956. *Trans. Assoc. Am. Physicians* 69: 41, 1956.

Wolff, H. G. Presentation of the George M. Kober Medal to Stanley Cobb. *Trans. Assoc. Am. Physicians* 69: 34, 1956.

128. Freedberg, A. S. Personal communication, 1977.

129. Harvey, *Interurban Clinical Club,* p. 203; see also Freedberg, A. S. Herrman L. Blumgart, 1895–1977. *Trans. Assoc. Am. Physicians* 90: 22, 1977.

Memorial Note. Herrman Blumgart. *N. Engl. J. Med.* 296: 1117, 1977.

130. Freedberg, Personal communication, 1977.

131. Altschule, M. D., and Volk, M. C. The minute volume output and the work of the heart in hypothyroidism. *J. Clin. Invest.* 14: 385, 1935.

Blumgart, H. L., Gargill, S. L., and Gilligan, D. R. Studies on the velocity of blood flow. XIII. The circulatory response to thyrotoxicosis. *J. Clin. Invest.* 9: 69, 1930–31.

Blumgart, H. L., Gilligan, D. R., and Swartz, J. H. The elimination of ethyl iodide after inhalation and its relation to therapeutic administration. *J. Clin. Invest.* 9: 635, 1930–31.

Ernstene, A. C., and Volk, M. C. Cutaneous respiration in man. IV. The rate of carbon dioxide elimination and oxygen absorption in normal subjects. *J. Clin. Invest.* 11: 363, 1932.

Gilligan, D. R., Berlin, D. D., Volk, M. C., Stern, B., and Blumgart, H. L. Therapeutic effect of total ablation of normal thyroid on congestive heart failure and angina pectoris. IX. Postoperative parathyroid function. Clinical observations and serum calcium and phosphorus studies. *J. Clin. Invest.* 13: 789, 1934.

Gilligan, D. R., Volk, M. C., and Blumgart, H. L. Observations on the chemical and physical relation between blood serum and body fluids. I. The nature of edema fluids and evidence regarding the mechanism of edema formation. *J. Clin. Invest.* 13: 365, 1934.

Rourke, M. D., and Ernstene, A. C. A method for correcting the erythrocyte sedimentation rate for variations in the cell volume percentage of blood. *J. Clin. Invest.* 8: 545, 1929.

132. Harvey, *Interurban Clinical Club,* p. 345.

133. Blumgart, H. L., and Gilligan, D. R. March hemoglobinuria; studies of clinical characteristics, blood metabolism and mechanism: with observations on three new cases and review of literature. *Trans. Assoc. Am. Physicians* 56: 123, 1941.

Blumgart, H. L., Riseman, J. E. F., and Davis, D. Results of total ablation of thyroid in cardiac patients operated upon one to two and a half years ago with particular reference to cardiac asthma, congestive failure and angina pectoris. *Trans. Assoc. Am. Physicians* 50: 294, 1935.

Blumgart, H. L., Schlesinger, M. J., and Davis, D. Studies on the relation of the clinical manifestations of angina pectoris, coronary thrombosis, and myocardial infarction to the pathological findings. *Am. Heart J.* 18: 1, 1940.

134. Dill, D. B. The Harvard Fatigue Laboratory; Its development, contributions and demise. *Circulation Res.* 20 (suppl. 1): 1, 1967.

Dill, D. B. L. J. Henderson—His transition from physical chemist to physiologist; his qualities as a man. *The Physiologist* 20: 1, 1977.

135. Bock, A. V., Dill, D. B., and Edwards, H. T. On the relation of changes in blood velocity and volume flow of blood to change of posture. *J. Clin. Invest.* 8: 533, 1929.

Bock, A. V., Dill, D. B., and Edwards, H. T. Lactic acid in the blood of resting man. *J. Clin. Invest.* 11: 775, 1932.

Dennig, H., Talbott, J. H., Edwards, H. T., and Dill, D. B. Effect of acidosis and alkalosis upon capacity for work. *J. Clin. Invest.* 9: 601, 1930–31.

Field, H., Jr., and Bock, A. V. Orthopnoea and the effect of posture upon the rate of blood flow. *J. Clin. Invest.* 2: 67, 1925–26.

Field, H., Jr., Bock, A. V., Gildea, E. F., and Lathrop, F. L. The rate of the circulation of the blood in normal resting individuals. *J. Clin. Invest.* 1: 65, 1924.

Lawrence, J. S., Hurxthal, L. M., and Bock, A. V. Variations in blood flow with changes in position in normal and pathological subjects. *J. Clin. Invest.* 2: 613, 1925–26.

Talbott, J. H., and Michelsen, J. Heat cramps. A clinical and chemical study. *J. Clin. Invest.* 12: 533, 1933.

# Chapter 13

1. The origins of medical education in St. Louis provide an interesting story that is important to the development of the present school of medicine. See the autobiography of George Canby Robinson (*Adventures in Medical Education,* p. 101. Cambridge, Mass.: Harvard University Press, 1957).

See also:

Fox, M. E. History of the Washington School of Medicine. (An authorized history, manuscript unpaginated.) Archives, Washington University School of Medicine.

Opie, E. L. Adoption of standards of the best medical schools of Western Europe to the United States. *Perspect. Biol. Med.* 13: 309, 1970. (Includes a description of the founding and reorganization of the Washington University School of Medicine.)

2. David Linn Edsall to David F. Houston (Chancellor of Washington University), December 24, 1909. In Aub, J. C., and Hapgood, R. K. *Pioneer in Modern Medicine: David Linn Edsall,* p. 69. Boston: Harvard Medical Alumni Association, 1970.

3. Opie, Adoption of standards of the best medical schools of Western Europe by those of the United States.

4. Dock, G. Autobiographical notes. Courtesy of the Barlow Society for the History of Medicine. Los Angeles, Calif.

Robinson, *Adventures in Medical Education,* p. 101.

5. Bibliography of the writings of Dr. George Dock. The Barlow Society for the History of Medicine. Los Angeles, Calif., 1950.

Blumer, G. George Dock, 1860–1951. *Trans. Assoc. Am. Physicians* 65: 16, 1952.

Burns, G. R. Men of medicine: A gifted and inspiring teacher, George Dock. *Postgrad. Med.* 8: 325, 1950.

Dock, G. Historical notes on coronary occlusion: From Heberden to Osler. Frank Billings Lecture. *J.A.M.A.* 113: 563, 1939.

Dock, G. Clinical pathology in the eighties and nineties. *Am. J. Clin. Pathol.* 16: 671, 1946.

6. Vaughan, V. C. *A Doctor's Memories,* p. 222. Indianapolis: Bobbs-Merrill, 1926.

7. Capps, J. A. The President's address. *Trans. Assoc. Am. Physicians* 49: 1, 1934.

8. Robinson, *Adventures in Medical Education,* p. 101.

9. The introduction of electrocardiography made it clear that certain cases of Stokes-Adams attacks were due to other disturbances of mechanism than classical heart block. Robinson and Bredeck (Ventricular fibrillation in man with cardiac recovery. *Arch. Intern. Med.* 20: 725, 1917) first reported syncopal attacks in connection with bouts of ventricular fibrillation.

10. Smith, D. T. Frederic Moir Hanes, 1883–1946. *Trans. Assoc. Am. Physicians* 59: 19, 1946.

11. Frawley, T. F. Ralph A. Kinsella, Sr., 1886–1966. *Trans. Assoc. Am. Physicians* 80: 13, 1967.

12. Kinsella, R. A. Points of difference and similarity in bacterial and rheumatic endocarditis. *Trans. Assoc. Am. Physicians* 51: 103, 1936.

Kinsella, R. A., and Muether, R. O. Studies of experimental streptococcal endocarditis. *Trans. Assoc. Am. Physicians* 49: 115, 1934.

13. Turner, T. B. Alan Mason Chesney, 1888–1964. *Trans. Assoc. Am. Physicians* 78: 17, 1965.

14. Dragstedt, L. R. Evarts Ambrose Graham (Mar. 19, 1883–Mar. 4, 1957). (See p. 226 for Shaffer's account); *Biog. Mem. Natl. Acad. Sci.* 48: 221, 1976. (Contains Graham's complete bibliography.)

15. Graham, E. A. Report of the Surgical Service, 1928–29. Archives, Washington University School of Medicine. (Includes a report to the Barnes Hospital.)

Wangensteen, O. H. The academic surgical arena; past and present. A tribute to Evarts Graham, great surgical leader and innovator. *Surgery* 64: 595, 1968.

16. Graham, E. A. The resistance of pups to late chloroform poisoning in its relation to liver glycogen. *J. Exp. Med.* 21: 185, 1915.

17. Announcement of Award of Gross Prize to Robert Elman. *St. Louis Post Dispatch,* October 13, 1945. Archives, Washington University School of Medicine.

Obituary of Robert Elman. *St. Louis Post Dispatch,* December 24, 1956. Archives, Washington University School of Medicine.

Elman, R. The effects of loss of gastric and pancreatic secretions and the methods for restoration of normal conditions in the body. *J. Exp. Med.* 50: 387, 1929.

Elman, R. Intravenous injection of amino acids in regeneration of serum protein following severe experimental hemorrhage. *Proc. Soc. Exp. Biol. Med.* 36: 867, 1937.

Elman, R., and Lischer, C. Experimental burns. II. Effect of elastic pressure applied to a burned area. *War Med.* 3: 482, 1943.

Elman, R., and McCaughan, J. M. On the collection of the entire external secretion of the pancreas and the fatal effect of total loss of pancreatic juice. *J. Exp. Med.* 45: 561, 1927.

18. The Reminiscences of David Preswick Barr, 1956, found in the Columbia Oral History Collection, is copyright by The Trustees of Columbia University in the City of New York, 1975, and is used by permission.

Rogers, D. E. David Preswick Barr, 1889–1977. *Trans. Assoc. Am. Physicians* 91: 15, 1978.

19. See p. 235 for the story of the Loomis Laboratory.

20. The Reminiscences of David Preswick Barr.

Rogers, David Preswick Barr.

21. Barr, D. P., and Peters, J. P., Jr. Studies of the respiratory mechanism in cardiac dyspnea. III. The effective ventilation in cardiac dyspnea. *Am. J. Physiol.* 54: 345, 1920.

Barr, D. P., and Peters, J. P., Jr. III. The carbon dioxide absorption curve and carbon dioxide tension of the blood in severe anemia. *J. Biol. Chem.* 45: 571, 1921.

22. Himwich, H. E., and Barr, D. P. Studies in the physiology of muscular exercise. V. Oxygen relationships in the arterial blood. *J. Biol. Chem.* 57: 363, 1923.

Loebel, R. O., Barr, D. P., Tolstoi, E., and Himwich, H. E. Studies of the effect of exercise in diabetes. II. Lactic acid formation in phlorhizin diabetes. *J. Biol. Chem.* 61: 9, 1924.

23. Barr, D. P. Studies in the physiology of muscular exercise. III. Blood reaction and breathing. *J. Biol. Chem.* 56: 171, 1923.

24. Moore, C. V. Harry L. Alexander, 1887–1969. *Trans. Assoc. Am. Physicians* 82: 24, 1969.

25. Alexander, H. L. Precipitin response in the blood of rabbits following sub-arachnoid injections of horse serum. *J. Exp. Med.* 33: 471, 1921.

26. Weaver, W. K., Alexander, H. L., and McConnell, F. S. Observations on the formation of wheals. IV. The influence of calcium concentrations on histamine wheals. *J. Clin. Invest.* 11: 195, 1932.

27.

Dr. Marriott has resigned and . . . the reason for his resignation is . . . serious. . . .

We share fully Marriott's opinion as to the gravity of the situation which has long been the main obstacle to progress in this school. . . .

The failure of the Corporation is that since Mr. Brookings' withdrawal, there has been no consistent effort to bring about a unity of purpose . . . The fault of the officers of the Barnes Hospital is that they have perpetuated an erroneous idea that originated in the early negotiations . . . out of which grew the contract between University and Hospital. As an inducement to persuade the hospital trustees to build an adequate hospital . . . Brookings offered that the University would supply all laboratory and general technical-scientific facilities. He did not then foresee the future increase in the elaboration and cost of such services. Unless a revision of this provision is reached it may yet bankrupt the Medical School . . . the hospital up to the present moment has continued its policy to object to and to block any modification. . . .

Another matter concerns the financial drain on the University caused by the custom of furnishing all laboratory examinations (except x-ray) free of charge to all patients in the Barnes Hospital. In the original agreement it was understood that the University should provide free of charge all laboratory service (except x-ray) to the *ward* patients. . . . This has been interpreted by the Hospital to mean that the University is expected to provide such service free of charge to all patients whether occupying *private rooms* or *beds in the wards.*

For the immediate future the relations with the Barnes Hospital and its attitude appear to us the most urgent problem. (Archives, Washington University School of Medicine.)

28. Barr, D. P., Ronzoni, E., and Glaser, J. Studies of the inhibitory action of an extract of pancreas upon glycolysis. II. Effect of the inhibitor upon glycolysis of malignant tumors. *J. Biol. Chem.* 80: 331, 1928.

29. Ronzoni, E., Glaser, J., and Barr, D. P. Studies of the inhibitory action of an extract of pancreas upon glycolysis. I. The effect of pancreatic inhibitors on the glycolysis of muscle tissue and muscle extract. *J. Biol. Chem.* 80: 309, 1928.

30. Bulger, H. A., Dixon, H. H., and Barr, D. P. The functional pathology of hyper-parathyroidism. *J. Clin. Invest.* 9: 143, 1930.

31. Bulger, H. A., Gausmann, F. Magnesium metabolism in hyperparathyroidism. *J. Clin. Invest.* 12: 1135, 1933.

Bulger, H. A., Peters, J. P., Eisenman, A. J., and Lee, C. Total acid-base equilibrium of plasma in health and disease. VII. Factors causing acidosis in chronic nephritis: A preliminary report. *J. Clin. Invest.* 2: 213, 1925–26.

Bulger, H. A., Stroud, C. M., and Heideman, M. L. Studies of the chemical mechanism of hydrochloric acid secretion. I. Electrolyte variations in human gastric juice. *J. Clin. Invest.* 5: 547, 1927–28.

Peters, J. P., Eisenman, A. J., and Bulger, H. A. The plasma proteins in relation to blood hydration. I. In normal individuals and in miscellaneous conditions. *J. Clin. Invest.* 1: 435, 1924-25.

32. Barr, D. P., Russ, E. M., and Eder, H. A. Protein-lipid relationships in human plasma. I. In normal individuals. II. In atherosclerosis and related conditions. *Am. J. Med.* 11: 469, 1951.

Mann, G. V. Diet-heart; End of an era. *N. Engl. J. Med.* 297: 644, 1977.

33. Veeder, B. S. William McKim Marriott, 1885-1936. *J. Pediatr.* 13: 619, 1938.

Veeder, B. S. Pediatric Profiles—William McKim Marriott, 1885-1936. *J. Pediatr.* 47: 791, 1955.

Veeder, B. S. William McKim Marriott. *Dict. Am. Biog.* 22 (suppl. 2): 432, 1958.

34. Archives, Washington University School of Medicine.

35. Marriott, W. M. The artificial feeding of athreptic infants. *J.A.M.A.* 73: 1173, 1919.

Marriott, W. M. *Infant Nutrition.* St. Louis: C. V. Mosby, 1930 (2nd ed., 1935).

36. Memorial for Alexis F. Hartmann, Sr.: From the agenda of the executive faculty of the Washington University School of Medicine, October 7, 1964, pp. 11, 383.

White, P. J. Alexis F. Hartmann, Sr. *J. Pediatr.* 64: 782, 1964.

37. Darrow, D. C., and Hartmann, A. F. Chemical changes occurring in the body as a result of certain diseases in infants and children. IV. Primary pneumonia in children. *Am. J. Dis. Child.* 37: 323, 1929.

Hartmann, A. F. and Senn, N. J. E. Studies in the metabolism of sodium R-lactate. *J. Clin. Invest.* 11: 327-45, 1932.

# Chapter 14

1. Bell, W. J. The medical institution of Yale College, 1810-1885. *Yale J. Biol. Med.* 33: 169, 1960.

2. Welch, W. H. Some of the advantages of the union of medical school and university. *N. Engl. Yale Rev.* 13: 145, 1888; idem, The relation of Yale to Medicine. *Yale Med. J.* 8: 127, 1901; idem, *Papers and Addresses of William Henry Welch,* vol. 3, p. 26. Baltimore: Johns Hopkins Press, 1920.

3. Klatskin, G. George Blumer, 1872-1962. *Trans. Assoc. Am. Physicians* 76: 14, 1963.

Lippard, V. W. The Yale School of Medicine in the twentieth century. *Yale J. Biol. Med.* 33: 184, 1960.

4. Paul, J. R. Dean Winternitz and the rebirth of the Yale Medical School in the 1920s. *Yale J. Biol. Med.* 43: 110, 1970.

5. Hoff, H. E. Thirty years after: In memory of L. H. Nahum. *Conn. Med. J.* 36: 483, 1972.

6. Keefer, C. S. Stanhope Bayne-Jones, 1886-1970. *Trans. Assoc. Am. Physicians* 83: 14, 1970.

7. Bayne-Jones, S., Francis, T., Jr., and Peters, J. P. Addresses delivered at the memorial exercises for Francis Gilman Blake. The Historical Library, Yale University School of Medicine, June 15, 1952.

Blake, F. G. Clinical investigation. *Science* 74: 27, 1931.

Blake, F. G. The President's address. *Trans. Assoc. Am. Physicians* 62: 1, 1949.

Harvey, A. McG. *The Interurban Clinical Club, 1905-1976. A Record of Achievement in Clinical Science,* p. 290. Philadelphia: W. B. Saunders, 1978.

Paul, J. R. Francis Gilman Blake, 1887-1952. *Yale J. Biol. Med.* 24: 435, 1951-52.

Paul, J. R. Francis Gilman Blake, 1887-1952. *Trans. Assoc. Am. Physicians* 65: 9, 1952.

Paul, J. R. Francis Gilman Blake. *Biog. Mem. Natl. Acad. Sci.* 28: 1, 1954. (Contains Blake's complete bibliography.)

8. H. M. Marvin had worked with Sir Thomas Lewis in London. In 1927 he studied (at

Yale) seventy-seven patients with severe heart failure, showing that digitalis acted best in failure due to nonvalvular disease. Slowing of the pulse in fibrillation was not synonymous with improved well-being for the patient; the majority of rheumatic valvular cases showed little relief from their symptoms. (Marvin, H. M. Digitalis and diuretics in heart failure with regular rhythm, with especial reference to the importance of etiologic classification of heart disease. *J. Clin. Invest.* 3: 521, 1927.)

9. Fulton, J. F. John Punnett Peters: Medical scientist. *Science* 123: 1023, 1956.

Harvey, *Interurban Clinical Club,* p. 138.

Paul, J. R., and Long, C. N. H. John Punnett Peters (Dec. 4, 1887–Dec. 29, 1955). *Biog. Mem. Natl. Acad. Sci.* 31: 47, 1957. (Contains Peters's complete bibliography.)

Strauss, M. B. Physician and citizen—John P. Peters, M.D. *N. Engl. J. Med.* 254: 1344, 1956.

Van Slyke, D. D. John Punnett Peters, 1887–1955. *Trans. Assoc. Am. Physicians* 59: 22, 1956.

10. Lavietes, P. H. John Punnett Peters: An appreciation. *Yale J. Biol. Med.* 29: 175, 1956.

Van Slyke, John Punnett Peters.

11. Peters, J. P. A critical estimate of the value of laboratory procedures in disorders of metabolism. *Bull. NY Acad. Med.* 10: 415, 1934.

12. Kydd, D. M. Salt and water in the treatment of diabetic acidosis. *J. Clin. Invest.* 12: 1169, 1933.

Lavietes, P. H. The metabolic measurement of the water exchange. *J. Clin. Invest.* 14: 251, 1935.

Lavietes, P. H., D'Esopo, L. M., and Harrison, H. E. The water and base balance of the body. *J. Clin. Invest.* 14: 251, 1935.

Peters, J. P. Alexander Woodward Winkler, 1908–1947. *Yale J. Biol. Med.* 20: 105, 1947. (Contains Winkler's complete bibliography.)

Peters, J. P., Kydd, D. M., and Lavietes, P. H. A note on the calculation of water exchange. *J. Clin. Invest.* 12: 689, 1933.

Peters, J. P., and Lavietes, P. H. The nature of "preformed water." *J. Clin. Invest.* 12: 695, 1933.

13. Atkins, E. John Rodman Paul, M.D. *Yale Medicine,* Fall/Winter: 9, 1971.

Miller, C. P. John Rodman Paul, 1893–1971. *Trans. Assoc. Am. Physicians* 85: 40, 1972.

Paul, J. R. Clinical epidemiology. *J. Clin. Invest.* 17: 539, 1938.

Paul, J. R. The advancement of scientific and practical medicine. *Trans. Assoc. Am. Physicians* 69: 1, 1956.

Paul, J. R. *Clinical Epidemiology.* Chicago: University of Chicago Press, 1958 (rev. ed., 1966, p. xiii).

Paul, J. R. From the notebook of John Rodman Paul. *Yale J. Biol. Med.* 34: 164, 1961–62.

14. Paul, J. R. A clinician's place in academic preventive medicine: My favorite hobby. *Bull. NY Acad. Med.* 47: 1262, 1971.

15. Paul, J. R. Clinical epidemiology. *J. Clin. Invest.* 17: 539, 1938.

16. Paul, J. R. *The Epidemiology of Rheumatic Fever.* New York: Metropolitan Life Insurance Co., 1930.

Paul, J. R. Age susceptibility to familial infection in rheumatic fever. *J. Clin. Invest.* 10: 53, 1931.

Paul, J. R., and Salinger, R. The spread of rheumatic fever through families. *J. Clin. Invest.* 10: 33, 1931.

Paul, J. R., Salinger, R., and Zuger, B. The relation of rheumatic fever to post-scarlatinal arthritis and post-scarlatinal heart disease: A familial study. *J. Clin. Invest.* 13: 503, 1934.

17. Paul, J. R., and Bunnell, W. W. The presence of heterophile antibodies in infectious mononucleosis. *Am. J. Med. Sci.* 183: 90, 1932.

18. Hoff, Thirty years after: In memory of L. H. Nahum.

19. Harvey, *Interurban Clinical Club,* p. 173.

Howard, J. E. Edwards Albert Park, 1877–1969. *Trans. Assoc. Am. Physicians* 83: 28, 1970.

Powers, G. F. Edwards A. Park, Yale professor, 1921–27. *J. Pediatr.* 41: 651, 1952.

20. Powers, Edwards A. Park.

21. Darrow, D. C. Grover Powers and pediatrics at Yale. *Yale J. Biol. Med.* 124: 243, 1952.

Harvey, *Interurban Clinical Club,* p. 188.

22. Harvey, *Interurban Clinical Club,* p. 184.

23. Yannet, H., and Darrow, D. C. Physiological disturbances during experimental diphtheritic intoxication. II. Hepatic glycogenesis and glycogen concentration of cardiac and skeletal muscle. *J. Clin. Invest.* 13: 779, 1933.

Yannet, H., and Goldfarb, W. Physiological disturbances during experimental diphtheritic intoxication. III. Respiratory quotients and metabolic rate. *J. Clin. Invest.* 13: 787, 1933.

24. Darrow, D. C., and Yannet, H. The changes in the distribution of body water accompanying increase and decrease in extracellular electrolyte. *J. Clin. Invest.* 14: 266, 1935.

Darrow, D. C., Yannet, H., and Cary, M. K. Physiological disturbances during experimental diphtheritic intoxication. IV. Blood electrolyte and hemoglobin concentrations. *J. Clin. Invest.* 13: 553, 1934.

25. Darrow, D. C., Hopper, E. B., and Cary, M. K. Plasmapheresis edema. II. The effect of reduction of serum protein on the electrolyte pattern and calcium concentration. *J. Clin. Invest.* 11: 701, 1932.

Elkinton, J. R. Daniel Cady Darrow, 1895–1965. *Trans. Assoc. Am. Physicians* 79: 26, 1966.

Harvey, *Interurban Clinical Club,* p. 244.

26. Darrow, D. C. Body fluid physiology: The relation of tissue composition to problems of water and electrolyte balance. *N. Engl. J. Med.* 233: 91, 1945.

27. Darrow, D. C. Congenital alkalosis with diarrhea. *J. Pediatr.* 26: 519, 1945.

Darrow, D. C. The retention of electrolyte during recovery from severe dehydration due to diarrhea. *J. Pediatr.* 28: 515, 1946.

Darrow, D. C. Therapeutic measures promoting recovery from the physiological disturbances of infantile diarrhea. *Pediatrics* 9: 519, 1952.

Darrow, D. C. The role of the patient in clinical research of a physiological problem. *Yale J. Biol. Med.* 30: 1, 1957.

28. Harvey, *Interurban Clinical Club,* p. 184.

29. Paul, J. R., and Trask, J. D. Observations on the epidemiology of poliomyelitis with particular inference to so-called "abortive" poliomyelitis. *Trans. Assoc. Am. Physicians* 47: 116, 1932.

Paul, J. R., and Trask, J. D. Immunity in "abortive" poliomyelitis. *Trans. Assoc. Am. Physicians* 48: 23, 1933.

# Chapter 15

1. Flexner, A. *Medical Education in the United States and Canada.* Bull. No. 4. New York: Carnegie Foundation for the Advancement of Teaching, 1910.

2. Youmans, J. B. Vanderbilt—Yesterday, today and tomorrow. *J. Tenn. Med. Assoc.* 59: 39, 1966.

3. Robinson, G. C. *Adventures in Medical Education,* p. 145. Cambridge, Mass.: Harvard University Press, 1957.

4. Harvey, A. McG. George Canby Robinson—Peripatetic medical educator. *Johns Hopkins Med. J.* 143: 84, 1978.

5. Youmans, Vanderbilt—Yesterday, today and tomorrow.

6. Burwell, C. S. Presentation of the Kober Medal to Dr. Ernest William Goodpasture. *Trans. Assoc. Am. Physicians* 58: 45, 1944.

Goodpasture, E. W. Reply to Kober Medal Award. *Trans Assoc. Am. Physicians* 58: 47, 1944.

Youmans, J. B. Ernest William Goodpasture. *Trans. Assoc. Am. Physicians* 74: 21, 1961.

7. Eppinger, E. C. Charles Sidney Burwell, 1893-1967. *Trans. Assoc. Am. Physicians* 81: 9, 1968.

8. Burwell, C. S., and Robinson, G. C. A method for the determination of the amount of oxygen and carbon dioxide in mixed venous blood of man. *J. Clin. Invest.* 1: 47, 1924.

Burwell, C. S., and Robinson, G. C. The gaseous content of the blood and the output of the heart in normal resting adults. *J. Clin. Invest.* 1: 87, 1924.

Dieuaide, F. R., and Burwell, C. S. Clinical experience with quinidine. *Arch. Intern. Med.* 31: 518, 1923.

9. Burwell, C. S., Neighbors, D., and Regen, E. M. The effect of digitalis upon the output of the heart in normal man. *J. Clin. Invest.* 5: 128, 1927.

Burwell, C. S., and Robinson, G. C. A note on the cardiac output of a single individual observed over a period of five years. *J. Clin. Invest.* 6: 247, 1928.

Burwell, C. S., and Smith, W. C. The output of the heart in patients with abnormal blood pressures. *J. Clin. Invest.* 7: 1, 1929.

10. Morgan, H. J. The inhibition zone in precipitin reactions with the soluble specific substance of pneumococcus. *J. Immunol.* 8: 449, 1923.

Morgan, H. J. The correlation of certain phenomena occurring during the growth of pneumococcus. *J. Exp. Med.* 39: 565, 1924.

Morgan, H. J., and Avery, O. T. The effect of the accessory substances of plant tissue upon growth of bacteria. *Proc. Soc. Exp. Biol. Med.* 19: 113, 1921.

Morgan, H. J., Binger, C. A. L., Hastings, A. B., and Neill, J. M. Blood reaction and blood gases in pneumonia. *J. Clin. Invest.* 1: 25, 1924.

11. Kampmeier, R. H. John B. Youmans, 1893-1979. *Trans. Assoc. Am. Physicians* 93: 25, 1980.

12. Dock, W. Medical research from Harvey to Harrison. *Arch. Intern. Med.* 104: 323, 1959.

Harrison, T. R. Acceptance of the Kober Medal. *Trans. Assoc. Am. Physicians* 81: 28, 1968.

Keefer, C. S. Presentation of the Kober Medal for 1968 to Tinsley Randolph Harrison. *Trans. Assoc. Am. Physicians* 81: 22, 1968.

13. Samuel Grant, while a medical student, measured the effect of chilling the skin on blood flow in the lining membranes of the nose and throat and discovered the alkalosis and tetany of overbreathing.

14. Grant, S. B. A study of the blood oxygen in diabetes mellitus. *Arch. Intern. Med.* 32: 764, 1923.

Grant, S. B. The role of anoxemia in the causation of tetany during hyperpnea. *Am. J. Physiol.* 66: 274, 1923.

Grant, S. B. Changes in the blood oxygen following therapeutic bleeding in cardiac patients. *J. Lab. Clin. Med.* 9: 160, 1923-24.

15. Dock, W., and Harrison, T. R. The blood flow through the lungs in experimental pneumothorax. *Am. Rev. Tuberc.* 10: 534, 1924-25.

Harrison, T. R., Dock, W., and Holman, E. Experimental studies in arterio-venous fistulae; cardiac output. *Heart* 11: 337, 1924.

16. Harrison, T. R. *Failure of the Circulation.* Baltimore: Williams & Wilkins, 1935.

17. Keefer, Presentation of the Kober Medal for 1968 to Tinsley Randolph Harrison.

18. The author is indebted to the late Tinsley R. Harrison for the information in this section.

19. Blalock, A., Harrison, T. R., and Wilson, C. P. Partial tracheal obstruction: An experimental study in the effects on the circulation and respiration of morphinized dogs. *Arch. Intern. Med.* 13: 86, 1926.

Harrison, T. R. and Blalock, A. Oxygen lack and cardiac output: Some clinical considerations. *J.A.M.A.* 87: 1984, 1926.

Harrison, T. R., and Blalock, A. Cardiac output in pneumonia in the dog. *J. Clin. Invest.* 2: 435, 1926.

Harrison, T. R., and Perlzweig, W. A. Alkalosis, not due to administration of alkali, associated with uremia: Report of a case. *J.A.M.A.* 84: 671, 1925.

Harrison, T. R., Wilson, C. P., and Blalock, A. The effects of changes in hydrogen ion concentration on the blood flow of morphinized dogs. *J. Clin. Invest.* 1: 547, 1925.

For other references see Leathers, W. S. Vanderbilt University School of Medicine. Report of Publications, Oct. 1925–Dec. 1938. Nashville, Tenn., 1940.

20. Blalock, A. Reminiscence: Shock after thirty-four years. *Rev. Surg.* 21: 231, 1964.

21. Blalock, A. Experimental shock: The cause of the low blood pressure produced by muscle injury. *Arch. Surg.* 20: 959, 1930.

22. See Harvey, A. McG. *Adventures in Medical Research,* p. 236. Baltimore: Johns Hopkins University Press, 1976.

23. Morgan, H. J. Edgar Jones, 1903–1951. *Trans. Assoc. Am. Physicians* 65: 24, 1952.

24. Wells, S. H., Youmans, J. B., and Miller, D. G., Jr. A formula and nomogram for the estimation of the osmotic pressure of colloids from the albumin and total protein concentrations of human blood sera. *J. Clin. Invest.* 12: 1103, 1933.

Youmans, J. B. Certain factors influencing the exchange of fluid between the blood and the tissues and their relation to the occurrence of edema in patients. *Trans. Assoc. Am. Physicians* 50: 118, 1935.

Youmans, J. B., Bell, A., Donley, D., and Frank, H. Endemic nutritional edema. II. Serum proteins and nitrogen balance. *Arch. Intern. Med.* 51: 45, 1933.

Youmans, J. B., and Trimble, W. H. Experimental and clinical studies of ergotamine. III. The effect of ergotamine on the oxygen consumption of normal trained dogs. *J. Pharmacol. Exp. Ther.* 38: 201, 1930.

25. Burwell, C. S. Hugh Jackson Morgan, 1893–1961. *Trans. Assoc. Am. Physicians* 75: 33, 1962.

26. Morgan, H. J. A contribution to the cellular pathology of experimental syphilis. *Trans. Assoc. Am. Physicians* 45: 67, 1930.

Morgan, H. J., Harris, S., Jr., Tompkins, E. H., and Cunningham, R. S. The effect of trypan blue on experimental syphilis in the rabbit. *Am. J. Syph.* 17: 522, 1933.

Thomas, C. S., and Morgan, H. J. Single cell inoculation with *Treponema pallidum. J. Exp. Med.* 59: 297, 1934.

# Chapter 16

1. Corner, G. W. *George Hoyt Whipple and His Friends: The Life Story of a Nobel Prize Pathologist.* Philadelphia: J. B. Lippincott, 1963.

*To Each His Farthest Star.* University of Rochester Medical Center, 1925–1975. Geneva, W. F. Humphrey, 1975. (A book of essays commemorating the fiftieth anniversary of the University of Rochester Medical Center.)

See Appendix C for an interview with Nolan Kaltreider.

2. Corner, *George Hoyt Whipple and His Friends.* (Contains a complete listing of Whipple's research papers.)

3. Whipple was strongly recommended by William Henry Welch and Simon Flexner.

Whipple, G. H. Autobiographical sketch. *Perspect. Biol. Med.* 2: 253, 1959.

4. Young, L. E. William Sharp McCann, 1889–1971. *Trans. Assoc. Am. Physicians* 85: 35, 1972.

5. McCann, W. S., Hannon, R. R., and Dodd, K. Studies of diabetes mellitus. III. The use of pancreatic extract insulin in the treatment of diabetes. *Bull. Johns Hopkins Hosp.* 34: 205, 1923.

McCann, W. S., Hannon, R. R., Perlzweig, W. A., and Tompkins, E. H. Studies of diabetes mellitus. II. The results of treatment by diet adjustment with reference to maintenance requirement and the ketogenic antiketogenic ratio. *Arch. Intern. Med.* 32: 226, 1923.

6. McCann, W. S. Unpublished memoirs. MS. Library. University of Rochester School of Medicine. (McCann was on the faculty at Johns Hopkins [1921–24] before assuming the chairmanship of medicine at the University of Rochester.)

7. Corner, *George Hoyt Whipple and His Friends.*

Young, William Sharp McCann.

On July 1, 1930, the strict full-time plan was abandoned and the "Harvard plan" was adopted. This allowed the clinical faculty to retain an agreed amount in patient fees.

8. McCann, W. S. University of Rochester School of Medicine and Dentistry. In *Methods and Problems of Medical Education*, vol. 7, p. 26. New York: Rockefeller Foundation, 1927.

9. Bassett, S. H., Killip, T., and McCann, W. S. Mineral exchanges of man. III. Mineral metabolism during treatment of a case of polycythemia vera. *J. Clin. Invest.* 10: 771, 1931.

Boak, R. A., Carpenter, C. M., and Warren, S. L. Studies on the physiological effects of fever temperatures. III. The thermal death time of treponema pallidum in vitro with special reference to fever temperatures. *J. Exp. Med.* 56: 741, 1932.

Hannon, R. R., and Lyman, R. S. Studies on pulmonary acoustics. II. The transmission of tracheal sounds through freshly exenterated sheep's lungs. *Am. Rev. Tuberc.* 19: 360, 1929.

Keutmann, E. H., and Bassett, S. H. Dietary protein in hemorrhagic Bright's disease. II. The effect of diet on serum proteins, proteinuria and tissue proteins. *J. Clin. Invest.* 14: 871, 1935.

Lawrence, J. S. Human elliptical erythrocytes. *Am. J. Med. Sci.* 181: 240, 1931.

Lawrence, J. S., and Todd, H. Variations in the characteristics of lymphocytes and supravital preparations. *Folia Haematol.* 44: 381, 1931.

Lyman, R. S. Ankle-clonus: The distinction of the organic and functional varieties. *Brain* 51: 168, 1928.

Lyman, R. S., and Ledig, P. G. An adaptation of the thermal conductivity method to the analysis of respiratory gases. *J. Clin. Invest.* 4: 495, 1927.

Rioch, D. M. Experiments on water and salt diuresis. *Arch. Intern. Med.* 40: 743, 1927.

10. Richard Lyman received his M.D. degree from Yale in 1921. Just before joining the staff at Rochester, he was a fellow in medicine and an assistant in psychiatry at Johns Hopkins (1922–25). He was in charge of the Laboratory of Internal Medicine in the Phipps Psychiatric Clinic of the Johns Hopkins Hospital.

11. With the exception of Paul Garvey and John S. Lawrence, all of the people in the department had been house officers who had stayed on as faculty members. McCann was opposed to people "going away" for postresidency training, according to Nolan Kaltreider. When anyone wished to do so, McCann was helpful, but made it clear that there would be no position to which to return. This practice was not changed until Lawrence Young became chairman of the department in 1957.

12. Hurtado, A., Kaltreider, N. L., and McCann, W. S. Studies of total pulmonary capacity and its subdivisions. IX. Relationship to the oxygen saturation and carbon dioxide content of the arterial blood. *J. Clin. Invest.* 14: 94, 1935.

Kaltreider, N. L., Hurtado, A., and Brooks, W. D. W. Study of the blood in chronic respiratory diseases, with special reference to the volume of the blood. *J. Clin. Invest.* 13: 999, 1934.

13. Yanagi, K. A clinical and experimental study of the stability of colloid osmotic pressure of serum protein. *J. Clin. Invest.* 14: 853, 1933.

Yanagi, K. The effect of posterior pituitary preparations upon the colloid osmotic pressure of serum protein, water and mineral metabolism of dogs. *J. Pharmacol. Exp. Ther.* 56: 23, 1936.

14. Dobriner, K. Urinary porphyrin in disease. *J. Biol. Chem.* 113: 1, 1936.

15. McCann, W. S. Effect of kidney on blood regeneration in pernicious anemia. *Proc. Soc. Exp. Biol. Med.* 25: 255, 1928.

McCann, W. S., Hurtado, A., and Kaltreider, N. Respiratory adaptation to anoxemia. *Am. J. Physiol.* 109: 626, 1934.

McCann, W. S., and Keutmann, E. H. Dietary protein in hemorrhagic Bright's disease. I. Effects upon the course of the disease with special reference to hematuria and renal function. *J. Clin. Invest.* 11: 973, 1932.

16. McCann, W. S. The present status of clinical investigation. *Am. Sci.* (The Sigma Xi Quarterly) 25: 150, 1937.

17. McCann, W. S., and Keutmann, E. H. The effects of high protein diets upon the course of chronic glomerulonephritis. *Trans. Assoc. Am. Physicians* 47: 80, 1932.

18. Bassett, S. H., Elden, C. A., and McCann, W. S. Mineral exchanges of man. I. Organization of metabolism ward and analytical methods. *J. Nutr.* 4: 235, 1931.

Bassett, S. H., Keutmann, E. H., van Zile Hyde, H., and van Alstine, H. Metabolism in idiopathic steatorrhea. II. Effect of liver extract and vitamin D on calcium, phosphorus, nitrogen, and lipid balances. *J. Clin. Invest.* 18: 121, 1939.

Bassett, S. H., and van Alstine, H. Mineral exchanges of man. VI. The effect of extirpation of a parathyroid tumor on the balances of electrolytes. *J. Nutr.* 9: 345, 1935.

Keutmann, E. H., and Bassett, S. H. Studies on the mechanism of proteinuria. *J. Clin. Invest.* 16: 767, 1937.

19. Stephens, D. J. Cyclical agranulocytic angina. *Ann. Intern. Med.* 9: 31, 1935.

Stephens, D. J., and Hawley, E. E. The relationship of vitamin C to the hemorrhagic diatheses. *J. Lab. Clin. Med.* 22: 173, 1936.

Stephens, D. J., and Tatelbaum, A. J. Elliptical human erythrocytes. *J. Lab. Clin. Med.* 20: 375, 1935.

20. Jones, E. The demonstration of collateral venous circulation in the abdominal wall by means of infra-red photography. *Am. J. Med. Sci.* 190: 478, 1935.

Jones, E., Stephens, D. J., Todd, H., and Lawrence, J. S. Studies in the normal human white blood cell picture. I. Variations in recumbent basal subjects and in individuals with change of posture. *Am. J. Physiol.* 105: 547, 1933.

Morgan, H. J. Edgar Jones, 1903–1951. *Trans. Assoc. Am. Physicians* 65: 24, 1952.

21. Lawrence, J. S., and van Wagenen, W. P. Hematopoietic changes associated with pituitary diseases. *Trans. Assoc. Am. Physicians* 53: 152, 1938.

22. Klatskin, G. On the action of crystalline vitamin $D_2$ (calcified) in chronic parathyroid tetany. *J. Clin. Invest.* 17: 431, 1938.

23. Kaltreider, N. L., Meneely, G. R., Allen, J. R., and Bale, W. F. Determination of the volume of the extracellular fluid of the body with radioactive sodium. *J. Exp. Med.* 74: 569, 1941.

24. Other source material for this chapter included the following:

McCann, W. S. *The First Decade: The University of Rochester School of Medicine and Dentistry and the Strong Memorial Hospital, 1926–1936.* Rochester, N.Y. University of Rochester, 1936. See the chapter on medicine.

McCann, W. S. Department of Medicine. In *The Quarter Century: A Review of the First Twenty-five Years, 1925–1950,* p. 76. Rochester, N.Y.: University of Rochester, 1950.

Annual Reports of the President of the University of Rochester. Reports of the Dean, School of Medicine and Dentistry, 1924–1950.

# Chapter 17

1. See Appendix D for an interview with Joseph T. Wearn.

2. Minutes of the Second Regular Meeting of the Section of Experimental Medicine. *Cleveland Med. J.* 2: 143, 1903.

3. Macleod, J. J. R. Organic chemistry in its relation to medicine. *Cleveland Med. J.* 9: 557, 1910.

4. The Cleveland *Plain Dealer* for November 21, 1906, quoted William Henry Welch as having said:

> In the movement in this country for higher education upon a university standard, the medical department of Western Reserve University has maintained an advanced position in its requirements for preliminary training and in its educational standard. Although the main emphasis in the work of this laboratory is to be upon original investigation, I deem it fortunate that it is connected with an important university and in close affiliation with an excellent hospital. The real home of science is the university and there science should find the most favorable atmosphere for its cultivation.

5. Stewart, G. N. *A Manual of Physiology, with Practical Exercises.* London: J. B. Baillière, 1895.

6. Archives, Western Reserve University School of Medicine.

7. Rogoff, J. M., and Stewart, G. N. The influence of adrenal extracts in the survival period of adrenalectomized animals. *Science* 66: 327, 1927.

8. Pike, F. H., Guthrie, C. C., and Stewart, G. N. Studies in resuscitation. IV. The return of function in the central nervous system after temporary cerebral anemia. *J. Exp. Med.* 10: 490, 1908.

Stewart, G. N. Studies on the circulation in man; The blood flow in the hands and feet in normal and pathological cases. *The Harvey Lectures* 8: 86, 1912.

Stewart, G. N. Studies on the ciruclation in man. XII. A study of inequalities in the blood flow in the two hands (or feet) due to mechanical causes (embolism, compression of vessels, etc.) or to functional (vasomotor) causes, with a discussion of the criteria by which the conditions are discriminated. *J. Exp. Med.* 22: 1, 1915.

9. Follis, R. H., Jr. Presentation of the Kober Medal for 1960 to David Marine. *Trans. Assoc. Am. Physicians* 73: 51, 1960.

Marine, D. Acceptance of the Kober Medal for 1960. *Trans. Assoc. Am. Physicians* 73: 58, 1960.

10. Marine, D. On the occurrence and physiological nature of glandular hyperplasia of the thyroid (dog and sheep) together with remarks on important clinical (human) problems. *Bull. Johns Hopkins Hosp.* 1l: 359, 1907.

Marine, D. Etiology and prevention of simple goiter. *The Harvey Lecture Series, 1923–1924,* pp. 96–122 (delivered January 19, 1924).

Marine, D., and Williams, W. W. The relation of iodine to the structure of the thyroid gland. *Arch. Intern. Med.* 1: 349, 1908.

11. Follis, R. H., Jr. Presentation of the Kober Medal for 1960 to David Marine. *Trans. Assoc. Am. Physicians* 73: 51, 1960.

Marine, D. Acceptance of the Kober Medal for 1960. *Trans. Assoc. Am. Physicians* 73: 58, 1960.

12. Marine, D., and Kimball, O. P. The prevention of simple goitre in man; a survey of the incidence and types of thyroid enlargement in the school girls of Akron, Ohio, from the fifth to the twelfth grades inclusive; the plan of prevention proposed. *J. Lab. Clin. Med.* 3: 40, 1917.

13. Warthin, A. S. The President's address. *Trans. Assoc. Am. Physicians* 43: 1, 1928.

14. Bean, W. B. Marion A. Blankenhorn. *Trans. Assoc. Am. Physicians* 71: 13, 1958.

Blankenhorn, M. A. Distribution of bile in certain types of jaundice. *Trans. Assoc. Am. Physicians* 32: 324, 1917.

Blankenhorn, M. A. Effect of sleep on normal and high blood pressure. *Trans. Assoc. Am. Physicians* 40: 87, 1925.

Blankenhorn, M. A., and Spies, T. Prevention, treatment and possible nature of peripheral neuritis associated with pellagra and chronic alcoholism. *Trans. Assoc. Am. Physicians* 50: 164, 1935.

15. Bean, W. B. Tom Douglas Spies, 1902–1960. *Trans. Assoc. Am. Physicians* 73: 36, 1960.

16. Hudson, C. L. Internal medicine and the scientific method. In *Medicine in Cleveland*

*and Cuyahoga County, 1810–1976,* ed. Brown, K. L., p. 128. Cleveland: Cleveland Academy of Medicine, 1977.

17. Hayman, J. M., Jr. Experiments on the patency of the blood vessels of nephritis kidneys obtained at autopsy. *J. Clin. Invest.* 8: 89, 1929.

Hayman, J. M., Jr., Halsted, J. A., and Seyler, L. E. A comparison of the creatinine and urea clearance tests of kidney function. *J. Clin. Invest.* 12: 861, 1933.

Hayman, J. M., Jr., and Johnston, S. M. Experiments on the relation of creatinine and urea clearance tests of kidney function and the number of glomeruli in the human kidney obtained at autopsy. *J. Clin. Invest.* 12: 877, 1933.

18. While at Western Reserve, Shibley studied the etiology of whooping cough. See: Shibley, G. S. Etiology of whooping cough. *Proc. Soc. Exp. Biol. Med.* 31: 576, 1933.

19. While in New York, Shibley worked on the common cold with Alphonse Raymond Dochez, and on the phenomenon of agglutination. See:

Dochez, A. R., Shibley, G. S., and Mills, K. C. Studies in the common cold. IV. Experimental transmission of the common cold to anthropoid apes and human beings by means of a filtrable agent. *J. Exp. Med.* 52: 701, 1930.

Shibley, G. S. Studies in agglutination. II. The relationship of reduction of electrical change to specific bacterial agglutination. *J. Exp. Med.* 40: 453, 1924.

20. Wearn, J. T. Wandering thoughts and observations on medical education. *Trans. Assoc. Am. Physicians* 67: 1, 1954.

21. Rammelkamp originally came to Cleveland as a member of Dingle's group in preventive medicine.

22. Wearn, J. T. Acceptance of the Kober Medal. *Trans. Assoc. Am. Physicians* 78: 48, 1965.

23. See chapter 8 for further biographical information on Carter.

24. Brown, ed. *Medicine in Cleveland and Cuyahoga County,* p. 168.

Rammelkamp, C. Roy Wesley Scott, 1888–1957. *Trans. Assoc. Am. Physicians* 71: 38, 1958.

Scott graduated from Western Reserve in 1913. After a year of internship at Lakeside Hospital under Charles Hoover, and another year of residency in medicine under Carter, Scott spent three years in the department of physiology under J. J. R. Macleod.

25. Brown, *Medicine in Cleveland and Cuyahoga County,* p. 169.

26. Goldblatt, H., Lynch, J., Hanzal, R. F., and Summerville, W. W. Studies on experimental hypertension. I. The production of persistent elevation of systolic blood pressure by means of renal ischemia. *J. Exp. Med.* 59: 347, 1934.

27. Brown, *Medicine in Cleveland and Cuyahoga County,* p. 560.

28. Page, I. H., and Helmer, O. M. A crystalline pressor substance (angiotonin) resulting from the reaction between renin and renin-activator. *J. Exp. Med.* 71: 29, 1940.

29. Ernstene, A. C. Russell Landran Haden. *Trans. Assoc. Am. Physicians* 65: 18, 1952.

30. Ernstene, A. C., and Gardner, W. J. The effect of splanchnic nerve resection and sympathetic ganglionectomy in a case of paroxysmal hemoglobinuria. *J. Clin. Invest.* 14: 799, 1935.

Pritchard, W. H. Carlton Ernstene, 1901–1971. *Trans. Assoc. Am. Physicians* 85: 13, 1972.

# Chapter 18

1. Sturgis, C. C. I. The period ending in 1908; Wilson, F. W. II. The years 1908–1927; Curtis, A. C. III. The period since 1927. The department of internal medicine. In *The University of Michigan: An Encyclopedic Survey,* ed. Donnelly, W. A., p. 833. Ann Arbor: University of Michigan Press, vol. 4, 1958.

2. Doolen, R. M. Founding of the University of Michigan Hospital: An innovation in medical education. *J. Med. Educ.* 39: 50, 1964.

3. Webb, G. B., and Powell, D. *Henry Sewall: Physiologist and Physician.* Baltimore: Johns Hopkins Press, 1946.

4. Vaughan, V. C. *A Doctor's Memories.* Indianapolis: Bobbs-Merrill, 1926.

5. Adami, J. G. *The Art of Healing and the Science of Medicine. Remarks at the opening of the new building. University of Michigan, 1901,* p. 47, n.p., n.d.

6. Dock, G. *Bibliography of the Writings of Dr. George Dock.* Los Angeles: Barlow Society for the History of Medicine, 1950.

7. Dock, G. Autobiographical notes. Courtesy of the Barlow Society for the History of Medicine, Los Angeles.

8. Cushny, A. R., and Edmunds, C. W. Paroxysmal irregularity of the heart and auricular fibrillation. *Am. J. Med. Sci.* 133: 66, 1907.

Cushny had for years been studying the physiology of irregularities of the pulse. In an early paper (Cushny, A. R. On the interpretation of pulse tracings. *J. Exp. Med.* 4: 327, 1899), he said: "A few words may be added in regard to the extreme irregularity of the heart known clinically as delirium cordis. . . . The clinical sphygmogram in these cases resembles exactly that obtained from dogs when the auricle is undergoing fibrillary contractions. I do not wish to assert that the clinical delirium cordis is identical with the physiological delirium auriculae, but the resemblance is certainly striking." In spite of this hint, clinicians seemed to pay no attention to the possibility of auricular fibrillation being the explanation of the rapid, totally irregular pulse of patients. [The case history of Cushny's patient is given by M. Block (The earliest correlation of clinical and experimental auricular fibrillation. *Am. Heart J.* 18: 684, 1939).] In his paper, Cushny observed a patient with paroxysms of total irregularity and analyzed the arterial pulse tracings. Cushny again compared this rhythm with atrial fibrillation in dogs, which was produced in the laboratory by induction shocks, overdosage with digitalis, and by other means. "The suggestion is made that in the patient described and in other cases of paroxysmal arrhythmia the condition is due to auricular fibrillation from inhibition of the vagus centre." (Bloomfield, A. L. *A Bibliography of Internal Medicine: Selected Diseases,* p. 6. Chicago: University of Chicago Press, 1960.

9. Harvey, A. McG. Albion W. Hewlett—Pioneer clinical physiologist. *Johns Hopkins Med. J.* 144: 202, 1979. (Contains a detailed description of Hewlett's research and an extensive bibliography.)

10. Hewlett, A. W., and Erlanger, J. A study of the metabolism in dogs with shortened small intestines. *Am. J. Physiol.* 6: 1, 1901.

11. Erlanger, J. A physiologist reminisces. *Ann. Rev. Physiol.* 26: 1, 1964.

12. Flexner, S. On the occurrence of the fat-splitting ferment in peritoneal fat necroses and the histology of these lesions. *J. Exp. Med.* 2: 413, 1897.

13. Hewlett, A. W. On the occurrence of lipase in the urine as a result of experimental pancreatitic disease. *J. Med. Res.* 11: 377, 1904.

14. Hewlett, A. W. The effect of the bile upon the ester-splitting action of pancreatitic juice: A preliminary communication. *Bull. Johns Hopkins Hosp.* 16: 20, 1905.

15. Hewlett, A. W. The effect of amyl nitrite inhalations upon the blood pressure in man. *J. Med. Res.* 15: 383, 1906.

16. Young, C. I., and Hewlett, A. W. The normal pulsations within the esophagus. *J. Med. Res.* 16: 427, 1907.

17. Hewlett, A. W. The interpretation of the positive venous pulse. *J. Med. Res.* 17: 119, 1907.

18. Hewlett, A. W. Clinical observations on absolutely irregular hearts. *J.A.M.A.* 51: 655, 1908.

19. Hewlett, A. W., and Van Zwaluwenburg, J. G. Method for estimating the blood flow in the arm: A preliminary report. *Arch. Intern. Med.* 3: 254, 1909.

20. Brodie, T. G. The determination of the rate of the blood flow through an organ. Reported at the Seventh International Physiological Congress, August 1907.

21. On March 13, 1973, William Dock wrote to William Hewlett, the son of Albion W. Hewlett, as follows:

Perhaps you have a bound copy of your father's reprints, but I thought you might like to see a few pages from his classic paper—"The First Quantitative Measurements of Blood Flow in a Limb." [This referred to the paper of Hewlett and Van Zwaluwenburg published in *Heart* in 1909.] In 1970 Eugene Braunwald, now head of medicine at the Peter Bent Brigham Hospital, reported using that method to demonstrate that arteriosclerotic narrowing could be reversed, flow to the leg increased and symptoms relieved by regimens which greatly lowered levels of blood cholesterol and triglyceride. I enclose xerox copies of that report, since Figure 7 is almost identical with Figure 4 in your father's paper. The changes in limb volume are now measured with a strain-gauge, introduced by Whitney in 1953. A late application is pulse measurement in the finger and in the penis of normal and impotent men [*Invest. Urol.* 8: 673, 1971]. Because our diabetic, two pack a day veteran smokers have leg problems and impotence at an early age, we became concerned about vascular disease causing both disabilities. This led me back to the 1909 paper.

Your father's selection of cases for study was as astute as his ingenuity in devising a method still in use. He found that in anemia the flow to the arm rose very little, and we now know blood is shunted to more vital areas. In the hyperthyroid patient, as shown on one of the sheets enclosed, flow is greatly increased, and we know this is needed to radiate the excessive heat produced by this disease. In 1925 I saw this method being used by Sir Thomas Lewis, the editor of *Heart*, and a very old friend of your father, to study flow in the hands of ladies with Raynaud's disease.

In the few weeks I was with your father, as resident physician, he showed me the Frank capsule he had just obtained for recording pulses with a synchronous electrocardiogram. He never had a chance to use it, but I put it to work, devised a way to record heart sounds with it, and thus set out on a path I still follow. (Archives, Stanford University School of Medicine)

22. Hewlett, A. W. Effect of room temperature upon blood flow in the arm, with a few observations on the effect of fever. *Heart* 2: 230, 1911.

23. Hewlett, A. W., Van Zwaluwenburg, J. G., and Agnew, J. H. A new method for studying the brachial pulse of man. *Trans. Assoc. Am. Physicians* 27: 188, 1912.

24. Hewlett, A. W. The pulse-flow in the brachial artery. IV. Reflections of the primary wave in dicrotic and monocrotic pulse forms. *Arch. Intern. Med.* 14: 609, 1914.

25. Hewlett, A. W. The effect of pituitary substance upon the pulse form of febrile patients. *Proc. Soc. Exp. Biol. Med.* 12–13: 61, 1914–16.

26. Hewlett, A. W. Eight years in the department of internal medicine. *Trans. Clin. Soc. Univ. Michigan* 7: 146, 1916.

27. Harvey, A. McG. *The Interurban Clinical Club, 1905–1976. A Record of Achievement in Clinical Science,* p. 118. Philadelphia: W. B. Saunders, 1978.

See Wilson, II. The years 1908–1927. In *The University of Michigan: An Encyclopedic Survey,* p. 841.

28. Means, J. H. Louis Harry Newburgh, 1883–1956. *Trans. Assoc. Am. Physicians* 70: 19, 1957.

29. Newburgh, L. H., and Minot, G. R. The blood pressure in pneumonia. *Arch. Intern. Med.* 14: 48, 1914.

Newburgh, L. H., Palmer, W. W., and Henderson, L. J. A study of hydrogen ion concentration of the urine in heart disease. *Arch. Intern. Med.* 12: 146, 1913.

Newburgh, L. H., and Porter, W. T. The heart muscle in pneumonia. *J. Exp. Med.* 22: 123, 1915.

30. Newburgh, L. H., and Clarkson, S. The production of atherosclerosis in rabbits by diets rich in meat protein. *Arch. Intern. Med.* 31: 653, 1923.

Newburgh, L. H., and Conn, J. W. Glycemic response to isoglucogenic quantities of protein and carbohydrate. *J. Clin. Invest.* 15: 665, 1936.

Newburgh, L. H., and Curtis, A. C. Toxic action of cystine on kidney. *Arch. Intern. Med.* 39: 817, 1927.

Newburgh, L. H., and Johnston, M. W. The determination of the total heat eliminated by the human being. *J. Clin. Invest.* 8: 147, 1930.

Newburgh, L. H., and Johnston, M. W. Nature of obesity. *J. Clin. Invest.* 8: 197, 1930.

Newburgh, L. H., Johnston, M. W., and Newburgh, J. D. *Some Fundamental Principles of Metabolism.* Ann Arbor: Edwards Bros., 1945.

Newburgh, L. H., and Lashmet, F. H. Comparative study of excretion of water and solids by normal and abnormal kidneys. *J. Clin. Invest.* 11: 1003, 1932.

Newburgh, L. H., Sheldon, J. M., and Johnston, M. W. Quantitative study of oxidation of glucose in normal and diabetic men. *J. Clin. Invest.* 16: 933, 1937.

Newburgh, L. H., and Squier, T. L. Renal irritation in man from high protein diet. *Arch. Intern. Med.* 28: 1, 1921.

Newburgh, L. H., and Wiley, F. H. Relationship between environment and basal insensible loss of weight. *J. Clin. Invest.* 10: 689, 1931.

Newburgh, L. H., Wiley, F. H., and Johnston, M. W. Note on calculation of water exchange. *J. Clin. Invest.* 12: 1151, 1933.

Newburgh, L. H., Wiley, F. H., and Lashmet, F. H. Method for determination of heat production over long periods of time. *J. Clin. Invest.* 10: 703, 1931.

31. Sheldon, J. M. *American Men of Science,* 9th ed., p. 1022.

32. Curtis, A. C. *American Men of Science,* 10th ed., p. 837.

Curtis, A. C., Horton, P. B., and Murrill, W. A. Vitamin A and carotene. I. The determination of vitamin A in the blood and liver as an index of vitamin A nutrition of the rat. *J. Clin. Invest.* 20: 387, 1941.

Curtis, A. C., Newburgh, L. H., Marsh, P., and Clarkson, S. The dietetic factor in the etiology of chronic nephritis. *J.A.M.A.* 85: 1703, 1925.

Curtis, A. C., Sheldon, J. M., and Eckstein, H. C. Experimental reproduction of lipemia. *Am. J. Med. Sci.* 86: 528, 1933.

33. Freyberg, R. H. *American Men of Science,* 10th ed., p. 1288.

In 1937, $1 million was appropriated from the Horace H. Rackham Fund, the interest on which was to be used for a period of not less than five years and not more than ten years, for the study of arthritis. This work was organized in the university hospital under the directorship of Freyberg.

34. Newburgh, L. H. Production of Bright's disease by feeding high protein diets. *Arch. Intern. Med.* 24: 359, 1919.

35. F. H. Lashmet received his M.D. degree from Michigan in 1927; during his first two years at Michigan he worked in physiology and received a M.S. degree in physiology in 1925. During his last two years he worked with Cowie in pediatrics, on the physiology of the gastrointestinal tract. He was a resident in medicine in 1928 and was appointed an instructor in 1929 and an assistant professor of internal medicine in 1933. He was also a member of the American Society for Clinical Investigation.

36. Newburgh, L. H., and Lashmet, F. H. Specific gravity of urine as a test of kidney function. *J.A.M.A.* 94: 1883, 1930.

37. Newburgh, L. H., and Marsh, P. L. Use of high fat diet in treatment of diabetes mellitus. *Arch. Intern. Med.* 26: 647, 1920.

38. Jerome Conn received his M.D. degree from Michigan in 1932, following which he had his residency training at the University of Michigan Hospital. He was appointed an instructor in medicine in 1934, an assistant professor in 1938, an associate professor in 1944, and a professor in 1950. Conn began his productive investigative career while with Newburgh, whom he succeeded as director of the endocrinology and metabolism section and of the metabolism research laboratories in 1943. His early work was mainly in the field of carbohydrate metabolism. Work during World War II for the U.S. Army on adaptation to hot climates led him into his fruitful studies on the role of the adrenal in regulating electrolytes and water balance, thus laying the basis for his later description of primary aldosteronism. On his retirement in 1973, he received the Distinguished Physician Award of the Veterans Administration, and he continued his work at the Ann Arbor Veterans Hospital until 1977. His publications include the following:

Conn, J. W. The advantage of a high protein diet in the treatment of spontaneous hypoglycemia. *J. Clin. Invest.* 15: 673, 1936.

Conn, J. W. *American Men of Science,* 12th ed., p. 1136.

Conn, J. W., and Conn, E. S. Hyperinsulinism: Extensive metabolic studies before and after removal of multiple pancreatic islet tissue adenomata. *J. Clin. Invest.* 19: 771, 1940.

Conn, J. W., Newburgh, L. H., Johnston, M. W., and Sheldon, J. M. Study of the deranged carbohydrate metabolism in chronic infectious hepatitis. *Arch. Intern. Med.* 62: 765, 1938.

39. Striker, C. L. Harry Newburgh. *Diabetes* 5: 408, 1956. (On this occasion, the Banting Medal of the American Diabetes Association was presented to Newburgh.)

40. Leaf, A. Personal communication, 1978.

41. Robinson, G. C. Louis Marshall Warfield, 1877–1938. *Trans. Assoc. Am. Physicians* 54: 2, 1939.

42. It was Warfield who recruited John B. Youmans for the Michigan faculty in 1922.

43. Wearn, J. T. Cyrus Cressey Sturgis, 1891–1966. *Trans. Assoc. Am. Physicians* 80: 24, 1967.

44. Sturgis, C. C. Angina pectoris as a complication in myxedema and exophthalmic goiter. *Boston Med. Surg. J.* 195: 351, 1926.

45. Wilson, II. The years 1908–1927. In *The University of Michigan: An Encyclopedic Survey*, p. 989.

46. Durant, T. M. Dr. Frank N. Wilson: A biographical sketch. *Trans. Stud. Coll. Physicians Phila.* 25: 160, 1958.

47. Herrmann, G. R., and Wilson, F. N. Ventricular hypertrophy, a comparison of clinical electrocardiographic and postmortem observations. *Heart* 9: 91, 1922.

Wilson, F. N., and Finch, R. The effect of drinking iced-water upon the form of the "T" deflection of the electrocardiogram. *Heart* 10: 275, 1923.

Wilson, F. N., and Herrmann, G. R. A new electrode for clinical and experimental electrocardiography. *Am. Heart J.* 1: 111, 1925.

Wilson, F. N., Hill, I. G. W., and Johnston, F. D. The interpretation of the galvanometric curves obtained when one electrode is distant from the heart and the other near or in contact with the ventricular surface. II. Observations on the mammalian heart. *Am. Heart J.* 10: 176, 1934.

Wilson, F. N., Johnston, F. D., Macleod, A. G., and Barker, P. S. Electrocardiograms in experimental myocardial infarction. I. Septal infarcts and the origin of the preliminary deflections of the canine levocardiogram. *Am. Heart J.* 9: 596, 1934.

Wilson, F. N., Wishart, S. W., and Herrmann, G. R. Factors influencing distribution of potential differences, produced by heart beat, at surface of body. *Proc. Soc. Exp. Biol. Med.* 23: 276, 1926.

48. Herrmann, G. R., and Wilson, F. N. An experimental study of incomplete bundle branch block and of the refractory period of the heart of the dog. *J.A.M.A.* 74: 1669, 1920; *Heart* 8: 229, 1921.

49. Barker, P. S., Alexander, J., and Macleod, A. G. Sensibility of the exposed human heart and pericardium. *Arch. Surg.* 19: 1470, 1929.

Barker, P. S., Shrader, E. L., and Ronzoni, E. The effects of alkalosis and of acidosis upon the human electrocardiogram. *Am. Heart J.* 17: 169, 1939.

50. Wilson, F. N., Macleod, A. G., and Barker, P. S. The T deflection of the electrocardiogram. *Trans. Assoc. Am. Physicians* 46: 29, 1931.

51. Barker, P. S., Macleod, A. G., Alexander, J., and Wilson, F. N. The excitatory process in the exposed human heart. *Trans. Assoc. Am. Physicians* 44: 125, 1929.

52. Wilson, F. N., Johnston, F. D., Hill, I. G. W., and Grout, G. C. The electrocardiogram in the later stages of experimental myocardial infarction. *Trans. Assoc. Am. Physicians* 48: 154, 1933.

Wilson, F. N. and Johnston, F. D. The occurrence in angina pectoris of electrocardiographic changes similar in magnitude and in kind to those produced by myocardial infarction. *Trans. Assoc. Am. Physicians* 54: 210, 1939.

53. Wilson, II. The years 1908–1927. In *The University of Michigan: An Encyclopedic Survey*, p. 998.

54. The address at the opening of the institute, entitled "The significance and relationship of the Thomas Simpson Memorial Institute for Medical Research" (*Science* 65: 359, 1927), was given by Henry A. Christian.

55. Isaacs, R., and Sturgis, C. C. Quantitative relationship between dosage and therapeutic response in 100 patients with pernicious anemia treated with liver extract or desiccated stomach. *J. Clin. Invest.* 10: 169, 1931.

Isaacs, R., Sturgis, C. C., Goldhamer, S. M., and Bethel, F. H. Purified liver extract administered intravenously in the treatment of pernicious anemia. *J. Clin. Invest.* 11: 808, 1932.

Isaacs, R., Sturgis, C. C., and Lodeesen-Grevinck, J. On the nature of the action of iron in "secondary anemia." *J. Clin. Invest.* 10: 686, 1931.

Isaacs, R., Sturgis, C. C., and Smith, M. The effect of the administration of liver to patients with various types of anemia. *J. Clin. Invest.* 6: 21, 1928.

Sturgis, C. C., and Farrar, G. E., Jr. Hemoglobin regeneration in the chronic hemorrhagic anemia of dogs (Whipple). I. Effect of iron and protein feeding. *J. Exp. Med.* 62: 457, 1935.

56. Doan, C. A. Raphael Isaacs, 1891–1965. *Trans. Assoc. Am. Physicians* 80: 11, 1967.

57. Isaacs, R. Properties of young erythrocytes in relation to agglutination and their behavior in hemorrhage and transfusion. *Arch. Intern. Med.* 33: 193, 1924.

Isaacs, R. A quantitative analysis of hemagglutination and hemolysis. *J. Immunol.* 9: 95, 1924.

Isaacs, R. The physiology of the leucocytes in the saliva in health and disease. *J. Clin. Invest.* 2: 616, 1926.

Isaacs, R., and Gordon, B. The effect of exercise on the distribution of corpuscles in the blood stream. *Am. J. Physiol.* 71: 106, 1924.

Minot, G. R., and Isaacs, R. Lymphatic leukemia: Age, incidence, duration and benefit derived from irradiation. *Boston Med. Surg. J.* 191: 1, 1924.

Minot, G. R., and Isaacs, R. Transfusion of lymphocytes: Their rapid disappearance from the circulation of man. *J.A.M.A.* 84: 1713, 1925.

58. Isaacs and Sturgis, Quantitative relationship between dosage and therapeutic response in 100 patients with pernicious anemia.

Isaacs, Sturgis, Goldhamer, and Bethel, Purified liver extract administered intravenously in the treatment of pernicious anemia.

Isaacs, Sturgis, and Lodeesen-Grevinck, On the nature of the action of iron in "secondary anemia."

Isaacs, Sturgis, and Smith, The effect of the administration of liver to patients with various types of anemia.

Sturgis and Farrar, Hemoglobin regeneration in the chronic hemorrhagic anemia of dogs (Whipple). I. Effect of iron and protein feeding.

59. Isaacs, R. The leukocytes in pernicious anemia; physiology, pathology and clinical significance. *J. Clin. Invest.* 6: 28, 1928.

Isaacs, R. Alterations of tissue cells in the blood stream. *Science* 68: 547, 1928.

Isaacs, R. The physiologic histology of the bone marrow. *Am. J. Physiol.* 90: 2, 1929.

Isaacs, R. Quantitative studies of the number of cells in the bone marrow. *J. Clin. Invest.* 9: 2, 1930.

Isaacs, R. On the fate of reticulocytes in the blood stream. *J. Clin. Invest.* 15: 469, 1936.

60. Bethel, F. H. Production of hepatic disease by dietary deficiency and its effect on the anti-pernicious anemia principle. *J.A.M.A.* 112: 878, 1939.

Bethel, F. H., and Goldhamer, S. M. Standards for maximum reticulocyte values following ventriculin and intravenous liver extract therapy in pernicious anemia. *Am. J. Med. Sci.* 186: 480, 1933.

Bethel, F. H., and Sturgis, C. C. The effect of vitamin B on hematology in the rat. *J. Clin. Invest.* 14: 721, 1935.

Bethel, F. H., Sturgis, C. C., and Isaacs, R. Relation between the reticulocyte production and degree of bone marrow involvement in pernicious anemia. *Proc. Cent. Soc. Clin. Res.*, pp. 41–42, October 1933.

61. Field, H., Jr. The effect of H-ion concentration on the utilization of insulin. *J. Clin. Invest.* 4: 447, 1927.

Field, H., Jr., Bock, A. V., Gildes, E. F., and Lathrop, F. L. The rate of the circulation of the blood in normal resting individuals. *J. Clin. Invest.* 1: 65, 1924.

Field, H., Jr., Henderson, L. J., Bock, A. V., and Stoddard, J. L. Blood as a physiochemical system. *J. Biol. Chem.* 59: 379, 1924.

Field, H., Jr., and Wise, E. C. Fatal probable riboflavin deficiency in man. *J. Clin. Invest.* 18: 474, 1939.

62. Smith, L. M. The determination of chlorides in trichloracetic acid filtrates from whole blood and plasma. *J. Biol. Chem.* 45: 437, 1921.

Smith, L. M. The minimum endogenous nitrogen metabolism. *J. Biol. Chem.* 68: 15, 1926.

Smith, L. M., Sturgis, C. C., and Isaacs, R. The treatment of pernicious anemia with a liver extract. *Ann. Intern. Med.* 1: 983, 1928.

63. Riecker, H. H. A study of experimental anemia in dogs; action of beef liver and iron salts on hemoglobin regeneration. *J. Clin. Invest.* 5: 141, 1927.

Riecker, H. H. The relation of chromatin to hemoglobin and bilirubin. *J. Exp. Med.* 49: 937, 1929.

Riecker, H. H. The relation of available iron to acid in alkaline diets. *J. Clin. Invest.* 10: 657, 1931.

Riecker, H. H., and Winters, M. E. Serum iron determinations applied to the study of experimental anemia. *Am. J. Physiol.* 92: 196, 1930.

64. Barnwell, J. B., and Adcock, J. D. Therapeutic pneumopericardium in tuberculosis pericarditis. *Univ. Mich. Hosp. Bull.* 6: 1, 1940.

Barnwell, J. B., Adcock, J. D., and Lyons, R. H. The circulatory effects produced in a patient with pneumopericardium by artificially varying the intrapericardial pressure. *Am. Heart J.* 19: 283, 1940.

65. Brown, C. L. *American Men of Science*, 10th ed., p. 472.

Brown, C. L., and Engelbach, F. Variations in the volume and in the acid content of gastric secretions of normal individuals following stimulation by histamin. *Ann. Intern. Med.* 6: 12, 1933.

Brown, C. L., and Meinenberg, L. J. The effects of pilocarpine on the volume, free and combined acid, total chlorides and pepsin of gastric secretion; and a comparison with the effects of histamin stimulation. *Ann. Intern. Med.* 7: 762, 1933.

66. Field, H., Jr., Melnick, D., Robinson, W. D., and Wilkinson, C. F., Jr. Studies on the chemical diagnosis of pellagra (nicotinic acid deficiency). *J. Clin. Invest.* 20: 379, 1941.

Robinson, W. D., Melnick, D., and Field, H., Jr. Urinary excretion of thiamine in clinical cases and the value of such analyses in the diagnosis of thiamine deficiency. *J. Clin. Invest.* 19: 399, 1940.

Robinson, W. D., Melnick, D., and Field, H., Jr. Correlations between the concentration of bisulphite binding substances in the blood and the urinary thiamine excretion. *J. Clin. Invest.* 19: 483, 1940.

67. Howell, W. H., whose words appear in *A Memorial of the Seventy-Fifth Anniversary of the Founding of the University of Michigan* (held commencement week, June 23–27, 1912), p. 80. Ann Arbor: University of Michigan, 1915.

# Chapter 19

1. Bonner, T. N. *Medicine in Chicago, 1850–1950.* Madison, Wis.: American History Research Center, 1957.

2. Irons, E. E. Ludwig Hektoen, 1863–1951. *Trans. Assoc. Am. Physicians* 65: 21, 1952.

3. Robinson, O. H. Frank Billings, 1854–1932. *Trans. Assoc. Am. Physicians* 48: 3, 1933.

4. Senn, N. Case of splenomedullary leukemia successfully treated by the use of the roentgen ray. *Med. Rec.* 64: 281, 1903.

5. Hektoen, L. Experimental measles. *J. Infect. Dis.* 2: 238, 1905.

6. Hektoen, L. Experimental measles. *J.A.M.A.* 72: 177, 1919.

7. Dochez, A. R., Avery, O. T., and Lancefield, R. C. Studies on the biology of streptococcus. I. Antigenic relationships between strains of Streptococcus hemolyticus. *J. Exp. Med.* 30: 179, 1919.

Stevens, F. A., and Dochez, A. R. Antigenic relationship between strains of streptococci from scarlet fever and erysipelas. *J. Exp. Med.* 43: 379, 1926.

8. Bliss, W. P. A biological study of hemolytic streptococci from the throats of patients suffering from scarlet fever. Preliminary report. *Bull. Johns Hopkins Hosp.* 31: 173, 1920.

9. Dick, G. F., and Dick, G. H. The etiology of scarlet fever. *J.A.M.A.* 82: 301, 1924.

10. Dochez, A. R., and Sherman, L. The significance of Streptococcus hemolyticus in scarlet fever. *J.A.M.A.* 82: 542, 1924.

11. Dick, G. F., and Dick, G. H. A skin test for susceptibility to scarlet fever. *J.A.M.A.* 82: 265, 1924.

Dick, G. F., and Dick, G. H. Scarlet fever. *Trans. Assoc. Am. Physicians* 39: 155, 1924.

12. Dick, G. F., and Dick, G. H. A scarlet fever antitoxin. *J.A.M.A.* 82: 1246, 1924.

Dick, G. F., and Dick, G. H. The prevention of scarlet fever. *J.A.M.A.* 83: 84, 1924.

Dick, G. F., and Dick, G. H. Therapeutic results with concentrated scarlet fever antitoxin. *J.A.M.A.* 84: 803, 1925.

13. Jacobson, L. O. George F. Dick, 1880–1967. *Trans. Assoc. Am. Physicians* 82: 32, 1969.

14. Ricketts, T. H., and Wilder, R. M. The transmission of the typhus fever of Mexico (Tabardillo) by means of the louse (Pediculus vestimenti). *J.A.M.A.* 54: 1304, 1910.

15. Colwell, A. R., Sr. Personal communication, 1976.

16. Snider, A. J. *The Otho A. Sprague Memorial Institute: First Fifty-Five Years* (*W. R. Odell, president*). Chicago: Ortho A. Sprague Memorial Institute, 1966.

17. Cannon, P. R. Harry Gideon Wells, 1875–1943. *Trans. Assoc. Am. Physicians* 58: 40, 1944.

18. Keeton, R. W. Rollin Turner Woodyatt. *Trans. Assoc. Am. Physicians* 67: 36, 1954.

19. Woodyatt's clinical research activities had, however, begun earlier, as he recorded:

In 1908 Doctor Billings privately paid me a salary to organize a division of research in the Department of Medicine at Rush Medical College. This established a position similar to that of an "assistant" in a German university medical clinic who divided his time between the research laboratory and the regular ward duties. I believe this arrangement, at that time, had no counterpart in the United States. It produced a group of physicians who later became heads of clinical departments, distinguished for their productivity. Doctor Billings was a regular visitor in this laboratory for research, keenly interested in the personnel and in the progress of their work. His personal magnetism aroused the best efforts from everyone. He was a devoted friend of the research investigator. (Hirsch, E. F. *Frank Billings: A Leader in Chicago Medicine,* p. 84. Chicago: University of Chicago Press, 1966.)

20. Woodyatt, R. T. Acidosis in diabetes. *Trans. Assoc. Am. Physicians* 31: 12, 1916.

Woodyatt, R. T. Objects and methods of diet adjustment in diabetes. *Arch. Intern. Med.* 28: 125, 1921.

Woodyatt, R. T. Principles underlying interpretation of blood-chemical data. *Trans. Assoc. Am. Physicians* 45: 283, 1930.

21. Colwell, Personal communication, 1976.

22. Capps, J. A. Robert Wood Keeton, 1883–1957. *Trans. Assoc. Am. Physicians* 70: 17, 1957.

23. Wangensteen, O. H. The academic surgical arena, past and present: A tribute to Evarts Graham, great surgical leader and innovator. *Surgery* 64: 595, 1968.

24. Graham, E. A. Late poisoning with chloroform and other alkyl halides in relationship to the halogen acids formed by their chemical dissociation. *J. Exp. Med.* 22: 48, 1915.

25. Irons, E. E. James Bryan Herrick, 1861–1954. *Trans. Assoc. Am. Physicians* 67: 15, 1954.

26. Herrick, J. B. *Memories of Eighty Years.* Chicago: University of Chicago Press, 1949.

27. Herrick, J. B. Peculiar elongated and sickle-shaped red corpuscles in a case of severe anemia. *Trans. Assoc. Am. Physicians* 25: 553, 1910.

28. Herrick, J. B. Clinical features of sudden obstruction of the coronary arteries. *J.A.M.A.* 59: 2015, 1912.

29. Herrick, J. B. Concerning thrombosis of the coronary arteries. *Trans. Assoc. Am. Physicians* 33: 408, 1918.

30. Herrick, J. B. An intimate account of my early experiences with coronary thrombosis. *Am. Heart J.* 27: 1, 1944.

31. Smith, F. M. The ligation of coronary arteries with electrocardiographic study. *Arch. Intern. Med.* 22: 8, 1918.

Smith made electrocardiograms before and after ligating the coronaries of dogs, some of whom survived the procedure for weeks. He described the T-wave changes. This work was followed by vast literature on the electrocardiogram after coronary occlusion. H. E. B. Pardee (An electrocardiographic sign of coronary occlusion. *Arch. Intern. Med.* 26: 244, 1920) began his article as follows: "The study of the form of the electrocardiogram continues to uphold the idea that when the muscular tissue of the heart is diseased, there will follow abnormal variations in the electrical currents due to the heart's contraction." By 1923 Smith (Electrocardiographic changes following occlusion of the left coronary artery. *Arch. Intern. Med.* 32: 497, 1923) felt able to conclude, after an electrocardiographic study of five cases, that "experimental and clinical observations justify the belief that the electrocardiograph may be employed to advantage in the diagnosis of coronary thrombosis in man."

32. Herrick, J. B. Acceptance of the Kober Medal. *Trans. Assoc. Am. Physicians* 45: 10, 1930.

Kober, G. Presentation of the Kober Medal to James B. Herrick. *Trans. Assoc. Am. Physicians* 45: 7, 1930.

33. Smith, F. M., Miller, G. H., and Graber, V. C. The effect of caffein sodio-benzoate, theobromin sodio-salicylate, theophyllin and euphyllin on the coronary flow and cardiac action of the rabbit. *J. Clin. Invest.* 2: 157, 1925–26.

Smith, F. M., Paul, W. D., and Rathe, H. W. Significance of coronary circulation in arteriosclerotic heart disease. *Trans. Assoc. Am. Physicians* 49: 163, 1934.

Watson, C. J. Fred M. Smith, 1888–1946. *Trans. Assoc. Am. Physicians* 59: 37, 1946.

34. Capps, J. A., and Coleman, G. H. *An Experimental and Clinical Study of Pain in the Pleura, Pericardium and Peritoneum.* New York: Macmillan, 1932.

35. Ricketts, H. T. Joseph Almarin Capps, 1872–1964. *Trans. Assoc. Am. Physicians* 78: 15, 1965.

36. Goodspeed, T. W. *A History of the University of Chicago, 1891–1916.* Chicago: University of Chicago Press, 1916.

McLean, F. C. University of Chicago Medicine in the Division of Biological Sciences. In *Methods and Problems of Medical Education,* 19th series. New York: Rockefeller Foundation, 1931.

Richter, R. B. A short history of the medical school at the University of Chicago. *Bull. Alumni Assoc. School of Med.* 22: 4, 1967.

Storr, R. J. *A History of the University of Chicago, Harper's University: The Beginning.* Chicago: University of Chicago Press, 1966.

Veith, I., and McLean, F. C. *Medicine at the University of Chicago, 1927–1952.* Chicago: University of Chicago Press, 1952.

37. Barker, L. F. Medicine and the universities. *Am. Med.* July 26, 1902. (Address delivered February 28, 1902, at a meeting of the western alumni of Johns Hopkins University.) See Cattell, J. M., ed. *Medical Research and Education,* p. 223, New York: Science Press, 1913.

38. Dobson, J. M. The modern university school; its purposes and methods. *J.A.M.A.* 39: 521, 1902.

39. Billings, F. Medical education in the United States. *J.A.M.A.* 40: 1271, 1903.

40. Hirsch, E. F. *Frank Billings: A Leader in Chicago Medicine,* p. 103, n.p., n.d.

41. McLean, University of Chicago Medicine in the Division of Biological Sciences, p. 1.

42. Hastings, A. B. Franklin Chambers McLean, 1888–1968. *Trans. Assoc. Am. Physicians* 82: 40, 1969.

Urist, M. R. Phoenix of medicine and physiology: Franklin Chambers McLean. *Perspect. Biol. Med.* 19: 23, 1975.

43. McLean, F. C. The sugar-content of the blood and its clinical significance. *J.A.M.A.* 62: 917, 1914; *Diabetes* 13: 193, 1964.

McLean, F. C. Physiology and medicine: A transition period. *Ann. Rev. Physiol.* 22: 1, 1960.

44. McLean, F. C. The numerical laws governing the rate of excretion of urea and chlorides in man. *J. Exp. Med.* 22: 212, 1915.

McLean, F. C. Clinical determination of renal function by an index of urea excretion. *J.A.M.A.* 66: 415, 1916.

McLean, F. C. The mechanism of urea retention in nephritis. *J. Exp. Med.* 26: 181, 1917.

45. Van Slyke, D. D., McLean, F. C., and Wu, H. Studies of gas and electrolyte equilibria in blood. V. Factors controlling the electrolyte and water distribution in the blood. *J. Biol. Chem.* 56: 765, 1923.

46. Veith and McLean, *Medicine at the University of Chicago*, p. 14.

47. Welch, W. H. Medicine and the university. Address at Convocation, University of Chicago, December 17, 1907. *J.A.M.A.* 1: 50, 1908.

48. Veith and McLean, *Medicine at the University of Chicago*, p. 14.

49. McLean, University of Chicago Medicine in the Division of Biological Sciences, p. 67.

Veith and McLean, *Medicine at the University of Chicago*, p. 41.

50. Leiter had trained under Van Slyke at the Hospital of the Rockefeller Institute, during which time he acquired his interest in renal disease.

Leiter, L. The surface tension of the blood serum in nephritis. *J. Clin. Invest.* 3: 267, 1926–27.

51. Landsteiner, K., and Miller, C. P. Serological studies on the blood of the primates. III. Distribution of the serological factors related to human isoagglutinogens in the blood of lower monkeys. *J. Exp. Med.* 42: 863, 1925.

Miller, C. P. Some observations on experimental meningococcal infection. *Trans. Assoc. Am. Physicians* 50: 237, 1935.

Miller, C. P., and Boor, A. K. Immunological characteristics of some substances obtained from gonococcus. *Trans. Assoc. Am. Physicians* 46: 223, 1931.

Miller, C. P., and Hawk, W. D. Experimental gonococcal infection. *Trans. Assoc. Am. Physicians* 55: 216, 1940.

52. Hastings, A. B. Franklin Chambers McLean, 1888–1968. *Trans. Assoc. Am. Physicians* 82: 40, 1969.

53. For a review of the controversy over the full-time plan at Chicago, which led to McLean's resignation, see Urist, Phoenix of medicine and physiology: Franklin Chambers McLean.

54. McLean, F. C., and Hastings, A. B. A biological method for the estimation of calcium ion concentration. *J. Biol. Chem.* 107: 337, 1934.

McLean, F. C., and Hastings, A. B. Clinical estimation and significance of calcium ion concentration in the blood. *Am. J. Med. Sci.* 189: 601, 1935.

55. Robertson, O. H., and Bock, A. V. Blood volume in wounded soldiers. II. The use of forced fluids by the alimentary tract in the restoration of blood volume after hemorrhage. *J. Exp. Med.* 29: 155, 1919.

Robertson, O. H., and Rous, P. The normal fate of erythrocytes. II. Blood destruction in plethoric animals and in animals with a simple anemia. *J. Exp. Med.* 25: 665, 1917.

Robertson, O. H., and Rous, P. Autohemagglutination experimentally induced by the repeated withdrawal of blood. *J. Exp. Med.* 27: 563, 1918.

Robertson, O. H., and Rous, P. Sources of the antibodies developing after repeated transfusion. *J. Exp. Med.* 35: 141, 1922.

56. Robertson, O. H., Coggeshall, L. T., and Terrell, E. E. Experimental pneumococcus lobar pneumonia in the dog. III. Pathogenesis. *J. Clin. Invest.* 12: 467, 1933.

Robertson, O. H., Graeser, J. B., Coggeshall, L. T., Harrison, M. A., and Sia, R. H. P. The relation of circulating antipneumococcal immune substances to the course of lobar pneumonia. III. Injected immune substances (antipneumococcus serum, types I and II). *J. Clin. Invest.* 13: 649, 1934.

57. Allen, E. V. Russell M. Wilder, 1885-1959. *Trans. Assoc. Am. Physicians* 73: 49, 1960.

Wilder, R. M. Recollections and reflections on education, diabetes and other metabolic diseases and nutrition in the Mayo Clinic and associated hospitals, 1919-1950. *Perspect. Biol. Med.* 1: 240, 1958.

58. George Dick to Dr. Bachmeyer, director of the University of Chicago Hospitals, November 3, 1938. University of Chicago Archives.

59. Byyny, R. L., Siegler, M., and Tarlov, A. R. Development of General Internal Medicine at the University of Chicago, Unpublished manuscript, 1976.

60. Jacobson, L. O. Alf Sven Alving, 1902-1965. *Trans. Assoc. Am. Physicians* 79: 16, 1966.

61. Bordley, J., III, and Harvey, A. McG. *Two Centuries of American Medicine, 1776-1976*, p. 678. Philadelphia: W. B. Saunders, 1976.

Huggins, C. Investigative approaches to the physiology of reproduction. *J. Urol.* 60: 812, 1948.

# Chapter 20

1. Myers, J. A. *Masters of Medicine: An Historical Sketch of the College of Medical Science, University of Minnesota, 1888-1966*. St. Louis: Warren H. Green, 1968.
See Appendix E for interview with Cecil J. Watson.

2. Flexner, A. *Medical Education in the United States and Canada*, p. 248. New York: Carnegie Foundation for the Advancement of Teaching, 1910.

3. A joint training program administered in the graduate school required that all medical residents at the Mayo Clinic, and at the University Hospital and affiliated teaching hospitals, register in the graduate school as medical fellows. Courses could be pursued, largely at the university in the basic sciences, for which the trainees paid tuition and which could lead to M.S. or Ph.D. degrees. A joint Graduate School Committee, composed of Mayo Clinic members and University of Minnesota faculty, conducted oral and written examinations for those seeking a degree. Although many of the Mayo Clinic candidates pursued basic science instruction on the Minneapolis campus, relatively few of the fellows from the university had training in Rochester. It was a relationship that allowed the fellows of the Mayo Clinic to earn a degree from the university. At the same time, scholarship was greatly encouraged at the clinic and at the university.

By the 1970s, the relationship with the Mayo Foundation had been greatly modified. In 1964 the Mayo Graduate School of the University of Minnesota was organized. In addition, medical fellows in clinical training at the University of Minnesota who desired to do course work in the graduate school were designated as medical fellow specialists.

4. The details of the stormy controversy over the setting up of the Mayo Foundation for Medical Education and Research, and its affiliation with the University of Minnesota School of Medicine, are described in Clapesattle, H. B. *The Doctors Mayo*, pp. 539-59. Minneapolis: University of Minnesota Press, 1941.

5. Keith, N. N., and Hench, P. S. Leonard George Rowntree, 1883-1959. *Trans. Assoc. Am. Physicians* 73: 31, 1960.

6. Abel, J. J., and Rowntree, L. G. On the pharmacological action of some phthaleins

and their derivatives, with special reference to their behavior as purgatives. *J. Pharmacol. Exp. Ther.* 1: 231, 1909.

7. Christian, H. A., Janeway, T. C., and Rowntree, L. G. On the study of renal function. *Trans. Cong. Am. Physicians Surg.* 9: 1, 1913.

Rowntree, L. G., and Fitz, R. Studies of renal function in renal, cardiorenal and cardiac disease. *Arch. Intern. Med.* 11: 121, 1913.

Rowntree, L. G., and Geraghty, J. T. An experimental and clinical study of the functional activity of the kidneys by means of phenolsulphonephthalein. *J. Pharmacol. Exp. Ther.* 1: 579, 1909–10.

Rowntree, L. G., and Geraghty, J. T. The phthalein test, an experimental and clinical study of phenolsulphonephthalein in relation to renal function in health and disease. *Arch. Intern. Med.* 9: 284, 1912.

8. Reimann, H. A. Solon Marx White, 1873–1966. *Trans. Assoc. Am. Physicians* 80: 30, 1967.

9. Fahr, G. Myxedema heart. *J.A.M.A.* 84: 345, 1925.

Fahr, G. Myxedema heart. *Am. Heart J.* 8: 91, 1932.

10. Berglund, H., Folin, O., and Derick, C. The uric acid problem: An experimental study on animals and man, including gouty subjects. *J. Biol. Chem.* 60: 35, 1924.

11. Reimann, H. Hilding Berglund, 1887–1962. *Trans. Assoc. Am. Physicians* 76: 9, 1963.

12. Berglund, H., Medes, G., Huber, C., Longcope, W., and Richards, A. N. *The Kidney in Health and Disease*. Philadelphia: Lea & Febiger, 1935.

13. Barron, M. The relation of the islets of Langerhans to diabetes with special reference to cases of pancreatic lithiasis. *Surg. Gynecol. Obstet.* 31: 437, 1920.

14. Ebert, R. V. Presentation of the Kober Medal for 1972 to C. J. Watson. *Trans. Assoc. Am. Physicians* 85: 51, 1972.

Watson, C. J. Concerning the naturally occurring porphyrins. III. The isolation of coproporphyrin I from the feces of untreated cases of pernicious anemia. *J. Clin. Invest.* 14: 116, 1935.

Watson, C. J. Acceptance of the Kober Medal for 1972. *Trans. Assoc. Am. Physicians* 85: 59, 1972.

15. Spink, W. W., and Augustine, D. L. Trichinosis in Boston. *N. Engl. J. Med.* 213: 527, 1935.

16. Spink, W. W., and Keefer, C. S. Studies of hemolytic streptococcal infection (three reports on erysipelas). *J. Clin. Invest.* 15: 17, 1936; 15: 21, 1936; 16: 155, 1937.

17. Spink, W. W. The pathogenesis of gonococcal infection. *Publication no. 11, American Association for the Advancement of Science*, p. 35, 1939; idem, *J.A.M.A.* 109: 1448, 1937.

18. Spink, W. W. *Sulfanilamide and Related Compounds in General Practice*. Chicago: Year Book Publishers, 1941.

19. Spink, W. W. *The Nature of Brucellosis*. Minneapolis: University of Minnesota Press, 1956.

20. Dr. Abraham I. Braude, professor of medicine, University of California, San Diego; Dr. Sydney M. Finegold, professor of medicine, University of California, Los Angeles; Dr. Wendell H. Hall, professor of medicine, University of Minnesota, Minn.; and Dr. Robert I. Wise, chairman and professor of medicine, Jefferson Medical College, Philadelphia, Pa.

21. Myers, *Masters of Medicine: An Historical Sketch of the College of Medical Science, University of Minnesota, 1888–1966*, p. 98.

22. Wangensteen, O. H. Glimpses of the University of Minnesota's surgery department. *Lancet* 83: 161, 1963.

23. Wangensteen to Spink. June 20, 1979. This letter was written at the request of the author.

24. Good, R. A., and Platou, E. S., eds. *Essays on Pediatrics in Honor of Irvine McQuarrie: Being a compilation of papers presented by his former students and associates*. Minneapolis: Lancet Publications, 1955.

McQuarrie, I. Autobiographic sketch. *Perspect. Biol. Med.,* Autumn 1962, p. 61.

25. Selected references of Irvine McQuarrie include:

McQuarrie, I. Isoagglutination in newborn infants and their mothers: A possible relationship between interagglutination and toxemias of pregnancy. *Bull. Johns Hopkins Hosp.* 34: 51, 1923.

McQuarrie, I. The department of pediatrics, University of Minnesota. *J. Pediatr.* 5: 365, 1934.

McQuarrie, I., Anderson, R. G., Wright, W. S., and Bauer, E. G. Familial hypoglycemosis of probable genetic origin. *Am. J. Hum. Genet.* 2: 264, 1950.

McQuarrie, I., Bauer, E. G., Ziegler, M. R., and Wright, W. S. The metabolic and clinical effects of pituitary adrenocorticotrophic hormone in spontaneous hypoglycemosis. *Proc. First Clin. ACTH Conference.* Mote, J. R., ed. New York: Blakiston, 1950.

McQuarrie, I., and Davis, N. C. Blood volume as determined by the change in the refractivity of the serum nonprotein fraction after the injection of certain colloids into the circulation. *Am. J. Physiol.* 51: 257, 1920.

McQuarrie, I., Hanson, A. E., and Ziegler, M. R. Studies on the convulsive mechanism in idiopathic hypoparathyroidism. *J. Clin. Endocrinol.* 1: 789, 1941.

McQuarrie, I., and Keith, H. M. Influence of acid-forming and base-forming constituents of ketogenic diet used in treatment of idiopathic epilepsy. *Proc. Soc. Exp. Biol. Med.* 25: 418, 1928.

McQuarrie, I., and Peeler, D. B. The effects of sustained pituitary antidiuresis and forced water drinking in epileptic children: A diagnostic and etiological study. *J. Clin. Invest.* 10: 915, 1931.

McQuarrie, I., and Ziegler, M. R. Mechanism of insulin convulsions. I. Serum electrolytes and blood sugar in relation to occurrence of convulsions. *Proc. Soc. Exp. Biol. Med.* 39: 523, 1938.

# Chapter 21

1. Clapesattle, H. B. *The Doctors Mayo.* Minneapolis: University of Minnesota Press, 1941.

2. Work in clinical pathology was begun in 1900 by Dr. Isabella Herb.

3. In 1910 Theodore Kocher, of Berne, wrote a paper (Ueber Jodbasedow. *Arch. f. klin. Chirurg.* 92: 166, 1910) that influenced the use of iodine in exophthalmic goitre. Kocher, who was confused by the frequency of simple goitre in Berne and the difficulty of always making a clear differentiation from Basedow's disease, concluded that "iodine medication remains a two-edged sword which cuts both ways in Basedow, and in practice the harm caused by iodine in all typical and atypical forms is much greater than the benefit." In 1922 Plummer was writing an account of thyroid disease for a new edition of *Oxford Medicine.* As he mulled over the various reports on the use of iodine, he realized where Kocher had erred—by not distinguishing between simple goitre accompanied by hyperthyroidism and true exophthalmic goitre. He decided that iodine should receive a thorough trial on his goitre service at St. Mary's (Clapesattle, *The Doctors Mayo,* pp. 634–35). Plummer and Boothby (The value of iodine in exophthalmic goitre. *J. Iowa Med. Soc.* 14: 66, 1924) gave large amounts of iodine to patients with hyperthyroidism. There was prompt alleviation of toxic symptoms and a fall in basal metabolic rate; it became possible to do a subtotal thyroidectomy without precipitating a thyroid crisis.

In their paper, Plummer and Boothby stated that a discussion of theories leading up to their trial was conducted at the meeting of the Association of American Physicians in June 1923. Nothing regarding this appears in the 1923 volume of the association's transactions, but in 1924 (*Trans. Assoc. Am. Physicians* 33: 178, 1924), in a discussion of a paper by E. H. Mason, Plummer gave a statement of his rationale in using iodine. Under the heading

"American Association of Physicians," there appeared in the *J.A.M.A.* (80: 1955, 1923) a brief note by Plummer. In it he said: "Acting on this plan, we administered 10 drops of compound solution of iodine for 10 days *following operation* [italics mine] with the result that we found there is no such thing as postoperative deaths from hyperthyroidism if this dosage has been administered with regularity. In other words, the patient is relatively short of iodine, and dies from lack of it. When we replace iodine, we do away with postoperative deaths."

Boothby soon published a confirmatory paper (The use of iodine in exophthalmic goitre. *Endocrinology* 8: 727, 1924).

The occasional development of myxedema after prolonged administration of iodine was reported by S. F. Haines (Exophthalmic goitre and myxedema; report of cases. *Endocrinology* 12: 55, 1928), raising questions as to the mechanism of iodine action on the thyroid in general and also in Graves's disease.

4. Louis B. Wilson was, for several years, assistant director of the Minnesota State Board of Health Laboratory and assistant professor of pathology at the University of Minnesota. Under his direction, the laboratory work in clinical pathology was developed. (*Sketch of the History of the Mayo Clinic and the Mayo Foundation*, p. 52. Philadelphia: W. B. Saunders, 1926.) This sketch was written by Mrs. Mead H. Mellish and Wilson and was based in part on William J. Mayo's account, as recorded by Mrs. Mellish.

5. Sprague, R. G. Development of Endocrinology at the Mayo Clinic, 1913–1951. This unpublished manuscript was kindly lent to me by Dr. R. G. Sprague.

Wilson, L. B. The pathological changes in the thyroid gland as related to the varying symptoms in Graves's disease. *Trans. Assoc. Am. Physicians* 23: 562, 1908.

Wilson, L. B. Pathology of nodular (adenomatous?) goitres in patients with and without symptoms of hyperthyroidism. *Trans. Assoc. Am. Physicians* 37: 68, 1922.

Wilson, L. B., and Kendall, E. C. The relationship of the pathological histology and the iodine compounds of the human thyroid. *Trans. Assoc. Am. Physicians* 30: 458, 1915.

6. Hench, P. S. Presentation of the Kober Medal to Edwin Calvin Kendall. *Trans. Assoc. Am. Physicians* 65: 42, 1952.

Kendall, E. C. The isolation of crystalline form of the compound containing iodine which occurs in the thyroid. *J.A.M.A.* 64: 2042, 1915.

Kendall, E. C. *Thyroxine.* New York: Chemical Catalogue Co., 1929.

Kendall, E. C. Acceptance of the Kober Medal. *Trans. Assoc. Am. Physicians* 65: 52, 1952.

7. Haines, S. F. Walter Meredith Boothby, 1880–1953. *Trans. Assoc. Am. Physicians* 67: 10, 1954.

8. Boothby, W. M., and Sandiford, I. Basal metabolism. *Physiol. Rev.* 4: 69, 1924.

Boothby, W. M., Sandiford, I., Sandiford, K., and Slosse, J. Effect of thyroxin on respiratory and nitrogenous metabolism of normal and myxedematous subjects. I. Method of studying reserve or deposit protein with preliminary report of results obtained. *Trans. Assoc. Am. Physicians* 40: 195, 1925.

9. Mellish and Wilson, *Sketch of the History of the Mayo Clinic and the Mayo Foundation*, p. 71.

Willius, F. A. *Henry Stanley Plummer: A Diversified Genius.* Springfield, Ill.: Charles C Thomas, 1960.

10. Kendall, E. C., and Keith, N. M. Louis Blanchard Wilson, 1866–1943. *Trans. Assoc. Am. Physicians* 58: 43, 1944.

11. Mann, F. C. To the physiologically inclined. *Ann. Rev. Physiol.* 17: 1, 1955.

Sprague, R. G. Frank Charles Mann, 1887–1962. *Trans. Assoc. Am. Physicians* 77: 22, 1964.

Visscher, M. B. Frank Charles Mann (Sept. 11, 1887–Sept. 30, 1962). *Biog. Mem. Natl. Acad. Sci.* 38: 161, 1964. (Contains Mann's complete bibliography.)

12. Clapesattle, *The Doctors Mayo,* p. 621.

13. Keith, N. M., and Hench, P. S. Leonard George Rowntree, 1883–1959. *Trans. Assoc. Am. Physicians* 73: 27, 1960.

14. Brown, G. E., and Craig, W. McK. Physiological effects of unilateral and bilateral

resection of major and minor splanchnic nerves in man. *Trans. Assoc. Am. Physicians* 48: 213, 1933.

Brown, G. E., and Horton, B. T. Clinical syndrome due to cold, with local and general systemic reactions suggesting those obtained by histamine. *Trans. Assoc. Am. Physicians* 47: 357, 1932.

Keith, N. M. A method for the determination of plasma and blood volume. *Trans. Assoc. Am. Physicians* 30: 102, 1915.

Keith, N. M., and Pulford, D. S., Jr. Chloride retention in experimental hydronephrosis. *J. Exp. Med.* 37: 175, 1923.

Rowntree, L. G., Greene, C. H., and Aldrich, M. Quantitative Pettenkofer values in blood with special reference to hepatic disease. *J. Clin. Invest.* 4: 545, 1927.

15. Allen, E. V. Russell M. Wilder, 1885–1959. *Trans. Assoc. Am. Physicians* 73: 49, 1960.

16. Woodyatt, R. T. George Elgie Brown, 1885–1935. *Trans. Assoc. Am. Physicians* 51: 3, 1936.

17. Rowntree, L. G. Water intoxication. *Arch. Intern. Med.* 32: 157, 1923.

Rowntree, L. G. and Brown, G. E. Studies in blood volume with the dye method. *Ann. Intern. Med.* 1: 890, 1928.

Rowntree, L. G., Osborne, E. D., Sutherland, C. G., and Scholl, A. J. Roentgenography of the urinary tract during the excretion of sodium iodide. *J.A.M.A.* 80: 368, 1923.

Rowntree, L. G., Weir, I. F., and Larson, E. E. Studies in diabetes insipidus, water balance and water intoxication. Study I. *Arch. Intern. Med.* 29: 306, 1922.

18. Pruitt, R. D. Norman M. Keith, 1885–1976. *Trans. Assoc. Am. Physicians* 89: 23, 1976.

19. Keith, N. M., Osterberg, A. E., and King, H. E. Excretion of potassium by normal and diseased kidney. *Trans. Assoc. Am. Physicians* 55: 219, 1940.

Keith, N. M., Wagener, H. P., and Barker, N. W. Some different types of essential hypertension: Their course and prognosis. *Am. J. Med. Sci.* 197: 332, 1939.

Keith, N. M., Wagener, H. P., and Kernohan, J. W. The syndrome of malignant hypertension. *Arch. Intern. Med.* 41: 141, 1928.

Keith, N. M., and Whelan, M. A study of the action of ammonium chloride and organic mercury compounds. *J. Clin. Invest.* 3: 149, 1926–27.

20. Woodyatt, George Elgie Brown.

21. Burchell, H. B. Edgar V. Allen, 1900–1961. *Trans. Assoc. Am. Physicians* 75: 13, 1962.

22. Burwell, C. S. Reginald Fitz, 1885–1953. *Trans. Assoc. Am. Physicians* 67: 12, 1954.

Harvey, A. McG. *The Interurban Clinical Club, 1905–1976. A Record of Achievement in Clinical Science,* p. 131. Philadelphia: W. B. Saunders, 1978.

23. Brown, G. E. Observations on the surface capillaries in man following cervicothoracic sympathetic ganglionectomy. *J. Clin. Invest.* 9: 115, 1930–31.

24. Brown, G. E. Calorimetric studies of the extremities. III. Clinical data on normal and pathologic subjects with localized vascular disease. *J. Clin. Invest.* 3: 369, 1926–27.

Brown, G. E., and Sheard, C. Measurements on the skin capillaries in cases of polycythemia vera and the role of these capillaries in the production of erythrosis. *J. Clin. Invest.* 2: 423, 1925–26.

Craig, W. McK., Horton, B. T., and Sheard, C. Thermal changes in peripheral vascular disease during sympathetic ganglionectomy under general anesthesia. *J. Clin. Invest.* 12: 573, 1933.

Sheard, C. Calorimetric studies of the extremities. I. Theory and practice of methods applicable to such investigations. *J. Clin. Invest.* 3: 327, 1926–27.

Sheard, C., Rynearson, E. H., and Craig, W. McK. Effects of environmental temperature, anesthesia and lumbar sympathetic ganglionectomy on the temperatures of the extremities of animals. *J. Clin. Invest.* 11: 183, 1932.

25. Clapesattle, *The Doctors Mayo,* pp. 639–42.

Rowntree, L. G., and Adson, A. W. Bilateral lumbar sympathetic neurectomy in the treatment of malignant hypertension. *J.A.M.A.* 85: 959, 1925.

26. Rowntree, L. G. *Amid Masters of Twentieth Century Medicine: A Panorama of Persons and Pictures*. Springfield, Ill.: Charles C Thomas, 1958.

Rowntree, L. G., Brown, G. E., and Roth, G. *The Volume of the Blood and Plasma in Health and Disease*. Philadelphia: W. B. Saunders, 1929.

27. Aside from the clinical research that Henry S. Plummer found time for, little was done at the clinic until the addition of the Rowntree unit. They promptly set up laboratories at St. Mary's for urine, blood, and gastric analysis and then acquired special laboratories for their investigative work, until each man had his own, complete with equipment and technicians. Stimulated by the incomparable opportunities the clinic practice provided, they were soon producing results that won favorable notice from the medical world.

Older internists on the clinic staff, some of whom had long wanted hospital services themselves, were irked by the attention given the newcomers and grumbled about the space and money spent on them and the time off allowed them for trips to medical conventions, where they were in great demand as speakers. The resentment spread until it threatened to reach disruptive intensity. The Rowntree unit rapidly developed into a little medical clinic within the clinic, drawing its financial support and its patients from the clinic, but otherwise being quite independent.

Several of the men were showing a tendency to let their younger associates do the work while they went off on one trip after another, only to claim the credit when the results were published. This discouraged the younger men, and that, above all else, William J. Mayo would not tolerate. He knew it to be a threat to the very life of the clinic, to the spirit that had made it and upon which its continued success would in large measure depend.

When the medical unit sought to establish its own laboratories for animal experimentation, it was decided to call a halt to the growing separatism. The Board of Governors voted to disperse the medical unit and distribute its staff and laboratories among the clinic sections.

The special service for clinical investigation came slowly to life again, as an unofficial outgrowth of the work of George E. Brown, one of the members of the former medical unit. He was a man of tact and had an undeniable flair for clinical research, so that soon some of the other clinicians were, of their own volition, referring obscure cases to his hospital service for the detailed study they themselves had no time to make.

The Board of Governors finally recognized this development by giving it official status as a clinical investigation laboratory, with Brown in charge. But the lesson of the previous experience had been well learned. It was clearly understood that the new laboratory belonged to no one person, but was open to all.

28. Allen, Russell M. Wilder.

Wilder, R. M. Recollections and reflections on education, diabetes and other metabolic diseases and nutrition in the Mayo Clinic and associated hospitals, 1919–1950. *Perspect. Biol. Med.* 1: 240, 1958.

29. Ricketts, H. T., and Wilder, R. M. The transmission of typhus fever (Tabardillo) of Mexico by means of the louse (Pediculus Vestimenti). *J.A.M.A.* 54: 1304, 1910.

Ricketts, H. T., and Wilder, R. M. The etiology of typhus fever, a further preliminary report. *J.A.M.A.* 54: 1373, 1910.

30. Boothby, W. M., and Wilder, R. M. Preliminary report on the effect of insulin on the rate of heat production and its significance in regard to the calorigenic action of adrenalin. *Med. Clin. North Am.* 7: 53, 1923.

Wilder, R. M., Boothby, W. M., and Beeler, C. Studies of the metabolism in diabetes. *J. Biol. Chem.* 51: 311, 1922.

31. Wilder, R. M., Allan, F. N., Power, M. H., and Robertson, H. E. Carcinoma of the islands of the pancreas. *J.A.M.A.* 89: 348, 1927.

32. Wilder, R. M. Hyperparathyroidism, with report of tumor of parathyroid. *Trans. Assoc. Am. Physicians* 44: 242, 1929.

33. Johnson, J. L., and Wilder, R. M. Experimental chronic hyperparathyroidism. I. Metabolic studies. *Am. J. Med. Sci.* 182: 807, 1931.

Wilder, R. M. Hyperparathyroidism: Tumor of the parathyroid glands associated with osteitis fibrosa. *Endocrinology* 13: 231, 1929.

Sprague pointed out, however, that the clinic physicians did not become really proficient in the diagnosis of hyperparathyroidism until 1942, when F. R. Keating returned from a six-month period of study, under Fuller Albright, at the MGH. Then the detection of hyperparathyroidism increased tenfold.

34. Mayo, C. Paroxysmal hypertension associated with tumor of retroperitoneal nerve. *J.A.M.A.* 89: 1049, 1927.

35. Pincoffs, M. C. A case of paroxysmal hypertension associated with suprarenal tumor. *Trans. Assoc. Am. Physicians* 44: 295, 1929.

36. Rowntree, L. G., and Greene, C. H. The treatment of patients with Addison's disease with the "cortical hormone" of Swingle and Pfiffner. *Science* 72: 482, 1930.

37. Hartman, F. A., MacArthur, C. G., and Hartman, W. E. A substance which prolongs the life of adrenalectomized cats. *Proc. Soc. Exp. Biol. Med.* 24: 69, 1927.

Swingle, W. W., and Pffifner, J. J. An aqueous extract of the suprarenal cortex which maintains the life of bilaterally adrenalectomized cats. *Science* 71: 321, 1930.

Swingle, W. W., and Pfiffner, J. J. Further observations on adrenalectomized cats treated with an aqueous extract of suprarenal cortex. *Science* 71: 489, 1930.

Swingle, W. W., and Pfiffner, J. J. The adrenal cortical hormone. *Medicine* 11: 371, 1932.

38. Rowntree, L. G., Greene, C. H., Ball, R. G., Swingle, W. W., and Pfiffner, J. J. Treatment of Addison's disease with the cortical hormone of the suprarenal gland. *J.A.M.A.* 97: 1446, 1931.

39. Greene, C. H. Clinical use of the extract of the adrenal cortex. *Arch. Intern. Med.* 59: 759, 1937.

40. Rowntree, L. G., and Snell, A. M. *A Clinical Study of Addison's Disease.* Philadelphia: W. B. Saunders, 1931.

41. Edwin J. Kepler came to Rochester in 1925 as a fellow in medicine. He had a rare insight into clinical physiology, which he applied with skill in diagnosis and therapy. He became a leader in the study of diseases of the adrenal cortex and was largely responsible for the clinic's pioneering work in the treatment of Cushing's syndrome by radical adrenalectomy.

42. Edward H. Rynearson entered the Mayo Foundation as a fellow in medicine in 1927 and, after his training was completed, worked for a period with Philip Hench. His major contributions were those concerning hyperinsulinism and diseases of the anterior pituitary.

43. Wilder, R. M., Kendall, E. C., Snell, A. M., Kepler, E. J., Rynearson, E. H., and Adams, M. Control of Addison's disease with a diet restricted in potassium. *Trans. Assoc. Am. Physicians* 51: 132, 1936.

44. Cutler, H. H., Power, M. H., and Wilder, R. M. Concentrations of chloride, sodium and potassium in the urine and blood. Their diagnostic significance in adrenal insufficiency. *J.A.M.A.* 111: 117, 1938.

45. Robinson, F. J., Power, M. H., and Kepler, E. J. Two new procedures to assist in the recognition and exclusion of Addison's disease: A preliminary report. *Proc. Staff Meet. Mayo Clinic* 16: 577, 1941.

46. The author has made extensive use, with permission, of Dr. R. G. Sprague's unpublished manuscript, Development of Endocrinology at the Mayo Clinic, 1913–1951, in recounting the events surrounding these classical studies.

47. Kendall, E. C., et al. Isolation in crystalline form of the hormone essential to life from the suprarenal cortex: Its chemical nature and physiological properties. *Trans. Assoc. Am. Physicians* 49: 147, 1934.

48. In many cases of rheumatoid arthritis, the disease rather relentlessly progresses, but Hench had noted that if patients with this disease develop jaundice or become pregnant, there might be a remission of the arthritis that is sometimes quite impressive. Hench

and his colleagues attempted to reproduce the effects of jaundice or pregnancy by various means. These included the transfusion of blood from jaundiced or pregnant donors to arthritis patients; the administration of female hormones and various biliary products; and the production of jaundice experimentally by the administration of several different chemical agents. None of these artificial procedures seemed to have any appreciable effect on the arthritis.

Hench also had been impressed by the fact that the weakness, fatigue, and low blood pressure exhibited by many patients with rheumatoid arthritis were similar to the symptoms of Addison's disease, and he began to wonder whether the antirheumatic substance might be an adrenal hormone. After consultation with Kendall in 1941, Hench decided to administer compound E to rheumatoid patients, but the amount of this substance then available was almost negligible; hence it was decided to try some of Kendall's rather crude extract, cortin. This had no beneficial effect.

Hench, P. S., Kendall, E. C., Slocumb, C. H., and Polley, H. F. Effect of the hormone of the adrenal cortex, cortisone and of pituitary adrenocorticotropic hormone on rheumatoid arthritis. *Trans. Assoc. Am. Physicians* 62: 64, 1949.

Sprague, R. G. Philip Showalter Hench, 1896–1965. *Trans. Assoc. Am. Physicians* 78: 26, 1965.

49. Sprague, Development of Endocrinology at the Mayo Clinic, 1913–1951.

50. Giffin, H. Z. Observations on treatment of myelocytic leukemia by radium. *Trans. Assoc. Am. Physicians* 32: 32, 1917.

Giffin, H. Z. Splenectomy following radium treatment for myelocytic leukemia. *Trans. Assoc. Am. Physicians* 33: 59, 1918.

Giffin, H. Z. Hemoglobinuria in hemolytic jaundice. *Trans. Assoc. Am. Physicians* 37: 452, 1922.

Giffin, H. Z. Ovalocytosis with features of hemolytic icterus. *Trans. Assoc. Am. Physicians* 54: 355, 1939.

Giffin, H. Z., Brown, G. E., and Roth, G. M. Blood volume preceding and following splenectomy in hemolytic icterus and splenic anemia. *J. Clin. Invest.* 7: 283, 1929.

Sprague, R. G. Herbert Ziegler Giffin, 1878–1969. *Trans. Assoc. Am. Physicians* 82: 33, 1969.

51. Snell, A. M., and Roth, G. M. The lactic acid of the blood in hepatic disease. *J. Clin. Invest.* 11: 957, 1932.

Wilbur, D. L. Albert M. Snell, 1895–1960. *Trans. Assoc. Am. Physicians* 73: 32, 1960.

52. Owen, C. A., Jr. The discoveries of vitamin K and dicumarol and their impact on our concepts of blood coagulation. *Mayo Clin. Proc.* 49: 912, 1974.

Snell, A. M., and Butt, H. R. Factors governing absorption and utilization of vitamin K. *Trans. Assoc. Am. Physicians* 54: 38, 1939.

53. Snell, A. M. Manfred Whitset Comfort, 1895–1957. *Trans. Assoc. Am. Physicians* 71: 20, 1958.

54. Comfort, M. W., Gambill, E. E., and Baggenstoss, A. H. Chronic relapsing pancreatitis; study of 29 cases without associated disease of biliary or gastrointestinal tract. *Gastroenterology* 6: 239, 1946.

55. Willius, F. A. Cardiology in the Mayo Clinic and the Mayo Foundation for Medical Education and Research. In *Methods and Problems in Medical Education*, Series 8, p. 193. New York: Rockefeller Foundation, 1927.

56. Pruitt, R. D. Arlie Ray Barnes, 1892–1970. *Trans. Assoc. Am. Physicians* 83: 12, 1970.

57. Barnes, A. R., and Whitter, M. B. Study of the R-T interval in myocardial infarction. *Am. Heart J.* 5: 142, 1929.

58. Feldman, W. H. Streptomycin: Some historical aspects of its development as a chemotherapeutic agent in tuberculosis. *Am. Rev. Tuberc.* 69: 859, 1954.

Hinshaw, H. C. Historical notes on the earliest use of streptomycin in clinical tuberculosis. *Am. Rev. Tuberc.* 70: 9, 1954.

# Chapter 22

1. Gonda, T. A. Stanford University School of Medicine. *Calif. Med.* 110: 74, 1969.

2. Blumer, G. Random recollections of Cooper Medical College (1889–91). *Stan. Med. Bull.* 6: 357, 1948.

3. See Harvey, A. McG. Arthur D. Hirschfelder—Johns Hopkins' first full-time cardiologist. *John Hopkins Med. J.* 143: 129, 1978.

4. Veysey, L. Ray Lyman Wilbur. *Dict. Am. Biog.* (suppl. 4): 891, 1946–50.

5. Bloomfield, A. Thomas Addis, 1881–1949. *Trans. Assoc. Am. Physicians* 63: 7, 1950.

6. Wilbur, R. L., and Addis, T. Urobilin: Its clinical significance. *Arch. Intern. Med.* 13: 235, 1915.

7. Addis, T. The number of formed elements in the urinary sediment of normal individuals. *J. Clin. Invest.* 2: 409, 1925–26.

Addis, T. The effect of some physiological variables on the number of casts, red blood cells and white blood cells and epithelial cells in the urine of normal individuals. *J. Clin. Invest.* 2: 417, 1925–26.

8. Addis, T. The ratio between the urea content of the urine and of the blood after the administration of large quantities of urea: An approximate index of the quantity of actively functioning kidney tissue. *J. Urol.* 1: 263, 1917.

Addis's important studies of renal function in disease were an outgrowth of his investigations on the rate of urea excretion. This paper gives Addis's rationale for the "urea ratio": "The ratio between the urea content of the urine and of the blood expresses the number of times by which the urea excreted in the urine during a certain period of time exceeds the amount of urea present in 100 cc. of the blood supplied to the kidney during this time." Addis (Renal function and the amount of functioning tissue. *Arch. Intern. Med.* 30: 378, 1922) later formulated more precisely the significance of the test: "Under certain special conditions, when the amount of secreting tissue in the kidney varies, the ratio urea in one hour's urine:urea in 100 cc. of blood is directly proportional to the amount of secreting tissue in the kidney." Addis, with C. K. Watanabe and J. Oliver (Determination of the quantity of secreting tissue in the living kidney. *J. Exp. Med.* 28: 359, 1918), showed that "under the strain induced by the administration of urea, it is possible to demonstrate the relation between the degree of anatomical damage in the kidney and the degree of defect in the urea-excreting capacity induced by uremia." This was shown further in another paper with B. A. Myers and J. Oliver (The regulation of renal activity. IX. The effect of unilateral nephrectomy on the function and structure of the remaining kidney. *Arch. Intern. Med.* 34: 243, 1924).

The Addis ratio was never widely adopted in clinical practice, as were the "maximum" and "standard" urea clearances of E. Møller, J. F. McIntosh, and D. D. Van Slyke (Studies of urea excretion. II. Relationship between urine volume and the ratio of urea excretion by normal adults. *J. Clin. Invest.* 6: 427, 1928; IV. Relationship between urine volume and rate of urea excretion by patients with Bright's disease. *J. Clin. Invest.* 6: 485, 1928).

9. When Addis described his urea ratio (mg. urea in 1 hr urine, divided by mg. urea in 100 ml. of blood), he gave the answer as a pure number—namely, the normal was 50.4. It was George Barnett who pointed out to him that 50.4 really represented the number of deciliters of blood freed of urea per hour. When Rytand told Homer Smith of this many years later (Addis had noted it as a footnote in his Harvey lecture), Smith recorded it in his famous monograph on the kidney, suggesting that had Addis used the word *cleared* instead of the word *freed*, renal physiology might have been advanced by several decades. (Rytand, D. Personal communication, 1978.)

10. Addis, T. A clinical classification of Bright's disease. *J.A.M.A.* 85: 163, 1925.

Addis, T. *Glomerular Nephritis: Diagnosis and Treatment.* New York: Macmillan, 1948.

Addis, T., and Oliver, J. *The Renal Lesion in Bright's Disease.* New York: Paul B. Hoeber, 1931.

In the above paper, clinician and pathologist united in a study directed at correlating clinical features with pathological findings. Many of the patients had been followed for years with careful studies of urinary sediment and with urea ratios.

While Addis and Oliver's monograph was being assembled, there appeared the important work of D. D. Van Slyke and his associates (Observations on the course of different types of Bright's disease and on the resultant changes in renal anatomy. *Medicine* 9: 257, 1930), who had similar aims.

Oliver (*The Architecture of the Kidney in Chronic Bright's Disease.* New York: Paul B. Hoeber, 1939) later dealt, in monographic form, with a correlation of ordinary stained sections with three-dimensional teased preparations of kidney from patients with Bright's disease.

11. Rytand, Personal communication, 1978.

12. Addis, T., and Raulston, B. O. A reversible form of experimental uremia. *Trans. Assoc. Am. Physicians* 45: 318, 1930.

13. Harvey, A. McG. *The Interurban Clinical Club, 1905–1976: A Record of Achievement in Clinical Science,* p. 544. Philadelphia: W. B. Saunders, 1978.

14. Harvey, A. McG. Albion Walter Hewlett—Pioneer clinical physiologist. *Johns Hopkins Med. J.* 144: 202, 1979.

15. Hewlett, A. W., and Alberty, W. M. Influenza at the Navy Base Hospital in France. *J.A.M.A.* 71: 1056, 1918.

16. Hewlett, A. W., and Kay, W. E. The effect of tyramin on circulatory failure during infections and during or after operations. *J.A.M.A.* 70: 1810, 1918.

17. Lewis, J. K., and Hewlett, A. W. The cause of increased vascular sounds after epinephrine injections. *Heart* 10: 1, 1922–23.

18. Hewlett, A. W., and Nakada, J. R. Recovery from the hyperpnea of moderate exercise: Recovery ratio. *Proc. Soc. Exp. Biol. Med.* 21: 207, 1923–24.

19. Hewlett, A. W. The vital capacities of patients with cardiac complaints. *Heart* 11: 195, 1923–24.

20. Hewlett, A. W., and Jackson, N. R. The vital capacity in a group of college students. *Arch. Intern. Med.* 29: 515, 1922.

21. Hewlett, A. W., Lewis, J. K., and Franklin, A. The effect of pathological conditions upon dyspnea during exercise. I. Artificial stenosis. *J. Clin. Invest.* 1: 483, 1924–25.

22. Hewlett, A. W., Barnett, G. D., and Lewis, J. K. The effect of breathing oxygen-enriched air during exercise upon pulmonary ventilation and upon the lactic acid content of blood and urine. *J. Clin. Invest.* 3: 317, 1926–27.

23. Hewlett, A. W., Barnett, G. D., and Lewis, J. K. The effect of training on lactic acid secretion. *Proc. Soc. Exp. Biol. Med.* 22: 537, 1925.

24. From the official minutes book of the American Society for Clinical Investigation.

25. Cox, A. J., Hilgard, E. R., and Rytand, D. A. Arthur L. Bloomfield, 1888–1962. *Stan. Med. Bull.* 20: 137, 1962.

Rantz, L. A. Arthur Leonard Bloomfield, 1888–1962. *Trans. Assoc. Am. Physicians* 76: 12, 1963.

26. Bloomfield, A. L. The fate of bacteria introduced into the upper air passages. *Am. Rev. Tuberc.* 3: 553, 1919.

Bloomfield, A. L. Variations in the bacterial flora of the upper air passages during the course of common colds. *Bull. Johns Hopkins Hosp.* 32: 121, 1921.

Bloomfield, A. L. The localization of bacteria in the upper air passages: Its bearing on infection. *Bull. Johns Hopkins Hosp.* 32: 290, 1921.

Bloomfield, A. L. The dissemination of bacteria in the upper air passages. II. The circulation of bacteria in the mouth. *Bull. Johns Hopkins Hosp.* 33: 145, 1922.

Bloomfield, A. L. The mechanism of elimination of bacteria from the respiratory tract. *Am. J. Med. Sci.* 164: 854, 1922.

Bloomfield, A., and Harrop, G. A., Jr. Clinical observations on epidemic influenza. *Bull. Johns Hopkins Hosp.* 30: 1, 1919.

27. Bloomfield, A. L., and Keefer, C. S. Studies on clinical physiology of the stomach. *Trans. Assoc. Am. Physicians* 41: 80, 1926.

28. Bloomfield, A. L., and Polland, W. S. Experimental referred pain from the gastrointestinal tract. II. Stomach, duodenum and colon. *J. Clin. Invest.* 10: 453, 1931.

Bloomfield, A. L., and Polland, W. S. *Gastric Anacidity.* New York: Macmillan, 1933.

Bloomfield, A. L., and Polland, W. S. The fate of people with unexplained gastric anacidity. Follow-up studies. *J. Clin. Invest.* 14: 321, 1935.

29. Bloomfield, A. L. *A Bibliography of Internal Medicine. I. Communicable Diseases* (1958); *II. Selected Diseases* (1960). Chicago: University of Chicago Press.

30. Dock, W., and Tainter, M. L. The circulatory changes after full therapeutic doses of digitalis, with a critical discussion of views of cardiac output. *J. Clin. Invest.* 8: 467, 1930.

Tainter, M. L., and Dock, W. Further observations on the circulatory actions of digitalis and strophanthus with special reference to the liver, and comparisons with histamine and epinephrine. *J. Clin. Invest.* 8: 485, 1930.

31. Dock, W., and Lewis, J. K. The effect of thyroid feeding on the oxygen consumption of the heart and of the other tissues. *J. Physiol.* 74: 401, 1932.

32. Lewis, J. K., and Dock, W. The origin of heart sounds and their variations in myocardial disease. *J.A.M.A.* 110: 271, 1938.

33. Dickson, E. C. Botulismus. *Oxford Med.* 5: 231, 1921.

Dickson, E. C. Mimicry of tuberculosis by coccidioidal granuloma. *Trans. Assoc. Am. Physicians* 44: 284, 1929.

34. Rytand, D. A. Lowell Addison Rantz, 1912–1964. *Trans. Assoc. Am. Physicians* 78: 35, 1965.

35. Rantz, L. A., Boisvert, P. J., and Spink, W. W. Etiology and pathogenesis of rheumatic fever. *Arch. Intern. Med.* 76: 131, 1945.

Rantz, L. A., Boisvert, P. J., and Spink, W. W. Hemolytic streptococcic sore throat: The post-streptococcic state. *Arch. Intern. Med.* 79: 401, 1947.

36. Rytand, D. A. The effect of digitalis on the venous pressure of normal individuals. *J. Clin. Invest.* 12: 847, 1933.

Rytand, D. A. The rate of excretion of urine in subjects with different amounts of renal tissue. *J. Clin. Invest.* 12: 1153, 1933.

Rytand, D. A. The number and size of mammalian glomeruli as related to kidney and to body weight, with methods for their enumeration and measurement. *Am. J. Anat.* 62: 507, 1938.

Rytand, D. A. The renal factor in arterial hypertension with coarctation of the aorta. *J. Clin. Invest.* 17: 391, 1938.

Rytand, D. A. Hereditary obesity of yellow mice: A method for the study of obesity. *Proc. Soc. Exp. Biol. Med.* 54: 340, 1943.

Rytand, D. A. The circus movement (entrapped circuit wave) hypothesis and atrial flutter. *Ann. Intern. Med.* 65: 125, 1966.

Rytand, D. A., and Dock, W. Experimental and concentric and eccentric cardiac hypertrophy in rats. *Arch. Intern. Med.* 56: 511, 1935.

# Chapter 23

1. Kerr, W. J. Herbert Charles Moffitt, 1867–1951. *Trans. Assoc. Am. Physicians* 64: 12, 1951.

2. Moffitt, H. C. Is pernicious anemia of infectious origin? *Trans. Assoc. Am. Physicians* 26: 288, 1911.

Moffitt, H. C. Studies in pernicious anemia. *Trans. Assoc. Am. Physicians* 29: 476, 1914.

3. Moffitt, H. C. Presidential address. *Trans. Assoc. Am. Physicians* 37: 1, 1922.

4. Whipple, G. Autobiographical sketch. *Perspect. Biol. Med.* 2: 253, 1959.

5. Whipple, G. A hitherto undescribed disease characterized by deposits of fat and fatty acids in the intestinal and mesenteric lymphatic tissues. *Bull. Johns Hopkins Hosp.* 18: 382, 1907.

6. Whipple, G., and Hooper, C. W. Hematogenous and obstructive icterus. Experimental studies by means of the Eck fistula. *J. Exp. Med.* 17: 593, 1913.

Whipple, G., and Hooper, C. W. A rapid change of hemoglobin to bile pigment in the circulation outside the liver. *J. Exp. Med.* 17: 612, 1913.

7. Corner, G. W. *George Hoyt Whipple and His Friends: The Life Story of a Nobel Prize Pathologist.* Philadelphia: J. B. Lippincott, 1963.

8. Whipple, G. H., Stone, H. B., and Bernheim, B. M. Intestinal obstruction. IV. The mechanism of absorption from the mucosa of closed duodenal loops. *J. Exp. Med.* 19: 166, 1914.

9. After Hooper's death, his wife offered to give the University of California redwood timberlands, conservatively valued at $1 million, the income from which was to maintain an institution defined as a "school of medical research." That this new institute was to be known as a school implied that the clinical division of the university medical school was not itself a center of medical research. This was indeed true, according to Corner, for neither the medical school building, which was erected in 1897, nor the small hospital nearby, had any facility for experimental investigation. The medical school had grown out of a small, privately owned institution, founded in 1864 by a pioneer doctor, Hugh H. Toland, which the university took over in 1873. This takeover resulted, however, in very little change in the clinical teaching. The part of the school in San Francisco looked after its own affairs, and the chairs of medicine and surgery were filled by members of the local medical profession who were in active practice.

In 1899, the university administration, presumably looking forward to concentrating its medical school on the main campus at Berkeley, began to build up preclinical departments both in Berkeley and San Francisco, under full-time investigators and teachers. A. E. Taylor, later a distinguished nutritional chemist, was a professor of pathology and physiological chemistry at San Francisco from 1899 to 1910, when he left for the University of Pennsylvania.

He did not, however, influence the clinical men among whom he worked. After the San Francisco earthquake and fire of 1906, the teaching of all preclinical subjects, except pathology, was discontinued in San Francisco, and all medical students took their preclinical work in Berkeley, where a distinguished group, including Frederick P. Gay, Samuel S. Maxwell, T. Brailsford Robertson, and Herbert M. Evans, was assembled. In San Francisco, however, the busy physicians who constituted the clinical faculty were content with teaching only. They had neither the time nor inclination for advancing medical knowledge by experimental investigation. There were, however, some distinguished early investigators at the school, including James Blake and Charles Brigham.

The Hooper Foundation was one of the earliest institutes for general medical research to be founded in the United States. Its only predecessor with equally broad scope was the Rockefeller Institute in New York. Two other institutes with similar, but less general, aims had been founded a little earlier, the McCormick Institute for Infectious Diseases (1903), in Chicago, and the Sprague Memorial Institute (1911), in the same city. The Hooper Foundation was an independent unit of the University of California, reporting directly to the regents through the president of the university. On its board were Dean Moffitt, William Henry Welch, and Henry S. Pritchett, president of the Carnegie Corporation of New York.

Welch was largely responsible for the Hooper Foundation being developed under the auspices of the University of California. The Hooper family wished to establish the foundation as a separate institute, similar to the Rockefeller Institute. Welch strongly advised against this, as a result of his experience at the Rockefeller. The Hooper Foundation thus became the first institute for medicine to be established under university auspices.

10. Walker, E. L. A comparative study of the amoebae in the Manila water supply, in the intestinal tract of healthy people, and in amoebic dysentery. *Philippine J. Sci.* 6B: 259, 1911.

Walker, E. L., and Sellards, A. W. Experimental amoebic dysentery. *Philippine J. Sci.* 8B: 253, 1913.

11. Cooke, J. V., and Whipple, G. H. Proteose intoxications and injury of body protein. V. The increase in non-protein nitrogen of the blood in acute inflammatory processes and acute intoxications. *J. Exp. Med.* 28: 243, 1918.

12. Hurwitz, S. H., Kerr, W. J., and Whipple, G. H. Regeneration of blood serum proteins. III. Liver injury alone: Livery injury and plasma depletion: The Eck fistula combined with plasma depletion. *Am. J. Physiol.* 47: 379, 1918–19.

13. Whipple, G. H., and Hooper, C. W. A rapid change of hemoglobin to bile pigment in the pleural and peritoneal cavities. *J. Exp. Med.* 23: 137, 1916.

Whipple, G. H., and Hooper, C. W. Bile pigment metabolism. I. Bile pigment output and diet studies. *Am. J. Physiol.* 40: 332, 1916.

Whipple, G. H., and Hooper, C. W. Bile pigment metabolism. II. Bile pigment output influenced by diet. *Am. J. Physiol.* 40: 349, 1916.

14. Whipple's complete bibliography may be found in Corner's biography.

15. Whipple, G. H., Dawson, A. B., and Evans, H. M. Blood volume studies. III. Behavior of large series of dyes introduced into the circulating blood. *Am. J. Physiol.* 51: 232, 1920.

16. Whipple, G. H., Rodenbaugh, F. H., and Kilgore, A. R. Intestinal obstruction. V. Proteose intoxication. *J. Exp. Med.* 23: 123, 1916.

Whipple, G. H., and Van Slyke, D. D. Proteose intoxications and injury of body protein. III. Toxic protein catabolism and its influence upon the non-protein nitrogen partition of the blood. *J. Exp. Med.* 28: 213, 1918.

17. Corner, *George Hoyt Whipple and His Friends,* pp. 73–114.

18. Good, R. A., and Platon, E. S., ed. *Essays on Pediatrics in Honor of Irvine McQuarrie.* Minneapolis: Lancet, 1955.

McQuarrie, I., and Whipple, G. H. II. Renal function influenced by proteose intoxication. *J. Exp. Med.* 29: 421, 1919.

McQuarrie, I., and Whipple, G. H. A study of renal function in roentgen ray intoxication. Resistance of renal epithelium to direct radiation. *J. Exp. Med.* 35: 225, 1922.

19. Warren, S. L., and Whipple, G. H. Roentgen ray intoxication. III. Speed of autolysis of various body tissues after lethal x-ray exposures. The remarkable disturbance in the epithelium of the small intestine. *J. Exp. Med.* 35: 213, 1922.

Warren, S. L., and Whipple, G. H. Roentgen ray intoxication. IV. Intestinal lesions and acute intoxication produced by radiation in a variety of animals. *J. Exp. Med.* 38: 741, 1923.

20. Kerr, W. J., Cannon, E. F., and Lagen, J. B. A new approach to the etiology and treatment of angina pectoris. *Trans. Assoc. Am. Physicians* 54: 225, 1939.

Kerr, W. J., and Hensel, G. C. Observations of the cardiovascular system in thyroid disease. *Arch. Intern. Med.* 31: 398, 1923.

Kerr, W. J., Mettier, S. R., and McCalla, R. L. The capillary circulation of the heart valves in relation to rheumatic fever. *Trans. Assoc. Am. Physicians* 43: 213, 1928.

Kerr, W. J., Sampson, J. J., Lagen, J. B., and Kellogg, F. The use of the Matthews oscillograph in phonocardiography. *Trans. Assoc. Am. Physicians* 47: 27, 1932.

Ralston, H. J., and Kerr, W. J. Vascular responses of the nasal mucosa to thermal stimuli with some observations on skin temperature. *Am. J. Physiol.* 144: 305, 1945.

21. Starr, P. Hans Lisser, 1888–1964. *Trans. Assoc. Am. Physicians* 78: 33, 1965.

22. Lisser, H., and Shepardson, H. C. A further and final report on a case of tetania parathyreopriva treated for one year with parathyroid extract (Collip), with eventual death and autopsy. *Endocrinology* 13: 427, 1929.

23. Gordan, G. S., Soley, M. H., and Chamberlain, F. L. Electrocardiographic features associated with hyperthyroidism. *Arch. Intern. Med.* 73: 148, 1944.

24. Gordan, G. S., Evans, H. M., and Simpson, M. D. Effects of testosterone propionate on body weight and urinary nitrogen excretion of normal and hypophysectomized rats. *Endocrinology* 40: 375, 1947.

25. Escamilla, R. F., and Lisser, H. Simmonds' disease: A clinical study with review of the literature: Differentiation from anorexia nervosa with statistical analysis of 595 cases, 101 of which were proved pathologically. *J. Clin. Endocrinol.* 2: 65, 1942.

26. Escamilla, R. F., Lisser, H., and Shepardson, H. C. Internal myxedema: Report of a case showing ascites, cardiac, intestinal, and bladder atony, menorrhagia, secondary anemia and associated acrotinemia. *Ann. Intern. Med.* 9: 297, 1935.

Goldberg, M. D., and Lisser, H. Acromegaly, a consideration of its course and treatment. *J. Clin. Endocrinol.* 2: 477, 1942.

27. Biskind, G. R., Escamilla, R. F., and Lisser, H. Treatment of eunuchoidism: Implantation of testosterone compounds in cases of male eunuchoidism. *J. Clin. Endocrinol.* 1: 38, 1941.

Lisser, H., Escamilla, R. F., and Curtis, L. E. Testosterone therapy of male eunuchoids. III. Sublingual administration of testosterone compounds. *J. Clin. Endocrinol.* 2: 351, 1942.

28. Escamilla, R. F., and Lisser, H. Induction of menarche and development of secondary sexual characteristics in a women aged 34 by injections of estradiol dipropionate. *Endocrinology* 27: 153, 1940.

29. Althausen, T. L. Hormonal and vitamin factors in intestinal absorption. *Trans. Assoc. Am. Physicians* 61: 54, 1948.

Althausen, T. L., Doig, R. K., Weiden, S., Motteram, R., Turner, C. N., and Moore, A. Hemochromatosis: An investigation of 23 cases with special reference to nutrition, to iron metabolism, and to studies of hepatic and pancreatic function. *Trans. Assoc. Am. Physicians* 63: 209, 1950.

30. Aggeler, P. M., White, S. G., Glendening, M. D., Page, E., Leake, T. B., and Bates, G. PTC factor deficiency; a previously undescribed hemophilia-like disease due to a deficiency of a heretofore unknown thromboplastin component. *Am. J. Med.* 13: 90, 1952.

31. Aggeler, P. M., and Lucia, S. P. *Hemorrhagic Disorders.* Chicago: University of Chicago Press, 1944.

# Appendix A

1. Ashford, B. *A Soldier in Science.* New York: William Morrow, 1934. (An autobiographical sketch.)

2. Baldwin, E. R. Antitoxic serum in tuberculosis. *Trans. Assoc. Am. Physicians* 13: 111, 1898.

Baldwin, E. R. Opsonins in tuberculosis. *Trans. Assoc. Am. Physicians* 22: 517, 1907.

Baldwin, E. R. Review of theoretical considerations and experimental work relative to opsonins with observations at the Saranac laboratory. *Trans. Assoc. Am. Physicians* 23: 48, 1908.

Baldwin, E. R. Acceptance of the Kober Medal. *Trans. Assoc. Am. Physicians* 51: 24, 1936.

Waring, J. J. Edward R. Baldwin, 1864–1947. *Trans. Assoc. Am. Physicians* 61: 7, 1948.

Webb, G. Presentation of the Kober Medal to E. R. Baldwin. *Trans. Assoc. Am. Physicians* 51: 23, 1936.

3. William Jephtha Calvert. *Who Was Who* 5: 110, 1969–73; idem, *J.A.M.A.* 127: 1144, 1945.

Calvert, W. J. Cause of pulsation in empyema. *Am. J. Med. Sci.* 130: 890, 1905.

Calvert, W. J. Acute dilatation of the arch of the aorta. *Interstate Med. J.* 13: 237, 1906.

Calvert, W. J. Position of the heart in pericarditis with effusion. *Bull. Johns Hopkins Hosp.* 18: 403, 1907.

Calvert, W. J. Displacement of the heart by pleural pressures. *Bull. Johns Hopkins Hosp.* 18: 444, 1907.

Calvert, W. J. Compensatory venous congestion. *Bull. Johns Hopkins Hosp.* 18: 447, 1907.

4. Cowie, D. M. A comparative study of the occult blood tests; a new modification of the guaiac reaction; its value in legal medicine. *Am. J. Med. Sci.* 133: 408, 1907.

Cowie, D. M. An experimental study of the action of oil on gastric acidity and motility. *Arch. Intern. Med.* 1: 61, 1908.

Cowie, D. M. A method of obtaining human plasma free from chemical action. Its effect on phagocytosis. *J. Med. Res.* 21: 327, 1909.

Cowie, D. M. Some clinical observations on blood pressure with special reference to the effect of prostatic massage. *Am. Med.* 5: 632, 1910.

Cowie, D. M., and Chapin, W. S. Experiments in favor of the amboceptor-complement structure of the opsonin of normal human serum for the staphylococcus albus. *J. Med. Res.* 17: 95, 1907.

Cowie, D. M., and Lyson, W. Further observations on the acid control of the pylorus. *Am. J. Child. Dis.* 2: 252, 1911.

5. Cole, R. Charles Phillips Emerson. *Trans. Assoc. Am. Physicians* 54: 11, 1939.

Harvey, A. McG. *The Interurban Clinical Club, 1905–1976. A Record of Achievement in Clinical Science*, p. 49. Philadelphia: W. B. Saunders, 1978.

6. Bolduan, C. Haven Emerson—The public health statesman. *Am. J. Pub. Health* 40: 1, 1950.

Emerson, H. Response. *Am. J. Pub. Health* 40: 4, 1950.

Harvey, *Interurban Clinical Club*, p. 91.

Paul, J. R. Haven Emerson, 1874–1957. *Trans. Assoc. Am. Physicians* 71: 23, 1958.

7. Fischer, M. H. False diverticula of the intestine. *J. Exp. Med.* 5: 333, 1900–1901.

Fischer, M. H. The toxic effect of formaldehyde and formalin. *J. Exp. Med.* 6: 487, 1901–2.

Fischer, M. H. Remarks on the treatment of nephritis. *Trans. Assoc. Am. Physicians* 27: 595, 1912.

Striker, C. *Medical Portraits*, p. 87. Cincinnati: Academy of Medicine of Cincinnati, 1963.

8. Richardson, M. W. On the presence of the typhoid bacillus in the urine. *J. Exp. Med.* 3: 349, 1898.

Richardson, M. W. On the value of urotropin as a urinary antiseptic with especial reference to its use in typhoid fever. *J. Exp. Med.* 4: 19, 1899.

Richardson, M. W. On the present status of vaccine and serum therapy. *Trans. Assoc. Am. Physicians* 23: 449, 1908.

9. Rosenow, E. C. Studies in pneumonia and pneumococcus infections. *J. Infect. Dis.* 1: 280, 1904.

Rosenow, E. C. The role of phagocytosis in the pneumococcidal action of pneumonic blood. *J. Infect. Dis.* 3: 683, 1906.

Rosenow, E. C. Virulence of pneumococci in relation to phagocytosis. *Science* 27: 657, 1908.

Rosenow, E. C. Immunological and experimental studies on pneumococcus and staphylococcus endocarditis. *J. Infect. Dis.* 6: 245, 1909.

10. Harvey, *Interurban Clinical Club*, p. 166.

Howard, C. P. President's address. *Trans. Assoc. Am. Physicians* 44: 4, 1929.

Sailer, J. Peptic digestion, inhibition of. *Trans. Assoc. Am. Physicians* 21: 438, 1906.

Sailer, J. Excessive acidity of the gastric contents. *Trans. Assoc. Am. Physicians* 22: 624, 1907.

Sailer, J. Acute pancreatitis. *Trans. Assoc. Am. Physicians* 23: 540, 1908.

Sailer, J. Further experiments in the toxemia of experimental acute pancreatitis. *Trans. Assoc. Am. Physicians* 26: 446, 1911.

11. Harvey, A. McG. Pioneer American virologist—Charles E. Simon. *Johns Hopkins Med. J.* 142: 161, 1978.

Simon, C. E. A contribution to the study of the opsonins. *J. Exp. Med.* 8: 561, 1906.

Simon, C. E. A further contribution to the knowledge of the opsonins. *J. Exp. Med.* 9: 487, 1907.

Simon, C. E., and Thomas, W. S. On complement fixation in malignant disease. *J. Exp. Med.* 10: 673, 1908.

12. Harvey, *Interurban Clinical Club,* p. 88.

Steele, J. D. Nucleus test in pancreatic disease. *Trans. Assoc. Am. Physicians* 21: 331, 1906.

Steele, J. D. Diagnosis of pancreatic disease. *Trans. Assoc. Am. Physicians* 21: 359, 1906.

Steele, J. D. Clinical examination of the feces. *Trans. Assoc. Am. Physicians* 21: 792, 1906.

Steele, J. D. Experimental observations upon the value of intestinal antiseptics. *Trans. Assoc. Am. Physicians* 22: 200, 1907.

13. Simmons, J. S. Richard Pearson Strong, 1872–1948. *Trans. Assoc. Am. Physicians* 62: 20, 1949.

Strong, R. P. Some questions relating to the virulence of microorganisms, with particular reference to their immunizing powers. *J. Exp. Med.* 7: 229, 1905.

Strong, R. P. President's address. *Trans. Assoc. Am. Physicians* 41: 1, 1926.

R. P. Strong and O. Teague (Studies on pneumonic plague and plague immunization. II. The method of transmission of infection in pneumonic plague and manner of spread of the disease during the epidemic. *Philippine J. Sci.* 7B: 137, 1912) studied in detail the transmission of pneumonic plague. They emphasized the importance of masks and other protective measures. They also (IV. Portal of entry of infection and method of development of the lesions in pneumonic and primary septicemic plague; experimental pathology. *Philippine J. Sci.* 7B: 173, 1912) believed that the primary point of infection was not the tonsil, but some part of the respiratory passages. "Having reached the lung tissue, the bacilli rapidly multiply and produce at first pneumonic changes of the lobular type and shortly afterward more general lobar involvement of the lung tissue." (Bloomfield, A. L. *A Bibliography of Internal Medicine: Communicable Diseases,* p. 55. Chicago: University of Chicago Press, 1958).

Strong and Musgrave made important studies on dysentery in the American forces in the Philippines simultaneously with those of the Flexner commission (see chapter 23).

14. Harvey, *Interurban Clinical Club,* p. 22.

Tileston, W. The blood in measles. *J. Infect. Dis.* 1: 551, 1904. Although it was noted many years before that there was absence of leukocytosis in measles (in contrast to scarlet fever) and, indeed, actually a leukopenia, Tileston gave comprehensive studies in twenty-eight cases. Tileston pointed out the now well-known drop in polymorphonuclear leukocytes toward defervescence with increase of lymphocytes. (Bloomfield, *A Bibliography of Internal Medicine: Communicable Diseases,* p. 435.)

Tileston, W. The diagnosis of complete absence of pancreatic secretion from the intestine with the results of digestion and absorption experiments. *Trans. Assoc. Am. Physicians* 26: 513, 1911.

Tileston, W. Total non-protein nitrogen and the urea of the blood in health and disease as estimated by Folin's method. *Trans. Assoc. Am. Physicians* 29: 260, 1914.

Tileston, W., and Underhill, F. P. Tetany in the adult, with special reference to alkalosis and calcium metabolism. *Trans. Assoc. Am. Physicians* 37: 87, 1922.

# Appendix B

1. Sturgis, C., and Wearn, J. T. I. The effects of the injection of epinephrine in soldiers with "irritable heart." *Arch. Intern. Med.* 24: 247, 1919.

# Appendix C

1. Merle Scott, W. J., and Morton, J. J. Sympathetic inhibition of the large intestine in Hirschsprung's disease. *J. Clin. Invest.* 9: 247, 1930–31.

Morton, J. J., and Merle Scott, W. J. The measurement of sympathetic vaso-constrictor activity in the lower extremities. *J. Clin. Invest.* 9: 235, 1930–31.

## Appendix D

1. Hoover expressed his views on this subject in a paper entitled "The Required Conflict between the Laboratories and Clinical Medicine," which was presented before the Cleveland Academy of Medicine. The paper was published in *Science* (71: 491, 1930) after his death.

2. Stetson, C. A., Rammelkamp, C. H., Jr., Krause, R. M., Kohen, R. J., and Perry, W. D. Epidemic acute nephritis: Studies on etiology, natural history and prevention. *Medicine* 34: 431, 1955.

That certain types of streptococci predominate in infections followed by nephritis was convincingly demonstrated by this group, who showed that acute nephritis occurred during convalescence from type 12 pharyngitis, but in no one convalescing from other types such as 3, 6, and 19. Certain strains are clearly *nephritogenic*.

# Indexes

# Name Index

# Subject Index